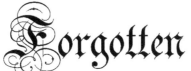 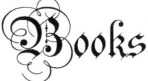

ISBN 978-0-260-23948-8
PIBN 11012688

1 MONTH OF
FREE
READING

at

www.ForgottenBooks.com

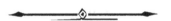

By purchasing this book you are
eligible for one month membership to
ForgottenBooks.com, giving you
unlimited access to our entire
collection of over 1,000,000 titles via
our web site and mobile apps.

To claim your free month visit:

www.forgottenbooks.com/free1012688

English
Français
Deutsche
Italiano
Español
Português

www.forgottenbooks.com

Mythology Photography **Fiction**
Fishing Christianity **Art** Cooking
Essays Buddhism Freemasonry
Medicine **Biology** Music **Ancient**
Egypt Evolution Carpentry Physics
Dance Geology **Mathematics** Fitness
Shakespeare **Folklore** Yoga Marketing
Confidence Immortality Biographies
Poetry **Psychology** Witchcraft
Electronics Chemistry History **Law**
Accounting **Philosophy** Anthropology
Alchemy Drama Quantum Mechanics
Atheism Sexual Health **Ancient History**
Entrepreneurship Languages Sport
Paleontology Needlework Islam
Metaphysics Investment Archaeology
Parenting Statistics Criminology
Motivational

ELEMENTS

OF THE

THEORY AND PRACTICE

OF

PHYSIC,

DESIGNED FOR THE USE OF STUDENTS.

BY

GEORGE GREGORY, M. D.

FIRST NEW-YORK,

FROM THE THIRD LONDON EDITION.

WITH NOTES, *100283*

BY

DANIEL L. M. PEIXOTTO, M. D.

Editor of the New York Medical and Physical Journal ; Vice President of the Medical
Society of the City and County of New-York ; Fellow of the College of Physicians and Surgeons of the University of the State of New York, etc.

AND A NEW AND COMPLETE VERSION OF THE CELEBRATED
PROPOSITIONS OF M. BROUSSAIS.

NEW-YORK:

PUBLISHED BY M. SHERMAN.
....
1830.

TO

JOHN B. BECK, M. D.

OFESSOR OF MATERIA MEDICA AND MEDICAL JURISPRUDENCE
IN THE COLLEGE OF PHYSICIANS AND SURGEONS IN THE
UNIVERSITY OF THE STATE OF NEW-YORK, &c. &c.

As a memorial of friendship, uninterrupted for years, and a
ble token of the esteem entertained for his talents, and of the
ardent wishes cherished for his prosperity in the professional ca-
reer which he has so auspiciously commenced, the present impression of the very popular work of Dr. GREGORY is respectfully
inscribed,

By

His Friend,

THE EDITOR.

ADVERTISEMENT

` TO THE AMERICAN EDITION.

THE present reprint has been undertaken, not from any invidi-
ous motives of interference with other editions extant, but from a
simple desire to present the student of medicine with a more complete and perfect text of Dr. Gregory's work than has yet appeared
in this country.

To render this edition more generally useful and acceptable
there has been appended a new version of THE PROPOSITIONS OF
M. BROUSSAIS, which contain a full view of the physiological doctrines, and of which no entire or accurate copy has before been
submitted to the English, or American reader.

THE NOTES have been added to supply a few important omis-
sions in the body of the work, and to diffuse more generally a
knowledge of certain *American* opinions and modes of practice,
which deserve to be embodied into a general system of medicine.

This volume exhibits, therefore, a condensed expose of some of
the most popular medical views of the theory and practice of physic entertained in Great Britain, France, and the United States
of America.

PREFACE.

THE object of the author, in the following pages, is to lay before the student of medicine an outline of the present state of the theory and practice of medicine, unbiassed by attachment to any professed principle, and to delineate those views of pathology which appear to direct the reasonings, and to give a tone to the language of medical writers at the present period. The idea of such a work was originally suggested by the necessity which he found of editing a short syllabus to the course of lectures, which he is delivering in the Metropolis, on the Theory and Practice of Physic: It seemed to him in the prosecution of this object, that a slight alteration of his plan would enable him to lay before the junior branches of the profession an elementary work, which might prove more extensively useful. It is no part of his design to present what has been called a *System of Physic*, that is to say, to digest all that has hitherto been written about diseases, or to explain their varied phæ-nomena on any one hypothesis, Such attempts have been made, but they have commonly proved fruitless ; and in this respect experience but corroborates what might reasonably have been expected from an attentive survey of the nature and extent of medical science.

The general design of the volume coincides very nearly with that of Dr. Cullen's First Lines, a work of which it is scarcely possible to speak in terms of adequate praise ; which for perspicuity of description, acuteness of reasoning, and elegance of language, will probably long continue unrivalled ; and which, for its various merits, is justly classed among the standard classical works in medicine. It cannot be concealed, however, that many of the theoretical speculations in which Dr. Cullen indulged are in a great measure forgotten ; that much which he thought important is now neglected, and much that he neglected has since risen into consequence. This must ever be the fate of medical authors, and their productions. In the progress of years, new views of disease will naturally arise, and the general aspects of the science be materially altered.

It has appeared to the author, that in the course of the last twenty years, the science of medicine has undergone so considerable a
change, as to justify an attempt to give a new view of the Elements
of Pathology and of the Practice of Physic. Without desiring to
inquire minutely to what particular causes this change is to be ascribed, or how far the science has profited by it, it will be sufficient
for his purpose to allude very generally to the influence which the
works of Baillie and Bichat have had in bringing it about. To the
former the greatest praise is due for directing the attention of the
profession to the investigation of Morbid Anatomy, more effectually than had been done by Morgagni, his laborious but diffuse
predecessor in the same branch of study. The *effects* of disease in
the alteration of structure have been, by his means, more clearly
developed, and in many cases the *seats* of disease more accurately
ascertained.

But it is to the labours of Bichat that medicine is peculiarly indebted for those changes in its aspect now adverted to, and which
must be obvious to all in the general tone and character of the
medical writings of the present time. His Anatomie Generale,
and Traite des Membranes, present new and beautiful views of
the animal œconomy, which are obviously fitted to become the basis of pathology, by illustrating the *origin* of disease in the different structures of the body. The influence of these views on medical reasonings is daily becoming more apparent, and is now felt,
if not acknowledged, by many who are yet strangers to Bichat's
works. In several parts of the present volume they will be found
alluded to, but it will be the work of time to extend them, by cautious deductions, to the more obscure parts of the science.

It is a supposition, borne out by the evidence of history, that the
progress of medicine is upon the whole, in the great road of improvement. It is unfair to argue that the science is retrograde,
because we occasionally recur to an ancient opinion or practice.
Considering the mass of books which have been written on medical subjects, it would appear scarcely possible to invent a practice,
or to offer an opinion, which may not be traced in the writings of
former authors : but it is not in this way that the value of any new
suggestion can be ascertained, or the state of medical practice at
any one period justly appreciated. To form an estimate of either,
it is necessary to look to the great body of pathology, and it is
here that we shall find those improvements which modern medicine may boast. Nor must it be supposed, that improvements in

In this work the main object of the author has been to unite general views of disease with the detail of symptoms and treatment. He has rather gone into greater length in the former department, because the works commonly in the hands of medical students do not, to the best of his knowledge, contain any exposition of those leading pathological doctrines which it is his object to inculcate, and which he believes to be essential to the successful treatment of disease, by those at least who have not yet enjoyed the advantages of experience.

In an elementary Treatise on the Practice of Physic, it is not to be expected that any new matter should find a place. If therefore the author has occasionally indulged in speculations of his own, he ought rather to offer some excuse for his presumption, than bring it forward as a recommendation of the work. It has been his object to incorporate into the volume all the latest and most approved views of his contemporaries, regarding both the pathology and treatment of diseases. He has freely availed himself of their observations, and in many instances retained their expressions. Much however that is important has no doubt been overlooked; for the great extent of the subject precluded all hope of studying, and comparing accurately, even the best writers upon the different topics of inquiry. The author is, indeed, perfectly conscious of the many imperfections of the work, and he submits it with much deference to the judgment of the public.

CONTENTS.

PART I. ACUTE DISEASES.

PART II.

INTRODUCTION.

THE diseases of the human body being very numerous, it becomes highly important to make such an arrangement of them as may assist the memory, and if possible contribute to a clearer comprehension of their analogies and peculiarities. The first and most simple distinction among diseases is founded upon their susceptibility of relief from manual operation. This has led to the division of the science of medicine into the two great branches of Physic and Surgery, which, though for the most part taught and practised separately, are yet so intimately connected, that neither can be appreciated in all its bearings, unless viewed in conjunction with the other. Such a survey points out that the diseases of the external and internal parts of the body are all regulated by the same laws, judged of by the same means, excited frequently by the same causes, and alleviated or removed on the same general principles. Under this impression, it would be unnecessary for me to attempt to trace the boundaries of Physic and Surgery, which, for all useful purposes, is sufficiently effected by the courtesy of the world.

Among the diseases which fall under the particular congnizance of the Physician, the first distinction is into such as are attended, or unattended by Fever; that is to say, into the *febrile* and *apyrexial*. The second is into the *acute* (by which physicians understand diseases running a short and defined course;) and *chronic*, or such as are lingering and of uncertain duration. A third distinction, equally elementary, is into constitutional and local diseases;—into those namely, in which the whole system equally partakes, and those which depend more obviously and immediately upon the læsion of some particular organ. These are not to be considered in any other light than as artificial boundaries; or as beacons which may direct the student while in the path of education, but which may and ought to be neglected when that object is attended. It will hereafter be shown, that acute and chronic, local and constitution-al diseases, are blended together in an infinite variety of ways, which it is vain to attempt to unravel by the most ingenious contri-vances of an artificial system. It is, in fact, a most important principle in Pathology, that an intimate connection is established between all the parts of the living system, which must necessarily baffle every attempt to give a *perfect* idea of diseases by *separate* investigations. With this understanding, however, thoroughly im-pressed upon the mind, such distinctions may safely and advantage-ously be made the groundwork of a nosological arrangement of diseases, well calculated to elucidate the first principles of the science ; and they are taken as the basis of that which is observed in the following pages.

An inquiry into any particular disease includes in the first place a detail of the *symptoms* by which it is characterized in its several stages ; and in particular of such as serve to distinguish it from other diseases with which it is in danger of being confounded ; or to direct the judgment of the physician as to its probable dura-tion and termination ; and, lastly, of the appearances found after death. This first branch of the subject, therefore includes what-ever can be learned regarding a disease by *clinical* observation, and it constitutes the *history* of the disease—the *Medicina Prima* of ancient authors.

The second object of inquiry is the *pathology* of the complaint, by which is to be understood whatever can be made out concern-ing it by a process of reasoning. It includes an investigation of the *predisposing* and *exciting* causes, and of the seat and *nature* of the disease, in as far as they can be ascertained. This is the most abstruse and difficult part of the inquiry ; and though, even if suc-cessfully prosecuted, it does not *always* lead to practical results, yet in most instances, it throws the surest light upon this object of research ; and where it fails to point out the means of relief, often . suggests the reason, why that is difficult, tedious, or impossible.

The third topic of inquiry in the account of a particular disease is the *treatment*. To this, of course, every other part of the subject must be considered as subordinate. As a general principle of the first importance, I would wish here to inculcate strongly upon the student, that the cure of all diseases must be effected by the pow. ers of the *living system* ; and that his remedies are merely to be employed with the view of placing the body under the most favour. able circumstances for resisting disease. The general principles upon which the treatment of any disorder is to be conducted can alone find a place in this work. A knowledge of the manner of adapting these to the infinitely varied circumstances under which disease occurs, must be the result of personal experience, as it will be the sure reward of diligent observation.

In an elementary work on the Theory and Practice of Physic, something more however is required than a mere detail of the in. dividual diseases to which the human body is subject. I have al. ready stated, that they have their points of *analogy* as well as of *dissimilarity* ; and it is an object of consequence to determine these analogies to show the great features of resemblance which all dis. eases bear, and to trace the almost insensible gradations by which · they run into each other, and which enable us, either to view them as separate objects of inquiry, or as the closely connected mem. bers of a great family. This beautiful mixture of uniformity and variety in the phænomena of disease presents one of the most for. midable obstacles which a work of this nature has to encounter, and it can only be surmounted, and that partially, by occasional di. gressions into the obscure doctrines of GENERAL PATHOLOGY. Up. on these the Science of Medicine may be said strictly to be found. ed. They will, of course, be more or less important, and applica. ble to practice, in proportion as they are supported by views more or less correct of Chemistry and Mechanics, and of those laws which regulate the vital actions of the Animal Economy. The ob. scurity which is acknowledged to pervade all parts of General Pa. thology, is, in some, only faintly broken in upon by the glimmer. ings of conjecture. These will in the present volume be simply

1*

noticed, without attempting to estimate, with any degree of nicety, their claims to our confidence.

The work is divided into two parts, of which the first treats of acute, and the second of chronic disorders. The arrangement of diseases follows in its general outline, and in many of its details, the Nosology of Dr. Cullen; a work of great value, to which I shall have frequent occasion to refer, and to whose various merits I shall find many opportunities of doing justice. The alterations in it which I have adopted are such as appear to be rendered necessary from the improvements which have lately taken place in Pathology. The great features, however, of Dr. Cullen's system are retained, which being founded on a close observation of the phænomena of disease, will probably continue for ever to be the surest basis of any elementary view of The Theory and Practice of Physic.

PART I.

ACUTE DISEASES.

CLASS I. FEVERS.

CHAP. I.

GENERAL DOCTRINE OF FEVER.

Importance of the Subject. Fever how characterized. Of Rigors and Heat of Skin. Frequency of Pulse. Loss of Muscular Power. Disturbance in the Functions of the Stomach. Other Functions disturbed in Fever. Leading Divisions of Febrile Diseases. Causes of Fever, predisposing and occasional. Nature of Fever. Periodic movements observable in Fever. Doctrine of Critical Days. Principles of the Treatment of Fever.

FEVER is the most important, because the most universal and the most fatal of all the morbid affections of which the human body is susceptible. Its presence characterizes a great number of diseases; and in others which are not for the most part attended by it, the physician must always be prepared to expect its occurrence. It is *that*, by the presence or absence of which all his views of treatment are to be regulated, whose rise, progress, and termination, he always watches with the closest attention, and by the degree of which present, he is enabled in a great measure to estimate the danger in each particular case. Some idea may be formed of the great mortality of fevers from the statements of Sydenham, who calculated that two-thirds of mankind die of acute diseases properly so called, and two-thirds of the remainder of that lingering febrile disease, consumption. Fever has proved a fertile theme, on which the ingenuity of physicians in all ages has been exerted. Indeed the attention which it has received from every medical author, both ancient and mod-

2

difficult.
ind. by
disputa-
tion

ern, would alone be sufficient to impress upon any one the importance of the doctrines it embraces. How *difficult*, lastly, is the
study of fever may be inferred from this, that though so much
has been written concerning it, there is no one subject in the
whole circle of medical science which still involves so many disputed points. In every view the doctrines of fever must be considered of paramount importance, and they constitute therefore,
with great propriety, the foundation of all pathological reasoning.

attack
consists in
what?

When a person is suddenly attacked by shiverings or rigors,
followed by a hot skin, a quick pulse, and a feeling of langour
and lassitude, he is said to have an attack of fever. With such
symptoms are usually present also a loss of appetite, and thirst,
restlessness, and diminished secretion. These constitute the
six leading symptoms of fever or pyrexia, the characteristic
features by which its presence may always be detected. Every
function of the body indeed is more or less disturbed, but we
select for the *definition* of *fever* those which are of the most
importance in the animal œconomy. The marks of disturbance
in them afford the *characters* of fever just enumerated, and of
which we now propose to treat in detail.

1. (Chilliness, succeeded by increased heat of skin, is the
first and leading feature of fever.) The chilliness or rigor is
sometimes so slight as almost to escape the notice of the patient. At other times it is exceedingly violent, so that he complains bitterly of cold. His teeth chatter. His limbs tremble.
The skin is pale, rough, and contracted. The features shrink.
A sensation is felt as of cold water trickling down the back.
(By degrees the chilliness subsides, and begins to alternate with
warm flushings. A heat of skin greater than natural succeeds,
and with it returns the colour of the skin.) The cheeks become
even flushed, and the eyes suffused. The features recover their
usual size, or appear more turgid than in health. The hot stage
of fever is then said to be formed, which may go off in a few
hours, as in the case of an ague, or may continue for days or
weeks, as in common *continued* fever.

The duration of the (cold stage) varies from an hour to two or
even three days. Though often very slight, it is perhaps never
entirely wanting ; (and it is at all times to be carefully inquired
for and noted by the physician, as marking the precise period

of the accession of fever.) This it is useful to know in all febrile diseases ; but in some, as small-pox and measles, it forms
the basis of our prognosis.   The coldness of which the patient
complains is sometimes, though not always, perceptible to the
touch of another, but never to the extent that might have been
anticipated from the sufferings and expressions of the patient.

2. (The second great feature denoting the presence of fever
is an increase in the frequency of the pulse.) This is one of the
earliest and most constant of all the symptoms of fever, and perhaps would scarcely ever be wanting, but for some accidental
circumstance, such as a congestion of the blood in the vessels
of the brain or liver.   The feverish pulse of an adult varies in
point of frequency, from the slightest increase above the natural standard, to that point at which it can with difficulty be num-
bered.* (In forming any judgment of diseases by the frequency of the pulse, great allowance must always be made)for the
age of the patient,—for sex, constitution, and temperament of
body,—for the kind and period of the disease,—for external circumstances ; such, for instance, as the state of the air surrounding the patient, and the irritations to which he is exposed,—
lastly, for the effect of diet and medicines, and even in some circumstances the position of the body.   The pulse of fever differs from that of health in other points, besides that of comparative frequency.   These characters of the febrile pulse are distinguished by the terms hardness, wiriness, fullness, softness,
and weakness ; but as they are not essential to the existence of fever, they will more properly come under consideration hereafter.

Of these leading characters of fever, rigor succeeded by heat
of skin, and increased frequency of pulse, it is curious to observe what different judgments have been formed.   The bulk
of mankind have almost uniformly and by common consent laid
the greatest stress upon the increased heat of the body, and ac-

---

* For practical purposes it may be advisable for the student to make
some rude divisions of feverish pulses. The first may have 84 in a
minute for its average, and range between the natural standard and
90. The second may have 100 for its average, and its range will be
from 90 to 110. The third 120, ranging between 110 and 132. The
last, which I would call the *rapid* pulse, has 144 for its average. It
is the kind of pulse which is familiar to all in the last stages of *hectic*
fever.

cordingly all the expressions for *fever* in different languages
are derived from words signifying heat or fire.   This was for a
long time the doctrine of the schools, Galen having taught that
the essence of fever was in *prœternatural heat*.   Boerhaave, who
investigated the phenomena of fever with great accuracy, and
acknowledged the importance of these leading symptoms, yet
imagined that the quickened pulse was the single *essential* symptom of fever, uniformly present from the beginning to the end
of the disease, and by which the physician judges of its presence or degree.   Dr. Cullen, on the other hand, placed the rig-
or and shivering in the first rank of febrile symptoms.   He imagined that as the hot stage of fever is so constantly preceded by the cold stage, the one was *caused* by the other, and the
cause of the cold stage therefore the cause of all that followed
in the course of the paroxysm.   These opinions we may be allowed to consider as upon a par in point of relative merit. They
may all be supported by specious arguments, but we must end
by confessing, that fever does not consist in *this* or *that* symptom, but in the co-existence and succession of many.

   3. Among the various evidences of the presence of fever, the
(loss of muscular power)was noticed, marked by the occurrence
of languor and lassitude, a sensation of fatigue, and great pain
referred to the muscles and joints, particularly of the back and
limbs.) This striking index of fever was elegantly illustrated by
Boerhaave, under the title of *debilitas febrilis*.   It is to be distinguished from that weakness of muscle which arises from great
exertion, the privation of nourishment, or the violence or long
continuance of an evacuation.   It is present in a greater or less
degree in all fevers, though it bears no proportion to the violence
or danger of the disease.   It is aggravated by the slightest exertions of muscular power, and in severe cases is but partially
relieved by the horizontal posture.*

   4. Disturbances in the functions of animal heat, circulation,
and muscular motion, afford them the most prominent marks of
fever ; but every other function of the body, animal, vital, and

   * In the most severe forms of yellow fever, and other malignant epidemic diseases, the strength of the muscular system is often preserved
entire even to the last moments of life. See Rush's Med. Inquiries
and Observations ; Mc Arthur on Yellow Fever ; Johnson, &c. &c.
                                                Editor's Note.

natural, is more or less deranged, and that of the stomach in so remarkable a degree, as to demand particular notice. *Loss of appetite, nausea, and vomiting,* are very common symptoms of fever, but they are of secondary importance, both because fever frequently subsists without them, and they without fever. Connected with the loss of appetite, we may mention the symptom of *thirst,* one of the most familiar of all the characters of fever, and yet one more frequently wanting than any other. The desire is almost invariably for cold drink, and doubtless this is a beautiful provision of nature. There is no ground for believing with Asclepiades, and the followers of his school, that any danger is to be apprehended from the indulgence of this appetite.

5. The *restlessness and want of sleep* which occur in febrile diseases, are characteristic symptoms which deserve notice. They are seldom wanting in the early stages of fever, and are peculiarly distressing to the patient, often continuing during the whole course of a long fever. The return of sleep is one of the surest indications of its decline.

6. Nothing more strikingly characterizes the presence of fever than a general diminution and depraved state of the secretions all over the body. This is exemplified in the dryness and clamminess of the mouth, and the white and furred tongue, which are so frequently observed in all febrile diseases. The skin is dry and parched from the cessation of cuticular transpiration. The urine is scanty and high coloured. The bowels are generally constipated. The evacuations which may be procured are for the most part dark and fœtid. These and several other phenomena of fever are referable to the important general principle now laid down.

The restoration of secretion is generally considered as the test of the decline of fever, and hence it is, that in Sauvage's definition of fever, we find the terms, *cum madore cutis in declinatione ;* this however is not applicable unless such change be general over the body. *Occasional* perspirations are rather evidences of the febrile state, and as such frequently become the direct guides of our treatment.

Having thus explained the characters of *pyrexia,* it will be proper to inquire, what are the leading divisions of febrile diseases, and to point out generally what are the chief predisposing and *occasional* (or exciting) causes of fever.

A very superficial observation of nature is sufficient to point out the first distinction among febrile diseases, I mean that into *idiopathic* and *symptomatic.** Fever is often observed to arise without any very obvious cause, and the patient is then said to have idiopathic fever. When it occurs after an injury, or when it is coupled with redness of the throat, or acute pain of the side, he is said to have symptomatic fever.† It requires a more extended observation of the phenomena of disease to remark the leading divisions of *idiopathic* fever, which may be considered as three fold. There are fevers which consist of paroxysms ; there are simple continued fevers, and fevers complicated with eruption. In other words, idiopathic fevers are divisible into three great classes of INTERMITTENT, CONTINUED, and EXANTHEMATOUS. Among the symptomatic fevers which fall under the cognizance of the physician, a distinction has been attempted between those which are connected with local inflammation, and those attended with hæmorrhagy. It is not one of much importance, although I have assumed it as a basis of arrangement in this work.

These are the leading divisions of febrile diseases ; but to understand in what endless varieties they are presented to us, it will be sufficient to cast a cursory glance over the great variety of local inflammations with which they may be combined, and to reflect on the extent of influence, which climate, season, peculiarities of soil, age, temperament, and condition of body, may be presumed to exert in modifying their symptoms.

Very little is known with certainty in regard to the predisposition to fever. It is observed under aspects the most various. Every age and condition of body is subject to it ; it occurs in every variety of season and climate ; but each of these circumstances modifies its character, and contributes to establish those minute shades of distinction among febrile diseases which it will be my object hereafter to point out and illustrate. It is, however, abundantly obvious, that some persons are more liable than others to attacks of fever. In common language, their constitutions are more easily lighted up into fever. The cir-

---

* See Appendix ; Note A.

† Provided the injury, or the local affection has *preceded* the fever.

ED.

cumstances which appear more especially to give this predisposition to fever are the following: 1. The sanguine temperament and irritable habit of body; 2. The period of youth; 3.
Depression of mind; 4. Peculiar conditions of the atmosphere.
These will come under special consideration hereafter.

The exciting causes of fever are very numerous, and apparently of very opposite characters. External injuries, irritations of various kinds existing *within* the body (such as worms,)
the free use of wine, and exposure to cold and moisture, are
among the most obvious. They have been called by pathologists
the *common* causes of fever, in contradistinction to others of a
more recondite nature which have been termed *specific : viz.*
marsh miasmata, contagion, and morbid poison. Much importance is properly attached to each of these causes of fever.
They open very wide fields of inquiry, which, in future chapters, will become the objects of separate investigation.

It has been a favourite topic of inquiry among all writers on
fever, What is its nature?—In what particular state of the fluids
or solids of the body does it consist? The subject has been prosecuted with great diligence, but the result of the investigation
is very unsatisfactory. The earliest opinion on the nature of
fever was that of Hippocrates, who imagined it to be a *salutary*
effort of nature to throw off some noxious matter; and it is remarkable that this opinion was entertained before the class of
eruptive fevers was known, the phenomena of which certainly
afford the greatest countenance to it. The same doctrine was
supported by Stahl, who acknowledged, however, that when the
morbific matter was too abundant, or the powers of the body
not sufficiently energetic, fevers were hurtful. Boerhaave assumed as the essence or proximate cause of fever, a *lentor*, or
viscid state of the blood, and he applied this principle very inge-
niously to the explanation of the phenomena of fever.

The most rational views of the intimate nature of fever are
those of Hoffman, who believed that fever consisted primarily
in *diminished energy of the nervous system.* Without following
this author through the minute explanation of the several symptoms of fever which he founded upon this doctrine, we may be
permitted to say, that as a general principle it is fairly admissi-
ble, and that it satisfactorily accounts for many of the first and
most characteristic among them. Dr. Cullen went a step farther,

and argued that the diminished energy of the brain brought on *spasm of the extreme vessels,* which spasm was the real *proximate* cause of fever.* Since Dr. Cullen's time there have been several ingenious attempts to explain the pathology of fever. Dr. Wilson Philip supports the doctrine that fever consists, not in a spasm of the extreme vessels, but in the præternatural distension, and consequent *debility of the capillaries.*

Each of these theories is open to many and strong objections. An insuperable difficulty indeed seems to hang over the pathology of fever, but it is fortunately of little moment.† No theory of the proximate cause of fever which has yet appeared has contributed in any material degree to improve the treatment; though several of them, especially the Hippocratic, have had the effect of misleading and confusing the practitioner. The phenomena of fever give evidence of diminished energy of the brain, with increased action of the heart and arterial system; and the difficulty in the pathology of fever consists in showing, in what manner these disturbances of function are connected with each other. The older pathologists supposed it was brought about by the *vis medicatrix naturæ,* for which in modern times we have substituted the principle of *reaction;* but the precise mode in which this reaction of the heart and arteries is effected appears to be altogether inscrutable.

To the diminished energy of the nervous system we ascribe the languor, lassitude, loss of appetite, general uneasiness and pain of the back, which mark the invasion of fever. The functions of the brain not being as yet thoroughly understood, it is doubtful whether or not we are authorised in attributing to the same source the diminished and depraved secretion which occurs in fever; but it is highly probable that the phenomenon is in some measure connected with it. The same thing may be said of the increased heat which attends fever, the physiology of animal heat being, like that of secretion, involved in much obscurity. It would appear, however that this is a mixed function, in which the brain and heart are both essentially concern.

* See Appendix, Note B.

Febris, si phænomena illius species, reliquis morbis est notior; si constitutionem et causam, omnium ignotissima.—Baglivi de Praxi Medica, cap. xiii, sect. 5.

ed. The restlessness, head-ache, delirium, and other disturbances of the animal functions, which occur in fever are certainly attributable to an increased flow of blood upon the delicate
structure of the brain. They neither depend upon inflammation,
as some have contended, nor upon debility. They are neither
connected with actual *congestion* within the brain, nor are they
referable to sympathy of that organ with the chylopoietic viscera, as others have imagined.

In any attempt to explain the phenomena of fever, the luminous views of Dr. George Fordyce should be constantly kept in
remembrance. "A fever," says this able writer,* "is a disease
which affects the whole system. It affects the head, the trunk
of the body, and the extremities. It affects the circulation, the
absorption, and the nervous system. It affects the skin, the
muscular fibres, and the membranes. It affects the body, and
likewise the mind. It is therefore in every sense a disease
of the whole system."

Many of the phenomena of fever, its progress, and termination, appear to be guided by one of those laws of the animal
œconomy, the influence of which is sufficiently manifest in a
state of health—I mean the principle of *periodic movement*. The
most obvious illustration of this which physiology affords is in
the periods of utero-gestation and menstruation; but the recurrence of our appetites, the disposition to motion, sleep, and
waking, and in many, the natural evacuations, are phenomena
regulated also by a principle of periodic movement. The regularity observable in the periods of the eruptive fevers, of which
we shall hereafter speak more fully, is unquestionably the most
beautiful and well marked illustration of the same thing which
pathology affords; but it is exemplified also in some of the
phenomena of gout, mania, epilepsy, and menorrhagia. To
this principle of periodic movement in the animal œconomy
have been ascribed the *types* of intermittent, and the *crises* of
continued fevers. Of the former we shall treat more fully hereafter. What is essential to be known concerning the latter may
find its place here.

The doctrine of critical days, that is to say, the supposition
that fevers are disposed to terminate favourably or unfavoura-

* Dissertations on Fever, No. 1, p. 28.

3

bly at certain periods of the disease more than at others, has found many advocates, and some opposers even from the earliest times. The very general reception which it has met with among mankind makes me unwilling to distrust it altogether; and if we bear in mind how many circumstances may contribute to disturb the regular course of a disease, we may admit the doctrine of critical days in fever without much risk of error. There has been some dispute about the precise days, but they are generally set down as the seventh, ninth, eleventh, fourteenth, seventeenth, and twenty-first, counting from the invasion of the cold fit. During the first week of fever no days of crisis can be ascertained. In the second week it happens on the alternate odd days, and the three first are therefore called the tertian crisis. In the third week the critical days follow the quartan type, and the three last are therefore called the quartan crises. It is seldom that these observations can be verified in the fevers of this country, which run their course with much less regularity than those of warmer climates.*

The last illustration of that principle of periodic movement observable in the diseased actions of the body, which I shall now notice, is the disposition in all febrile diseases whatever to evening exacerbation and morning remission. This is strikingly manifested in *hectic* and *infantile* fever: but it is equally to be traced in all the more common forms of continued fever. Severe as the symptoms may have been during the day, they will generally be found aggravated about six or seven o'clock in the evening. Restless as the patient may have been during the night, he will generally obtain some rest, or relief from his complaints, soon after daylight. These circumstances are important in reference to the proper period for the exhibition of medicines.

A few general remarks on the principles which should regulate our treatment of idiopathic febrile diseases will conclude what is to be said regarding the general doctrine of fever.

1. The most important feature in this view of the subject is, the natural tendency in all febrile diseases to run a certain course, and to terminate in the restoration of health. It is this circumstance which forms so prominent a distinction be-

* See Appendix; Note C.

tween acute and chronic disorders. It is observable in many local affections attended with fever, but it is very strikingly il. lustrated in the case of continued fevers, and the exanthemata. The latter will always, and the former will very frequently run their regular course, notwithstanding all the efforts of art. In ancient times, nay even at no very distant date, it was made a question, whether it was safe and proper to cut short a fever. The question is set at rest with regard to the *propriety* of doing so, but the possibility of it is still very questionable. It may sometimes be practicable, but it can never become the founda. tion of our treatment in febrile diseases. The natural tendency of fever to come to a crisis, or to work its own cure, may on the other hand be often kept in view with the best advantage; and though the extravagancies of a *medecine expectante* are just. ly blameable, the spirit of the doctrine should never be disre-garded.

2. We might lay infinitely more stress on this principle in the general treatment of fever, and act up to it with much more freedom, were it not that a second interferes with it, of at least *equal* importance, but leading to a practice diametrically oppo-site. This is the disposition which exists in all febrile states of the system to local congestions and inflammations, and other ir-regular distributions of blood, which end in very serious distur-bance of function, or actual disorganization of structure. Such a principle appears to have been overlooked by several of the old school of medicine, or at least never to have attracted that attention, which its importance in practice merits. It shows the necessity of using every endeavour to cut the fever short, before such local congestions or inflammations have taken place, or at any rate before they have attained any dangerous height.

3. The third circumstance of importance in regulating the treatment of fever is the necessity of studying symptoms, and of deducing from them the indications of cure. The pathology of fever is so obscure, that it affords but little help in determi-ning the plan of treatment. In many diseases, apoplexy for ex-ample, or dropsy, individual symptoms are of little practical importance, for we treat them by a consideration of their cause; but in fever the alleviation of particular symptoms is often a matter of the highest consequence. The variations too in the

symptoms of a fever are often great and rapid ; and with them
must vary our views of the actual condition of the body, and
consequently the plan of our treatment. It will be seen hereafter, that this point of doctrine applies to all the forms of idiopathic fever.

4. The necessity of attention to the nature of the prevailing
epidemic is the next point which I would urge. Epidemic diseases are with very few exceptions febrile ; and it is a curious
but well ascertained fact, that the epidemics of particular seasons acquire a particular character, the knowledge of which
assists very materially in forming a judgment as to the treatment proper to be pursued in any individual case. Sydenham
was among the first authors who directed their attention to
the *epidemic character of seasons.* He pointed out, not only
that different febrile diseases prevailed in different years, but
that the same form of febrile disease assumed in different years
different characters, and required corresponding changes of
treatment. "I have difficulty," he states, "on the breaking
out of any new epidemic, in providing, that one or two of those
who first employ me are not hurried off before I can trace the
genius of the disease, so as to fix the cure of it." This important doctrine might be illustrated, not only by the phenomena
of continued fevers, whose characters are so infinitely varied,
but by those also of agues, and the inflammatory affections of
the thorax and abdomen. (The principle is observable even
in the phenomena of eruptive fevers, such as small-pox and
measles, which are but little modified by the influence of other
causes.)

5. There are two principal modes of treating fever, the evac-
uating, and the stimulating. The first includes bleeding, vomiting, purging, saline diuretics, and diaphoretics. The second
comprises the employment of ether, wine and brandy, aromatics and cordials, bark and bitters, opium. The skill of the physician is eminently displayed in determining under what circumstances of fever, in what stages of fever, in what kinds of fever,
these several modes of treatment are respectively applicable, to
what extent they should be carried, and how and when they may
be advantageously blended with each other.

CHAP. II.

Nosological Divisions of Continued Fever. Circumstances modifying the Symptoms of Continued Fever; Climate and Seasons; the State of the Air; Constitution and Habits of Body. Symptoms of Inflammatory Fever. Of common Continued Fever. Of Typhus. Of Fever complicated with local Affection. Causes of such Complication. Of the Organs and Structures affected in the Course of Fever. Nature of the local Affection. Morbid Appearances from continued Fever. Period of Fevers at which local determinations take place. State of oppression in Fever. Principles of Prognosis. Of Malignancy and Putrescency. Favourable Symptoms. Average Mortality by Continued Fever.

IDIOPATHIC FEVER was stated in the last chapter to admit of a three-fold division; *viz.* into intermittent, continued, and eruptive fevers. We shall begin by the consideration of continued fevers, and in the present chapter confine our attention to the various *appearances* which they exhibit.

The views of physicians with regard to continued fevers have undergone a number of very remarkable changes, to which nothing has more essentially contributed than the infinite diversity of symptoms by which they are characterised. Nosologists have been at great pains to note minutely these different symptoms, and have founded upon them their divisions of continued fever. Boerhaave has three, Linnæus four, Sauvages five, and Macbride five-and twenty species of continued fever. Some (as Sauvages) have assumed as the basis of their arrangement, the comparative duration of the disease; but the generality of authors have made the difference of symptoms the ground-work of their distinctions. From the very earliest periods it was observed, that some fevers showed symptoms of strong inflammatory action, while others exhibited marks of depressed nervous energy, and, as it was said, of *putrescency.* One of the first distinctions therefore among fevers was into the *febris ardens* and the *febris putrida.* There being however a variety of fevers, which shewed first the one, and then the other of these sets of symptoms, nosologists added a third class, or that of *mixed fevers.* Such is the arrangement of Dr. Cullen ; and the terms Synocha, Typhus, and Synohcus, were employed by him to express these fundamental divisions of continued fever.

Of late years, a different view of the varieties of continued fever has been gradually gaining ground. An increased importance is attached to the *exciting cause*, and the term *typhus* is employed to designate a particular form of continued fever, which we shall presently describe, one of the distinguishing features of which is, that it is communicable by contagion.* To that kind of fever which arises from cold, excess in wine, or other common sources of irritation, we apply the term *common continued.*

A third important distinction among continued fevers is now derived from the circumstance of their affecting all organs and functions equally, when they are called *simple fevers*, or implicating one organ or structure more particularly than another, and deriving from it some peculiarity of character. Fevers of the latter class (called *complex* fevers) are infinitely diversified, and have received the several denominations of brain fever, catarrhal fever, gastric fever, mesenteric fever, miliary fever, bilious fever. These distinctions among fevers, though apparently vague, are yet sufficient for all practical purposes. They do not withdraw the mind from the important consideration, that the nosological divisions of fever are arbitrary, and calculated, not so much to direct the method of cure, as to increase the facility of instruction.

Continued fevers have all a common character, which various circumstances serve in a remarkable manner to modify. What

* Dr. John Armstrong, the author of the most able and popular work extant on Typhus Fever, was originally a believer in its contagiousness. With a candor and honesty, which reflects honor on his scientific independence, he has since publicly recanted this belief.— See N. Y. Edition of Armstrong on Typhus, and Mc Gill on Typhus Fever in 30th Number of N. Y. Med. and Phys. Journal.— ED.

these are, and the extent of their influence, is a subject worthy of accurate investigation.

1. The most important of them all is climate. Its effects upon the general character of man, the structure of his body, his stature, his intellectual faculties, his habits, and dispositions, it is the province of the physiologist, the natural historian, and the political œconomist, to unfold. Its influence upon the morbid conditions of the body, we shall have frequent opportunities of illustrating. We shall see it exemplified in the phenomena of hepatitis, gout, scrofula, dysentery. Of all states of disease, as fever is the most general, so is it that, over which climate has the greatest modifying influence. The important principle to be kept in view is, that a hot climate is favourable to the developement of inflammatory fever; while the low, or nervous form of fever prevails chiefly in cold or temperate climates.

2. Season may be considered as modifying the character of continued fever much in the same manner as climate. The spring and summer seasons favour the prevalence of inflammatory fever; autumn and winter of the putrid or nervous fever. (Warm climates and seasons give a tendency to complications of abdominal disease with fever; cold climates and seasons, on the other hand, to affections of the thoracic viscera. ˋ The evidences of this point of doctrine will appear when we come to treat of the diseases of particular organs.

3. The next of those circumstances which strikingly modify the symptoms of continued fever, is the condition of the air. The influence of the atmosphere on febrile diseases is a subject that opens a very wide and difficult field of investigation. It appears, that of those states of the air which affect the origin, diffusion, progress, and character of fever, some are obvious to our senses, and some not. Sydenham has described these under the appropriate designations of the *temperies aeris manifesta*, and *occulta*. The condition of the air, in regard to heat and cold, dryness and moisture, must obviously exert an important influence; but it has further been always observed, that the most dangerous fevers are those which prevail where the atmosphere, in its chemical composition, is impure from the neglect of proper ventilation. Such a vitiated state of the air (very liable to occur in camps, jails, ships, crowded and small apartments) gives occasion to those symptoms which are called

low or putrid; while, on the other hand, a free circulation of cool and pure air conduces to the developement of those which are now generally called the symptoms of *excitement*. This is sometimes exemplified in a remarkable manner, in the sudden removal of a patient labouring under continued fever from an impure atmosphere into the spacious wards of a well regulated hospital. The symptoms have under such circumstances been observed to alter so materially, and the constitution to undergo such a change, as to require, and to enable the practitioner to carry into effect, measures which were previously inadmissible, But besides these *obvious* qualities of the air which modify the symptoms of fever, there are certain others undiscoverable by any of our senses, which appear to have great influence over them. A few conjectures have been hazarded by Sydenham and others, with the view of throwing some light on the nature of these *occult* qualities of the air; but the subject is involved in a degree of obscurity, which will probably for ever continue to baffle our researches. Their existence, however, can hardly be doubted, and to them we must in a great measure attribute the prevalence of *epidemics*, still more decisively that curious phenomenon alluded to in the last chapter, the *diversity* in the character of the epidemic diseases of different years.*

4. The last which I shall mention, in an enumeration of the important circumstances which modify the symptoms of fever, is confined in its operation to the affected individual ;—I mean, constitution and habit of body. The extent of influence which peculiarities of constitution and habit of body exert over the symptoms and character of fever is, however, less than might naturally have been expected. The important fact indeed is, that under circumstances the most opposite, fever often shows the most striking uniformity—that the young and the old, the robust and the delicate, the active and the idle, the dissolute and those of regular lives, exhibit, when attacked by fever, the same series of symptoms. Still a certain degree of allowance must always be made for the constitution and habit of body of the individual affected ; and it has been found, that a number of minute circumstances referable to this head, tend in differ- ent ways to the modification of fever. Of these the principal

---

* See Appendix ; Note D.

are, the period of life, the temperament of body, the tone of the fibre, the kind of diet on which the individual had been previously nourished, and the state of the mind.

The period of infancy enjoys a very remarkable exemption from idiopathic continued fever, although abundantly susceptible of fever in other forms. The period of youth, the sanguine temperament, and a full diet of animal food, with a proportion of wine or distilled spirits, give a tendency to an inflammatory character in the fever. On the other hand, weakness of body and flaccidity of fibre, whether the effect of original formation, or of previous diseases, or of great exertion, or long watchings, or deficient nourishment, conduce to the low and typhoid form of fever; and it is therefore in individuals of this habit of body, that the purest cases of typhus are observed. The state of mind is universally found to have great influence over the susceptibility of the body to the reception of continued fever. The depressing passions, anxiety, fear, despair, dispose to the propagation and add to the malignity of fever; while hope and confidence serve, in a manner no less remarkable, to ward off its attack, or to stem its violence.

I have already attempted to explain, that though continued fever should be considered as a single *genus*, yet for the convenience of illustration and description, it is useful to make some broad distinctions among its various forms. I pointed out a division into inflammatory, common continued, and typhus fever, as one that was well adapted for an elementary view of the subject. The symptoms commonly presented by these different forms of fever may next come under our notice.

1. Inflammatory fever (the *Synocha* of Dr. Cullen) is not often met with in its exquisite form in this country. It is that, however, which fever assumes in all hot climates where there is no *peculiarity of soil* to interfere with its development. It is instanced in the summer fever of Sicily and the Mediterranean, as described by Dr. Irvine, Dr. Burnett,* and others. Its invasion, which is generally very sudden, is marked by excessive prostration of strength, with some shivering, soon succeeded by a violent heat of skin, pain of back, head-ache, giddiness,

---

* Irvine's " Observations on Diseases chiefly as they occur in Sicily,"—Burnett's " Account of the Fever of the Mediterranean Fleet."

and general uneasiness. The head-ache is very acute, the eyes are suffused, the countenance flushed. The temporal and carotid arteries beat violently. There is often copious bleeding at the nose, with restlessness; and occasionally, but not constantly, delirium. The tongue becomes rapidly coated with a thick fur. Nausea, vomiting of bile, great thirst, and a costive state of bowels prevail. The pulse varies from 100 to 120, strong, full, and regular. The respirations are quick ; the skin hot and excessively dry ; the urine scanty and high coloured. Violence in the degree of symptoms, and rapidity of progress, are the prevailing characters of inflammatory fever. If suffered to run its course, it may prove fatal in less than twenty-four hours. If proper measures are pursued, the disease will often yield, but unless they are speedily resorted to, lingering convalescence will be found to follow, attributable in all probability to a degree of local mischief in the delicate structure of some organ, particularly the brain, occasioned by the violence of the first attack.

2. The common continued fever of this and most other temperate climates (the *Synochus* of Cullen) is less sudden in its invasion, less rapid in its progress, and all its symptoms are less violent. The patient is generally under its influence several days before he is confined to bed. The pulse at first is frequent and strong, but by degrees it loses strength without diminishing in frequency. The duration of the disease is very various ; but when once the symptoms of fever have subsided, the convalescence is usually rapid.

3. To the severest cases of continued fever which occur in temperate climates, which have their origin, as we shall presently explain, for the most part in contagion, which commence insidiously, and present in their progress a set of symptoms which denote great depression of nervous energy, rather than high excitement of the heart and arteries, physicians apply the name of *typhus*. This form of fever begins with a slight feeling of indisposition, succeeded by chilliness, languor, depression, sighing and oppression in breathing, and loss of appetite. These symptoms increase for several days, till the patient becomes so weak that he cannot sit up without great exhaustion. The disease is then fairly set in, having its exacerbation in the evening, and declining in violence towards the morning.

Many of the characters of typhoid fever are unsusceptible of accurate description ; and of these the most remarkable is the *expression of countenance*, so uniform as to make all typhoid patients, in a great degree, resemble each other. It is a very peculiar expression of *anxiety*, joined to a flushed appearance of the cheeks. It is seldom wanting, and constitutes, in fact, a striking characteristic of typhus. The pulse in this form of fever is very frequent, generally averaging from 120 to 130, small and weak. The tongue, at first very much coated, becomes in the progress of the disease brown, or almost black ; it it is dry and parched ; occasionally, instead of being coated, it appears smooth and præternaturally red. Black sordes collect around the teeth. The evacuations from the bowels are exceedingly fœted, and often black, or mixed with blood. As the disease advances they are passed involuntarily. The urine is in like manner fœtid, turbid, and in small quantity. The skin is hot and dry. From an early period of the disease delirium occurs, of a low muttering kind ; and tremors, subsultus tendinum, with total want of sleep, and great uneasiness or *restlessness*, supervene. Sometimes however there is *stupor*. Typhus is further characterised by extreme weakness of muscular fibre. The slightest exertion, such as rising in bed, aggravates all the symptoms, or even brings on a fit of syncope. The body emaciates rapidly. Effusions of blood underneath the skin take place and appear in the form of livid spots or streaks, called petechiæ and vibices. The duration of the disease varies from two to three, or even four weeks ; when, unless some favourable change or crisis takes place, the countenance collapses, the features shrink, the eye loses its lustre, the pulse sinks ; and hiccup, rattling in the throat, coldness of the extremities, and profuse clammy sweats, with a cadaverous odour of the body, indicate the approach of death.

Such are the leading characters of typhus fever. When only the mildest of these symptoms are present, the disease is call-*typhus mitior*. When the same occur in their highest state of intensity, and when to them are added the more formidable of the above recited symptoms, such as are supposed to denote a malignant and putrescent state of the body (especially hæmorrhages and petechiæ,) the disorder assumes the character, and with it the name of *typhus gravior*. The students will of

course understand that these two varieties of typhus fever run
into each other by imperceptible degrees, and neither admit of
, nor require any very precise distinctions. Both the one and
the other occasionally exhibit marks of inflammatory action at
the onset, but a fever is always named from the character of the
predominating symptoms.

From the detail which has been now given, it is obvious that
inflammatory and typhoid fever, however they may differ in
some points, yet agree in affording evidence of deranged function in every organ of the body,—the brain, the heart, the lungs,
the stomach and bowels, the liver, the kidneys, and the skin.
Cases both of inflammatory and of typhus fever have been
observed, which follow the progress I have now attempted to
describe, implicating equally every organ and function. These
are cases of *simple* fever, but they are comparatively rare. It
is much more common to see one or other of these organs particularly affected. What the circumstances are which direct
the violence of the febrile action upon one organ or structure in
preference to another, does not always appear, but it can sometimes be satisfactorily explained.

Peculiar conformations of body, hereditary predispositions,
or the weakening of parts by previous diseases, have a decided
influence. A stout young man, with a short neck, and of a full
habit of body if attacked by fever, will be more likely, *cæteris
paribus*, to have symptoms denoting determination to the head,
than a tall thin young man, with a narrow chest, and subject to
cough. The latter, during the progress of fever, may very prob.
ably have difficult breathing, with pain of side, and purulent expectoration. Much may be attributed also to the influence of climate and season ; heat favouring the disposition to abdominal,
and cold to thoracic affections. But it must be confessed there
is something more than this required to account for the phenom.
enon. What the exact pathological principle is, upon which it
further depends, has not indeed been hitherto explained, although some attempts towards elucidating it have been made.
It appears, from numerous observations, that various states of
disease of the brain and its coverings, both acute and chronic,
such as blows on the head, fractures of the cranium, lacerations
of the dura mater, tumours and abscesses within the substance
of the brain, are not unfrequently attended by disease of distant

organs; such disease being attributable simply to a state of disordered circulation in the encephalon, and disturbance in the
functions of the nervous system. To the same cause, whatever
be its precise nature, we refer many of those local affections
with which fever is so frequently complicated.

It is a point of some importance to determine what the organs and structures are, most liable to become affected in the
course of fever,—what is the nature of these local affections,
—and at what periods of the fever they chiefly occur.

1. Of the organs liable to become more particularly implicated in fever, the most important is the brain. The symptoms
by which we judge of this having taken place, will be hereafter
described in detail when treating of phrenitis and apoplexy.
The principal are head ache, giddiness, suffused eyes, delirium,
coma. The second in point of importance is the mucous membrane of the stomach and bowels. The symptoms denoting a
particular affection of this structure are now usually called the
gastric symptoms. They are, pain in the epigastrium, nausea
and vomiting, a sense of fulness in the bowels, diarrhœa or
dysentery. The liver may next be mentioned as liable to suffer in the course of fever. It is not observed to any great extent in this country, but it is very commonly met with in hot
climates, and gives a character to the endemic fevers of those
regions. The peculiar character of hepatic or bilious fever is
given by the concurrence of jaundice, irritable stomach, and
pain or fullness of the right hypochondrium, with the usual
symptoms of pyrexia. The pleura and peritonæum are also
occasionally attacked; but next to affections of the head, by
far the most frequent of all the local complications with fever,
is disease of the mucous membrane of the bronchia, appearing
in the form of cough, difficult breathing, increased (sometimes
purulent) expectoration, and general diffused pain over the
chest.*

2. Much controversy has taken place regarding the nature of
the affection, under which the different organs labour when at-

* Dr. Crampton, in an essay, entitled "Medical Report, containing
a brief account of the late Epidemic in Dublin," has given (page 48)
an estimate of the relative proportions in which different organs were
there pressed in fever. Out of 755 cases, 550 complained of the head,

tacked in the course of fever. Dr. Clutterbuck, who urged the
importance of these local determinations in fever, believed that
it was *inflammation*; and seeing how much more frequently the
brain was affected than any other part of the body, maintained
that continued fever was essentially inflammation of the brain.
Others have argued, that in a large proportion of cases, the
vessels of the affected part are in a state not of inflammation, but of distention, or *congestion*. A distinction has even
been attempted between *inflammatory typhus*, in which the seat
of disease is in the system of arterial vessels, and *congestive typhus*, in which the branches of the venous system are concerned. It has been supposed that this distinction between the inflammatory action of arterial capillaries, and the congestion of
blood in veins, explains the diversities of morbid appearances
found after death, and may serve as a guide in directing us to
the proper methods of treatment. Now allowing the possibility
of such a state of congestion in the venous system (which however is not proved in this case,) it still remains to be shown,
that it may not, and does not run into the other. Until this is
done, we cannot attach any great degree of pathological or
practical importance to the distinction. The appearances on
dissection in those who die of fever sufficiently point out, that
danger is chiefly to be apprehended from the occurrence of inflammation; and that against such a state the measures of the
physician are to be directed, when he has evidence of local disease complicated with continued fever.

Morbid anatomy, it must be confessed, throws but little light
on the pathology or *nature* of fever; but it points out its *effects*,
and illustrates in particular those local affections which we
have mentioned as so often coupled with fever. The most common morbid appearance, in cases of fever, is a gelatinous effusion upon the surface of the arachnoid membrane. Serum is
sometimes found in the ventricles; besides which we perceive
in many instances a fulness of the vessels of the brain, as if
they had been subjected to a fine anatomical injection. Occasionally we meet with extravasations of blood, or the deposition

129 of the chest, and 76 of the abdomen. The proportions however
will of course vary in different places, in different seasons, and in different years.

of purulent matter. In the thorax we find marks of an inflamed pleura. Pus is sometimes effused into the cavity of that membrane. Also, redness of the lining membrane of the bronchia, with increased mucous or purulent secretion. In the abdomen there are occasional evidences of peritonæal inflammation; but the most usual appearance is that of ulceration, more or less extensive, of the mucous coat of the intestines.

3. The last topic to which I proposed to advert in this division of the subject, was the period of fever at which these local determinations are most usually observed to take place. In a few cases it is at the very onset of the disease; and this circumstance is important, as leading to the distinction between the states of *oppression* and *collapse*. The attack of fever is always attended by weakness; but if the blood be at that period particularly determined to the brain, a state of apparently extreme debility is brought on, which has often intimidated the practitioner, and prevented the adoption of those decisive measures which might then be *safely* had recourse to, and which alone could ensure a favourable termination. In a large proportion of cases where great weakness attends the *onset* of the disease, the symptom is to be attributed to a load oppressing the brain, to a state of *oppression*, and not of weakness, exhaustion, or, as it is called, *collapse*. Local congestions, however, take place in the progress of fever more frequently than at its commencement. They have even occurred when the febrile symptoms have subsided, and the patient been considered convalescent. · To decide, whether the symptoms which then supervene are referable to a state of oppression or collapse, is one of the most difficult points in the practice of physic. It can be effected only by a close attention to particular symptoms. The pulse is for the most part the safest guide; but the appearance of the countenance, the position of the body, and other minutiæ which *clinical* observation can alone teach, assist materially in the decision of the question.

The judgment of the physician regarding the probable course, duration, and termination of any particular case, is founded, in a great measure, on the observation of *symptoms*. This, in medical language, is the *prognosis*; and the principles by which it is regulated apply to a certain extent to all diseases.

1. There is, in the first place, a *general prognosis* founded

on an extensive view of disease, which enables us to give an opinion regarding the probable course of particular cases, without any minute attention to symptoms. Thus, we can confidently predict, that a case of catarrh or sore throat will end favourably, that a case of acute rheumatism will prove tedious, a case of croup hazardous, of consumption hopeless. In treating of diseases in detail, some allusion to general prognosis will always be made.

2. There is a prognosis applicable only to individual cases, and this is to be regulated by an attention to a number of minute circumstances, in detecting which, and estimating their relative importance, the skill of the physician is eminently called forth. This part of his duty can be but imperfectly taught in books. It is generally said to be guided by the presence or absence of certain *symptoms,* which are set down under the heads of *favourable* and *unfavourable* symptoms. These have been collected together with great industry by various authors, but taken singly they are not of that consequence which might have been imagined. It is impossible, indeed to lay down with strict accuracy the rules of prognosis. In actual practice, it is commonly determined by several considerations of a *general* nature ; and of these, it will be found that one of the most important is the period of the disease at which a particular symptom occurs. To be able to draw legitimate conclusions therefore with reference to prognosis, from the observation of such a symptom, it is necessary to be well acquainted with the usual train in which the phenomena of the disease manifest themselves, and the causes upon which each depends. The age and habits of the patient, the natural strength of his constitution, the circumstances in which he is placed, the period of time which has elapsed before medical treatment is resorted to, and the possibility of employing medicines effectually, have also a most important influence over the course and probable termination of the disease. They must all, therefore, be taken into consideration in determining the prognosis ; but they are obviously much too indefinite for particular investigation.

The *symptoms* which denote danger in continued fever are those, first, of excessive inflammatory excitement ; secondly, of topical congestion ; and thirdly, of great depression, or irregular action of the nervous power. Among the latter are inclu.

ded those which the older writers were in the habit of designating as the symptoms of *malignancy and putrescency*, a state of body, the notion of which has been, in latter times, the frequent subject of dispute. That the powers of the living body, in checking the putrescent tendency of all animal matter, should be diminished in certain states of disease, does not, however, appear to be an unreasonable supposition. The following may be enumerated as the chief symptoms which denote *malignancy* and the putrescent diathesis. They are of course the symptoms most to be dreaded in typhus gravior. A loose or very imperfect coagulation of the blood ; fœtor of the evacuations ; a squalid appearance of the skin, and a cadaverous odour of the body ; hæmorrhages from the mouth, nose, stomach, rectum, or urethra, the blood being of a very loose texture, and quickly putrefying ; petechiæ and vibices ; a disposition to gangrene in the skin, wherever it has been accidentally wounded, or abraded, or exposed to long pressure ; the speedy putrefaction of the body after death. It would be necessary to clear up many of the difficulties in which the doctrines of the blood are involved, before we could arrive at a satisfactory explanation of these phenomena ; but in the mean time there are sufficient grounds for believing, that malignancy and putrescency in acute diseases depend principally upon the functions of the brain becoming *early* and *deeply* implicated. The vitiated condition of the fluids which results may be viewed as the great pathological distinction between typhus gravior and typhus mitior.

The most alarming symptoms in the milder form of typhus may be thus enumerated : a dilated pupil ; involuntary evacuations ; hiccup ; low muttering delirium continuing through the day as well as night ; constant watchfulness ; picking of the bed-clothes ; subsultus tendinum.

A variety of symptoms are mentioned by writers on continued fever as favourable ; such as deafness, tumours behind the ears, miliary eruptions, diarrhœa, sediments in the urine, the breaking out of a sweat, and the formation of abscesses. Upon the latter, much stress has been laid. They have been considered as *critical* discharges, that is to say, as serving to carry off noxious humours generated during the fever. This point of doctrine we do not now insist upon ; and upon the whole it may be remarked, that there is no single symptom occurring in the course of fever, which can be set down as decidedly favourable ; but that the probability of recove-

5

ry must always be estimated by the character of the symptoms when viewed in connection with each other.

The *general* prognosis in continued fever is certainly favourable. Under proper management, a large proportion of cases recover. This is a point which has been made an object of inquiry by different writers and a very curious coincidence has been traced in the extent of mortality occasioned by continued fever under circumstances considerably different*. The average of deaths in the hospitals of this country appears to be in the ratio of about one to twelve, which is believed to be considerably *below* the ordinary scale of the mortality of fever, when it occurs in private habitations, even with access to medical assistance. It varies of course with the general character of the epidemic, the period of the disease at which it is first submitted to medical treatment, and other circumstances of nearly equal importance, the influence of which has been already adverted to.†

* Consult Bateman's " Succinct Account of the Contagious Fever of this Country."—London, 1818.   Page 75.

† See pages 26 and 27.

CAUSES OF CONTINUED FEVER.

Exciting causes of Fever. Of common causes leading to Ephemeral Fever. Of Cold as the cause of Disease in general. Of Fever in particular. Alternations of Atmospheric Temperature. Of Contagion. First accounts of Contagion. General Doctrines of Contagion. Of Fomites. Other supposed causes of Fever.

It was stated in the first chapter (page 16,) that the exciting causes of continued fever admitted of a division into the two great classes of *common and specific.* The first of these are, in a measure, obvious to our senses; and their operation, is to a certain degree intelligible. The second are more recondite in their nature, and their mode of operation is very obscure, if not altogether inscrutable. Another well-marked line of distinction between them may be drawn from the circumstance of the first, or the common causes of fever, inducing this state of disease *rapidly*, while the latter require a certain, and generally a defined length of time before their influence is apparent. Feverishness suddenly brought on by any of the more common kinds of irritation, is for the most part transient in its course, and has accordingly received from nosologists the name of *Ephemera.*

Any irritating causes are capable of engendering fever in the human body; but this they will more particularly do, when the frame is *predisposed* to fever, either by peculiarity of temperament or habit, or by the state of the mind and nervous system, or by certain conditions of the air. Those which are most frequently observed to operate as exciting causes of fever, are, external injuries, cold, the presence of worms, difficult dentition, an overloaded stomach, the free use of wine or distilled spirits, excessive fatigue, insolation (or exposure to the direct rays of the sun), long watching, or long protracted pain. Of all these *common* causes of con-

tinued fever, the most frequent is *cold*; and as cold will hereafter
be mentioned as an occasional cause of several other diseases, besides fever, both acute and chronic, we shall direct our attention
in a more particular manner to this branch of the subject.

It becomes, in the first place, a matter of some importance to
determine, in what manner cold is to be considered as the cause
of disease, and particularly of febrile disease.   In a healthy condition of body the extremes of heat and cold, though continued for
a great length of time, are borne without injury ; but in feeble
frames, and in irritable habits of body, the case is different. With
them the simple reduction of atmospheric temperature predisposes
to, and at length excites various forms of disease, but in most cases
disease of a *chronic* kind, such as dyspepsia, scrofula, chorea, and
hysteria, It is seldom that we observe *fever* arising from such a
cause. Fever consequently is not more common in northern than
it is in tropical latitudes. But though cold applied to the body
under common circumstances does not create fever, the case is
widely different when it is associated with moisture, when it operates after a long continuance of hot and close weather, or where it
is applied suddenly, partially, irregularly, or when the body is overheated and perspiring profusely, either from the nature of the climate, or from great exertion, or exposure to artificial heat.

The importance of the function of perspiration in regulating the
uniformity of animal heat, and the actions of other organs, is well
known to the physiologist, and is illustrated by him in various ways.
It seems probable that it is through the medium of this function
that cold operates in the production of fever. It closes the pores,
checks perspiration, and drives the blood in increased quantity upon the internal organs. When we look to the vast *extent* of the skin,
and reflect on the immense quantity of blood with which it is supplied, it is not difficult to understand that this disturbance in the
operations of the animal œconomy, should be occasionally productive of bad effects, and experience shows that of these the most usual is *fever*.

When once fever is excited, it may assume different appearances. In many cases the mischief falls upon some particular organ
of the body, the tonsils, the lungs, the liver, the bowels, or joints ;
and is directed upon them, sometimes without any apparent cause,
at other times in consequence of some cognizable circumstance,
such, for instance, as weakness in the structure of the organ, or a

predis.
7 par.
ticular
organ

liability brought on by previous disease. This is an important law of the animal œconomy, which serves to explain many points in pathology, and which therefore will be frequently referred to. There are few constitutions indeed which have not some one organ more disposed to disease than another. Original conformation, age, mode of life, habits, diet, climate and season, and disposition left by previous disorders, with many others, contribute to this, and it is one great source of the varieties of disease. According to the constitution then of the individual, will in many cases be the result of exposure to cold. When a general disturbance of all the func. tions of the body takes place, cold is said to generate *idiopathic fever.*

Closely allied to cold in the mode of its operation is *sudden al. ternation of atmospheric temperature.* This has been observed in all countries to be a fruitful source of febrile diseases, and of none more than continued fever. Nowhere is it better exemplified than in this country, so remarkable for the unsteadiness of its climate, which in the course of four-and-twenty hours not unfrequently exhibits the succession of the four seasons. These sudden changes of atmospheric temperature are particularly favourable to the production of fever; and are, *per se*, capable of exciting it. In this way we account for the greater comparative frequency of continued fevers, hæmoptysis, and inflammatory affections of various kinds in spring and autumn than at any other period of the year.

Continued fever, however, has another and a very important exciting cause, which frequently operates where neither cold nor alternations of atmospheric temperature can be suspected, as where fevers attack persons shut up in close rooms with others labouring *conta-gion* under the disease. When fever appears under such circumstances, it is said to have its origin in *contagion.** A number of the most important doctrines of the science of pathology are closely associated with the subject of contagion. From the earliest periods at which it became an object of inquiry, this has been acknowledged; but the investigation is obscure and difficult, and has proved a source of endless controversy. Many of the disputed points in medicine are interesting only to the man of science; but the doctrines of contagion are of general interest, because involving practical considerations of the highest importance. Without attempt.

* See Appendix ; Note E.

to clear up all the difficulties in the way of the inquiry, I shall be
satisfied with a brief enumeration of its leading positions, and of
the principal points in dispute.

1. Attempts have been made to throw discredit upon the doctrine of contagion as the cause of fever, by showing that it was for
a long time either unknown to, or disregarded by physicians.   It
is certainly a curious fact, that for the first dawnings of information concerning it, we are indebted, not to Hippocrates or Galen,
but to ancient poets and historians.   Thucidydes, in his account of
the epidemic fever or plague that raged in Athens during the Pelo-
ponnesian war shows that he understood contagion in the sense in
which we now use the term ;—noxious matter from one morbid
body producing a similar disease in another.   In Plutarch's life of
Pericles we read, that whilst that commander was laying siege to
the city of Epidaurus, a distemper prevailed in his army, which not
only carried off his own men, but *all that had intercourse with them.*
Livy, in the account of a camp fever which affected the armies of
the Romans and Carthaginians at the siege of Syracuse, distinctly
states that it was propagated by contagion.   Virgil and Lucretius
employ the term *contagion* to express the manner in which a disease of sheep spread among the flock.

Medical writers were, for the most part, very inattentive to contagion until the time of Sydenham, in whose work (sect. ii, chap. 2),
a distinct reference to contagion may be met with.   Boerhaave and
the followers of his school were very incredulous on the subject of
contagion.   Their ideas about it too were imperfect and confused,
from the circumstance of their blending the notion of contagion
with that of marsh miasmata.   Dr. Huxham, Dr. Lind, and Sir
John Pringle, are the great original writers on contagion, particularly on that of continued fever.   Since their time the subject has
undergone the most rigid examination, and, as we have said, has
given rise to the most discordant opinions.

2. Much confusion has been introduced into the doctrine of contagion by the employment of the term *infection*, and by the different acceptations in which contagion and infection have been taken.
The facts are simply these.   Febrific miasms, emanating from the
bodies of those labouring under disease, are sometimes diffusible
through, or soluble in, atmospheric air ; and in this state operate
upon the animal œconomy, probably through the respiration.   Of
this kind are the miasms of measles, of scarlet fever, and typhus

fever. Some again attach themselves to the natural or diseased secretions of the body, and operate by direct application to the unbroken surface ; of this kind are the miasms of plague, itch, lues,
gonorrhœa, Egyptian ophthalmia, and tinea capitis. Thridly, some
contagions, soluble like the last in the secretions, are apparently
of a more fixed kind, and exert an agency only when the skin is
wounded. Of this kind are the miasms of hydrophobia, and cow-
pox. Lastly, there are some which will operate in all the three
modes now described ; of which small-pox offers the most striking
illustration. To the first of these modes of communication, the term
infection has been usually appropriated ; to the second *contagion*, (*a
contactu*) ; and to the third, inoculation ; but they are all intimately
allied, and no advantage is gained by too closely limiting the acceptation of the two former terms.

The difficulties hence arising have been farther increased by the
want of a proper distinction between common contagion and specific contagion. Diseases which cannot be produced in any other
way than by contagion, are said to have their origin in *specific contagion*. Of this kind are small-pox, cow-pox, measles, the plague,
hydrophobia, and syphilis. Diseases which, occasionally produced
by contagion, are yet sometimes owing to the operation of other
causes, and said to arise from *common contagion*. Of this kind are
catarrh, cynanche parotidæa, erysipelas, ophthalmia, typhus, and
·scarlatina. The laws of common and specific contagion are in
many respects similar, but they have also their points of difference.
To illustrate these, and to determine the peculiarities of each individual contagion, will be an important object in future parts of the
work.

3. In the last paragraph I have assumed as an established principle what has been, and what is still made the subject of keen dispute ; viz. that typhus fever does originate from contagion, and
that it is of the kind which we have called *common*, in opposition to
specific contagion. Both these points have been called into question. By a few, and happily a very few, it has been contended,
that the notion of a contagious origin of typhus fever is altogether
unwarranted ; but the views of these *anti-contagionists* are so completely at variance with the generally received opinions of medical
men, and so irreconcileable with facts obvious to all mankind, that
any formal refutation of them is unnecessary. On the other hand,
there have been, and there continue to be, physicians who believe

in the *exclusive* origin of typhus from contagion ; who maintain that
no disease can propagate itself by contagion which had not its own
origin in contagion ; in other words, who deny that common continned fever, under any, the most adverse circumstances, can ever
spread by contagion. This opinion involves the difficult, but for
the most part idle question, how contagious fevers ever originated ;
but setting this aside, it may fairly be argued that it is neither borne
out by observation nor by reasoning. There is nothing improbable in the supposition, that what originated in cold may be afterwards
propagated by contagion. It violates no established law of the animal œconomy. Experience on the other hand appears to favour it ;
and it may therefore be laid down as an important practical principle, that fever which originated in the first instance from *common*
causes, may, under certain circumstances, either of local situation
or constitution of body, spread by contagion*. What those particular circumstances are, which thus concur to favour the development
of febrile contagion, may be anticipated from remarks already offered. The principle of them are, crowded and ill-ventilated apartments, want of cleanliness and comfort, and previous weakness of
the affected individual, whether owing to excessive fatigue, or an
unwholesome or scanty diet.

4. Many of the controverted points in the doctrine of contagion
hinge upon this question ; but there is another fundamental one, of
almost equal importance. Sydenham long ago urged it with great
force of argument, and a due attention to his observations might
have prevented much of the controversy which has lately taken
place on the subject of the plague and yellow fever :—I mean that
particular constitution of the atmosphere, which disposes to, or which
checks, the *diffusion* of all febrile contagions, whether common or
specific. It is well ascertained, that a contagious disease, even of
the most malignant kind, which may have gained footing in a popu-
lous city or district, does not necessarily attack every one within
its sphere, or go on progressively to the destruction of all the inhabitants. Several circumstances contribute to this ; first, peeu-
liarities of constitution, which secure certain individuals *completely*
from the influence of the contagion ; and, secondly, the immunity
from future attacks, which in several instances of febrile contagious

* This view of the question is now generally known by the name of the
doctrine of contingent contagion, and it has received the support of the most
able contemporary pathologists.

disease is afforded by once undergoing it. To this last law of contagion, we shall have occasion to refer more particularly, when the
eruptive fevers come under consideration ; but for the present it
may be stated, that it applies, although with some exceptions, to
typhus fever. These two circumstances assist in explaining the
fact just mentioned, but they are not *fully* adequate to the effect.
A certain constitution of the air, therefore, sometimes favouring,
but sometimes checking the diffusion of contagion, must be admitted as a third general principle upon which it depends.

Some physicians have pretended to find fault with this multiplication of causes for explaining a single phenomenon, and have argued that a peculiar, or, as Sydenham says, an *epidemic constitution*
of the air, is of itself capable of explaining what others refer to
the combined operation of it, and of the principle of contagion.
As well might they argue, that the tree could be reared without a
seed, because a peculiar condition of the soil is required for its
reception and growth. Several of the most important facts in the
histories of great epidemics, particularly the plague, will hereafter
be illustrated by a reference to the foregoing fundamental doctrines
in the laws of contagion.

5. Much speculation has taken place among medical authors,
regarding the mode in which contagion produces its effects on the
animal œconomy. It has been observed of a number of diseases
notoriously arising from contagion, that they exhibit, even from an
early period, symptoms of great depression of nervous energy, or
of *collapse.* This is exemplified in the case of plague, typhus, cynanche maligna, influenza, erysipelas ; and it has hence been imagined, that there is in the nature of contagion something which is
directly *sedative,* or depressing to the nervous energy. A more
extended view of disease would show the fallacy of this as a general principle. Measles and ophthalmia, which yet exhibit all the
marks of genuine inflammatory *excitement,* are diseases as obviously
arising from contagion, as plague or typhus. The first operation
of contagion may be, and probably is, upon the brain and nerves,
but its *precise* effect upon them is altogether inscrutable. Still,
while I offer a caution against assuming as a principle of pathology
any thing sedative in the nature of contagion, I am not insensible to
the importance of the fact, that cases of disease arising from *common* contagion, above all continued fevers, are more likely to be of

6

the low or typhoid kind, than such as are attributable to cold, or , other causes independent of contagion.

6. Of the intimate nature of the contagious particles which arise from morbid bodies, and which produce a like disease in others, we know nothing; but there are a few particulars known or con- jectured regarding the *manner* in which their influence is exerted on the animal œconomy, which it will be proper to notice.

7. Great attention has been paid by Dr. Haygarth and others, to determine the *distance* to which the noxious effluvia extend, and at which they operate in exciting disease. There is reason to be- lieve that this varies in different cases, and that the plague, typhus, and small pox, have, in this respect, each their several laws. The subject, however, does not appear to have been yet investigated with sufficient accuracy, to enable us to lay down any established points of doctrine with regard to it. It is not exactly known, how far the sphere of contagious influence is affected by ventilation. In the case of *continued fever*, we are warranted in saying, that a free circulation of a pure and cool air renders the contagious par- ticles comparatively inert, and that *concentration* is nearly, if not altogether, indispensable to the activity of contagion*. Some phy- sicians have extended their views farther, and have maintained that there are certain chemical substances which have the power of decomposing contagious effluvia, or, at least, of rendering them, in some way or other, innoxious. Of these, the principal are acid vapours, particularly those of the nitric and acetic acids, and chlorine. *Fumigation* therefore has been recommended as a pow- erful means of counteracting contagion. The theory upon which it has been introduced is exceedingly doubtful, and the practice far from being generally applicable, acid vapours of all kinds being more or less injurious to breathing. If fumigation is adopted as a substitute for thorough ventilation, it may prove injurious; if only superadded, it is perhaps superfluous; but on a point of such *prac- tical* importance it is right to speak with much caution.

8. Attempts have been made to ascertain the exact period at which contagion begins to exert its influence; and it has been sat- isfactorily shown, that in this respect each particular contagion ac- knowledges a different law. (The *latent period* of typhus (that is to

---

* On this subject consult, " Facts and Observations regarding Infection," by Sir G. Blane, in the " *Transactions of a Society for the Improvement of Medical and Chirurgical Knowledge,*" vol. iii, page 425.

say, the time which elapses between exposure to the contagion, and first sympton of fever) is generally from ten days to a month, but it has been known to extend to six weeks, or even two months.) Physicians have also attempted to determine at what particular period of a disease its contagion is the most active, and when the body ceases altogether to afford contagious matter. This point it would be of much importance to ascertain, as it would indicate when a patient might safely be permitted to mix in society ; but unfortunately there do not appear to be sufficient data to enable us to decide the question with any degree of accuracy.

9. The last subject of inquiry which the general doctrine of con- tagion offers, is the attachment of contagious particles to certain bodies, thence called *Fomites*, where they lurk, often for a very long period of time, and subsequently renew the disease with all its former, or even with increased virulence. It is the most curi- ous fact in the history of contagion, and one established upon the most unquestionable evidence. The principle too appears to be of more general application than any other which the doctrine of con- tagion involves. The plague and typhus, small-pox and scarlet fever, ophthalmia and porrigo, afford the most familiar illustrations of it ; but it is doubtful if there is any species of contagious dis- ease, which may not be communicated through the medium of fomites. They may be either hard or soft bodies. The walls and wainscoting of the room, beds and bed-furniture, the furniture of the room, and the clothes of the patient, are those against which we are chiefly to be on our guard. It is well ascertained, that the clothes of an individual, who is himself unsusceptible of the dis- ease, may become the fomites of its contagion. In this manner typhus, small-pox, and plague, are not unfrequently disseminated.

Such are the most important topics which the general doctrine of contagion embraces. They are brought forward in this place, because contagion, as a cause of continued fever, demanded par- ticular notice. It remains however for me to observe, that besides those exciting causes of continued fever which have now been mentioned, there are some others to which this form of disease has been attributed, which at least deserves to be enumerated. Of these the first is a vitiated state of the air, in consequence of the accumulation of persons in a confined space. The second is the putrefaction of animal and vegetable matters. The third is a state of famine or scarcity. The prevalence of fever at particular periods has been often attributed to one or other of these sources, and many occurrences in history favour the opinion. That they powerfully *contribute to the diffusion of fever* when once generated, cannot be questioned; but they have all been so frequently observed to exist without fever ensuing, that their power of *exciting, per se,* this state of disease, must still be considered among the doubtful points in medical science.

TREATMENT OF CONTINUED FEVER.

Necessity of Treatment in Fever. Indications of Cure. The antiphlogistic Regimen. Possibility of cutting short a Fever. Remarks on the different Means resorted to in the Treatment of continued Fever. The Abstraction of Blood. Cold Affusion. Emetics. Saline and antimonial Medicines. Purgatives. Cordials. Bark. Opiates. Blisters.

IT is well remarked by Dr. Cullen, that though in every fever which runs its full course, there is an effort of nature of a salutary tendency, and though from hence it might be inferred that the cure of fevers should be left to the operations of nature, or that our art should be directed only to support and regulate them, it yet requires but a moderate share of observation to understand that these are very precarious, and often wholly insufficient to overcome the disease. Permanent derangement of the function or structure of an organ is sometimes occasioned before such operations are set up, and a reliance upon them therefore often leads to negligent and inert practice. The necessity of treatment in fever is now indeed generally ackowledged. Occasionally, the natural tendency of fever to terminate favourably may be kept in view with great advantage ; as, for instance, in the latter stages of *simple fever,* where measures of depletion are unnecessary, and wine and cordials would be doubtful remedies. In a large proportion of cases, however, the operations of nature may be superseded by the well-directed exertions of art. To point out what these are, to what extent they may be carried, and how they must be varied to meet the varying forms in which fever presents itself, is my object in the present chapter. It is to be regretted that the nature of the subject is such as to render it impossible to lay down any specific directions for the guidance of the student, as we may hereafter do, when explaining the treatment proper in pneumonia, colic, or jaundice. All that is now pro-

posed is to notice the principal means that are resorted to in the
cure of fever, and to add such observations as may throw light on
the objects for which they are employed, and point out the necessary cautions in their administration. (In no disease is so much left
to the discretion of the practitioner as in continued fever.)

The general objects to be kept in view in the treatment of any
disease are called, in medical language, the *indications of cure*. In
the case of fever, they have, for the most part, been drawn from
the hypothetical views of authors regarding the nature and proximate cause of fever ; but such indications of cure are little calculated to direct us in the choice and application of remedies. The
views which have been here taken of the varieties of continued fever, and of the circumstances which modify its symptoms, suggest
the following as the simplest indications of cure in fever :—

1st. To moderate the violence of arterial excitement.
2d. To obviate local inflammations and congestions.
3d. To support the powers of the system.
4th. To relieve urgent symptoms.

An important step towards the attainment of all these objects is
a strict attention to the ANTIPHLOGISTIC REGIMEN, under which
term physicians include a great variety of details proper to be observed not only in continued fevers, but in all febrile affections whatever. This regimen is of itself sufficient to cure a number of the
slighter kinds of febrile, disease, such as catarrh, and sore throat.
It consists in avoiding or moderating those irritations, which in one
degree or another are almost constantly applied to the body. Dr.
Cullen has divided them into three classes :—impressions made upon our senses ;—the exercise of the body and mind ;—the taking
in of aliments. In all fevers therefore, care is to be taken to guard
against external heat, and such impressions upon the eye and ear,
as would prove painful to the patient and aggravate the symptoms
of his disease. The popular prejudice against the admission of fresh
air ; the use of cold washing, and the frequent changes of linen and
bed-clothes in cases of fever, is now gradually giving way; but for
a great length of time it exerted a most pernicious influence over the
treatment of fever. All exertions of body and mind are to be forbidden. Their continued operation tends manifestly to exhaust the
nervous power ; already sufficiently reduced by the mere presence

of fever. The horizontal posture is to be enforced. The presence of aliment proving always a stimulus to the system, abstinence is to be recommended, particularly from animal food in the shape of broths and jellies, which are too often had recourse to in the early stages of fever. They load the stomach, increase the disposition to nausea and vomiting, accelerate the pulse, augment the heat of the skin, and occasion head-ache, flatus, tormina, and many other unpleasant symptoms. The diet therefore should consist of roasted apples, sago, arrow root, tapioca, and gruel. Grapes, oranges, and ripe fruits in their season may also be permitted. Thirst is to be allayed by light, cool, and subacid drinks, such as tea, apple tea, barley water, toast water, and lemonade. The utmost cleanliness is to be observed in the patient's person, and in every thing around him.

Before proceeding to a detail of the other means which are re-sorted to in the treatment of continued fever, it is necessary to in-quire, how far it is possible, by a vigorous employment of measures in the early stages of a fever, to cut it short. The question has been much agitated, and there are many authors who contend that it can frequently be effected. It may fairly be admitted, that there are mild attacks of fever, particularly such as occur in young per-sons, where a prompt evacuation appears to have the effect of in-terrupting that chain of morbid action, which ends in the full de-velopment of fever ; but it may reasonably be doubted, whether any of the severer cases of continued fever could have been *cut short* by any exertion of art ; those, for instance, either arising from con-tagion or from common causes, which extend to fourteen or twen-ty-one days. Were it possible to do so in a few cases, it should yet be borne in mind, that active treatment in the majority of cases of continued fever, even though early resorted to, is chiefly ser-viceable, not in shortening the course, but in moderating the *vio-lence* of the disease. It was the remark of a very shrewd physi-cian, that the skilful pilot does not pretend to *quell* the storm, but is content with steering his ship in safety through it.

Of the different means of fulfilling the indications of cure former-ly laid down, the most powerful is the *abstraction of blood*. Every part of the treatment of fever has been the subject of controversy, but the employment of blood-letting is that, which of all others has been the most keenly disputed. As it is however of the greatest importance to have clear ideas regarding it, I shall make an attempt to estimate the utility of blood-letting in fever, and to point out the circumstances under which it may be proper to employ it*.

There cannot exist a doubt as to the necessity of blood-letting in the genuine inflammatory fever, the *endemic* of warm climates. The violence of that disease, the rapidity of its progress, and the high degree of arterial excitement which characterize it, call for the adoption of a system of measures, at once powerful and immediate in their effects. On the first attack, therefore, blood is to be taken from the arm to the extent of twenty or thirty ounces, and in a full stream. This it is frequently necessary to repeat in the course of a few hours ; the extent of the evacuation being always regulated by the violence of the symptoms, particularly by the degree of head-ache, and the fulness and tension of the pulse. These must be diminished without delay ; and though other means are not to be neglected, it is upon venesection that our chief reliance is to be placed. The removal of pain, faintness, the pulse becoming steady, and weakening, are the signs of a sufficient bleeding. Some have urged opening the temporal artery in preference to bleeding at the arm, but without sufficient reason ; and here it may once for all be said, that opening the temporal artery is not an operation to be recommended, except under particular circumstances. It often fails, even when practised by skilful hands. The requisite quantity of blood cannot always be obtained speedily, or estimated accurately. There is, lastly, often considerable difficulty in securing the artery, nor does it appear that there is any peculiar benefit resulting from the operation to counterbalance these obvious disadvantages.

Common continued and typhus fever do not necessarily require the adoption of blood-letting. A large proportion of cases, especially of the latter, would be hurt by it ; and in many, to say the least, it is uncalled for. But, on the other hand, there are some, and those among the most formidable which fall under our observation, which as imperiously require it.

The objects for which blood-letting is instituted in the common continued fevers of this country, and in genuine typhus, are various. Some recommend it very early in the disease, in the hope of cutting it short at once. This is a fortunate result of the prae-

* Nowhere have I seen this subject more clearly stated than in the writings of Baglivi, chap. vi, section 3.

tice occasionally witnessed ; but it is one which can seldom be anticipated. The legitimate object of blood-letting in these diseases, is the checking those dispositions to inflammatory action which are so often met with in severe cases, which sometimes come on insidiously, and at other times suddenly, and are productive in either way of serious mischief to the affected organ. This applies with peculiar force to those conditions of the brain which are supposed to depend on congestion *sub-acute* inflammation ; for the delicacy of its structure exposes it readily to injury ; and injury of the brain, even of the slightest kind, is always to be dreaded. It is frequently observed, that a judicious abstraction of blood in the early stages of fever not only diminishes the head-ache, the great sensibility to light and sound, the delirium, the cough, the pain and fulness of the abdomen, but it apparently shortens the course of the disease, and more obviously still, the period of convalescence.

It is at the onset of the fever, that is to say, between the first and fourth day, when the good effects of blood-letting are most unequivocally exhibited. At this period of the disease the powers of life may be *oppressed*, but it is not probable that they are yet much *exhausted*. From this they will recoil, if the oppressive load of the disease be quickly removed.* But blood-letting may sometimes be resorted to with the best effects at more advanced periods of the disease. Great nicety indeed is required in distinguishing the symptoms that demand it, and in apportioning the evacuation to the extent of local disease, and the general powers of the constitution ; but, for the most part, it will be found preferable to employ *local bleeding*, when the object in view is the relief of an urgent symptom. Of the comparative advantages resulting from general and local bleeding, in the continued fevers of this country, it is difficult to speak with precision. I have frequently had occasion to see affections of the head, in fever, yield speedily to the application of leeches, where the loss of blood from the arm appeared only to weaken the body, without influencing the local affection. Leeches I believe to be, upon the whole, preferable in fever to the application of cupping-glasses as occasioning less irritation.

* See Bateman on " the Contagious Fever of this country," page 102; a work containing a most judicious exposition of the principles and details of the treatment of continued fever, upon which it would be difficult to improve.

7

The appearance of the blood drawn in cases of continued fever varies considerably. To a certain extent, it may serve as a guide to us, in indicating the propriety of further depletion. It is sometimes buffy, and the coagulum firm; but in genuine typhus the coagulum is commonly loose and the buff gelatinous, an appearance supposed to contraindicate the employment of bleeding. In a case of great oppression of the brain, however, amounting almost to apoplexy, but connected with the *invasion* of fever, I once saw the most marked good effect from general blood-letting, and yet the blood drawn scarcely coagulated at all.

Cold affusion, upon which great reliance was at one time placed in the treatment of fever, is attended with so much inconvenience and fatigue to the patient, that in this climate it is now very generally superseded by the employment of cold or tepid sponging. From, this in most cases, much benefit is derived. It is grateful to the patient; it diminishes the heat of the body, takes off that dryness of the skin which occasions so much irritation, and is sometimes succeeded by a quiet slumber, and a gentle perspiration. It may be repeated whenever the skin is *hot and dry*, and it is often useful even at very advanced periods of the disease. In those exquisite forms of inflammatory fever which are met with in hot climates, the cold affusion, in the manner recommended by the late Dr. Currie,* is a powerful means of diminishing the high excitement that prevails. We may form some idea of this, from the well-marked good effects of cold lotions applied to the head, in diminishing head-ache, delirium, and restlessness, in the common continued fevers of this country.

When the opportunity offers of administering remedies in the first days of the fever, an emetic should never be omitted. A grain or two of emetic tartar, or the draughts 1 and 2, in the APPENDIX, may be recommended for this purpose. An emetic has the double advantage of clearing the stomach of sordes (whether undigested aliment, bile, or vitiated mucus,) and of determining the blood to the surface, and in this way relieving the oppressed state of internal organs. Saline medicines, such as the citrate of potash and acetate of ammonia, according to the forms Nos. 39 and 40, are very useful throughout the early and middle periods of the disease. They allay thirst and appear to exert some influence in controlling

* See Currie's "Medical Reports," 2 vols.

the action of the heart and arteries, directing the fluids to the kidneys, and relieving the general tension of the system. They should constitute the basis of our treatment in most cases; and in the milder forms of *simple* fever, little else is required.

Antimony was long distinguished as a *febrifuge* of great virtue; but latterly an opinion has prevailed, that its efficacy in the treatment of fever is rather a matter of tradition than the dictate of experience. To this I cannot subscribe, having had frequent opportunities of satisfying myself of its claims upon our confidence. It occasionally acts upon the stomach and bowels; but independent of this, antimony proves useful in fever, (apparently by some power of diffusing and equalizing the circulation.) The protoxyd, as we find it in the *pulvis antimonialis* of the London Pharmacopœia, is, I believe, the best form in which it can be administered. In combination with small doses of calomel, and given either at night, or every six hours, according to the urgency of the symptoms, its efficacy is often manifested by an improved appearance of the tongue and alvine evacuations. The antimonial wine is also a valuable remedy in fever, and coinciding in its effects with the saline draughts already adverted to, is usually administered in combination with them, as in formula No. 41.

No doubt can be entertained respecting the propriety of exhibiting purgative medicines during the whole course of continued fever.* Combinations of antimony, jalap, and rhubarb, with calomel, as in the forms Nos. 6, 7, 8, and 12, are well adapted for the commencement of fevers. The milder formulæ, Nos. 19, 21, and 24, for its middle and later periods. Purgative medicines are serviceable in different ways. They diminish, in an early period of the disease, the mass of circulating fluids; lower the *tone* of the whole system; and expel from the body aliment, the fermentation or putrefaction of which would necessarily aggravate the sufferings of the patient. At a more advanced stage, they evacuate those morbid secretions of the liver and intestines, which are continually taking place, and the lodgment of which in the bowels would tend greatly to *oppress* the nervous system, and, therefore, increase the danger. It is not to be imagined, however, that the administration of purga-

* See "Observations on the utility and administration of Purgative Medicines in several Diseases," by Dr. James Hamilton; a work of great merit.

tives in fever is altogether devoid of risk. They should never be prescribed without duly considering the circumstances of the case, nor without some adequate motive. It is indispensably requisite to watch the degree to which the abdominal viscera are affected, and cautiously to refrain from them (or at all events from the most active of them, such as jalap, colocynth, or calomel) whenever inflammatory action is present, or any *disposition* to it, as evinced by diarrhœa, or tenderness of the abdomen. If the symptoms are such as appear to demand relief by the bowels, and the practitioner is fearful of latent inflammatory action, he will have recourse to castor oil, or rhubarb, which experience has shown to be the least irritating of the aperients in common use.

The great weakness which prevails in fever naturally suggests the free employment of cordial and tonic medicines, more particularly wine, ether, camphor, musk, bark, and aromatics; but it is now generally acknowledged, that the indiscriminate use of stimulant remedies in fever is highly pernicious; that they have a tendency to aggravate many of those local determinations, from which danger is chiefly to be apprehended; and, therefore, that their employment is to be regulated by circumstances, no less than that of blood-letting. The period of the fever, the particular situation in which it appears, its exciting cause, the age, constitution, and former habits of the patient, are of course to be taken into account; but we are chiefly to be guided by the *character of the symptoms,* and the *effects of the remedies.*

1. In the state of true collapse, marked by cold and clammy sweats, a feeble wavering pulse, oppressive breathing, the supine posture of the patient, and a moist, brown, and loaded state of the tongue, stimulants, especially wine or brandy, are not only beneficial but absolutely necessary. Such symptoms are clearly indicative of a failure of the powers of life, and unless stimulants are duly supplied in quantities proportioned to the exigencies of the case, the patient rapidly sinks. Those cases of typhus which are accompanied by petechiæ, or the large livid blotches called vibices, in short, by what we have denominated the symptoms of putrescency, are benefited by the steady and moderate exhibition of wine, bark, and aromatics. There is a third class of symptoms which has been supposed to indicate the propriety of a similar plan of treatment; I mean those which denote irregularity in the action of the nervous power, such for instance as subsultus tendinum, picking

of the bed-clothes, and a tremulous tongue. These are distinctly symptomatic of cerebral irritation, of a state which is indeed some-times relieved, but not unfrequently aggravated, by wine and cor-dials. If these symptoms are present along with a parched tongue, a hot and dry skin, and any degree of *sharpness* of the pulse, wine even in small quantity is generally hurtful. It is a state which may often be better combated by local bleeding, blistering, and laxa-tives. Wine is indeed at most times a doubtful remedy in fever, which should never be persevered in, unless the signs of improve-ment are very unequivocal.

2. The effects of all stimulant remedies are to be carefully watched. Even when most essentially required, as in the lowest state of collapse, they will sometimes occasion a degree of excite-ment, from which danger may be apprehended. If the tongue un-der their exhibition becomes dry, and delirium increases, they should be immediately diminished, or altogether withdrawn. If the patient is upon the whole improving, this should satisfy us. Any attempt to accelerate his recovery by increasing the stimulus will only risk his safety.

In the progress of simple fever, where no derangement of partic-ular organs interferes with the general plan of treatment, it is often desirable to afford the patient the comfort of some gentle stimu-lant, and *ether* is that which may be most safely and advantageous-ly resorted to. It may at first be united to saline draughts, as in R No. 42 ; and afterwards given in the more powerful form, R No. 61. Bark may sometimes be administered towards the close of a continued fever with manifest advantage. The formulæ Nos. 68 and 69, and more especially those containing the sulfate of quinine, Nos. 72 and 73, merit a preference.

From the want of sleep and restlessness which so generally pre-vail in fever, and prove so distressing to the patient, opiates might be expected to be useful, but experience teaches otherwise. In the early stages of the disease they are quite inadmissible ; and even in the latter, their employment is often followed by an aggravation instead of a relief of the symptoms. Opium frequently augments the heat and thirst, constipates the bowels, and increases delirium. In some few cases indeed, given at bed time, and combined with a diaphoretic, as in the form No. 52, an opiate is adviseable ; as for instance, when, after purging and local bleeding, great restlessness continues, attended with a low muttering delirium, aggravated to-

wards night. If on the following morning the tongue appears dry
and smooth, the opiate was probably injurious ; if moist, it may
safely be repeated.

In particular states of fever, the efficacy of blisters has been
long acknowledged, and several different explanations of the fact
have been offered. They have been supposed to act as stimulants,
or to have a power of relieving spasm, and they have accordingly
been recommended by some at any period of continued fever   By
others, they have been principally resorted to in the latter stages,
of the disease, their good effects being then traced to a principle of
revulsion, and they have been chiefly applied by such practitioners
to the calves of the legs, and the soles of the feet. It is now, however generally agreed, that blisters are only useful in obviating
those local congestions and inflammations which occur in the course
of fever, and more particularly within the head, bringing on that
state of cerebral irritation which is marked, sometimes by delirium
accompanied with much restlessness and attempts to get out of bed,
and occasionally by the opposite, but no less formidable symptom
of *stupor*. Under these circumstances, great benefit is experienced
from the application of a blister to the nape of the neck ; besides
which, the head should be shaved, and cloths dipped in a cold lotion constantly applied to it. In cases of local determination to any
organ of the thorax or abdomen, a blister over the affected part will
prove equally advantageous.

In the progress of continued fever, some symptoms occasionally
arise, which from their urgency demand particular attention ; and I
may select as one peculiarly meriting the attention of the student,
diarrhœa. It usually indicates an inflammatory condition of the
bowels, and should be always treated by soothing and emollient remedies, such as the draughts Nos. 48 and 49. *Vomiting* is a very
troublesome symptom, best combated I believe (at least in this climate), by totally abstaining from medicine, and even from nourishment of the mildest kind, for a considerable time. *Hiccup* is another very distressing and often alarming symptom, usually treated
by antispasmodics (opium, ether, and musk) ; but I have found it to
yield with more certainty to gentle purging. During the convalescence, the diet of the patient must be strictly regulated ; but in
the way of medicine, little else is required at this period than an occasional laxative (R Nos. 28, 30, 36,) and the exhibition of a light
tonic, such as the infusion of cascarilla bark, cusparia, or columba. O
(R Nos. 34, 77, 78.)

CHAP. V.

Its nosological Character. Origin and History. Symptoms of the Plague. Mild Form of Plague. Effects of different Remedies. Of the Contagion of Plague. Its peculiarities. Circumstances tending to render the Plague epidemic.

THE Plague, classed by **Dr.** Cullen among the exanthemata, is yet, in strict nosological language, a continued fever closely allied to typhus, and therefore demanding notice more particularly in this place. It may be viewed, indeed, without over refinement, as the link which connects the two great classes of idiopathic fevers. In its mode of propagation, it resembles the exanthemata. In its symptoms and progress, we shall trace an obvious resemblance to those of typhus.

The historical details connected with this very singular disease are highly interesting. The ancients do not appear to have been acquainted with it, but it must be confessed that its origin and early history are involved in much obscurity. For many centuries past it has been *endemic* on the shores of the Mediterranean ; and though it has occasionally shown itself in other latitudes, as at Moscow in 1771, and in this country in 1665, yet in that situation only is it at all times to be met with. Grand Cairo may be considered as the great *nidus* of the contagion of plague, and from this point, at particular seasons, it spreads with a malignity scarcely to be estimated. The interest with which such a disease must at all times be viewed, has been much heightened of late years from the circumstance of its having appeared in our own settlements (in 1813 at Malta, in 1816 in the Ionian Islands), and been subjected there, as well as in Egypt in 1800, to the observations of our countrymen. The symptoms of this disease, the peculiarities in the laws of the contagion of the plague, the circumstances which appear to favour its diffusion, and the consequent appearance of the disease as an *epidemic*, are the points to which my attention will in this chapter be principally directed.

A feeling of great languor and lassitude ushers in the attack of plague, which for the most part happens towards evening. There is always a cold stage, though it is seldom of long duration. Heat of skin, head-ache, and giddiness succeed. The pain of the head is referred to the temples and eye-brows. The eyes appear heavy, dull, and muddy. The expression of countenance changes in a remarkable manner. Sometimes there is a wild and furious look ; sometimes a look claiming commiseration, with a sunk eye and contracted feature. The most striking of all the early symptoms of plague is the *staggering*, and the sudden extreme prostration of strength. A strong tendency to void the urine is generally noticed. The stomach is very irritable, and rejects almost every thing presented to it. The tongue is white and moist. The bowels are sometimes torpid, and at other times loose, the evacuations being always highly offensive. The speech falters. The pulse is at first small, hard, and quick ; but after the appearance of buboes it often becomes fuller and softer. It is sometimes intermittent. In point of frequency, its average may be stated at 100. The heat of skin is seldom very intense. The head is occasionally perfectly clear and collected. At other times, stupor occurs immediately after the formation of the hot fit. Some cases of the disease are ushered in by a violent fit of mania. The greatest indifference with regard to recovery prevails, and is always reckoned a most unfavourable symptom.

After one, two, or at farthest three days, pains in the groins and axillæ announce the formation of *buboes*. These pains are often highly acute, and unless speedily followed by the swelling of the gland, the patient dies delirious. In women the axillae, in men the groins are chiefly affected. Carbuncles appear at the same time, but indifferently on all parts of the body. Petechiæ and vibices are much more frequent than carbuncles, which it appears do not oc. cur above once in twenty cases. The fatal termination is some. times preceded by violent hæmorrhages from the mouth, nose, or in. testines.*

---

* This detail of the symptoms of Plague is abstracted, by permission of Sir J. M'Grigor, from the official reports of the epidemic of 1816, trans-

The duration of the disease is very various. A few cases are on record, where the patient died within a few hours from the invasion. To many it proves fatal during the first paroxysm or period, which includes the time from the evening of the attack to the close of the following night. (The third and fifth days are, however, upon the whole, those of the greatest danger.) The former is the usual period of the appearance of bubo ; the latter, of the abatement of the febrile symptoms. If the patient survives the fifth day, and the bubo is fully formed, he may be considered as nearly out of danger. The convalescence indeed is always very tedious, from the extreme debility which the disease leaves ; and the patient's life is not unfrequently again put into imminent hazard from the occurrence of gangrene in the extremities.

Such is the train of symptoms which characterize this disease. Some idea of the extent of the mortality which it occasions may be formed from the fact, that out of 700 persons attacked by it in the district of Leftimo in Corfu 1815, seventy only were saved, and 630 died. It is curious, however, to observe, that occasionally this very formidable disease assumes a totally different character. The *mild* form of plague is not peculiar to any families, or classes of persons, or districts, or periods of the epidemic. It is more commonly met with towards its decline, but it is observed occasionally even from the very first. Buboes form in this variety of the disease about the usual period, generally with a good deal of inflammation, and go on to suppuration. Carbuncles and petechiæ, however, are never observed to attend it. It is marked by the same set of febrile symptoms as characterize the malignant form of the disease but they are all milder in degree. It terminates occasionally by a critical discharge, but does not appear to require, or to be at all affected by, any kind of medical treatment. A few cases have been recorded of plague appearing in the form of buboes, without any constitutional affection.

A circumstance of some importance, as tending to point out the analogy between the plague and other forms of continued fever, has been taken notice of by Sir James M'Grigor, in his Medical Sketches of the Expedition from India to Egypt ;—I mean the effect of season, ventilation, and peculiarities of soil, in modifying the

mitted to the Army Medical Board by the officers in charge of the Plague Hospitals in the Ionian Islands.

8

character of the symptoms. The cases of plague which occurred in the cold months of the year were marked by an inflammatory diathesis. Those which were sent in from crowded hospitals were attended from the very first with low or malignant symptoms. Those which occurred when the army was encamped near the marshes of El-Hammed, showed a kind of remittent or intermittent type.

Some dissections have been made of the bodies of persons who have died of the plague, but they afford little or no instruction. The few morbid appearances noticed, were met with in the cavity of the abdomen.

In the malignant form of plague, every variety of treatment has been tried, but with so little effect, that it may be considered as a disease nearly beyond the reach of medicine. The violent headache which occurs during the first twenty-four hours, seems to point out the propriety of blood-letting, and it is recommended by the general custom of Turkish practitioners; but in the hands of English surgeons it proved of no avail. In the cases in which it was tried, it did not appear, however, to make matters worse. The blood first drawn was generally sizy, but never afterwards.

Where mercury can be brought to affect the mouth, it appears to be of some service, but it is seldom that sufficient time is afforded for this specific effect of the remedy. Ether and laudanum are valuable medicines in allaying the irritability of the stomach. Wine and opium are of no use during the violence of the disease, and bark can seldom be retained. This is much to be regretted, for wherever it can be made to stay on the stomach, even in those severe cases where carbuncles and vibices appear, its good effects are conspicuous. Camphor, bark, and wine are given with much advantage during the period of convalescence. Emetics, purgatives, and the cold affusion have been tried, but it does not appear that they are of any particular service. Diaphoresis can seldom be produced, owing to the disposition to vomit; but wherever it can be procured, the symptoms seem to be mitigated by it.

Great attention is always paid to the local treatment of the buboes. They seldom go back, and it is usual, therefore, to employ means with the view of accelerating their suppuration. For this purpose the Turks are in the habit of applying the actual cautery, but it did not answer in the practice of our army surgeons. The irritation occasioned by it was excessive, so as sometimes to hasten the patient's death. Blisters and poultices are certainly preferable; but, upon the whole, it is quite obvious, that as little can be done in the way of surgical treatment in the plague, as by internal medicines.

The general resemblance which plague bears to those malignant forms of typhus fever, which are occasionally witnessed in cold countries, must be abundantly obvious. The great distinction between them lies in the occurrence of buboes; in other words, in the tendency which plague has to effect the lymphatic system. This line of distinction however is so broad, that plague is to be viewed as a continued fever, allied indeed to typhus, but differing from it in the important circumstance of having its origin in specific contagion. That the plague is a highly contagious disease cannot for a moment be made a matter of dispute; but some physicians have maintained that it is not a fever *sui generis*, generated by a specific contagion, but only an aggravated form of typhus; in support of which opinion it has been argued, that cases of typhus complicated with buboes have sometimes been observed in this country*. This idea, however, is entertained only by a few, and the doctrine of a specific contagion in plague is that which is now generally received. Its laws have been investigated with some accuracy, and the following seem to be the most important of those which have hitherto been ascertained.

1. The *latent period* of the contagion of plague, or that between communication with an affected individual, and the appearance of symptoms, varies in different cases. It is scarcely ever less than three days, and it seldom exceeds six. Instances indeed are recorded of the disease not appearing until the tenth day, but these cases are rare.

2. The contagion spreads to a very small distance only from the body of the patient. The consequence of which is, that the disease is seldom, if ever, communicated except by actual *contact*.

3. The dead body does not communicate the disease so readily as the living. This appears to be well understood in Turkey; but that the contagion is sometimes received from the dead body, cannot, I apprehend, be doubted.

4. The contagion of plague is readily imparted to *fomites*, in

* See Minutes of Evidence taken before the House of Commons, on the Question of Plague. 1819.

which it may lurk for a very long time, more particularly if seclu-
ded from the air.

5. Re-infection is occasionally observed, but, upon the whole, is
not common. The individuals throughout Turkey, who are employed about the persons of plague patients, have, with very few
exceptions, undergone the disease. Sufficient instances, however,
are met with of persons taking the disease a second time, and even
dying of the second attack, to make all who have previously had
it, cautious in their intercourse with the affected.

6. Plague, like the small-pox, may be taken by inoculation. The
experiment has been tried in several instances, but in none has it
succeeded in mitigating the disorder. Dr. Whyte in 1801, and Mr.
Van Rosenfeldt in 1817, paid with their lives the forfeit of their te-
merity. The former died on the fourth, the latter on the second
day of the disease.

Plague I have stated to be endemic in Egypt ; and both at Cairo
and Constantinople cases of the disease are almost always to be
met with. In other words, they occur *sporadically* in those places.
While the English army was in Egypt in 1801, cases of plague
were continually occurring ; but the judicious regulations then
adopted, coupled with the state of the air, prevented the disease
from spreading, and the troops suffered but very little. At Malta
however, in 1813, and in the Ionian Islands during the years 1815-
16, the plague raged epidemically ; and from early times it has been
observed, that at certain seasons the plague disseminates itself with
extraordinary malignity. To this nothing can give any effectual
check but the enforcement of severe measures by the strong arm of
military power. At Marseilles in 1720, at Messina in 1743, at
Grand Cairo in 1759, and on various other occasions, when the
plague was suffered to advance without any such control, the ravages which it committed were of incalculable magnitude. The establishment of a cordon around the whole of the affected district,
the rigid seclusion of families, the immediate removal of all suspected cases into quarantine, and of all decided cases to the laza-
ret, are the preventive measures of most obvious importance. By
these, promptly and vigorously exerted, the extension of the plague
in the Ionian Islands has been several times, in the course of the
last five or six years, prevented ; and it is now no longer questionable, that it might in the same manner be effectually checked in
every part of the Turkish Empire.

Many inquiries have been instituted with the view of determining, if possible, what the circumstances are which render the plague epidemic at certain seasons. Some particular constitution of the air is generally supposed to occasion it; but what that is, never has been, and probably never will be ascertained. The extremes both of heat and cold are said to be unfavourable to the propagation of plague, but this opinion must be taken with some limitations. The Plague raged in summer at Malta, in the winter months at Corfu. Nor is it clear, that it is upon any pecnliar state of dryness or moisture in the atmosphere that the phenomenon depends; though indeed there is a popular belief all over the Levant, that the heavy dews which begin to fall about St. John's day check the advance of the plague. To this circumstance is attributed the curious but well-ascertained fact, that though the disease had been previously raging in the town, the inhabitants may after that day leave their homes and mix in society with comparative security.

It is a common remark in the Levant, that the advances of the plague are always from south to north. When the plague is at Smyrna, the inhabitants of Aleppo handle goods without precaution, and have no fears of contagion. When the disease, on the other hand, is at Damascus, great precautions are observed, and all the Frank families hold themselves in readiness to *shut up* or to leave the town. An epidemic pague, therefore, nearly always begins at Grand Cairo, spreads to Aexandria, and from thence through Syria to Smyrna and Constantinople.

The seeds of the plagte being always present in Turkey, if it were not for these peculiarities in the laws of its contagion, that country must have been long since depopulated. Whether the genuine Levant plague could spread in this climate, is a point upon which physicians are not agreed. The general opinion is, that it might so spread under particular circumstances; and therefore, that the quarantine regulations established by the legislature are absolutely necessary for the protection of these countries.

Train of Symptoms in the Paroxysm of an Intermittent. Primary Types
of Ague. Of the Remittent Fever. Consequences of Ague. Prognosis.
Causes of Ague, predisposing and occasional. Of Marsh Miasmata and
Malaria. Treatment of Intermittent Fevers. During the Paroxysm.
During the Interval. Bark. Arsenic. Of the Bilious Remittent Fever
of warm Climates. Endemic Fever of Sierra Leone.

INTERMITTENTS are readily distinguished from every other form of
idiopathic fever by their occurrence in paroxysms, each of which
may be considered as an epitome of a febrile disease, exhibiting in
the course of about eight hours all the stages of fever—its rise, progress, crisis, and termination in the recovery of health. This circumstance has contributed to give to intermittent fever a large share
of the attention of pathologists. By an accurate investigation of
its phenomena, they have endeavoured to arrive at a knowledge of
the nature of febrile action, and have imagined they could apply to
the more varied appearances of other diseases, those general views
which the consideration of agues suggested. Distrusting in some
measure this principle, I commenced the inquiry by a sketch of
the more frequent, and, in this country at least, far more important subject of continued fever.

The symptoms which occur in the paroxysm of an intermittent
fever divide themselves in the first place into the two great classes
of *regular* and *superadded*. The former admit of an obvious subdivision into three stages,—the *cold*, the *hot* and the *sweating*, in the
course of which the different functions of the body undergo very
remarkable changes. The phenomena of the *cold* fit have been
already in part described. Nausea and vomiting, great lassitude
and weakness, and a sense of weight and oppression about the

præcordia, accompany this stage of the disorder. The hot stage is usually attended with a full and active pulse, scanty and high-coloured urine, a hurried breathing, considerable head-ache, throbbing of the temples, confusion of thought, or even delirium. A moisture at length breaks out on the face and neck, which gradually extends over the whole body, and the febrile symptoms then rapidly diminish. The pulse sinks to its natural standard; the feeling of weakness goes off; the heat of skin, head-ach, and thirst abate; the appetite returns; the secretions are restored to their healthy condition, the urine depositing a *lateritious* sediment. Such are the *regular* symptoms of an ague. Many others however are occasionally superadded, varying of course with the climate, the season, and the idiosyncracies or peculiarities in habit of the individual affected. They are stupor and coma, pleuritic or rheumatic pains, diarrhœa, inflamed liver and bowels, vomiting, jaundice, cramps, hœmorrhages, and the like.

The paroxysm of an ague varies considerably in its duration. It may, upon an average, be estimated at about six or eight hours. After a certain interval, the same train of symptoms is renewed; and the period of recurrence gives what is called the *type* of the fever. From very early times three primary types of intermittent have been observed—the QUOTIDIAN, the TERTIAN, and the QUARTAN, in which the febrile paroxysm completes its revolution in the respective periods of twenty-four, forty-eight, and seventy-two hours. Of these the most common is the tertian, and this therefore is always considered as the *primary* type of fever. Several irregular types of intermittent fever have been taken notice of by authors, such as the double tertian, the semitertian, and the double quartan, but they are not of frequent occurrence. When the febrile symptoms, instead of ceasing *entirely* the interval between the paroxysms, abate only to a greater or less degree, the fourth, or REMITTENT type of fever, is present. Aggravated and masked as this often is by visceral congestions, it is difficult to trace its connection with the common intermittent of this country. Nevertheless their mutual relations are undeniable.

In the course of the disease it is frequently observed that the type changes; tertians and quartans into quotidians, quotidians into remittents. Under more favourable circumstances, the remittent shows the character of an intermittent; and, generally speaking, the change into a type of less frequent repetition indicates an abatement in the severity of the disease; physicians have remarked, that the tertian type of fever has its invasion in the forenoon, the quartan in the afternoon, and the quotidian in the morning. The quartan which has the longest interval, has the longest and most violent cold stage, but upon the whole, the shortest paroxysm. The hot fit of the tertian is comparatively the longest. The quotidian, with the shortest interval, has, at the same time, the longest paroxysm.

Upon what particular circumstances the type of intermittent fever depends, has never been ascertained; but that climate and season have great influence over it, and also over the general character of the symptoms, cannot be disputed. Vernal agues generally assume the tertian type, and are marked by an inflammatory diathesis. They are however mild, and usually run their course quickly. Quartan agues prevail chiefly during the autumn and winter months, and they are the most obstinate of all the forms of intermittent fever. Great as is the influence of season, it is yet inferior to that of climate. The remittent type occurs almost exclusively in hot countries; but to form an adequate idea of the extent to which the symptoms of ague can be modified by climate, and of the extreme violence which under certain circumstances of the soil and situation they are found to exhibit, it is necessary to consult the works of Dr. Cleghorn and Dr. Lind,* authors of the highest repute on the subject of intermittent and remittent, in other words, of *endemial* fever.

An ague sometimes continues, particularly in cold climates, to affect the body for a very long period, without producing any permanent derangement of function or structure; but this is a very rare occurrence in hot countries. There endemial fever rapidly induces inflammatory affections, especially of the abdominal viscera, dysentery, cholera, dyspepsia, or chronic *obstructions* of the liver and spleen. The tendency of this kind of fever to produce an enlarged state of the spleen has long been observed, but the cause of this peculiarity is as yet undetected. From these organic derangements, results, as another consequence of ague, *dropsy.*

No general prognosis in intermittent and remittent fever can be given, which is not qualified by reference to the climate in which the disease appears. In this country, and in Holland, ague is not

* Cleghorn on the Diseases of Minorca, 1751. Lind on the Diseases of Hot Climates, 1768.

a disease of danger; but at Sierra Leone, and along the neighbouring coast of Guinea, at Batavia, and various other situations between the tropics, the malignity of the endemic fever is quite ap-
palling.   Season also, as I have already stated, affects the general
prognosis.   It is influenced in like manner by the previous duration of the disease.   An ague which has been present a consider-
ble time, has so far riveted itself in the constitution, that its removal becomes tedious and difficult.   Relapses under such circumstances are frequent, and tend materially to injure the constitution.
An ague is more or less dangerous, in proportion as it is complicated with more or less of permanent derangement of the function or
structure of an organ.   Enlargements of the spleen from ague are
sometimes removed, but they require great vigilance on the part
of the practitioner. (Agues particularly as they occur in hot climates, are lastly to be judged of, in reference to prognosis, by the
character of the *superadded* symptoms, and by the *degree* of their
violence.)

The circumstances which predispose the body to an attack of intermittent fever have been detailed by authors with great minuteness, but there are only a few which are of any practical importance.   Certain states of the air favour the disposition of the body
to receive ague, rivet it in the constitution, baffle us in our attempts
to cure the disease, and induce a tendency to relapse from the application of slight causes.   Of these the most remarkable are the
concurrence of a cold with a moist state of atmosphere, the prevalence of an easterly wind, and the night air.   Of the last of these,
it is highly important in a practical point of view to appreciate the
full influence.   Dr. Lind, whose opportunities of observation were
very extensive, lays much stress upon it.   He urges the danger of
sleeping, or remaining all night in unhealthy situations; and in his
Essay on the Diseases of Hot Climates, illustrates this important
principle by many apposite examples.

Weakness of the body, whether owing to a poor and unwholesome diet, long watching, fatigue, severe evacuations, or previous
diseases, augments the disposition to ague.   Hence it is that it
prevails with so much greater frequency and virulence in camps
than in any other situation; particularly after a severe campaign,
when the men have been hard worked, and exposed to great privations.   There is reason to believe, that the disposition to take ague
is affected by certain states of the mind; anxiety and inactivity in-

9

creasing it, while hope and confidence, and whatever can excite the energy of the mind, lessen the susceptibility. An army is generally most free from fever while actively engaged in military pursuits.

habit

In an enumeration of the predisposing causes of ague, *habit* merits especial mention, or (that tendency which previous attacks give to a recurrence of the complaint.) In this circumstance, intermittent fevers differ from continued, where one attack lessens the liability to a second; but it is a principle in pathology, which, though inapplicable to continued fevers, is yet found to influence the phenomena of several other febrile diseases; sore throat, for instance, erysipelas, and dysentery. So powerful is its effect in ague, that very slight causes are sufficient to renew the paroxysm, when long habit has left a predisposition in the system. It even serves to give an intermitting character to other diseases.

malaria

The great important *occasional* cause of intermittent and remittent fevers are exhalations from soil, especially from marshy, swampy, and low grounds, and hence called by physicians MARSH MIASMATA. It should be well understood however, that the existence of a *marsh* is by no means essential to the production of an ague; and therefore the term *malaria* which simply implies the tainting or vitiation of the air by noxious exhalations, is preferable, as involving less theory, and being of more general application. It is certainly a curious fact, that this pathological principle, so obvious, and so important in its practical tendency, should have been unknown to, or at least unnoticed by, the older medical authors. Lancisi is the original writer on marsh miasmata*. Since his time the subject has been occasionally but not very fully discussed, and we are still, it must be owned, much in the dark respecting many of the circumstances upon which the production of febrific miasms depends. It is presumed, however, that they arise from the combination of earth and moisture with putrescent vegetable matter, and that they are the result for the drying process in particular soils. Moisture alone, though ever so abundant, will not produce ague, for it is a rare disease at sea, even upon the foggy banks of Newfoundland. When the marsh is covered by water, agues are less frequent. Of the exact nature of these febrific miasmata we are

---

* His Treatise is entitled " De Noxiis Paludum Effluvis ; Rome, 1717."

ignorant; but some points have been noticed with regard to them, which it will be proper to advert to.

The most elevated parts of a marsh being always the healthiest, it is imagined that the miasmata are comparatively heavier than atmospheric air. There is reason too to believe, that they cannot be wafted by currents of air to any great distance from the spot where they were generated, but on this point some differences of opinion have lately prevailed. The calm months of the year being the most productive of agues, it is reasonable to suppose that the mias. mata are most powerful when concentrated, and that diffusion by a brisk wind renders them comparatively inert. Culture and proper draining prevent their formation, and hence it is that intermittent fevers are so much less frequent in England at present than they were formerly. A very short exposure to the exhalations of an unhealthy country is sufficient to affect the system. Travelling through the Pontine Marshes has often been followed by an attack of ague. There is considerable diversity in the period which elapses between exposure to malaria and the invasion of disease. It sometimes does not exceed a few days; but there is reason to believe that the *latent period* has occasionally extended to several weeks, or even months.

That the exhalations from marshy grounds are peculiarly liable to produce intermittent fever is abundantly obvious; but agues prevail extensively in certain districts where there are no marshes. There however it will always be found that there is something equivalent to a marsh, either a subsoil of such a nature as does not allow water to percolate easily through it; or an extent of wood impeding thorough ventilation and the action of the sun's rays; or excessive dampness with heat; or a total inattention to drainage and culture. In one or other of these ways, we may readily explain the prevalence of endemial fever in the uncultivated parts of America, at Sierra Leone, on the shores of the Black Sea, and in many districts of Italy and Sicily.

Febrific miasmata then may arise, under particular circumstances, from almost any soil that retains surface water, the disease which they excite having I believe, in nearly all cases, a tendency to exhibit the phenomena of *intermission*, or at least of well-marked *remission*. Persons residing in the very centre of London, are occasionally attacked by intermittent fever. In the time of Sydenham, agues were common in every part of the metropolis. To the

great attention which is now paid to the sewers, we are probably,
in a considerable degree, indebted for the present healthiness of
the town, and particularly for our exemption from ague.

These *conditions of the soil* are not merely the occasion of *agues,*
but they serve to modify the character of continued fever, and of
any other febrile disease which may happen to occur in such a situation. This principle in pathology we have already had occasion
to allude to, when treating of continued fever. A tendency is thus
given to *exacerbation* and *remission* in the symptoms of the disease ;
and it is not improbable, that many cases of what might be considered genuine remittent fever from marsh exhalation, are, in fact,
cases of common continued fever from cold, modified by peculiarities of soil. This consideration involves the question of the relation
in which intermittent and continued fevers stand to each other;
and before entering on the method of treatment in intermittents, I
may shortly advert to it. It is contended by some, that all fevers
are closely allied to each other, in their nature, in the operation of
their exciting causes, and in their method of cure. Other pathologists again maintain, that intermittent and continued fevers are *essentially* different from each other, and that *essential* differences
exist in the principles of their treatment. Our knowledge of the
pathology of fever is hardly sufficient to authorize a *decided* opinion
on the speculative question at issue, but it is certainly better for
the student to view them as *distinct* classes of disorders.

It has been made a question whether agues ought to be cured.
An idea has prevailed in many aguish countries, that there was
something salutary in the endemic fever. Boerhaave himself, a
physician of great genius, was misled by this prejudice ; and not
satisfied with the negative merit that agues do no harm, and may
therefore be suffered to continue, speaks of their positive advantages.* These opinions no longer prevail ; and the only question
which they now suggest is, whether, under certain circumstances,
it may be proper to allow the *type* of the fever clearly to develope
itself before measures are taken for its suppression. Another erroneous notion respecting the treatment of agues has frequently
been avowed ; namely, that their management requires little or no
exercise of professional skill. So far is this from being the case,

---

* Cæterum, nisi malignæ, corpus ad longævitatem disponunt, et depu-
rant ab inveteres malis. BOERHAAVE, *Aphor.* 754.

that agues often baffle the best directed exertions of our art. They become complicated with other diseases; their symptoms are modified by climate, season, and habit of body ; nor can their treatment be properly adapted to these different circumstances, except under the guidance of pathology. It is true, indeed, that the hypothetical views of authors, regarding the proximate cause of intermittent fever, give us no assistance whatever in determining the treatment ; but the pathology which is subservient to practice, is altogether of a different character. The practice in agues then, it may be observed, is to be regulated in many respects by the same principles which direct us in the treatment of continued fever.

In considering the method of cure in intermittent fevers, their tendency to spontaneous termination must be borne in mind. Hippocrates, in the very dawn of medical science, took notice that tertians particularly in the month of July, often terminated, without the aid of medicine, within five, seven, or at most nine revolutions ; and modern experience has confirmed the observation.* Mild vernal tertians will frequently go off spontaneously ; but though this tendency is to be kept in view, that the practitioner may feel he is working with nature, and not against her, it is by no means to check his efforts to put a speedy period to the disease.

The treatment of ague divides itself into two parts, the palliative and the curative ; in other words, the treatment during the paroxysms, and in the intervals between them. During the paroxysm, the object of the practitioner is to hasten its different stages, and to relieve urgent symptoms. In the interval, the indication of cure is to prevent its return : and this either by strengthening the body, or more properly, by producing such an effect upon it, and particularly upon the nervous system, as may prevent the development of fever. As we are altogether unacquainted with the manner in which malaria and miasmata produce agues, so in like manner must we profess our ignorance of the exact modus operandi of our true febrifuge medicines.

In the cold stage, stimulants, especially æther (R No. 61), and the volatile alkali (R No. 82), warm diluents, and the pediluvium, may be had recourse to, in addition to the external warmth which hot bricks and blankets afford. In the hot stage, cold acidulated drink and saline diaphoretics are advisable. Two practices how-

* Vide Cleghorn on "the Epidemical diseases of Minorca," page 205.

ever of a peculiar nature have been recommended in this stage of the disease, which require particular notice. The first is the employment of blood-letting, and the second that of opium. With respect to blood-letting, much controversy has taken place as to its propriety, even from the time of Celsus. We have the assurance of Pringle and Cleghorn,* that in warm climates and hot seasons it is a safe and proper practice, rendering the intermission or remission more complete, taking off that inflammatory diathesis which counteracts the beneficial effects of bark, and removing those pleuritic and rheumatic affections, and those symptoms of congestion in the liver and brain, which are often complicated with fevers of endemic origin. The blood drawn in the hot fit of an ague frequently exhibits the buffy coat.

Dr. Lind speaks in the most favourable terms of the exhibition of *opium* in the hot stage of ague. He recommends the opiate to be administered about half an hour after its commencement, and he states, that it shortens and abates the fit, relieves the head-ache (which is always an urgent symptom in this period of the disease), and brings on a profuse sweat with an agreeable softness of the skin, ending in a refreshing sleep. Dr. Lind is entitled to great confidence, for he was an accurate observer, and his opportunities of seeing the disease under all its modifications were very extensive.

In the interval, as I have already remarked, the *indications of cure* are more obscure. It is commonly stated, that the object is to give *tone* to the system ; but the acknowledged efficacy of arsenic in the cure of agues does not countenance such an opinion. The precise effect produced upon the body by those drugs which are the most powerful in curing agues has not been ascertained. They appear to concur in producing some strong impression upon the nervous system, which prevents the development of fever. This idea is corroborated by the consideration, that the nearer they can be given to the expected period of the paroxysm the more certain is their effect. An emetic (R No. 1,) administered immediately before the accession of the cold stage is very serviceable. A strong opiate, especially in combination with æther, as in the antispasmodic draught (R No. 83,) has frequently succeeded in checking the

* Pringle on the diseases of the Army, page 200. Cleghorn on the Diseases of Minorca, page 197.

paroxysm, when given on its first approach. The volatile alkali may be used with the same intention. Various remedies of a similar kind, consisting principally of combinations of spirit and aromatics, have acquired great reputation with the vulgar. They agree in producing some strong impression either upon the stomach or external senses. The most generally successful, however, of all the means which have been resorted to for the cure of intermittent fever, is the exhibition of bark and of arsenic.

Bark is most effectual, when recent and of good quality, when given during a state of perfect *apyrexia*, in the form of powder carefully prepared, in large doses, and as near as possible to the expected paroxysm. (One or two drachms may be taken every hour, for six or eight hours previous to the fit.) Much certainly depends on the *quantity* administered in a short space of time. All means therefore should be taken to prevent its disagreeing with the stomach, or running off by the bowels. For this purpose it may sometimes be advantageously united with an aromatic, or with opium, or a few grains of rhubarb ; or the form of decoction and extract (as in R Nos. 70 and 71,) may be substituted for the powder. Modern pharmacy has given us a most efficient and elegant preparation of bark, in the sulfate of quinine, which in doses' of three or four grains (R Nos. 72 and 73), frequently repeated, may be fully relied on. The effects of the cinchona in the cure of ague are materially aided by its combination with some diffusible stimulant, especially the subcarbonate of ammonia, port wine, brandy, or strong aromatic tincture. But there are certain states of the constitution which are found to interfere with the exhibition of bark in any form, and to counteract any good effects from it. The principal of these are, an inflammatory diathesis prevailing in the system, disorders of the primæ viæ, obstructions of the liver and spleen, and the presence of other diseases. Hence arises the necessity of blood-letting, of purgatives, of saline and antimonial medicines, and of alteratives, particulaly mercurials, either previous to, or combined with bark, according to the circumstances of the case.

Various substitutes for the cinchona bark, native and foreign, have been introduced into the Materia Medica, belonging to the class of bitters and astringents. Among the best may be reckoned the barks of cusparia, of different species of salix and quassia, and the roots of the acorus calamus, bistort, and rhatany. They are all very inferior however in point of efficacy to the cortex cinchonæ, arising doubtless from their want of that peculiar vegetable alkali (quinine and cinchonine,) which is the efficient ingredient in the latter drug. Of the mineral substances employed in the cure of agues, the most powerful by far is arsenic, the efficacy of which has been ascertained by the most ample experience. It is best given in the form of the liquor arsenicalis, and in the dose of five drops, gradually augmented. After a certain length of time, sometimes indeed from the very first, it will produce nausea and vomiting, when its exhibition must be suspended, and a few grains of rhubarb given. Under proper management, arsenic will be found, next to bark, the most generally useful of all medicines in the treatment of agues; but its administration requires to be regulated in the same manner as that of bark. The best mineral substitute for it is the sulfate of zinc, which is largely employed in the fenny counties of England. In doses of one or two grains, three times a day, and in conjunction with a small proportion of opium, it has proved eminently serviceable.*

Remittent fever arises, as I have already stated, like the intermittent, from malaria. It is a type of fever very frequent in hot climates, where it occasionally occurs under a highly aggravated form. Its symptoms vary with the nature of the climate, the season, the constitution of the patient, and many *local* circumstances, so that it is difficult to give any precise detail of them. They bear a general resemblance to those of intermittent fever; but some formerly mentioned as occurring in the course of *continued* fever, are met with also in the remittent, and materially affect the character of the disease, the prognosis, and the method of cure. The most important are those which indicate severe *gastric* derangement; and this combination of remitting fever from noxious exhalation, with high vascular excitement, and inflammation, or congestion, or simple disturbance of function in some of the abdominal viscera (the consequence no doubt of atmospheric heat,) constitutes that formidable disease known by the name of *the billious remittent of hot climates.*

The endemic fever of Sierra Leone, by which so many lives have

* See Appendix; Note F.

Endemic fever

Symp.

recently been lost, is a true remittent fever. The symptoms which characterize its onset, are violent pain in the region of the liver, increased on pressure, and a sense of fulness with pulsation in the præcordia. In a short time evidences of strong determination of blood to the head take place, and by this the patient is commonly carried off. If he survives, enlargement of the spleen almost uniformly succeeds, and this state of disease is accompanied by paroxysms of *intermitting* fever, not assuming however any fixed type. In some instances disorganization of the spleen has occurred without any prior attack of the fever. Its source cannot be questioned. There is indeed no marsh whose palpable exhalations defy scepticism, but its place is amply supplied by the excessive and almost unvarying humidity of the atmosphere, the rank luxuriance of the vegetation, and the extreme heat, which causing a continual evaporation from the soil and rivers, serves also to enervate the human frame, and predispose it to the noxious influences of a tainted atmosphere.

The treatment of this, as of every other variety of remittent fever, is to be regulated, partly by those principles which have been laid down as applicable intermittents, and partly also by those which guide us in continued fever.

Treatment

Free evacuations by blood-letting, leeches, and cupping, with active aperients (especially calomel,) and saline diaphoretics, must precede the administration of bark in any of its forms. To determine the extent to which these evacuant remedies should be pushed, constitutes the great and acknowledged difficulty in the management of remittent fever, and this knowledge must be the result of extensive and often dear-bought experience. In a large proportion of cases, it is also requisite to affect the system with mercury.*

* See Appendix ; Note G.

10

OF THE YELLOW FEVER.

Controversy on this Subject. Varieties of Fever in the West Indies. Symptoms of the Epidemic Yellow Fever. Its Analogy to Typhus. Treatment of the Disease. Notice of the principal controverted points in the History of the Yellow Fever. Question of Foreign Origin. Of propagation by Contagion. Of Exemption from a second Attack.

ALTHOUGH we presume, that the observations already made have explained the most important principles involved in the pathology of fever, and though the discussion might therefore be expected to terminate here, still it may be found advisable to pay some special attention to the subject of *yellow fever.* It is one which has excited a great deal of interest in this and other countries, during the last thirty years. It has given rise to the most singular differences of opinion among persons, to all appearance, equally qualified to form a correct judgment regarding it ; nor has the controversy yet entirely subsided. Little doubt can remain, that this has arisen from the want of correct views of the pathology of fever; and it surely cannot be an useless task to attempt to elucidate a subject, confessedly so obscure, by applying doctrines already laid down, to an explanation of the principal points in dispute.

The disease of which I propose here to treat under the title of the *yellow fever* is that which, under the name of Maladie de Siam, or Bulam fever, has been frequently observed to prevail in the West Indies, along the shores of North America, particularly at New. York and Philadelphia, and more lately in the southern parts of Spain. It has spread *epidemically* in those regions, and been pro-ductive of very great mortality in particular seasons.

It is scarcely necessary to apprize the student, that hot countries are subject, no less than cold, to the occasional visitations of epi. demic disease. They have also, of course, their peculiar endem-

ics, and the term yellow fever is currently applied, in the West Indies, to express modifications of fever different from that which I
am now about to describe. To the want of precision in the naming
and classing of fevers, and to carelessness in tracing the analogies
and distinctions of epidemic and endemic diseases, may be attributed in a great measure the dispute to which the subject of yellow
fever has given birth.

Most of the genuine febrile diseases of hot climates appear to
have a *bilious* tendency. The inflammatory as well as the intermittent and remittent endemics of those countries, are frequently
accompanied with a yellow colour of the skin, and other symptoms
supposed to denote that the functions of the liver are materially disturbed. The symptoms and treatment of these forms of endemic
disease, however, it is not my intention to discuss. The present object of inquiry is the epidemic yellow fever, such as raged in the
West India Islands and at Philadelphia in 1793 ; at Cadiz in 1800 ;
at Malaga in 1803; at Gibraltar in 1804 and 1813 ; and at Ascension Island in 1823. As this particular form of fever exhibited in
all these situations very much of the same defined and in several
respects peculiar character, I shall give a short account of its symptoms and progress, of the appearances found on dissection, and of
the most approved system of treatment.*

The attack of yellow fever is ushered in, in the usual way, by
langour and rigors. There is sometimes a peculiar dejection of
countenance observed, with a remarkable aversion to the least motion ; at other times there is an appearance of inebriation. The
face is flushed ; but the most prominent of the early symptoms of
the disease is head-ache, of a very peculiar kind. It is exceedingly
severe, and referred to the forehead and bottom of the orbits. The
eyes appear dull, glassy, suffused, and protruded. The tongue, is
at first furred and moist, and trembling, but by degrees it becomes
dry and black, or sometimes of a fiery red colour. The heat of skin
is but little increased. The patient sometimes lies in an almost insensible state, but extreme restlessness has also been noticed.

To this succeeds the second striking feature in the symptoms of
the disease, great irritability of the stomach. The matter rejected

* For many of the remarks contained in this chapter, I beg to express
my obligations to Dr. Fraser, late Inspector of Hospitals at Gibraltar, who
obligingly gave me access to his voluminous and valuable documents on
the yellow fever.

is very seldom bilious, or if it is so at first, it speedily loses that character. For the most part it is slimy and tasteless, and adheres in small flakes to the sides of the containing vessel. As the disease advances, it assumes a dark colour, and comes to have the appearance of coffee-grounds. This is the *black vomit*, which may be considered the characteristic feature of this disease, as much as buboes and carbuncles are of the plague. The dejections have a tarry appearance. There is often noticed a total suppression of urine, which like the black vomit, is a fatal symptom. Hiccup, hæmorrhages, and petechiæ have been observed in some cases, even from an early period.

I have retained to the last, the mention of that symptom which gives name to the disease—yellowness of the skin, but it is not of that importance which might have been anticipated. Many cases indeed run through their whole course without exhibiting it ; but when it appears early, or when the skin assumes a leaden or livid cast, it is to be considered an unfavourable symptom. A few other peculiarities in the disease are all that remain to be noticed. The yellow fever is occasionally attended with an ulcerated state of the throat. A fatal termination has often happened in the most unexpected manner; a very singular remission of all the symptoms taking place about sixty hours from the first attack, and raising hopes which are soon to be disappointed. Death is sometimes preceded by a degree of low muttering delirium ; at other times the patient sinks exhausted, but with the intellect quite unimpaired. The usual duration of the yellow fever is from five to seven days. If the patient passes the sixth day without the occurrence of black vomit, or suppression of urine, his chance of recovery is much increased ; but even then symptoms like those of common typhus occasionally supervene, and prove fatal. Relapses in this fever are very rare.

Upon dissection, very few appearances present themselves which can be considered as throwing light on the pathology of the disease. The body has been observed speedily to become livid. Yellowness of the skin has sometimes been first noticed to occur after death. A state of turgescence of the cerebral veins has been described, and occasionlly there has been observed a peculiar redness of the inner coat of the stomach. The gall-bladder is generally found distended with dark and viscid bile. The structure of the liver is not found to be altered. It sometimes assumes an ash colour.

Such are the most usual symptoms of the yellow fever. They will be seen to bear some resemblance to those of the plague, and the analogy between these diseases has been urged with much force by Sir J. M' Grigor. A more important analogy may be traced between the epidemic yellow fever and the genuine typhus fever of this country ; and there can be no doubt, that the former bears the same relation to the endemic fever of the West Indies, that typhus does to the common *synochus* of Europe. It is properly called therefore the *typhus icterodes*. It is the *malignant* fever of tropical climates, characterized, like the malignant fevers of temperate climates, by deep-seated affection of the brain, and extreme irritability of the stomach, but in a higher degree of *intensity*.

The cause of the yellow colour of the skin in this fever has been made a subject of inquiry. By some this appearance has been attributed to disordered function of the liver ; by others, to bile absorbed from the intestinal canal without hepatic derangement. Sir Gilbert Blane has thrown out the idea, that it may be owing rather to a depraved state of the red globules of the blood. In whatever way this question may be decided, it is perfectly clear that the state of the *biliary* organs has very little to do with giving a character to this formidable disease, which is to be viewed as one of the most aggravated forms of typhoid fever. In respect of mortality, the yellow fever may even take precedence of the plague. At Gibraltar in 1804 the disease raged among the inhabitants, uninfluenced by any distinction of age, sex, or condition.* The deaths amounted to somewhat more than one in three ; a proportion, according to Sir Gilbert Blane, considerably above the devastation of the pestilence of the Levant.

The treatment of the epidemic yellow fever is a point which has attracted great attention from all classes of inquirers : but their observations tend only to show that it is a disease of so singularly malignant a nature, as in a large proportion of cases, to bid defiance to all the efforts of art. This is particularly exemplified when the disease first makes its appearance in any town or district. The peculiar combination of circumstances, whether in re-

* Of a population of nine thousand civilians, only twenty-eight persons escaped an attack of the disease.

bloodletting not beneficial except in plethoric habit

spect of local situation, or of the state of the atmosphere, or of the constitution of the inhabitants, which gives the peculiar feature of malignity to the symptoms of the disease, operates also against the practitioner, and deprives him of the usual powerful means of combating fever. The severe head-ache which characterizes the early stages of the disease, naturally suggests blood-letting as a probable means of relief; but experience has proved that, though occasionally, it is not generally beneficial. The blood, when drawn, separates very imperfectly; upon exposure to the air, it does not acquire its usual florid colour, and scarcely ever exhibits a buffy appearance. In determining however the propriety of having recourse to blood-letting in yellow fever, the *habit of body* is certainly to be studied. In a plethoric habit, where the pulse is firm, a single bleeding will probably be beneficial. All that I wish to urge is, that venesection is useful rather with reference to the individual attacked than to the nature of disease.

calomel aloes gamboge

The principal object which it is found necessary to keep in view in the treatment of yellow fever, is the allaying that excessive irritability of the stomach, which leads to the black vomit. Calomel, given at first in a smart dose, so as to operate freely as a purgative, and repeated in smaller doses at intervals of three or four hours, so as to keep up this effect, was the most approved practice among the English practitioners at Gibraltar in 1813. To the calomel were occasionally united aloes and gamboge. In the exhibition of these medicines no time was to be lost; for it was only by their speedy and full effect, that the prevention or relief of the vomiting could be ensured. Pediluvia, and tepid sponging were found beneficial. Under certain circumstances, the warm bath was administered with good effect. Cold applications to the forehead and hands occasionally served to relieve the urgent head-ache. When the powers of life appeared to fail, it is unnecessary to say that stimulants and cordials were had recourse to. Subacid drinks were given, and a strict antiphlogistic regimen pursued through the whole disease. The same rigid attention to diet and regimen were required during the period of convalescence.

I have stated, that among the points in dispute regarding the yellow fever, is the question of the identity of the epidemic yellow, or Bulam fever, with the endemic fevers of the West Indies. Upon this question an opinion has already been given. The other topics of controversy are, first, whether the disease be always imported, or whether it can ever be generated by a combination of *common* or endemic causes ;—secondly, whether, being once received into a town, it propagates itself by contagion ; and thirdly, whether those who have passed through the disease are susceptible of it a second time. These are all important questions, the replies to which are not so obvious as to that of its pathological affinity, which has already been noticed ; and they involve the most difficult parts of the controversy.

The first question is undoubtedly one which should be answered with some caution. Many circumstances connected with the early appearance of the epidemic yellow fever at Philadelphia in 1793, and at Gibralter in 1804, strongly favour the idea of its having been in those situations an imported disease. Several other facts however might be adduced, which militate against the universality of this doctrine ; and there is nothing inconsistent in allowing, that, though it is sometimes imported, the genuine malignant yellow fever may, under circumstances favourable to its development, be generated in any warm climate by a combination of endemic causes. With regard to the second question, no reasonable doubt can surely be entertained by any candid, intelligent, unbiassed man, that this disease, being once received into a town, is contagious. The evidence in favour of this opinion is certainly as strong as for that of the contagion of typhus, or of plague. Whether the yellow fever bears the greater analogy to the former or latter of these diseases, may indeed be disputed. We may deny that there is any thing specific in the contagion of yellow fever ; but that the disease is propagated by contagion of some kind, cannot be questioned, after the ample experience which has been had, both in America and Europe. If any doubts could have been entertained while the disease occurred only in the West Indies, in consequence of the resemblance of the epidemic to the endemic fevers of those islands, they must have yielded to the obvious arguments suggested by its appearance in Cadiz, Gibraltar, and still more lately at the Island of Ascension.* The contagious nature of the disease, it may be remarked, is a question which is perfectly distinct from that of its foreign or endemic origin.

* Consult Dr. BURNETT's " Official Report of the Fever which appeared in his Majesty's Ship Bann, and the Island of Ascension, in 1823." London, 1824.

latent period

Some of the laws of the contagion of yellow fever appear to be ascertained with tolerable accuracy. Its latent period varies from two to eight days. Ten days is, I believe, the longest period recorded of yellow fever appearing, after exposure to the contagion, and removal to a freely ventilated atmosphere. The contagion of yellow fever has a peculiar range of atmospheric temperature, but on a higher scale than that of the plague. It has never been known, but in those countries and at those seasons when tropical heats, that is, of eighty degrees Fahrenheit's, or upwards, prevail. It never fails to disappear as the winter approaches. It is certainly a singular circumstance in the history of the yellow fever, that it has never prevailed to any remarkable extent at a distance from the sea, and that its principal ravages have been on the shores of the Atlantic Ocean.

not generally taken a second time

The last circumstance which it is of importance to notice in the history of the yellow fever and the laws of its contagion, is the question whether it can be taken a second time. The answer is a very short one. Although a few well attested instances to the contrary have been recorded, still a most extensive experience has satisfactorily proved, that the immunity from second attacks is nearly complete, and that it forms one of the most striking characteristics of this remarkable disease.*

* See Appendix ; Note H.

CLASS II.

THE EXANTHEMATA, OR ERUPTIVE FEVERS.

CHAP. I.

THE EXANTHEMATA IN GENERAL.

Objects of Inquiry in this Chapter. Character of this Order of Diseases. Their Relation to simple Fevers. Defined Character and Course of Exanthematous Fever. Defined Character of the Eruption. Their Occurrence but once in Life. Exceptions to this Law, and Attempts to explain them. Their Origin from Specific Contagion. Relation of the Exanthemata to the other Morbid Poisons. Peculiarities of Specific Contagions. Communication by Inoculation. Latent periods. Incompatibility with one another, and with other Diseases. Criticism on Dr. Willan's Arrangement of the Exanthemata. Their connection with Disease of Mucous Membrane.

THE class of exanthemata, or eruptive fevers, is that to which our attention is next to be directed ; and as the diseases which it comprises present many points of analogy, and several peculiarities which distinguish them from other complaints, it may be advantageous to offer some general remarks upon the class, previous to examining its component parts in detail. My object on this occasion will be to point out the pathological relations of the exanthemata, and to give a general idea of the objects of investigation in the five following chapters. With this view, I shall direct my attention to the relation which they bear to simple fevers, to one another, to other diseases arising from morbid poisons, and to cutaneous complaints. These objects of inquiry involve the consideration of some of the most important laws which regulate the phenomena of disease, but they can only be very briefly touched upon in this place.

11

Idiopathic fevers were formerly stated to be of three kinds,
continued fevers, intermittents, and the exanthemata. The latter
may be viewed as continued fevers to which an eruption is superadded ; and a great deal of what has been said regarding the general doctrine of simple fever, particularly all that part which relates
to the prognosis and principles of treatment, will be found equally
applicable to the case of fever complicated with eruption. The
consideration of the exanthemata naturally follows that of fevers
strictly so called, for by such an arrangement we shall be able to
exhibit, in a connected view, all the leading doctrines of febrile
disease.

The genuine exanthemata are small-pox, chicken-pox, cow-pox,
measles, and scarlet fever. There are a few other diseases of lesser
importance, which, as allied in some respects to these, may be arranged in this division of the work, under the title of the minor
exanthemata ; but our attention in this chapter will be exclusively
directed to the former. The following is the common character of
the exanthemata. 1st. They are marked by the presence of fever,
which runs a defined course. 2d. They are attended with an eruption, which, like the accompanying fever, goes through a regular
series of changes. 3d. They occur to every individual once, and
only once, during life. 4th. They arise from specific contagion.

1. The first peculiarity of the exanthemata is the defined character and steady course which the accompanying fever exhibits,
under almost every variety of external circumstances and habit of
body. Here we trace a very marked and obvious distinction between exanthematous and common continued fever. It is a feature
however in the character of the exanthemata, which, though applicable as a general principle, requires to be received with some
qualification. It is strikingly illustrated indeed by the phenomena
of small-pox and measles, but it is less distinct in the scarlet fever ;
and in the cow-pox and chicken-pox, very little fever is discernible
at any time. The *character* of exanthematous fever, except in the
case of one form of scarlatina, is inflammatory, and this it assumes
in the young and the old, and in all varieties of climate, season,
and situation. The regularity in the *course* of exanthematous fever
is well shown in the three days of the eruptive fever of variola,
and the eight days of its fever of maturation. These curious facts
form a striking illustration of the doctrine of critical days in fever,
and of that principle of periodic movement in the animal œconomy,

regulating many phenomena both in a state of health and disease, to which we formerly referred. It is a singular circumstance, that this corroboration of the doctrine of critical days, should not have been known till above a thousand years after that principle in pathology had been inculcated.

· 2. The second character of the exanthemata is drawn from their being attended with an eruption which goes through a, regular *eruption* series of changes. This is another of those remarkable facts in the animal œconomy, for which we may find some analogies, but which we shall never succeed in explaining. The appearance of the eruption in each of the diseases of this class is peculiar, and except in some severe cases of chicken-pox, can hardly admit of any doubt. The progress of the eruption in each disease is also peculiar, but it is uniform. That of scarlet fever shows itself on the second day, and declines on the fifth. The eruption of measles shows itself on the fourth day, and fades on the seventh. The eruption of small-pox shows itself on the third day, and maturates on the tenth. To this regularity of progress in the febrile eruptions there are a few, and but a very few exceptions. In the inoculated small-pox the eruption is sometimes postponed from the ninth to the twelfth day; in the measles from the fourth to the sixth, or even later. The most remarkable exception is that enjoyed by the cow-pox, which has the characters of an *exeanthema* without the occurrence of any eruption; but the regular progress of the vesicle and areola are sufficient to entitle it to its present place in the nosology. Even this sometimes varies, for without any obvious cause the vaccine pimple occasionlly remains dormant for four or five days, and is not elevated before the sixth or seventh day. These cases however are rare, and they only serve to teach us caution in framing our general positions. An inquiry into the course of each particular eruption will form a prominent feature in our account of the respective diseases. The exact nature of the eruption is not always well understood, as in the case of measles and scarlet-fever; but in that of small-pox it is genuine pustular inflammation.

3. The occurrence of the exanthemata to every individual once, *occur once* and once only, in the course of life, is the most curious and characteristic feature in the history of these diseases. That every race of man, under every possible variety of climate, age, and constitution, should be susceptible of the same disease, that this disease

should present everywhere the same character, and run through the same stages, and having once occurred, should never again appear in the same individual, though exposed to the utmost malignity of infection, are facts in the history of the animal œconomy which may well excite our curiosity. Their general accuracy is unquestionable, at least so far as the constitution of the human body allows us to acknowledge any such widely extended proposition. Here indeed, as in every other part of pathology, exceptions occur. A few constitutions have been met with, which appear to be completely insensible to the contagion of small-pox. Some individuals, who cannot be made to take the small-pox or scarlet fever at one age, are yet susceptible of it at another. In like manner it is established on undoubted evidence, that small-pox and measles may occur twice in the same individual. Some pathologists have refused to acknowledge the truth of this exception to the general law of the exanthemata, and have attempted to explain away the cases of secondary small-pox, by presuming on the ignorance or the carelessness of the practitioner in attendance. These and similar frivolous arguments do not admit of serious refutation. Such exceptions have undoubtedly occurred ; and it is our business to watch nature, and not prescribe to her the course which she is to pursue.

No doubt whatever can be entertained with regard to the occasional occurrence of second and even third attacks of scarlatina. They are sometimes milder, sometimes severer than the primary. Attempts have been made by pathologists, to explain the causes to which secondary attacks of the exanthemata are to be referred. Sir Gilbert Blane believes, that the first attacks are always or nearly always severe ; and he argues therefore, that the secondary attack is owing to the susceptibility of the constitution to the disease being in such individuals *stronger* than in others. Dr. Wells, on the other hand, apprehends, that where a secondary attack occurs, the first will be found to have been mild ; that the susceptibility therefore is not greater in these cases than in others, but that the primary attack had not been sufficient to *saturate*, as it were, the constitution. The phenomena of modified small-pox, which have lately attracted so much attention, hinge upon this question. Perhaps it will be found, that neither of these explanations is altogether satisfactory, and that the occurrence is attributable to some peculiarity in the constitution of the individual, the precise nature of which does not admit of being developed.

4. The last feature in the general character of the exanthemata is their origin from specific contagion. I have already (page 44) explained the difference between the several kinds of contagion, and pointed out a few of the most important principles involved in the doctrine, more particularly such as relate to the operation of *common* contagion, and are subservient to the pathology of fever. An origin from specific contagion is a character of eruptive fevers, but they possess it in common with many other complaints—the plague, psora, syphilis, and hydrophobia. It is this character indeed which associates the exanthemata with that tribe of diseases which have been designated by the title of the *morbid poisons.* This phrase has been invented to distinguish these disorders from such as arise from mineral or vegetable poisons, the bites of venomous animals, or the exhalations of marshes. It is supposed that the poison in all the diseases now alluded to, is produced from an animal body already in the state of disease, and therefore it is called a *morbid* poison. The plague has been considered by some authors as an exanthematous disease, but we have elsewhere given our reasons for believing that it is more nearly allied to the typhoid fevers. The yaws or framboesia is a peculiar disease, which, arising from a morbid poison, and running a defined course, may perhaps be admitted into this class.

Of the nature of the specific contagion in each of the exanthematous diseases we are completely ignorant, and the subject is altogether inscrutable. It is quite clear, however, that it is something of an exceedingly subtile nature. A single vesicle of cow-pox contains sufficient of the specific matter of contagion to communicate the disease to an incredible number of persons. A single drop is sufficient for each, perhaps a small portion of a drop, and of that there is reason to believe that the bulk consists of the common serum of the blood. The multiplication of this morbid poison in the body of the affected individual is wholly inexplicable. The older physicians applied the analogy of vegetable ferments to the explanation of the phenomenon, and certainly with much ingenuity. The doctrine a *materies morbi* is satisfactorily proved in the case of small-pox, cow-pox, plague, and syphilis, and the old humoral doctrines have doubtless therefore some foundation in nature. Whether they can be extended so as to explain the phenomena of other eruptive complaints, and of diseases whose pathological relations to the exanthemata are not so obvious, may in future times become an object of inquiry.

The exanthematous contagions were for a long time confounded. Small-pox and measles were for many centuries believed to arise from the same contagion. The measles and scarlet fever were considered by Morton to be the same disease, nor was the diagnosis clearly established until lately. Some pathologists at present believe there is an affinity between the contagions of small-pox and cow-pox ; and within the last few years, the notion of the indentity of small-pox and chicken-pox has been revived. The origin of all these contagions is involved in obscurity ; but though we cannot form the most distant idea how they first got into the world, we can yet in many instances trace, with some precision, the periods when they first began to spread as epidemics. It is a very remark-able circumstance, that the exanthemata, and the several morbid poisons associated with them, were unknown to the ancient physi-cians, and did not appear in Europe till after the birth of Christ. To ascertain the countries in which these diseases originally ap-peared, and from which they were propagated over the rest of the world, will prove an interesting subject of investigation.

Among the peculiarities of *specific* contagions, communication by inoculation has been mentioned. This however is not a general law. Measles, chicken-pox, and scarlet fever, cannot be given in this way ; and the remaining diseases of the class share this prop-erty with several other affections,—syphilis, gonorrhœa, psora, and Ægyptian opthalmia. The uniformity in the *latent period* of most of the specific contagions, whether febrile or chronic, deserves some notice in a general view of the pathological relations of the exanthemata. It appears to be often as accurately defined as the periods of the fever, and this by an unknown law of the animal œconomy. It admits, however, of some variety, though apparent-ly not so great as in the case of *common* contagion. The latent pe-riod of typhus for instance is considered to vary from a week to two months ; that of small-pox and plague certainly does not vary more than a few days.

It has always been reckoned a very striking feature in the his-tory of the exanthemata, that they are not compatible with each other, or with any other disorder. In most cases, if another dis-ease be present, the exanthemata will not advance. Thus diar-rhœa and fever prevent the success of inoculation. Eruptions on the skin, retard and modify the appearances of the vaccine vesicle. Cases have been mentioned, where the small-pox and measles oc. curring together, the small-pox has been delayed until the latter has run its course. This law however is subject to numerous exceptions. It has been proved for instance that small-pox and measles, as well as cow-pox and measles, may coexist. Measles and hooping-cough frequently proceed together. In like manner small-pox and cow-pox, chicken-pox and cow-pox are sometimes observed to advance, each vesicle preserving its own character. The principle nevertheless, is an important one; and it may perhaps be illustrated by the well-known fact, that during the prevalence of an epidemic plague or yellow fever (the one notoriously, and the other very probably arising from specific contagion,) all other disorders disappear.

In Dr. Willan's arrangement of cutaneous affections, it will be found that the natural connections of the exanthemata are broken, and these diseases thrown into other pathological relations, to which they do not appear to have any claim. This has been done under an idea that there is some essential difference between a pimple and a rash, a vesicle and a pustule. These I believe to be little more than modifications of each other, and by no means so distinct as to become the foundation of nosological arrangement. The same disease is vesicular at one period, and pustular at another. A slight accident may at any time convert the vesicle into a pustula. Indeed, as a general principle in pathology it may be stated, that the pustular or vesicular character of an eruption depends upon and is determined by, the quantity of inflammation existing in the cutis, and the degree of strength in the general system. Upon the whole there can be little doubt, that Dr. Cullen's classification of exanthemata is pathologically more correct, and in practice more applicable, than that suggested by Dr. Willan; and we shall follow it therefore in the subsequent pages.

The pathology of the eruptive febrile diseases is confessedly as obscure as that of the simple fevers; but latterly an attempt has been made to clear up some of the difficulties in which it is involved, by showing that disease of the great mucous membranes of the body is implicated in them, as intimately, and to almost as great an extent, as the skin itself.) The structure and functions of the skin and mucous membranes bear a close resemblance to each other, and many pathological considerations tend to prove that

there exists also a very close analogy in their diseases.   It would
be a rational conjecture therefore, that in fevers where the skin is
extensively concerned, the mucous membranes would participate,
and observation favours the opinion.   The principle appears to be
of very general application, and is illustrated not merely by the
symptoms which the different exanthemata present in their different stages, but by the appearances also found after death.   There
is reason to suspect, that upon this intimate connection between
exanthematous fevers and disease of mucous membrane, depend
several of the most important varieties and anomalies which have
been observed; such, for instance, as the recession of the eruptions, and the occasional recurrence of the disease.   As we proceed in the separate examination of the diseases of this order, we
shall have frequent occasion to refer to these, as well as to the other
general views of the exanthemata which have been taken in this
chapter, and which, though avowedly obscure, may yet give us
some assistance in explaining their several phenomena.

CHAP. II.

Introduction of the Small-Pox into Europe. Ravages committed by it. Symptoms of the Disease. Distinct and Confluent Small-Pox. Malignant Small-Pox. Coherent Small Pox. Prognosis. Morbid Appearances. Structure of the Pock. Peculiarities of the Contagion of Small-Pox. Causes of Confluence. General Plan of treatment. Practice of Inoculation.

It is a commonly received opinion, that the small-pox first appeared in China and Hindostan, and that it was known in those countries from a very remote period. Such an opinion is certainly countenanced by a number of strong arguments and very curious considerations ; by the mythology, the religious institutions, the sacred and historical records, the medical works, and the uniform traditions of those countries. In the account of Southern India, however, by Colonel Wilks, an ingenious and plausible attempt has been made to overthrow this long-established belief, to prove that the small-pox was first introduced into India in the sixth century, and to reconcile all the foregoing arguments with such a supposition. Without entering into the discussion of a question which has no practical bearing to recommend it, it will be sufficient for my purpose to state, that inoculation was practised in India long before it became general in Europe ;* and that we are unquestionably indebted to Asiatic ingenuity for the first efficacious means of combating this formidable disorder.

Whatever opinion may be entertained regarding the antiquity of small-pox in the East, no doubt exists as to the period when it first appeared in the West. This happened in Arabia, somewhere about the æra of the Hegyra, A. D. 622. From this point, as from a

* Consult Mr. Moore's very valuable and interesting work, entitled "*History of the Small-Pox.*"

12

centre, the small-pox gradually spread into Europe and Asia Minor. It appears to have reached England towards the close of the ninth century. All authors concur in representing the dreadful mortality occasioned by this pestilence wherever it appeared, and the consequent terror which it everywhere excited. Never was this more strikingly manifested than early in the sixteenth century, when some of the successors of Columbus carried the disease to America. The record of the desolation that followed in its track, it is painful to contemplate.

The general introduction of inoculation was brought about in 1722, by the acute observation and spirited efforts of Lady Mary Wortley Montague. For a long time, however, the practice was viewed with great distrust, nor were its merits fully appreciated till towards the latter period of the last century. This change in the ideas of the world concerning the value of inoculation, may be dated from the general adoption of the Suttonian practice in 1766.

For the first description of the small-pox we are indebted to Rhazes, one of the earliest of the Arabian authors, who flourished in the tenth century. The increasing prevalence, and almost incredible malignity of the complaint, rendered it an object of investigation to almost all succeeding authors. Sydenham, in particular, studied the disease with an attention to minutiæ, which can scarcely be parallelled in the history of medicine. In consequence, a mass of facts has been collected together concerning the small-pox, which does not admit of being detailed in the compass of an elementary work; nor, under present circumstances, does it appear necessary to devote to it that degree of attention which it received in earlier times. I shall content myself, therefore, with an attempt to give a general notion of the effects of the variolous poison upon the animal œconomy. I shall then point out how far they admit of being moderated; and conclude with a few remarks on the modification which small-pox undergoes from the mode of its reception into the system.

The contagion of small-pox has a latent period of from ten to fourteen days, at the end of which time it begins to show its deleterious effects upon the system. These vary both in *kind* and in *degree*; and attempts have been made to ascertain if possible, the sources of the different forms which small-pox assumes. By some, the mildness or malignity of the disease have been attributed to differences in the *contagion* from which it emanated. Innumerable facts, however, are upon record disproving this notion, and show-ing that the severest kind of small-pox may be taken from a case of the mildest sort. That other circumstances concur, I shall hereaf-ter point out; but the student should remember, that the great principle is *idiosyncracy*, or peculiarity of habit. As there are cer-tain constitutions that suffer more than others from lead, mercury, and the venereal poison, so are certain systems unusually irritable under the operation of the variolous virus. Many children suffer in this manner; and consequently an epileptic fit is, in early life, a frequent symptom of the accession of small-pox. It was very justly remarked, however, by Sydenham, that this does not necessarily denote, in them, a severe disease. The case is different when head symptoms accompany the attack of small-pox in more advanced life, and in robust habits. Early delirium, occurring under such circumstances, marks a deep implication of the brain and nervous system, from which, in the progress of the disorder, much is to be dreaded.

The eruptive fever of small-pox lasts in general forty-eight hours, and is, in very many cases, not to be distinguished from an attack of inflammatory, or of common continued fever. The suddenness of the seizure is the best guide; but the severe pain of the back, the vomiting, and pain of the epigastrium on pressure, assist in the diagnosis. The nature of the disease is put beyond a doubt by the eruption, which is first observed about the forehead and wrists, and, extending gradually over the other parts of the body, is usually completed in twenty-four, or at farthest in thirty-six hours. On the appearance of eruption, the febrile symptoms abate, and in ve-ry mild cases are never renewed. In the severer kinds of small-pox, they only experience at this period a slight remission. The further progress of the disease depends so much on the *quantity* of the eruption, that nosologists have assumed this as a basis of dis-tinction, and accordingly divide small pox into two species; the *distinct* and the *confluent*. This arrangement, however, does not seem to me sufficient for practical purposes; and I therefore pre-fer a fourfold division, into the *distinct*, the *simple confluent*, the *ma-lignant confluent*, and the *coherent*. The peculiarities in each of these forms of the disease I shall now shortly advert to; premising that, in all, the disease divides itself into three stages; the first ter-minating by the appearance of the eruption; the second by the maturation of the pustules; and the third by the falling off of the scabs.

1. The distinct small-pox shows itself in the form of elevated papulæ. On the third day a small vesicle, having a *central* depression, may be observed on the summit of each pimple. It contains, at this period, a minute portion of a thin transparent lymph. An inflamed margin, or *areola*, now forms around it; which, when the vesicles are tolerably numerous, diffuses considerable inflammation over the neighbouring skin, so as to give it a damask rose colour, and as the eruption advances, to occasion swelling of the face. About the sixth day the vesicles lose their central depression, and assume a spheroidal form. Suppuration has now taken place, and the pustules will be found to contain a thick matter of a yellowish colour. On the succeeding day, those which first appeared upon the face burst, and upon the eighth from the date of the eruption, scabbing commences over the body generally. The swelling of the face then subsides, and all fever is at an end. In about ten days more the crusts fall off; and the skin, though left for a time of a dark brown colour, is ultimately restored to its natural condition.

Such is the usual course of the eruption of distinct small-pox, but it is subject to considerable variety. Upon the face it is sometimes more rapid, while upon the extremities it is commonly more tardy, the pustules on the feet and legs being seldom fully ripened until the tenth or eleventh day from their first appearance. Their contents too vary in point of consistence, and hence have arisen those distinctions of vesicular, vesiculo-pustular, crystalline, horny, and water-pocks, which have been noticed by authors.

2. When the papulæ are very numerous, and exceedingly close set upon all parts of the body, more especially on the face, we call the disease *confluent*. For the first day or two no differences are perceptible between this and the preceding species, except that the patient is more languid and oppressed; on the third, however, still more upon the fourth, the change becomes apparent. The vesicles on the face run together into one continuous bleb, which, instead of a thick yellow pus, contains a thin brownish ichor. The face looks pale and doughy. On the trunk and extremities, the vesicles, although not actually *confluent*, are without areola, pale and flaccid. When the pustules break, extensive black or brown scabs are formed, attended with intolerable *fœtor*. At this period, the febrile symptoms undergo a remarkable exacerbation, constitu-

ting what is called *Secondary Fever*. But the mischief does not rest here. The violent action which has taken place in the skin, not having come to its natural crisis, is kept up. Ulceration of the cutis vera goes on beneath the scabs, and, if the patient survives, occasions pits and scars. In other cases, boils, abscesses, tedious ulcerations of the legs, and inflammations of the eyes harass the patient, wear out his strength, and perhaps ultimately destroy him.

Hitherto I have chiefly directed my attention to the effects of the variolous poison upon the skin ; but it is further to be remark. ed, that in some cases of distinct small-pox, and in almost all cases of the confluent variety, the mucous membrane of the mouth, larynx, and trachea is occupied by a peculiar eruption, which fol. lows a regular course, and has a most material influence on the progress of the disorder. Though present in a greater or less de. gree in all severe cases, it is by no means in exact correspondence with the quantity of eruption on the skin. The extent of vesicles upon the tongue, indeed, constitutes the only true index of the de. gree to which the trachea is affected. The symptoms to which it gives rise, are hoarseness, difficulty of swallowing, an increased secretion of saliva, cough, copious and viscid expectoration, and dyspnœa. In many cases of severe confluent small-pox, these symptoms are of the utmost importance, and absorb the whole at. tention of the patient.

3. Such are the phenomena of *simple confluence*. The student may imagine in how great a degree its dangers are aggravated, when to them are superadded the symptoms of malignancy and putrescency. Of these, one has been already mentioned, viz. early fierce delirium. The remaining are, hæmorrhage from the stom. ach, bowels, or uterus, petechial vesicles, gangrene of the extremi. ties, purulent ophthalmia, diffuse cellular inflammation, and erysi. pelas. These cases sometimes prove fatal as early as the fifth, and seldom survive beyond the tenth day of the disease (the eighth of eruption.)

4. It must be obvious, that in nature there can be no exact line of separation between the distinct and confluent kinds of small-pox. They run into each other by insensible degrees. Now to those ca. ses which are intermediate between the perfectly distinct and con. fluent, we give the name of coherent, or semiconfluent. This term applies, first, to cases where the eruption is uniform, but where the papulæ are not sufficiently numerous to coalesce before the fifth

or sixth day; and, secondly, to those where the eruption is in patches, confluent in one part, and distinct in another.

The appearances on dissection in those who die of small-pox, are confined, as far as my observation extends, to the mucous membrane of the trachea and the pleura. I have never been able to trace any morbid appearances in the head, even where cerebral affection was most decisively marked during life; and the abdominal viscera appear to be singularly exempt, under all circumstances, from the influence of the variolous virus. No vestiges of pustules have been ever traced at the Small-pox Hospital in the cavity of the abdomen.

When small-pox proves fatal about the tenth day, it is common to find evidences of active inflammation in the larynx and trachea. A copious, dark-coloured, and viscid secretion (quite peculiar to this complaint) lines their inner membrane, which is highly vascular. At a later period of the disease, one cavity of the thorax is occasionally found loaded with purulent effusion, the pleura having become implicated in the course of the disease. The substance of the lungs is then consolidated by the pressure of the effused fluid. Variolous pleurisy (as it may be called) is rare, and by no means well marked in any of its stages.

The prognosis in small-pox is regulated almost entirely by the form which the disease assumes; but of course the strength of the patient's constitution is, to a certain extent, to be taken into account. Distinct small-pox is a disease of little or no danger; while the confluent variety is attended, even under circumstances comparatively favourable, with imminent hazard to life. When malignancy and confluence are associated, the case is utterly hopeless. The mortality in small-pox simply confluent is about three in five. Coherent cases prove fatal in the proportion of about one in four. Upon the whole, it is computed, that of every six persons who receive small-pox in the natural way, one dies. The most unfavourable symptoms are those which indicate affection of the brain, larynx, and bronchia, violence of fever, and strong determination of blood to the skin. The most favourable are, quiet of mind, a tongue free from vesicles, swelling of the face, but above all a small, soft, and yielding pulse. From the tenth to the thirteenth day is the period of the greatest danger; but to feeble constitutions, and especially to scrofulous children, the sequelæ of the disease are scarcely less formidable than the violence of its crisis.

Before proceeding to the method of treatment in small-pox, I may notice a few circumstances connected with the disease, which are either objects of pathological curiosity, or of interest, as suggesting the means of lessening its violence.

The seat and structure of the pock has been a frequent subject of inquiry, and by some is supposed to be still involved in obscurity. The *rete mucosum* appears to be the true seat of the small-pox pustule, but the inflammation sometimes dips down into the cutis vera. The pock, when minutely examined, exhibits in its early stages a cellular structure, the walls of which are perfectly transparent, and appear to secrete the fluid which distends them. At the bottom of each pock a small slough of the cutis may be observed from the fifth to the eighth day, of a circular form, and about the thickness of writing paper. By several eminent pathologists this slough is considered the certain test of small-pox, and to be owing, not so much to the intensity, as to the peculiar *kind* of the inflammation.

The disposition to receive small-pox is so general throughout the human race, that few persons are met with who resist it during their whole lives, when fully exposed to its influence. All ages are alike susceptible of it. It is communicable by the mother to the fœtus in utero, but under such circumstances it has almost invariably proved fatal to the child. There is even reason to believe that a mother who has already passed through the disease may communicate it to the fœtus. The deleterious effects of the small-pox virus upon the gravid uterus are very remarkable. It seldom fails to occasion abortion, especially in the early months of pregnancy. In general, one attack of small-pox secures the system from the disease for ever after. Yet some exceptions to this law have been met with. Unequivocal cases of what are called *secondary* small-pox are recorded in the writings of authors, as having occurred in all ages and countries; and the second attack, though generally mild and modified, has proved in some instances severer than the primary. Even fatal cases of secondary small-pox have been recorded by authors of undoubted veracity.

I have already remarked, that the comparative mildness or violence of the disease depends principally upon some peculiar susceptibility of the system to the variolous poison; but some other circumstances concur. Delicacy in the structure of the skin is probably concerned in the phenomenon; for in this way only can we account for the greater disposition to confluence upon the face than on other parts. The rete mucosum is there loaded with vessels, which have manifestly a greater disposition than common to receive red blood. Further, whatever encourages the blood to the surface of the body has a tendency to produce confluence. Hence it is that a long succession of close and moist weather, exposure to great heat (as in the trade of the sugar baker,) the free use of ardent spirits, diaphoretic medicines, the warm bath, and stimuli applied to the skin, aggravate the disease in a high degree ; while cold, and frost, and light clothing, and the antiphlogistic regimen, tend greatly to lessen its severity.

The general principles of treatment in small-pox were for a long time misunderstood, and measures were consequently adopted which greatly increased the mortality of the disease. In the distinct small-pox very little is requisite ; and the danger in confluent cases is urgent under any system of management ; yet the advantages of a well regulated treatment are as obvious in small-pox as in any other disease.

During the eruptive stage the object is to moderate inflammatory excitement generally, and to lessen the quantity of eruption. For this purpose the patient is to be freely exposed to a cool atmosphere, and the strictest antiphlogistic regimen is to be pursued. Great diversities of opinion have prevailed regarding the propriety of blood-letting in this and the other stages of small-pox. There is no reason to believe that it lessens the *number* of pustules ; and it has been supposed to impair that strength of the body which is indispensable throughout the latter stages of the disease, when extreme weakness so often exists with extensive ulceration and gangrene. In forming a judgment however on this point, it is necessary to bear in mind, that these symptoms, though they sometimes arise from real debility of the powers of life, yet are often attributable to excessive inflammation of the skin, which might have been prevented by a judicious employment of the lancet. It is to be remembered also, that in small-pox, fully as much as in any other form of fever, there is a tendency to congestions and inflammations in the head and thorax. These must be treated upon the same principles as have been already urged with regard to fever generally.

Attention should be paid therefore to the concomitant symptoms, and the character of the pulse ; and where there is evidence of local determination, it must be obviated, according to its urgency, by *local or general bleeding* at any period of the disease, without refer-ence to the affection of the skin. Occasional purging and the usu-al antiphlogistic treatment are advisable during the whole period of febrile excitement. When the vesicles do not rise, or are filled only with a bloody serum, when the pulse is weak and the skin purple, marking a failure of the vis vitæ, the tone of the system is to be supported by wine, brandy, bark, camphor, and aromatics, with the occasional exhibition of gentle laxatives. When the pus-tules are nearly maturated, and throughout the latter stages of the disease generally, great benefit is experienced from *opiates*, in re-lieving the irritation of the skin and procuring sleep. There is a remarkable resemblance in the symptoms of the latter stages of small-pox to those of extensive burns and scalds, where the good effects of opium are well ascertained. While the scabs are sepa-rating, a cordial plan of treatment is often necessary, but it is re-quisite also in many cases, to look to, and counteract by laxatives and a proper diet, the tendency to local inflammation, which may continue even to the very latest period of the disease.

Considerable difficulty has always been experienced in the man-agement of the many severe sequelæ of confluent and coherent small-pox; but to meet these cases no express rules can be laid down. When the constitution is much enfeebled, and scrofula brought into action, tonics are of some service; and I have deri-ved considerable benefit from the decoction of sarsaparilla. A gen-erous diet, with an allowance of wine or porter, should be permit-ted; but change of air is the measure of most decided efficacy. The disposition to boils cannot, I believe, be counteracted by any medi-cinal treatment.

INOCULATION.

When the matter of small-pox is inserted under the skin, a pimple appears on the third day, followed by swelling in the axilla. The pimple then becomes surrounded by a jagged areola, in which small vesications are observable. On the seventh or at farthest the eighth day from the insertion of the virus, rigors occur, and in for-

13

ty-eight hours afterwards the eruption appears.* In a large majority of cases, the eruption proves to be of the *mild* and *distinct*
sort; and in very many instances the number of pustules over the
whole body does not exceed one hundred. The further progress
of the disorder differs in no respect from that of the distinct *casual*
small-pox as already described.

Nothing has ever been suggested calculated to throw the smallest light on the curious fact, that the mode of reception into the
system should thus influence the *quantity* of eruption. To so great
a degree does this take place, that the mortality by inoculated
small-pox, without any restriction as to age or strength of constitution, does not exceed one in five hundred. We select for the
period of inoculation that season of the year, and that time of life,
when inflammatory tendencies are least to be expected. It is sufficiently ascertained that beyond a few doses of a cooling aperient,
no preparatory course of *medicine* is requisite. A spare vegetable diet, cool air, and subacid drinks, will contribute to render the
disease mild and safe. Improper management may of course increase the quantity of eruption, and with it the danger of the patient. Some attention, therefore, ought always to be paid to the
treatment of inoculated small-pox; but the principles already laid
down are equally applicable in the present case, and will be sufficient without further detail for the guidance of the student.

---

* To this it is owing, that the inoculated small-pox takes percedence of
the natural disease.

CHAP. III.

Early Opinions regarding Varicella. Controversy respecting its Identity with Small pox. Varicella Lymphatica. Varicella Variolodes. Diagnosis of these disorders. Of Cow pox. Its Introduction by Jenner. Progress of the Vesicle. Surgery of Vaccination. Small-pox and Cow-pox occurring together, or after each other. Characters of modified Small-pox. Causes of Small-pox after Vaccination.

FROM the earliest periods at which small-pox was noticed, we read of a mild eruptive disease, liable to be confounded with it, but not preventing it; and consequently demanding attention with reference to diagnosis. This has gone by the several names of chrystalli, variolæ lymphaticæ, spuriæ, volaticæ, and pusillæ. By Riverius it was called varicella. Morton adopted from the vulgar, and introduced into medical language the term *chicken-pox*. The descriptions of this disease, which have been given by different authors, and their pathological views concerning it and its relation to small-pox, differ materially from each other.* It is clear, that acknowledging the necessity of diagnosis, they have yet failed in establishing it satisfactorily; for after the lapse of nine hundred years, the subject is declared to be so obscure as to demand fresh investigation.

For the last fifty years, authors have been in the habit of drawing their notions concerning varicella from the paper published by Dr. Heberden, in the first volume of the Transactions of the College of Physicians of London. The points of doctrine which he principally set forth were, that the chicken-pox arose from a specific contagion, affected the same individual but once during life, afforded no pro-

---

* See Cross on " The Variolous Epidemic of Norwich" in 1819. Part 2, Chap. 2. Sketch of the History of Varicella.

tection from small-pox, and was capable of being communicated by inoculation. It does not appear, indeed, that he ever witnessed inoculation in this disease; but in his description it is implied that it has been so propagated, although by mistake, and that an eruption followed which has passed with inexperienced and hasty observers, for the small-pox, from which however it does not secure the constitution. Dr. Willan, in 1806, bore testimony to the general accuracy of Dr. Heberden's description. He detailed the appearance of the eruption with more precision, but coincided in opinion that it is a contagious disease, affording no protection from small-pox, and communicable by inoculation.

More recent observations have tended to show that some mistake has crept into the views of these authors concerning the pathology of varicella. It has been rendered highly probable that the genuine varicella is not communicable by inoculation; but it has at the same time been shown, that many cases of *supposed* varicella do produce a disease by inoculation, which is not chicken-pox, but small-pox. Reasoning from these data, some modern authors have retained the notion of the specific disease varicella, but have given it new characters; while others have revived a doctrine which prevailed very generally in former times, and was distinctly avowed by Sauvages; *viz.* that chicken-pox and small-pox originate in one and the same contagion, and that *varicella* is indeed what its name imports, a mild, imperfect, or *modified* form of variola. In support of the latter opinion, many ingenious arguments have been brought forward in a work, which has certainly thrown much light upon the history of the eruptive diseases, connected in their origin or symptoms with variola.[†] The true solution of the difficulties which have encumbered this branch of pathology, appears to be this. There are two diseases distinct from each other in their origin and character, both of which have been designated by the title of *varicella*. The one is the varicella lymphatica, the true or genuine varicella, as described by Mr. Bryce. The other is the varicella variolodes partaking more decidedly of the nature of small-pox, and from which true small pox may be obtained by inoculation. These distinctions I shall keep before me in the remarks now to be offered.

* BRYCE. Ed. Med. and Surg. Journal, vol. xiv, p. 467.
† THOMSON's "Account of the Varioloid Epidemic of Scotland," London, 1820.

clear lymph is evacuated, and they neither exhibit a cellulated structure nor a central depression. The eruption commences on the breast and back, and subsequently extends to the face, scalp, and extremities. On the second and third days of eruption, an irregular circle of inflammation surrounds each vesicle. The disease is attended, especially in children, with an incessant tingling or itching, which leads them to rub off the tops of the vesicles, so that the characteristics of the disorder are often destroyed at an early period. Even if the vesicle remains unbroken, the contained fluid becomes opaque about the fourth day, at which time the disease is in many cases with difficulty distinguished from small-pox by the eye alone. The vesicles are nearly always distinct. One case of confluent varicella, however, has been described by Mr. Ring. On the fifth day the vesicles appear covered with slight crusts which are yellowish, scaly, and irregular, lying flat upon the surface of the body. In a very few instances only, have they been succeeded by pits. Dr. Willan and others have noticed that the vesicles of the chicken-pox do not all appear in one day, but follow each other in successive crops. This, however cannot be urged as a diagnostic mark of the disease, for it occurs also in the modified small-pox.

Such are the distinguishing characters of *varicella lymphatica*. If the eruption, instead of being vesicular, exhibits in its early stages the appearance of indurated basis,—if the vesicles have a central depression,—if, after discharging their contents, on the third day, a firm tubercle be found below,—and if the crusts which succeed are compact, defined, of a clear horny smoothness, and elevated, the disease was the varicella varioloqdes, and arose from the contagion of small-pox. All authors are agreed that the former, or genuine varicella, affords no protection from small-pox. It is generally admitted also that it sometimes spreads epidemically (as in schools ;) and hence some are inclined to attribute it to *specific contagion*. It is not now however contended by the best authors, that this contagion is communicable by inoculation, or that the disease affects an individual once only during life. I am not aware that varicella, in this its vesicular or genuine form, has ever been met with in adult persons. It would appear as if the delicate cuticle of infantile life was indispensable to its development.

The chicken-pox being a very slight disease, it is unnecessary to add any thing respecting its treatment.

COW-POX.

The introduction of cow-pox into general notice, is an event in the history of medicine too interesting to be passed over without some comment. The merit of the discovery rests wholly with Dr. Jenner, who made his first decisive experiment in 1796, and two years afterwards published his account of the *variolæ vaccinæ*.* The practice of vaccination was eagerly adopted by all classes of persons in this country, and has since spread with astonishing rapidity over every quarter of the globe. The consequence has been the almost complete extermination of the small-pox from some countries, and a most important diminution of its malignity in others, where that desirable event has been impeded.

It has been satisfactorily shown, that there is an affection of the hoof of the horse in every respect the same with that of the udder of the cow, from which the term cow-pox has been derived. Both the one and the other are communicable to man by inoculation. The disease thus produced has the curious property of so modifying the human constitution, as in many cases to remove altogether the susceptibility of small-pox contagion, or, failing in this, to secure at least the individual from the *dangers* of that formidable malady.

The cow-pox is a disease deserving of investigation, on account of its great importance to mankind. It has its laws, characters, and anomalies, as well as other diseases of more urgency; nor can a practitioner judge correctly of the progress of vaccination, or pronounce with any confidence as to the security which it gives, unless he has studied the subject in its various details, and inquired into the sources of fallacy, and the modifications of which the disease is susceptible. Our experience in cow-pox is indeed still very

* The date of this publication is June, 1798.

limited. It has been only known for about thirty years, and it would be hazardous to say, that we are even yet acquainted with all its peculiarities. Viewed in this light, it cannot therefore be a matter of surprise, that the opinions now entertained by patholo-gists on the influence of vaccination differ, in some respects, from those of the early writers.

The cow-pox is communicable only by inoculation, and has sel-dom been known to occur twice to the same individual in that reg-ular form, such as it is my object now to describe. After twenty-four hours the punctured point begins to inflame, and by help of a microscope, a small vesicle with a regularly rounded edge may be observed to arise. This on the third day appears to the naked eye as an elevated point. By the fifth day the vesicle is quite distinct, and lymph may be procured from it. The lymph is transparent, and like the matter of small-pox, is inclosed in little cells. On the eighth day, an *areola* or inflamed circle of about an inch and a half radius, begins to form around the vesicle, which is now in its most perfect state. On the tenth day the areola is at its height, and the vesicle is pearl-coloured, perfectly circular, and well elevated. As the inflammation fades, it leaves one or two concentric red circles, which continue visible for two or three days. On the fifteenth day the vaccination may be considered as completed. The lymph in the mean time becomes muddy and dark, and ultimately desiccates into a mahogany-coloured crust, which drops off towards the end of the third week, leaving behind it a small, circular, cellulated, and indented eschar, with a well defined border.

During the formation of the areola, it is often stated that symp-tomatic fever may be observed in children, and this has been held out as a *test* of perfect vaccination ; but the fact is questionable ; and in vaccinating adults, it is certainly not met with. The true test of the constitution being affected is the regular progress of the vesicle. But this may be interrupted in several ways. It may pass through its stages too quickly to saturate the system effectually. The vesicle may be injured by accident, or by being rubbed. An erysipelatous inflammation may come upon the arm, and take place of the true areola, and pus may be formed instead of vaccine lymph. The system may be pre-occupied by some chronic cutaneous dis-ease, by diarrhœa, fever, or some active internal inflammation. Lastly, there exists in some children a constitutional indisposition to the cow-pox, not to be anticipated. Under such circumstances great difficulty is experienced in infecting the arm, and the vesicle, when produced, is slow in its progress, of small size, and sur-rounded by an imperfect areola.

Of the interference of different febrile diseases with the progress of the vaccine vesicle, numerous instances have been recorded. The *suspension* of its progress might have been anticipated from the known facts of the reciprocal action of contagious fevers upon each other ; but not only is vaccination retarded by these disorders (mea-sles, scarlatina, chicken-pox, typhus, pneumonia, and the influen-za,) but it is occasionally rendered by them altogether inefficient.

These considerations point out the propriety of paying minute attention to the progress of vaccination, of preparing the body. in some instances, for its reception, and of keeping the system, during its progress, free from inflammatory action, in the manner formerly practised in inoculation for the small-pox. It requires no argu-ment to prove, that a process which is to *free* the constitution from a poison so active and subtle as that of small-pox, should be con-ducted with at least as much attention as was paid to its introduc-tion *into* the system.

The following appear to be the most important circumstances which merit attention in conducting the process of vaccination. The child should be in perfect health, and not less than two, nor more than six months old. The lymph should be taken from a ve-sicle of the seventh or eighth day. It is desirable in all cases to insert six or eight punctures in the arm, as the system is probably thereby more completely *saturated*, without any risk of severer in-flammation ensuing. An ample supply of lymph is thus ensured ; 'and it is a good practice not to inoculate above two or three children from the same vesicle, lest the *frequent* application of the lancet should cause the exudation of common serum, unimpregnated with the specific matter of the disease.' The skin should be perfectly tense, and the lancet sharp. When the areola is beginning to sub-side, it is advisable to exhibit a few doses of rhubarb and magnesia. Great care should be taken that the vesicle be not rubbed nor in-jured in any period of its course.

I proceed to detail the phenomena presented by the occurrence of small-pox, natural or inoculated, with cow-pox. They appear to point out some analogy existing between these diseases, which, coupled with other circumstances, may well justify Dr. Jenner in having given to the latter the title of *variolæ vaccinæ*.

Dr. Willan found, that by inoculating with variolous matter at different periods, not exceeding a *week*, from the insertion of the vaccine lymph, small-pox followed. The eruption thus produced may appear as late as the fifteenth day of the vaccination, but the disease is milder and shorter in its course than usual, and it is *modified* in its appearances. In the case of *natural* small pox, the sixth is the latest day at which it can appear after vaccination, so as to go through a severe and regular course. If it occur at a later period than this, it is generally modified ; and this modified or imperfect variolous eruption was, in the early history of vaccination, often mistaken for an eruption from the vaccine virus. Many errors, indeed, have arisen from an ignorance of the phenomena that attend the combination of these two diseases. Their influence is reciprocal. If the eruption of the small-pox takes place before the areola begins to form around the vaccine pock, the latter loses its regular character, while the eruption of small-pox follows its usual course. If vaccination be practised immediately preceding or subsequent to the eruption of small-pox, the vaccine vesicle does not come forward. By inoculation with vaccine and variolous matter at the same time, both diseases run their usual course.

Such are the principal phenomena which are presented by small-pox and cow-pox occurring together in the same individual. A superior interest has lately attached to the occurrence of these diseases after each other, at distant periods, particularly to that of *small-pox after vaccination*.

The cow-pox had not long been introduced, before it was ascertained that the preventive power of the vaccine virus was not perfect ; and every years experience serves more and more to show, that a certain proportion of those who have undergone vaccination will take small-pox at a subsequent period of their lives. The circumstances under which this occurs, the causes to which it may be ascribed, the proportion of vaccinated subjects thus affected, and the characters of the disease so produced, have lately excited much attention, and they will require to be rapidly sketched in this place.

14

The characters which small-pox presents when it occurs subsequent to vaccination, have been detailed with great minuteness by various authors, chiefly with the intention of establishing the diagnosis between it and varicella; but the view which we have taken of that disease will preclude the necessity of equal precision here. Small-pox has sometimes occurred after vaccination in its most perfect and genuine form, but in by far the larger proportion of instances, it is *modified* either in the aspect or progress of the pustules. So *completely* altered indeed is the appearance of the eruption, on some occasions, by the influence of previous vaccination, and so extremely mild is the character both of the fever and of the eruption, that the true nature of the disease could never have been suspected by one who had not observed it in a variety of instances, and marked the insensible gradations by which its characters run into each other. The *initiatory* fever is generally severe, but in almost all cases recedes entirely on the appearance of the eruption. The pustules are often hard or *horny*, but scarcely ever fail to exhibit the diagnostic mark of variolous eruption, depressed centres. They run through their stages with rapidity, maturing for the most part on the fifth day.

That this disease is a modified form of variola there can be no doubt, and in strict conformity with the language of the old authors we may call it the *varicella variolodes*. It follows exposure to variolous contagion; in its severer form it is capable of communicating the *casual* small-pox, and even the mildest varieties of it will, in the unprotected, produce genuine small-pox by inoculation. The danger attending it is very small. Mild as the inoculated small-pox is, small-pox after well conducted vaccination, in the great majority of cases, is even milder. In the few instances where it has ended fatally, the result is attributable to some accidental circumstance, such as its occurrence with diseased lungs, inflamed bowels, or scrofula rather than to the common and acknowledged effects of small-pox. It may occur at any period subsequent to vaccination. It has been taken by persons who had previously exposed themselves with impunity to the full influence of the variolous contagion. It may be communicated by inoculation, but it is received for the most part in the natural way.

The disease has been by some ascribed to incomplete vaccination, and the notion is probably in a great degree correct; for
though it has been observed in a few cases where the progress of
the vaccine vesicle was to all appearance regular, yet it has rarely occurred to me to witness it in a severe form, where the cicatrix
was perfect, that is, of moderate size, well defined, *perfectly circular* and *indented*. Deterioration of the vaccine virus from successive inoculations has been brought forward by other pathologists
as calculated to explain the occurrence of small-pox after vaccination. This opinion, however, is unsupported by any arguments;
and is quite irreconcileable with the phænomena of variolous inoculation. As little foundation is there for the hypothesis of a *spurious*
cow-pox, once formed to explain some of the anomalies which this
disease presents. (Taking all the evidence that has been afforded us
repecting small-pox after vaccination, it appears that we must seek
for its cause partly in the imperfect saturation of the system with
the vaccine influence, and partly in that law of the animal œconomy which regulates the susceptibility of variolous contagion.) Natural small-pox in its severest form does not always afford protection from a subsequent attack of the disease. To that *peculiarity
of constitution* which favours secondary small-pox, we must be content to refer those cases in which small-pox occurs subsequent to
perfect vaccination.

The proportion of the vaccinated who are subsequently affected
by small-pox in a *well-marked* form (for we may safely leave out of
consideration the cases of mild varicella,) is a point of the utmost
consequence to determine, but no satisfactory conclusions can be
drawn from the calculations which have hitherto been made. Upon
this indeed must ultimately depend the fate of vaccination; but no
reasonable doubt can be entertained from the facts now before the
world, that the proportion is such as not to affect, in any sensible
degree, the credit of vaccination; which must continue therefore
to uphold the fame of Jenner, and the triumph of medical art.*

* See Appendix; Note I.

First Appearance and early History of the Measles. Symptoms and Se-
quelæ of the Disease. Pneumonia. Phthisis. Cancrum oris. Putrid or
malignant kind of Measles. Peculiarities in the Contagion of Measles.
Treatment of the Disease.

THE measles was introduced into Europe about the same time as
the small-pox, and followed in its track. For a long time it was
supposed to be only a variety or modification of that disease, and
as such it is described by Hali Abbas and Rhazes. Diemerbroeck
in 1687, and Morton in 1696, maintained the *identity* of small-pox
and measles, nor was it until lately that the diagnosis was fully established. Sydenham described accurately the measles which prevailed in London in 1670, and to his history of the disease very
little has been added by more modern authors. For the few additions which have since been made, we are chiefly indebted to Dr.
Watson in 1763, and to Dr. Willan in 1800. Several *species* of
measles have been described by nosologists, but they are all referable to one,— the *rubeola vulgaris* of Dr. Cullen ; the other forms
which measles assumes being only modifications of this, arising either from a peculiar condition of the atmosphere, or the constitution of the individual affected.

The measles commences with the usual symptoms of *pyrexia* ;
nor is it at first to be distinguished from an attack of common continued fever. The diagnosis is to be effected by a knowledge of
the prevailing epidemic, and attention to those catarrhal symptoms,
which are the constant concomitants of the eruptive fever of measles. The mucous membranes of the head and chest are alike affected ; the tunica conjunctiva, the Schneiderian membrane, and
the mucous membrane of the larynx and bronchia. The eyelids are
swelled, and the eyes suffused, watery, and morbidly sensible to

light ; there is a copious thin secretion from the nose, with sneezing ; and lastly, a dry cough, with hoarseness and some degree of
dyspnœa. Besides these catarrhal symptoms, the eruptive stage
of measles is-marked by considerable heaviness of the head, and
drowsiness, amounting in some cases almost to coma. The heat of
the skin is great, the pulse frequent and hard, and the general
marks of pyrexia severer than what occur in cases of common catarrh. The eruption usually shows itself on the fourth day from
the occurrence of rigors, but it is sometimes delayed a day or two.
Cases indeed have occurred where the previous catarrhal symptoms continued for eight days, or even a fortnight.

The eruption of measles first appears on the forehead, and gradually spreads over the whole body. It shows itself in the form of
distinct, red, circular spots, which afterwards coalesce into patches of an irregular figure. The colour of the eruption is of a dingy
red, very different from the *vivid* redness of scarlet fever. It is sensibly elevated upon the face, and often also upon the breast and
back, but scarcely ever upon the extremities. Upon the first appearance of the eruption, the catarrhal symptoms and the accompanying fever sometimes subside completely, but this is by no
means a frequent occurrence. Indeed they are often aggravated,
so that upon the second or third day of the eruption it is not uncommon to meet with severe cough and dyspnœa, the measly catarrh merging, in fact, in acute pneumonia. The stomach too, in
severe cases, is often very irritable during the first days of measles, with vomiting of bile, and excessive restlessness. On the second day the eruption on the face is most vivid, and as it declines
on the face, is at its height on the extremities. In about five days
it completely disappears from the whole body. A slight discoloration of the skin commonly remains for a short time, which in some
cases goes on to desquamation.

The decline of the eruption is not always followed by the subsidence of the other symptoms. A considerable degree of cough, or
difficulty of breathing, frequently remains, marking the continuance of that inflammatory disposition which characterizes the former stages of the disease. The pulse continues frequent, and full ;
and in scrofulous habits of body this state of disease occasionally
ends in hæmoptysis, hectic fever, and genuine consumption. All the
sequelæ of measles have an inflammatory character. Upon the decline of the eruption diarrhœa often comes on, and Sydenham was,

I believe, the first to take notice that this frequently yielded to blood-letting. (Among the other consequences of measles may be enumerated ophthalmia, swellings of the lymphatic glands of the neck, chronic eruptions of a porriginous character discharges behind the ears, or affection of the bowels ending in *marasmus*. Inflammatory symptoms of an urgent kind often supervene when the practitioner is least prepared for them, and therefore a caution should be given to watch the patient attentively during the whole period of convalescence.)

Among the irregular forms of measles may be first noticed that species of the disease, called by Dr. Willan (*rubeola sine catarrho*.) It is a very rare variety, and only interesting in a pathological point of view. (The diagnosis is here, as might be expected, very difficult, and seldom satisfactory until it has produced in another child the common measles, which it is capable of doing.) The most remarkable anomaly which the history of measles presents, is its occasional occurrence in a very highly aggravated or (*malignant* form;) and this, not merely in individual cases, but even as an epidemic. Such a form of measles prevailed at Plymouth in 1745, in London in 1763, and at Edinburgh, from September to December 1816.* The symptoms of the eruptive stage, in these epidemics, were unusually severe. Extreme debility quickly supervened, with restlessness, or sometimes coma, a disposition to vomiting, a dry, hard, or black tongue, and a deep red colour of the fauces,—typhoid symptoms, that is to say, with great irritability of the stomach. In these cases too, the eruption did not exhibit its usual appearances. It frequently receded in the course of the first twenty-four hours; and when it first appeared was less elevated than usual, and of a dark and livid colour. A large proportion of these cases proved fatal; and on dissection, mucus was found collected in considerable quantity in the bronchia, with other marks of inflammation or congestion within the thorax. In the epidemic of Edinburgh, in 1816, the recession of the eruption was the worst symptom; few recovering in whom this occurred. It was neither attributable to cold, nor to the too free use of cathartics. It is commonly said, under these circumstances, that the energy of the system does not prove sufficient to *throw out* the eruption. The more correct ex-

---

* Consult the Works of Huxham, and the Observations of Dr. Watson in the 4th vol. Med. Obs. and Enq.—See also the Ed. Med. and Surg. Journal, January 1817.

pression seems to be (and the phenomena of small-pox and scarlet-fever give countenance to this view of the case) that when the
mucous membranes are violently attacked in the first instance, that
metastasis to the skin does not take place, which under common
circumstances relieves them.)

The measles arises from a specific contagion, the latent period
of which is about eight days, varying however to ten, or even
fourteen. It has been disputed whether measles can be taken a
second time. By some of the older authors its occasional recurrence was admitted, but of late years the fact has been most satisfactorily established. Dr. Baillie has described eight instances of
the kind, and it is a singular circumstance that they occurred in
individuals of the same family.* Dr. Willan has thrown out the
suggestion, that where there are no catarrhal symptoms, the susceptibility of the disease· is not removed. The measles prevails
generally during the spring months, and often along with small-
pox. The circumstances which determine the severity of the disease in particular individuals are not very well ascertained, but it
is certain that in scrofulous habits, and in those of a plethoric disposition, it is principally to be dreaded.

The danger in measles principally arises from pneumonic inflammation, but in very feeble frames, and in the lowest ranks of society, where cold and poverty combine with disease in reducing the
powers of life, the dreadful spectacle of gangrenous erosion of the
cheek is sometimes witnessed. This affection, commonly called
cancrum oris, begins in the inside of the cheek by a hard swelling.
The gums ulcerate and the teeth loosen and fall out ; a black spot·
next appears on the cheek, or at the corner of the lip, which rapidly spreads, and the child dies miserably. Such a complaint sometimes accompanies the latter stages of small-pox, and infantile fever, and sometimes it occurs idiopathically, but its pathology is always the same. Medicine furnishes but very imperfect means of
combating it. Tonics and local stimulants are indicated, but their
influence is very trifling.

Dr. Home, of Edinburgh, informs us, that he succeeded in inoculating the measles, by applying over an incision in the skin cot-
ton dipped in the blood of a patient labouring under the disease.'

---

* Transactions of a Society for the Improvement of Med. and Chir.
Knowledge, vol. iii, pages 258 and 263.

He states that the eruptive fever followed in six days, that the symptoms were mild, and the lungs not affected as in the casual disease. It does not appear however that these observations have been verified by any later experiments. (It is satisfactorily ascertained that the measles delays the progress of vaccination, and of the pustule of the inoculated small-pox.) Two cases however are recorded, by Dr. Russell, of the small-pox and measles running their regular course in the same individual, at the same time.*

The treatment of measles, in its common form, must be regulated chiefly by the symptoms which mark the tendency to thoracic inflammation. It is well ascertained that these are often aggravated by a free exposure of the body to cold, either during or previous to the eruption ; and some have remarked, that this aggravation of the catarrhal symptoms is occasionally attended by a *recession* of the eruption. Moderate warmth therefore is on all accounts advisable in measles. It has been imagined that active purging during the early stage has contributed to repel the eruption, and thus to increase the danger of the patient. This observation I have never been able to verify. On the contrary, saline purgatives seem well adapted to diminish the inflammatory excitement which prevails throughout the whole course of the disease. In mild cases nothing further is required than promoting a gentle perspiration, and exhibiting an occasional laxative.

Where pneumonic symptoms prevail, a more vigorous practice is necessary ; but a distinction is here to be made, which Dr. Willan has placed in a very clear point of view. The oppression of the respiration, and the cough which accompany the first appearance of this and of other eruptions, do not appear to depend on true inflammation, for they often go off suddenly, and they may, at any rate, generally be left to their natural termination. But it is upon the third day of the eruption, when the dyspnœa and cough become aggravated while the eruption is declining, when the cough in particular is hard, and accompanied by pain in the chest, that an active system of treatment is required. Bleeding from the arm is then indispensable, and must be repeated in proportion to the urgency of the symptoms. Even children of a tender age require in measles this evacuation, for which leeches and cupping afford but

* · See also " Case of the simultaneous occurrence of Small-pox and Measles," in the Med. Chir. Transactions, vol. xiii, page 163.

an imperfect succedaneum. (Children do not bear general blood-letting well, but they bear it better in measles than in almost any other disease.) The immediate danger from pneumonia, and the more distant but not less alarming risk of phthisis, make it advisa-ble to check the pneumonic symptoms in the speediest and most effectual way.

Saline and demulcent medicines are useful. Opiates may be given with much advantage after bleeding and aperients, if the cough continues troublesome. The warm bath every night is de-cidedly useful. A blister should be applied to the chest, but not until the strength of the pulse has been considerably reduced by local or general blood-letting. In the inflammatory sequelæ of measles, blistered parts have frequently a strong disposition to sloughing and gangrene. Upon the decline of the disease, if the pulse remains frequent, it will be proper to confine the patient to a very mild diet, and to direct a saline draught, with a few drops of tincture of digitalis, to be taken every six hours. The convales-cence of measles does not bear the exhibition of bitter and tonic medicines, like that of many other febrile diseases.

When the measles assumes that malignant or typhoid form which we formerly described, recourse must be had to the warm bath, blis-ters, wine, and *cordials* (aromatics, serpentaria, ammonia, ether.) The observations of Dr. Watson on the treatment of this form of measles are judicious, and applicable to disease in a very extend-ed view. If bleeding under these circumstances be resorted to, as this author remarks, the patient loses more by the debility which is brought on, than is gained by the relief afforded to the circula-tion within the thorax. It may be remarked indeed generally, that, in all typhoid fevers it is a point of great difficulty to determine, how far local congestions and inflammations are to be relieved, at the risk of reducing too much the tone and powers of the system. The malignant form of measles sometimes shows itself *sporadical-ly*, that is to say, in individual cases, while the general character of the epidemic is inflammatory. The circumstance may gener-ally be traced to the weakened condition of the child, the result probably of fever, hooping cough, scrofula, or some other preced-ing disease. Such cases seldom end happily, notwithstanding the most judicious practice.

15

First Notices of the Disease. Nosological Distinctions. Description of the different Varieties of Scarlatina. Prognosis. Pathology. Principles of Treatment. Nature and Treatment of the Dropsy succeeding Scarlatina.

THE scarlet fever is probably a disease of very modern origin. No mention of it is made by the ancient or Arabian authors, and the first time it is distinctly noticed is but little more than two hun-dred years ago. It has been suspected that the contagion came originally from Africa. Be this as it may, it first showed itself in a severe form in Spain in 1610, from whence it spread to Naples, where it raged epidemically in 1618. In 1689 the same disease made its appearance in London, and was described by Dr. Mor-ton, though not with the accuracy of the first Spanish and Italian authors. In 1735 it broke out in North America, and spread grad-ually but slowly over that continent. One of the most curious cir-cumstances in the history of the disease, is the slowness of its dif-fusion.

When the scarlet fever first appeared in Europe, it was in a very malignant form; but between the years 1660 and 1670, a febrile complaint attended with scarlet eruption was observed by Syden-ham in a degree so singularly mild, that nosologists have doubted its being really the same disease with that which had previously occurred. Dr. Cullen believed it was specifically different. Dr. Withering states, that in his early practice he considered scarlet fever, and putrid sore throat distinct diseases, requiring distinct me-thods of treatment. More enlarged experience however compelled him to renounce that opinion; and he says, that after paying the most assiduous attention to the subject, by observing the complaint in every difference of season, exposure, age, and temperament, he

was satisfied, that they constitute but one species of disease ; ___.
that they own there existence to the same specific contagion ;—that
the variations in their appearance depend upon contingent circum.
stances, and their greatest differences not greater than those of the
distinct and confluent small-pox.

The scarlet fever attacks the skin, the tonsils, and the mucous
membrane in their neighbourhood. In mild cases there is *efflores-*
cence, with little or no affection of the fauces. This constitutes
the scarlatina simplex. In very severe cases there is extensive
ulceration of the fauces, attended with typhoid fever, but with little
or no efflorescence. This is the extreme grade of the disorder,
and is called cynanche, or scarlatina maligna. In the common
·or intermediate cases both structures are implicated, and the disease is then denominated scarlatina anginosa.

1. The scarlatina simplex commences with slight febrile symptoms. The eruption appears on the second day, first about the
neck and face, in the form of innumerable red points, which in
twenty-four hours or less cover the whole body. On the limbs, but
especially about the fingers, there is a diffuse and continuous efflorescence, but on the trunk of the body the rash is distributed in irregular patches. The colour of the eruption is a bright scarlet, being always most distinct about the loins, and bendings of the joints.
On the breast and extremities, in consequence of the great determination of blood to the miliary glands and papillæ of the skin, the
surface is often rough, and there is an appearance of papillæ or
even minute vesicles, as in miliary fever. This is very liable to
happen when the patient is confined in a small room and loaded
with blankets. The efflorescence spreads over the surface of the
mouth and fauces ; and the papillæ of the tongue, which are always elongated, extend their scarlet points through a white fur,
thus affording one of the simplest diagnostics of the disease. (The
face is often sensibly swelled about the third day.) The febrile
symptoms are in some cases very slight. At other times there is
considerable heat of skin, restlessness, and frequency of pulse. The
eruption continues about three or four days, after which a desquamation of the cuticle takes place.

2. In the more common form of the disease, the *scarlatina angi-*
nosa, the precursory symptoms are more violent, and together with
the cutaneous efflorescence, an inflammation of the fauces appears,
going through its progress of increase and decline along with it.

Among the first symptoms of this disease is an uneasiness in the throat. The voice is thick, and deglutition difficult. The tonsils and fauces appear red and swelled, as in cynanche tonsillaris. For the most part this goes on to the formation of superficial ulcerations or specks. When these are numerous, they cause an unpleasant fœtor, and the throat is much clogged up with a viscid phlegm.

In this more aggravated form of the disease (the efflorescence seldom appears before the third day.) It chiefly comes out in scattered patches, always very distinct about the elbows. Frequently too it vanishes, and reappears partially, and at uncertain times. About the fourth or fifth day from its first appearance it is generally gone, and extensive exfoliation of the cuticle begins soon afterwards to take place, and continues for ten days or a fortnight. About the seventh day, it is not uncommon to find the patients complaining of considerable pain in their hands.

The febrile symptoms in this form of scarlet fever are usually very severe, and of a highly inflammatory character. The heat of of skin is more intense in this than in any other fever of our climate. The pulse generally averages 120. There is always much restlessness, languor, and oppression of the breathing. The countenance is expressive of very peculiar anxiety. The eyes are suffused. Head-ache is often a very urgent symptom. The decline of the disorder is usually attended with marks of great debility; and not unfrequently permanent deafness is left by it.

3. The third or *malignant* form is that which the scarlet fever assumed in London 1745, and which is so accurately described by Dr. Fothergill. It is ushered in by rigors, attended with giddiness, acute head ache, restlessness, faintness, a sense of heat and soreness of the throat, vomiting or purging. An efflorescence appears at irregular periods from the second to the fourth day, but is seldom permanent. A remarkable tumefaction of the fingers sometimes takes place, which, with the erysipelatous tinge they soon acquire, is often of itself sufficient to characterize the disease. In the throat appear dark sloughs surrounded by a livid base, and occasioning intolerable fœtor. The parotid glands swell, and become painful to the touch. The mouth is encrusted with a black or brown fur, and a viscid phlegm clogs up the fauces, so as even to threaten suffocation. The inside of the nostrils appears of a deep red or livid colour, from which a corrosive sanies flows, excoriating the angles of the mouth and cheeks. These symptoms are often accompanied

by severe diarrhœa, with hæmorrhages from the nose, mouth, and bowels. Those who escape these dangers have afterwards to struggle through the extreme weakness left by the disease, and the diarrbœa, or hectic, which often supervene. The accompanying fever is typhoid. The pulse is small, feeble, and irregular ; and often, from the very commencement, there is delirium or coma.

(The only disease with which scarlet fever is liable to be confounded is measles.) From this it is to be distinguished by the character of the eruptive fever, the colour of the efflorescence, and the affection of the fauces. Where measles however occurs complicated with cynanche tonsillaris, as I have occasionally witnessed, the diagnosis may be difficult. The prognosis in scarlet fever, when it assumes either of the latter forms, should always be guarded. It varies of course with the degree of violence of the febrile and local symptoms. The malignant scarlet fever is a disease of the utmost danger. Some die as early as the third or fourth day. Some linger on till the second or even the third week ; but generally it may be said that the patient is safe, if he passes the ninth day. (The recession of the eruption is always an unfavourable symptom) but the whole history of scarlet fever proves that it is more a disease of mucous membrane than of the skin, and the danger is therefore to be estimated by the extent to which that structure is implicated. Swelling of the parotid gland sometimes aecompanies the period of convalescence, and proves both painful and tedious.

Scarlet fever arises from a specific contagion, which has a latent period of from four to five days. There is a peculiar susceptibility of it in infancy and youth. Sir Gilbert Blane observes, that he never saw a person turned of forty affected by it. It is not however in this respect upon the footing of small-pox and measles ;— a disease, that is to say, which almost every one passes through ; for many individuals resist it, though exposed to the full influence of the contagion. But though specific contagion is the generally acknowledged, and certainly the most prevalent source of scarlatina, there is yet abundant evidence that fever, attended with scarlet eruption, and possessing all the other characters of this disease, does occasionally arise from exposure to cold.

A great controversy has taken place upon the question of secondary attacks of scarlet fever. Dr. Withering and Dr. Willan never witnessed a recurrence of the disease. It has been satisfac-

torily shown however that this does occur, and second attacks have
often proved severe. Scarlet fever is commonly said to prevail
chiefly in autumn, but it has been observed in all seasons of the
year. The *form* which it assumes in particular cases is partly to
be attributed to the character of the epidemic, partly to external
circumstances, and in part also to the constitution of the individual
affected. It has been made a question, to what causes we are to
ascribe the malignity of a particular epidemic. Season is said to
have some influence, the inflammatory form of scarlet fever appearing in spring and summer, and the typhoid in autumn and winter;
but no stress can be laid on this, for the complaint has been observed at the same time in all its forms, in individuals of the same
family. Upon the whole we must acknowledge, that the circumstances which determine the severity of this, or indeed of any
other febrile disease, have never been satisfactorily explained, and
perhaps they are really inscrutable. It is not accurately known at
what period a convalescent ceases to be capable of communicating
the infection. (The power of infecting appears to continue a very
considerable time) certainly a fortnight from the decline of the
efflorescence, and probably as long as any desquamation of the cuticle takes place.

Nothing need be said regarding the treatment of the scarlatina
simplex; but the principles which are to guide us, when the disease occurs in either of its two severer forms, require considerable
attention. They have given rise to much controversy, and were
certainly not satisfactorily explained till within these few years.
The treatment of scarlet fever is to be regulated in the first place
by the character of the accompanying fever. Where inflammatory symptoms prevail, they are to be moderated ; where the typhoid
disposition is manifest, the system is to be supported. To a certain extent, indeed, it must be allowed, that the character of the
fever is under the control of the practitioner, who, by vigorous
treatment at the onset, may prevent many symptoms of malignancy or putrescency ; but this principle is only of partial application,
for he has no control over the character of the epidemic. The
other extreme, however, is equally to be avoided, which is regulating altogether the early treatment by a consideration of the *possible* symptoms which may arise. In a disease assuming such different forms as scarlet fever, *existing* symptoms must be the guide of
practice.

To allay the high vascular and especially the cutaneous excitement which prevails in the early stage of scarlatina anginosa, affords us a second general principle of treatment. At one time it
was supposed that blood-letting was necessary ; but experience has
proved, that in the cold affusion we possess a means of controlling
this state of disease, safer, and for the most part (though certainly
not always) equally effectual. We are indebted to Dr. Currie of
Liverpool for this improvement in practice. The great heat of
skin renders the cold affusion grateful to the patient. The disorder prevails chiefly among children, in whom it can be applied with
facility. In common cases of scarlatina there is not that degree
of febrile weakness which the fatigue of a cold affusion would
augment. There is no tendency to affection of the chest, as in
measles, which the application of cold to the surface might aggravate. An ulcerated state of the throat forms no objection to its
use. On the contrary, the cold affusion frequently checks this
symptom in the most remarkable manner. The repetition of the
remedy at intervals, proportioned to the urgency of the symptoms,
is indispensable (it may be safely applied whenever the skin is *hot*
and *dry.*) It cools the skin, abates thirst, diminishes the frequency
of the pulse, the head-ache, and the languor, and disposes to sleep.

Blood-letting is sometimes indispensable, especially when the
disease attacks adults of full habit of body. An apprehension has
been entertained regarding the debilitating effects of this practice
in scarlet fever, which may safely be disregarded. Head-ache and
general oppression are the symptoms which most urgently call for
its adoption. Leeches to the temples are occasionally sufficient.
These may also be applied with great advantage to the *throat*, when
the swelling of the tonsils is very great. They commonly bleed
freely in this disease, in consequence of the excited state of the
cuticular circulation.

Emetics have been strongly recommended throughout the *whole*
course of scarlet fever ; but they are not advisable, except at the
very onset of the disease. Moderate purging is greatly to be preferred, and yet a prejudice against it was long entertained, probably in consequence of observing the danger of supervening diarrhœa. This symptom is however often prevented by laxatives, and
it is perhaps occasionlly dependent upon inflammatory action of
the mucous membrane of the bowels. Gargles of infusum rosæ
are useful at an early stage to wash away the vitiated mucus ;

when the sloughs are separating, barley water is preferable. In severe cases a blister may by applied to the throat.

In the malignant form of scarlet fever, treatment of any kind is of course less efficacious ; but several of the measures already recommended may be had recourse to with a prospect of success. An emetic at the commencement of the disease has often proved of great service, and in some cases appears to have completely broken its force. Stimulant gargles as of port wine, or of decoction of bark with tincture of myrrh, are of considerable use. The bowels should be cleared by gentle doses of castor oil, but severe purging is dangerous. Draughts with camphor, serpentaria, and ether, may be given at first every four hours ; but as the disease advances, it becomes necessary to support the patient with decoction of bark and acids, wine, opium, and aromatics. In the severe epidemic which prevailed in the West Indies in 1787,* capsicum taken internally, and employed as a gargle, proved very serviceable. The cautions however formerly laid down, when explaining the treatment of typhus, apply here. Symptoms must be watched, nor must tonics be given upon the mere *theory* of their necessity. The convalescence from this disease is always very tedious, but may sometimes be shortened by a judicious administration of bitters and cordials. At the same time it should be observed, that an excited and feverish state of the system frequently accompanies the process of desquamation, requiring the long continued use of *saline* as well as of active *aperient* medicines.

I have delayed to this period all mention of a very remarkable phenomenon in the history of scarlet fever ;—I mean the dropsy, which frequently succeeds it.† It generally takes the form of anasarca, but ascites has also been noticed. It as often succeeds the *mildest* as the severest cases. It occurs, on an average, upon the twenty-second day from the decline of the eruption, seldom earlier than the sixteenth, or later than the twenty-fifth. It is preceded for several days by languor, costiveness, and sickness. These symptoms frequently continue, accompanying a quick pulse. The urine is scanty, and often coagulates on heating. This species of dropsy sometimes proves dangerous from the occurrence of coma, but

* Vide Medical Communications, vol. ii, page 363.

† The reader will find a classical paper on this subject, from the pen of the late Dr. Wells, in the Transactions of a Society for the Improvement of Med. and Chir. Knowledge, vol. iii. page 167.

more commonly from thoracic symptoms indicating effusion in the chest.

In speculating on the nature of this affection, Dr. Wells decided-ly inclines to the idea of its being inflammatory, and in this he is supported by the opinions of later pathologists. He argues, that it is not owing to debility, for it often attacks those who are strong, and passes by those who are weak ; its occurrence is confined to a particular period, though great weakness may exist before and af. ter ; and lastly, it is often attended with a white tongue and a bound-ing pulse. But it must be admitted that its precise causes have never been clearly explained. (The common method of treating this form of dropsy is by purging, squills, and digitalis.) Some cases have lately been published, pointing out the efficacy of bleeding. I have met with several cases, however, which appeared to indicate the propriety of bleeding and purging, but which resisted both, and ultimately yielded to bark and aromatic confection.

Herpes. Urticaria, or Nettle-rash. Lichen. Roseola. Erythema. Fram-
bœsia, or the Yaws. Its symptoms and Progress. Peculiarities in the
Contagion of this Disease. Principles of its Treatment.

In the present chapter I propose to treat of those lesser febrile
eruptions, which do not, under any circumstances, go to the extent
of affecting life, and are chiefly interesting with reference to diagnosis. They are herpes, urticaria, lichen, roseola, erythema, and
frambœsia.

1. Of all the lighter varieties of cutaneous eruption complicated
with fever, HERPES is that which is most distinctly entitled to the
character of an *exanthema.* The term herpes is appropriated to a
vesicular disease, preceded by febrile languor, and other marks
of constitutional disturbance. The vesicles pass through a regular
course of increase, maturation, and decline, terminating, in most
cases, in about a fortnight or three weeks. Herpetic vesicles are
distinguished by their occurring in distinct but irregular clusters,
appearing in quick succession, being set near together, and upon an
inflamed base, which extends some way beyond the margin of each
cluster. The most frequent form of the disease is the herpes zos-
ter, or *shingles,* in which the eruption appears on the abdomen,
but is observed also in some cases on the extremities, or breast.
Young persons, from fifteen to twenty-five years of age, are commonly the subjects of this disease. Very little is known regarding
its causes. Anxiety of mind, change of climate, and irregular
modes of life, are the circumstances which principally *predispose* to
it. It is most frequent in summer and autumn, and seems in some
cases to arise from exposure to cold after violent exercise. It is
always slight, seldom confining the patient to the house, or occasioning any debility. Its course cannot be shortened by internal

medicine, and it does not require any external applications. In *self-limited* hot countries, herpetic *ringworms* (herpes circinatus) often prove both tedious and severe, but in this country they follow the usual progress. That variety of the disease termed herpes *labialis*, occa.sionally appears as an idiopathic affection, originating from cold and fatigue. It is then preceded for two or three days by nausea, lassitude, languor, and sometimes severe feverish symptoms. It is frequently symptomatic of some internal disorder.* The common purgative draught No. 21, repeated as circumstances may require, seems to comprise every thing that is really necessary in regard to the treatment of herpes. The decoction of bark is certainly use-ful in the severer cases, and may be given in combination with the liquor ammoniæ acetatis, if the secretions of the kidney are scanty.

2. There are several kinds of eruption attended with fever, *Urticaria* which have occasionally been mistaken for measles and scarlatina. They are all very trifling diseases, but they deserve some attention on the score of diagnosis. One of these is the febrile URTICARIA, or nettle rash, a rare disease, of which a very scanty notice will suffice. It is preceded for two or three days by feverish symptoms. The eruption appears in the form of white elevations of the cuticle, *wheals* similar to those produced by the stinging of nettles, and denomina.ted *wheals*. It is very itchy, especially during the night, or on *itchy* exposing the skin to the air while undressing. It continues about a week, occasionally fading during the day. In children it is brought on by the irritation of teething, and at different ages by disordered states of the stomach and bowels. Modifications of the febrile nettle-rash are induced in particular constitutions by certain articles of food, shell-fish, almonds, or cucumbers. These cases are commonly attended with considerable disturbance of the stom. *emetic* ach, languor, and oppression. A gentle emetic, followed by a common opening draught, is all that is requisite in the treatment of the febrile urticaria.

3. A disease much more frequently mistaken for the genuine *Lichen* exanthemata is LICHEN; and in some cases the diagnosis is by no means easy. The characters of the affection may be thus descri- *papular* bed. Lichenous eruption is papular, of a reddish colour inclining *reddish* to purple, and exhibits in many instances, the crescentic forms of *purple*

* For more copious information concerning this and the other diseases treated of in this chapter, consult Bateman's " Practical Synopsis of Cuta-neous Diseases." London, 1813.

measles. It is in clusters, and for the most part very copious about the hands and bendings of the wrist and elbow. It never advances to the formation of vesicles, but terminates generally at the end of three or four weeks, by slight desquamation of the cuticle. There is considerable variety however in the progress of lichenous eruption, as well as in the symptoms accompanying it. In many cases, the constitution appears quite unimpaired. At other times, severe febrile symptoms have been observed to usher the disease in, and to attend it for four or five days. There is always an unpleasant tingling and itching of the skin in lichen, increased by the warmth of bed, and whatever else determines the blood with unusual force to the surface. It is not a contagious disease. It is taken indiscriminately by those who have, and those who have not, passed through measles and scarlet fever. Eruptions of a lichenous character arise from various causes; sometimes from the heat of the atmosphere (constituting lichen tropicus, or the prickly heat of hot climates,) sometimes from the venereal poison, but more frequently still, in this climate at least, from circumstances ill defined or altogether unknown. The disease, being wholly devoid of danger, may often be left to follow its own course; but saline aperients, low diet, and a cool regimen, are plainly indicated.

4. A rash has been described by different authors as occasionally occurring in connection with febrile complaints, to which Dr. Willan has given the name of RoSEOLA. It differs from lichen in being a mere efflorescence, of a rose colour, without papulæ. One of the most common varieties of it, is that which precedes in many cases for one or two days the eruption both of the *modified* and *in*oculated small-pox. Occurring under such circumstances, roseola has frequently given rise to much discordance of opinion concerning the real nature of the case. A similar eruption has been very often observed during the summer months, in persons (especially females) of irritable constitution.

5. Closely allied to roseola, and scarcely indeed distinguishable from it, is the eruption called by Dr. Willan *erythema*. It is characterized by a nearly continuous redness of some portion of the skin, with a slight elevation of the surface, speedily subsiding. The disease is not contagious, and the accompanying febrile symptoms are very slight. The principal species of the disorder is called erythema nodosum. The eruption is here confined to the fore part of the leg, and takes the form of large oval patches, which run par-

allel with the tibia, and rise into painful protuberances, much resembling nodes. The eruption subsides in ten or twelve days, but
usually leaves the patient languid. Mild laxatives, followed by the
mineral acids, are sufficient for its cure. It is a singular circumstance, that this variety of erythematous eruption is seldom witnessed, except in females. It occurs principally in the months of June
and July.

6. FRAMBŒSIA, or the Yaws, deserves to be placed amongst the
exanthemata, first, because it can be taken but once in life; and,
secondly, because it is propagated by specific contagion. It differs
from them however in having no fixed course, but wearing itself
out in a longer or shorter time. It may be considered, therefore,
as the link uniting the febrile exanthemata to the chronic cutaneous diseases, porrigo, scabies, and lepra. Frambœsia is endemic
in Africa and the West Indies prevailing chiefly among negroes;
but Europeans sometimes take it. It is preceded by a degree of
constitutional disturbance, amounting, in some instances, to fever.
An eruption of small pimples then follows, increasing for ten days,
when pustules form. To these succeed loose irregular crusts, beneath which, foul sloughy ulcers are to be found, which gradually
shoot out a fungus, resembling in size and appearance a mulberry.
This occurs at irregular periods, sometimes as early as one month,
sometimes as late as three from the appearance of the eruption.
The disease in about eight months wears itself out. The fungus
contracts, and except where the inflammation ran very high, cica-
trizes, without leaving any scar. The general health is but little,
sometimes not at all, impaired in the progress of the complaint. It
is not a disease of danger.

The yaws arises from a specific contagion, the latent period of
which is seven weeks.* It may be propagated by inoculation, but
the disease is not thereby rendered milder or shorter. In Africa,
it is usually undergone, like the measles in this country, during
childhood. It is altogether beyond the reach of medicine. Like
the small-pox, it must run its course, and will leave the constitution,
when, after completing its various stages, it removes the susceptibility to future infection. Towards its decline it appears to be somewhat benefited by sarsaparilla, bark and acid, and a generous diet.

* See Edinburgh Medical and Surgical Journal, July 1819, article by
Dr. Thompson.

CLASS III.

PHLEGMASIÆ, OR INFLAMMATORY DISEASES.

CHAP. I.

GENERAL DOCTRINE OF INFLAMMATION.

Universality of Inflammation. Symptoms of external Inflammation. Pain, Heat, Redness, Swelling. Symptoms of internal Inflammation. Pain, disturbed Function. Fever, buffy Blood. Terminations of Inflammation. Resolution, Effusion, Suppuration, Gangrene. Predisposition to Inflammation. Causes of internal Inflammation. Mechanical and Chemical Irritants. Cold. Morbid Poison and Contagion. Metastasis. Prognosis.

EVERY organ and structure of the body is liable to inflammation; and, next to fever, this is the most important subject of inquiry in the wide extent of medical science. It involves several considerations of a general nature, which it will be for the advantage of the student to begin by pointing out. There are certain phenomena, for instance, observed to attend it in its progress and decline, whatever be the organ or structure attacked. The causes of inflammatory action also are very much the same, whatever part of the body be its seat. The *symptoms*, *terminations* and *causes* of inflammation, therefore, constitute its fundamental doctrines, and this chapter will be devoted to their consideration. In the next I shall advert to the *varieties* of inflammation, whether occasioned by differences of cause, or function, or texture of the part affected. Some remarks on the *theory* of inflammation, and the principles of its treatment, will conclude the inquiry into the general doctrine of *acute* inflammation. Much interest, however, has lately attached to the subject of *chronic* inflammation; and it may not be foreign to our purpose to offer, in conclusion, a few remarks on that state of disease, such as may be sufficient to point out its principal pathological features.)

When any part of the body which is obvious to our senses becomes inflamed, such as the skin, the tonsil, or the eye, there are four alterations from the healthy state of the part which become manifest. These are pain, heat, redness, and swelling. It is not any one of these symptoms singly, but their combination, which marks the existence of inflammation. The stomach may be painful from distension. The skin may be hot from fever. The cheek may be red from blushing. The breast may be swelled from the flow of milk. To determine how far each of these symptoms is to be considered an evidence of inflammation is an object of some importance.

1. A certain degree of pain attends every deviation from health. Pain arises from spasm, fatigue, distension, sympathy, irritation, and along with other symptoms it is an important criterion of inflammation. At first the pain attending inflammation is acute, or lancinating; afterwards it is a *throbbing* or pulsatile pain, and these varieties of pain indicate different stages in the process of inflammation. The kind and degree of pain in particular cases appears to be proportioned rather to the facility of distension in the part than to the quantity of nerves with which it is supplied.

2. The heat of an inflamed part is the least important and the most frequently wanting of all the characters of inflammation. It never can exceed that of the blood at the heart. It is most conspicuous, therefore, when inflammation attacks a part at the greatest distance from the centre of circulation; such as the great toe in gout, or the point of a finger in whitlow. There is reason to believe, that in the inflammation of internal organs, the heat of the part is not materially augmented.

3. Increased redness of a part, if permanent, is nearly decisive of the existence of inflammation. We find it after death to have occurred equally in cases of internal inflammation. It is obviously owing to one of two causes, or perhaps to both; the enlargement of old vessels, or the growth of new ones.

4. Swelling is an accidental symptom of inflammation, attributable to the degree of looseness in the structure and connections of the part. Generally speaking, therefore, where there is least

swelling there is most pain. Some structures of the body apparently inflame without any swelling at all.

Such are the signs of external inflammation, or phlogosis ; but
the physician has not, for the most part, the advantage which the
surgeon possesses, of judging by the eye of the existence of this
state of disease. The symptoms of *internal inflammation*, or of
phlegmasia, are more obscure, and require more minute investigation. Its presence is judged of in two ways,—by local and by
constitutional symptoms. The local symptoms are pain, increased on pressure, and disturbance of function ; constitutional fever,
and buffiness of blood.

1. Pain is the most important of them all ; but in order to characterize it as the pain of inflammation, it must be *increased on
pressure.* The test of pressure cannot, however, be applied in all
cases ; as in inflammation of the brain and bronchia, where a bony
or cartilaginous case defends the inflamed structure. Pain again
is not essential to constitute inflammation. Where the affection
exists in an organ of very loose texture, there is little or no pain
felt, as in peripneumony. Cases have even been recorded, of inflamed brain and pericardium proving fatal without any such inconvenience being produced, as warranted the suspicion of inflammatory action.

2. Disturbance of function is almost a necessary concomitant
of inflammation ; and wherever the function of an organ is understood, we may judge of the extent of inflammation in it by the degree of disturbance which its function undergoes. The particular
symptoms referable to this head are of course as various as the
organ attacked. Delirium marks inflammation of the brain. Impatience of light, ophthalmia. Hoarseness, inflammation of the larynx ;
and dyspnœa, that of the lungs. There are only a few cases on
record of inflammation existing in a part without disturbing its
function.

3. Fever, more or less urgent, accompanies every kind of internal inflammation. In degree it varies, from the slight febricula
which attends catarrh to the highest grade of inflammatory fever,
such as is witnessed in phrenitis. It differs no less in kind than in
degree. At one time it is inflammatory, at another typhoid ; in
one instance it has a *hectic* in another a *remitting* character. It may
be held as a general rule, that the degree of local inflammation
may be estimated by the violence of the constitutional symptoms ;

but at the same time it must be borne in mind, that the degree of fever present in any individual case, does not always bear a proportion to the importance of the organ affected, or the extent of local disease. It may run as high in cynanche tonsillaris, as in a severe attack of pleurisy, and frequently appears to be measured by peculiarity of constitution. Some persons, from these data, have argued, not without an appearance of reason, that the fever accompanying local inflammation is not always a secondary affection ;— that in cynanche tonsillaris, for instance, it is not the swelling of a small and insignificant gland which raises the pulse to 120 ; but that fever is the primary affection, which from some unknown cause induces the local inflammation. Where neither the constitutional nor the local symptoms are urgent, it is common with some physicians to employ the term *sub-acute inflammation.* In a pathological point of view nothing is gained by its adoption, but practically it is of some use ; as for instance, in distinguishing and directing the treatment of some cases of bronchial and rheumatic inflammation.

4. The last proof of the existence of internal inflammation is derived from the appearance of the blood drawn. All ages and countries have agreed in looking upon buffiness of the blood as a test of inflammatory action ; but different ideas have been entertained as to the degree of importance which should be attached to it. Boerhaave and the followers of his school considered it as the decisive argument in favour of that *lentor* or spissitude of the blood, on which they believed inflammation to depend. Of late, physicians have rather been inclined to undervalue it as a symptom of inflammation. Upon a careful review, however, of all the arguments which bear upon this question, I am satisfied that buffy blood is a very important criterion of the presence of inflammation. Gennine inflammation, indeed, sometimes exists without it ; and the first cup of blood may be buffy when the last is not. These and other anomolies are interesting in a practical point of view, but they do not affect the general question of the pathological importance of buffiness of blood. The cause of this appearance has been a frequent subject of investigation. It has been supposed to depend upon the slower coagulation of the blood ; but this is obviously insufficient, for blood may coagulate slowly and not be buffy. That blood will prove buffy, may often be predicted from the bluish appearance which it exhibits while flowing from the arm. Some

17

pathologists imagine, that the relative proportion of fibrine in the blood is augmented in a state of inflammation. Others attribute the phenomenon merely to increased rapidity in the blood's motion ; forgetting that the blood is often deeply buffed with the pulse at eighty. The subject, it must be confessed, is still involved in great obscurity.*

The progress of inflammatory action, generally described under the title of the *terminations* of inflammation, next claims attention ; and here I must begin by observing, that whatever opinion may be formed regarding the *precise* condition of the blood-vessels in inflammation, it is obvious, from the general tenour of the phenomena now described, that they are loaded with an unusual proportion of blood. Of this they must be *relieved*, before the vessels can be restored to their natural healthy condition. The terminations of inflammation therefore consist for the most part of the several modifications of *effusion.*

1. When an inflamed part gradually regains its healthy state without any derangement of its structure, or any *sensible* effusion from its vessels, the disease is said to terminate by *resolution.* This is invariably the object of the physician, but the surgeon is often baffled by it, because he occasionally excites inflammation with a view of profiting by some of its subsequent stages. Resolution may happen, first, without medical aid, when the inflammation is very slight ; and, secondly, when the requisite *unloading* of the diseased vessels has taken place by means of *local* or *general* bloodletting, or in milder cases by local cold and purging. We judge of the tendency to resolution by the *gradual* giving way of the symptoms of inflammation, particularly by the diminution of pain and of fever.

2. The second termination of inflammation is an increase of the natural secretions of the part. In membranes which have an external outlet, such as the several mucous membranes, this is almost equivalent to resolution. In the shut cavities, as those of the pleura, pericardium, and peritonæum, such a termination of inflammation is more to be dreaded ; but in many cases the fluid thus effused is gradually absorbed, and health ultimately restored.

3. The third mode by which inflammation terminates is *effusion* from the vessels of the part, either of blood or of some of its con-

* See Appendix ; Note J.

stituent parts. The mucous membrane of the bowels, when inflamed, frequently relieves itself by a discharge of pure blood. In
some cases the *serum* of the blood is effused, as in hydrocephalus
and inflammation of the tunica vaginalis testis. In other cases the
coagulating lymph of the blood is effused; forming adhesions, as in
pleurisy and peritonitis. A peculiar gelatinous fluid is thrown out
in rheumatism, and a saline matter in gout. The consequences of
these effusions vary according to the violence of the inflammation,
and the situation and structure of the part affected. Adhesions from
pleuritic inflammation are productive of little or no inconvenience;
occurring in peritonæal inflammation they lead to incurable marasmus or ileus. The effusion of serum from inflamed vessels forms
a part, and a very important part, of the general pathology of *dropsy*, to which we shall hereafter have occasion to refer. When effusion takes place in the substance of the solid viscera, they become hardened, and are rendered more or less unfit for the due
performance of their functions. This is a frequent effect of *chronic*
inflammation, and will be further noticed when discussing that
branch of the subject.

4. The fourth termination of inflammation is the effusion of a
new product of the blood, called *pus*, a bland fluid, of the colour
and consistence of cream. When this is poured out into some cavity formed during the process of inflammation, an *abscess* is said to
exist; when the purulent matter forms upon an exposed surface,
ulceration is said to be established. This subject opens an extensive field of inquiry; but it falls more properly within the province
of surgery. By John Hunter and others the different topics which
it embraces, more particularly the nature of *ulcerative action*, have
been investigated with great success; and among other points, that
remarkable analogy has been explained which subsists between
pus and a secreted fluid, between an ulcerating and a secreting
surface. The formation of pus by internal inflammation exhibits
nothing different from what occurs when the inflamed texture is
in contact with the air. The symptoms by which we judge of suppuration having taken place in an internal organ are the following;
—1. A change from the lancinating to the throbbing pain. 2. A
sensation of weight or fulness in the inflamed part. 3. The pulse
continuing frequent, but becoming soft and full. 4. The occurrence of rigors and of night sweats,—in other words, the development of *hectic fever*.

5. The last and the most formidable of all the terminations of inflammation is sloughing, *sphacelus*, gangrene, or mortification, which are only different *degrees* of the same morbid condition. This happens, first, from the excessive violence of the first stage of inflammation, rendering it impossible for the vessels to restore themselves by any kind or degree of effusion. But as the tendency to gangrene often shows itself early, and without any particular violence of the first stage, it must be ascribed, secondly, to a *septic* tendency in the disease itself, as in the case of plague. The malignity of that contagion so overpowers the nervous system, that the vessels of the inflamed part are unable to resist the shock of the disease, and the part itself dies. Thirdly, the disposition to gangrene is, in many instances, independent both of the *nature* and of the *violence* of the inflammation, and is referable simply to the weakness of the patient's habit, which is such as to be unable to oppose resistance even to a mild attack. The symptoms of internal gangrene are :—1. The sudden cessation of pain. 2. A sinking and irregular pulse. 3. A change in the expression of countenance from that of febrile anxiety to exhaustion. 4. Delirium.

It remains to be stated, that several of these terminations of inflammation may be going on at the same time. Thus a mucous membrane may throw out a muco-purulent fluid. Flakes of coagulable lymph may float in the serum which an inflamed peritonæum has thrown out. The destruction of the part may be gradual and partial, and it is then eaten away by sloughy, or what has been called *phagedænic* ulceration.

Proceeding next to investigate the causes of inflammation, I shall first direct my attention to the circumstances which predispose to internal inflammation ; and shall then point out the principle exciting causes of that state of disease.

Inflammatory affections occur in all climates, and to all ages, temperaments, and conditions of body ; and there is consequently no small difficulty in determining the true nature of the *diathesis phlogistica*, or that particular state of body in which inflammatory action is most easily lighted up. Dr. Cullen states, that the inflammatory diathesis chiefly prevails in systems of the greatest vigour. A full habit of body, a plethoric state of vessels, and *tension of fibre*, are the terms usually employed to express the state of the system, when predisposed to acute inflammation. It cannot be disputed, that in such habits we often meet with genuine inflammatory diseases; but the student must bear in mind that this is neither the only state of body in which they occur, nor is it even the most common. He will find, that when the constitution is *below par*, when it has been weakened by previous diseases, by low living, by anxiety of mind, by excessive bodily fatigue, continued for a long period of time, inflammation of the most acute kind is often excited, which runs as rapid a course, and is attended with symptoms as violent, as inflammation occurring in persons full of blood, and of the most robust habit. The state of *weakness* then, of *irritability*, and of *atony*, is at least as favourable to the development of inflammation as that of *plethora* and *tension*. The state intermediate between these two is that which affords the surest preservative against the attack, not only of inflammatory, but of every other description of disorder. To that kind of inflammation which occurs in robust habits, the term *entonic* has been applied; *atonic* to that which takes place in a reduced state of the system. As expressive of a pathological principle, these terms are not objectionable; but the student must remember that they are inapplicable in *practice*, inasmuch as the several kinds of inflammation are to be treated on the same general principles. It is only with reference to prognosis, and the *extent* to which measures of depletion are to be pushed, that the study of the predisposition to inflammation is practically useful.

With respect to the *exciting* causes of internal inflammation, it may be first stated, that occasionally we can form no conjecture as to the true cause of the complaint; but at other times we can define it with considerable certainty; and among the most important causes of internal inflammation will be found the following;—mechanical and chemical irritants; cold; a peculiar habit of body, formerly characterised as a depraved state of the blood and humours; the presence of a morbid poison; contagion; and metastasis.

1. Mechanical and chemical irritants. The phrenitis of infants has been traced to the irritation of teething; gastritis to poison; enteritis to the presence of hardened fæces; nephritis to calculus in the kidney; ophthalmia to dust and sand; erysipelas to leech-bites, or the distension of the skin from dropsy.

2. Cold is the most important of all the exciting causes of internal inflammation. There is scarcely any form of it which does not occasionally owe its origin to cold; and many inflammatory

affections, as rheumatism and pleurisy, have no other cause of the smallest practical importance. The period of time that elapses between the application of cold and the occurrence of inflammatory symptoms is subject to great variety. In the case of sore throat, it often follows in the course of a few hours. In that of acute rheumatism, a week, or even a fortnight, has been known to elapse. What the circumstances are which direct the inflammation upon one organ or structure rather than another, may be gathered, to a certain extent, from what has already been stated when treating of fever (page 41.) In what manner cold operates as the cause of internal inflammation, has been a constant subject of inquiry with all pathological writers, but it is still involved in the greatest obscurity.

3. Some forms of inflammation, which to a superficial observer might appear to arise without any assignable cause, have their origin in a peculiar state of body, the nature of which is not always understood, but which the older physicians supposed to consist in some _morbid state of the fluids or humours_. This piece of pathology is exemplified in the phenomena of gout; in the inflammation of absorbent glands occurring in scrofulous children on the approach of winter; and in the pustular eruptions, called _acne_, to which young persons are subject about the age of puberty. The mere presence of fever unquestionably leads to local inflammation; and hence it is that in the progress of typhus, thoracic or abdominal inflammations so frequently supervene.

4. The existence of a morbid poison in the system is a frequent occasion of internal inflammation. This principle we have already had ample opportunities of illustrating in the phenomena of the plague, small-pox, measles, and the other exanthemata. It is equally exemplified in those of secondary syphilis, where the inflammation of the fauces, or of the iris, or of the joints, is obviously attributable to the presence of a morbid poison. The bite of the rattlesnake excites a peculiar kind of inflammation in the cellular membrane. Anatomists frequently suffer from the absorption of matter formed in the course of disease, especially of _acute_ disease, such as peritonitis. In irritable habits this induces not merely inflammation of the glands and cellular membrane, but also of the pleura and peritonæum, often of the most acute and dangerous kind. Closely allied to this, in a pathological view, is the important but well-ascertained fact of the origin of many inflammatory

affections from *contagion*. There is a species of contagious catarrh. Two species of cynanche are contagious. There is a contagious form of ophthalmia. Erysipelas is contagious under certain
circumstances ; so in all probability is dysentery. There is reason
to suspect that one of the forms of peritonæal inflammation is occasionally propagated in the same way.

5. The last cause of internal inflammation which it will be necessary to notice in this general view of the subject, is *metastasis*,
or the translation of inflammation from one organ or structure to
another. This is a very curious point in pathology, sufficiently
established indeed as a matter of fact, but the reasonings concerning which are hitherto very obscure and imperfect. It is exemplified in the ophthalmia which succeeds gonorrhœa ; in the inflammation of the testicle which succeeds the mumps ; in the inflammation of the pericardium which succeeds rheumatism ; in the inflammation of the brain which succeeds erysipelas of the face. In what
manner the metastasis is effected has never yet been developed. It
appears, however, that to *sympathy from similarity of structure*
something may be referred ; for in most cases of metastasis, it will
be found that the structures primarily and secondarily affected have
an affinity to each other.

In forming an estimate of the degree of danger in any case of
internal inflammation, the student will keep chiefly in view the *nature of the organ attacked*, the *strength of the patient's constitution*,
and the *length of previous illness*. Inflammations which arise suddenly and unexpectedly, occur for the most part in structures not
essential to life, and are comparatively of little danger. Of this
kind are inflammations of the pleura, of the tonsils, of the joints,
and of the testicle. On the other hand, all those inflammations
which are preceded by a long course of previous languor and ill
health, occur in organs which are essentially necessary to life—
such as the larynx, the pericardium, the bowels, or the brain ; and
these are attended with the utmost danger. Attention therefore to
the previous history of the patient is an indispensable step towards
forming a just notion of the degree of danger, as well as of the
necessity that may exist for prompt and active remedies.

Varieties of Inflammation. From the situation and function of the part affected. From Differences of Texture. By whom first investigated. Inflammation of Cellular Membrane and Parenchyma. Of Serous Membrane. Of Mucous Membrane. Of the Skin. Of Fibrous Membrane. Varieties of Inflammation from Differences of Cause. Theories of Inflammation. Agency of Blood vessels. Of Nerves. Question as to Differences in the Nature of inflammatory action. General System of Treatment in Acute Inflammation. In the states of Suppuration and Gangrene.

THE study of the varieties of internal inflammation is no less important, in a practical as well as pathological point of view, than that of the great features of *resemblance* which all inflammations bear. Some of these have been long known to, and amply described by medical writers. Others have only attracted attention in the course of the last twenty or thirty years, and are not yet described with that accuracy of which the subject is susceptible, and which, from its immediate application to practice, it deserves. The specific distinctions among inflammations may be reduced to the three following :—1. The situation and function of the part inflamed. 2. The structure of the part inflamed. 3. The exciting cause.

1. The first source of variety in inflammatory affections is the situation and function of the organ inflamed. This is an obvious practical distinction ; and it was accordingly noticed by all the oldest writers on physic. It is but of small importance however in a pathological view ; for an organ is composed of different parts or textures, and each of these is liable to an inflammation which exhibits some peculiarities. Though on common occasions therefore it is sufficient to speak of inflammation of the eye, or of the lungs, or of the bowels, yet in a scientific inquiry, it is necessary

to be more precise, and to speak of inflammation of the conjunctiva, or of the iris, or of the tarsi ; or to mark a distinction in the
other cases by the terms, pleurisy, peripneumony, inflammation of
the peritonæum, or of the mucous membrane of the intestines.

2. The second, and by far the most important of all the sources
of distinction among inflammations, is to be found in the structure
of the part inflamed. Every part of an animal body, the cuticle
and hair excepted, is subject to inflammation, and according to its
structure, is inflammation occurring in it, modified both in symptoms and termination. It is an important and well-ascertained fact,
that inflammation, in by far the larger proportion of cases, is confined to one texture ; that it spreads along that one, without affecting other contiguous textures ; and that almost all extensions of it
from one tissue to another are to be viewed as casual exceptions
to a general law. For a long time this subject was either altogether overlooked, or but very slightly attended to by pathologists.
Dr. Carmichael Smyth has unquestionably the merit of being the
first who thought deeply and wrote expressly upon it.* The views
which he took of this great question are highly ingenious, extensive, and accurate. Subsequent observation, indeed, has corrected
some and enlarged others ; but, upon the whole, they may be considered as constituting the basis of all our reasonings concerning
the varieties of inflammation. John Hunter and Bichat pursued
the same track of inquiry. It was the fault of the latter author
that he perhaps *refined* rather too much upon it.

Physiologists reduce the fundamental textures of the body to
five :—*viz.* cellular membrane, serous membrane, mucous membrane, skin, and fibrous membrane ; and, accordingly, there are
five varieties of inflammation founded on peculiarity of structure :
—*viz.* phlegmonous, serous, mucous, erysipelatous, and rheumatic.
A very brief sketch of the distinguishing characters of each of
these forms of inflammation is all that is consistent with the plan
of this work.

1. That texture of the body which is the most generally diffused
is cellular membrane, under which head physiologists include, not
merely the membrane strictly so called, but the parenchyma of the
different solid viscera and glands, which consist of cellular membrane connecting a congeries of minute blood-vessels and nerves.
The inflammation of cellular membrane is called phlegmonous or

* Vide " Medical Communications," vol. ii. page 168. London, 1788.
18

common inflammation, and its peculiarities are probably referable to the lax texture of the part, and the size of its arteries. Phlegmonous inflammation is distinguished by the great swelling which attends it, by its throbbing pain, and by its tendency to circumscribe itself and ultimately to form *abscess*. The process by which phlegmonous inflammation is circumscribed appears to consist in the effusion of coagulable lymph, uniting the cells together, and becoming afterwards the walls of the abscess. To this order of inflammations belong peripneumony, cynanche parotidœa, nephritis, hepatitis, and some others. Phlegmonous inflammation which terminates by sloughing is called *carbuncle*.

In particular habits of body, and under circumstances not always well understood, cellular membrane inflames without showing any disposition to circumscribe itself. This constitutes what has been called *diffuse cellular inflammation*, which has lately attracted much attention from pathological writers.* It occurs principally in debilitated states of body, or from some unusual *malignity* in the exciting cause.

2. Serous or diaphanous membranes are distinguished by a degree of transparency, by their firm and close texture, and by their function—the secretion of a serous fluid. The great serous membranes of the body are the tunica arachnoides, the pleura, pericardium, and peritonæum. Though possessed of little sensibility in the healthy state, these membranes are the seat of acute pain when inflamed. Lancinating pain, therefore, is the first character of *serous inflammation*. It is attended by a *hard* and *wiry* pulse, and a remarkable whiteness of the tongue, but for the most part without corresponding febrile debility. The peculiar terminations of this variety of inflammation are, the exudation of coagulable lymph forming præternatural adhesions,—the effusion of serum into the cavities lined by the membranes, forming dropsy ;—and occasionally the secretion of pus. It was at one time a matter of doubt whether pus could be formed, except by the sides of an abscess, or by an ulcerated surface ; but it is now well understood, that both serous and mucous membranes in a state of inflammation occasionally throw out true purulent matter.

3. The mucous membranes are those which line the various passages and cavities of the body which have an external outlet,

---

* See a valuable paper, by Dr. Duncan, junior, in the first volume of the Transactions of the Medico-Chirurgical Society of Edinburgh.

They secrete a mucus for the protection of their surface from the air, or the acrimony of the fluids which may come in contact with them. Their surface is *villous*, and interspersed with the orifices of glandular follicles. There are three great tracts of mucous membrane,—those, *viz.* of the nose, larynx, and bronchia ; of the mouth, stomach, and intestines ; of the urethra and vagina.

When a mucous membrane inflames, its natural secretion either ceases, or becomes depraved, appearing thin, acrid, *puriform*, or even purulent. It acquires an increase of irritability ; but the pain which is present is slight in comparison with that experienced from the inflammation of a serous membrane. The fever which attends it is, in like manner, seldom of so acute a kind, but it is sometimes accompanied with a remarkable degree of *debility*, which continues through a protracted period of convalescence. In respect of ter-mination, a curious difference exists in the different tracts of mu-cous membrane, attributable probably to some peculiarity in their anatomical structure. The intestinal tract is remarkably prone to ulceration, and the rapidity with which it runs into this state is worthy of note. The membrane lining the trachea throws out, du-ring inflammation, coagulable lymph ; that of the urethra pus. These and other characters of *mucous inflammation* we shall after-wards illustrate more fully, when treating of ophthalmia, catarrh, bronchitis, and dysentery.

4. Closely allied to a mucous membrane, in point of texture and function, is the skin ; and the inflammation of this structure is attend-ed with some interesting peculiarities. The phenomena of small-pox prove that the skin is susceptible of phlegmonous inflammation ; but the genuine inflammation of the skin has peculiar characters, which have acquired for it the name of erythematous, or more properly of *erysipelatous* inflammation. It is characterized, like phlegmon, by pain, heat, tension, and redness ; but instead of a ten-dency to circumscribe itself, its disposition is to spread ; instead of abscess, it goes on to the formation of *vesicle* ; and it occurs, much more frequently than other kinds of inflammation, in weak, irrita-ble, relaxed, and exhausted states of constitution.

The membrane lining the mouth and fauces being covered by a cuticle may be considered as a continuation of the skin. It is equal-ly susceptible of erysipelatous inflammation, leading, especially in children, to the formation of those vesicles known by the name of *aphthæ*. The inflammation produced by blisters, burns, and scalds, and the areolæ of small-pox and cow-pox, are instances of erysipelatous inflammation ; closely allied to which also, are the eruptions of measles and scarlet fever. The true seat of the redness in all these cases is the vascular net-work called *rete mucosum*, the vessels of which in the healthy state do not carry red blood. In the facial capillary system, however, the *disposition* of these vessels to receive red blood is very great, as is manifest in the phenomena of blushing. On this principle we account for the fact that the exanthematous eruptions begin about the face and neck ; that erysipelas is so much more common and dangerous in the face than in any other part ; and, as was formerly mentioned, that small-pox is most liable to become *confluent* on the face.

5. The last structure which demands attention is that of *fibrous* membranes, a class of membranes whose physiological relations were first investigated by Bichat. It must be admitted, that in this arrangement there is some mixture of hypothesis, but still there appears to be a foundation for it in nature. Fibrous membranes have a dense structure, and they do not exhale. They have the periosteum for their base. The dura mater, tendinous and aponeurotic expansions, and capsular ligaments, come under his head. Synovial membranes are usually classed by physiologists with the serous, but in a *pathological* view they may without impropriety be arranged here.

Inflammation of fibrous membranes is commonly called arthritic, or *rheumatic inflammation*, the peculiarities of which have been very long known. It differs from common inflammation in several points. 1. It never terminates in abscess, or adhesion, or gangrene, though the local symptoms be ever so severe ; but it is followed by gelatinous exudation, or earthy or saline depositions about the sheaths of tendons, and the ends of bones, impeding motion in the parts. 2. It is generally slower in its progress than the inflammation of other structures. 3. It has a remarkable tendency to sudden shiftings, or metastases. 4. The accompanying fever has a peculiar character, which will hereafter be pointed out : the functions of the brain, for instance, are never affected in it. 5. It rarely proves fatal.

Such are the chief structures of the body, and such the respective charcters of the inflammation which attacks them. It remains to be stated, that the exciting causes of inflammation exert a considerable influence over the character of the disease. Thus inflammation of the tunica conjunctiva exhibits different appearances, according, as it originates from cold, or from contagion. Inflammation of the tonsils has a different aspect when it arises from the presence of the venereal virus in the system, from that which it assumes when it is owing to cold, or the contagion of scarlatina. The practitioner of experience can indeed often ascertain the cause, by observing the *appearances* of the disease.

Many theories of inflammation have been proposed ; many attempts, that is to say, have been made to explain the precise nature of inflammatory action. But inflammation is an action peculiar to life. It is on a par with secretion and absorption ; and if we cannot unfold the nature of the healthy vital actions, it is not surprising that pathologists have failed in explaining those which occur in disease. It is pretty well agreed, that inflammation is a morbid action of capillary vessels. This portion of the great circulating system appears to act a very important part in almost all the operations of the animal body. The capillaries are probably the organs mainly concerned in secretion and the growth of parts, and possibly also in absorption ; but the whole subject of the functions of the capillary system is exceedingly obscure. Bichat appears to have considered it as altogether beyond our reach. Uninfluenced by these considerations, many modern pathologists have attempted to define accurately the state of the capillary vessels during inflammation. All are agreed, that under such circumstances the blood-vessels of the part carry an unusual proportion of blood ; but some attach to this the notion of an *increased* action of their coats ; others imagine, that in *some* part at least of their course, there is a spasmodic constriction ; while a third class of pathologists maintain, that during inflammation the action of capillary vessels is *diminished*. Into the merits of these different theories I have no intention to enter, after the opinion which I have expressed as to the almost impenetrable obscurity of the subject. The theory of *increased action* of the capillaries is upon the whole, that which is likely to prove the most useful guide in practice ; and, though by no means free from objections, will, with these reservations, be employed hereafter, wherever the nature of the subject may lead to theoretical discussions.

In the common theories of inflammation, every thing is attributed to the agency of blood-vessels. It is a matter, however, deserving of some inquiry, how far the nerves are concerned in inflammatory action. Several circumstances tend to the notion, that a buffy state of the blood is a phenomenon depending on nervous influence ; but it would be out of place to enter upon the consideration of such obscure and difficult questions here. Nor do these comprise the only point concerning inflammation on which pathologists have differed. A doubt has been expressed, whether differences of anatomical structure are sufficient to explain all the diversities which we observe in inflammatory action. It has been suggested, that is to say, that there may be differences in the *nature* of inflammatory action; that the same set of vessels may at one time be in a state of phlegmonous, and at another of erysipelatous, or rheumatic inflammation. This refinement, however, appears to be unnecessary.

The general principles of treatment in inflammation admit of being laid down with some accuracy; but they are of course varied by many circumstances, among which the most important are, the period or stage of the disease; the habit of body; the exciting cause; and the structure of the part inflamed.

The indications of cure in the early periods of internal inflammation are, first, to unload the vessels; secondly, to lessen the *vis a tergo*, the force of the heart's action; thirdly, to excite the vessels to a more healthy action; and, fourthly, to alter, if possible, the inflammatory condition of the blood. These indications are to be fulfilled by the nicely-regulated employment of blood-letting, general and local; purging, refrigerant medicines, and the local application of cold; occasionally by blisters and warm fomentations; and, in a few cases, by stimulants and tonics. The choice of the particular means best adapted to the different inflammatory affections of the body, will be a principal object of inquiry hereafter.

When suppuration is established, moderate evacuations may sometimes be proper, and even rendered necessary by the urgency of a particular symptom; but the mischief being now done, the object of the practitioner is rather to support the strength of the patient, than to risk, by further depletion, its complete exhaustion. A nourishing diet, therefore and tonic medicines will often be requisite, in conjunction with such means as diminish local action, and lessen the quantity of purulent secretion. Internal gangrene being so rarely an object of treatment by the physician, it is only necessary to remark in this place, that it requires the exhibition of wine and other cordials. For the treatment of external gangrene, and for the treatment of external inflammation generally, I must refer to works on surgery, where this subject is fully treated; it being the most important of all those which occupy the attention of the surgeon.

2. The treatment of internal inflammation is to be regulated, in

some degree, by a consideration of habit of the body in which it occurs. *Entonic* inflammation demands blood-letting from the general system, full purging, and active measures of depletion. Inflammation occurring in *weakened* habits is, in many cases, more effectually relieved by the *local* abstraction of blood, by blisters, and
such other means as lessen the action of the part, without impairing that strength of the general system which is so indispensable
for the repair of injury.

3. The treatment of internal inflammation is modified in the
third place by the nature of the exciting cause. Scrofulous inflammation of the absorbent glands, and inflammation of the periosteum
or fauces from the venereal virus, require a peculiar treatment,
adapted to the circumstances of each case. Tonics in the one, and
mercury in the other, must be superadded to the general system of
management already adverted to.

4. To a certain degree, the structure of the part inflamed affects
the treatment. Inflammation of a serous membrane demands the
copious and rapid abstraction of blood. That of mucous membrane
does not bear the same extent of evacuation, nor does it so often
require it. Erysipelatous inflammation is often successfully treated
by bark and acids. Rheumatic inflammation is under the control
of certain drugs, which have comparatively but little effect upon
common inflammation; colchicum, for instance, mercury, and
opium.

The convalescence from all the severer kinds of inflammation,
such as inflammation of the brain, lungs, larynx, or bowels, is very
tedious, being often protracted for three or four months, and this,
whether bleeding had been largely or sparingly employed. The
system receives a shock from the occurrence of inflammation in
any organ necessary to life, from which it recovers with great difficulty; nor does it appear that these subsequent efforts of nature
can be at all assisted (as in the case of fever,) by the employment
of bitter or other tonic remedies.

Such are the general outlines of the management of acute inflammation, under its several modifications. The subject is as important as it is extensive; for in inflammatory diseases the value
of medical treatment is more unequivocally manifested than in any
other class of disorders, and the skill and resources of the physician are here put to their severest trial.

CHAP. III.

CHRONIC INFLAMMATION.

Diversity of Structures affected by Chronic Inflammation. Chronic Inflammation, primary and secondary. State of the Constitution in this Affection. Causes of primary Chronic Inflammation. Its Nature and Seat. Effects of Chronic Inflammation. Thickening of Structure, Schirrus, Tumors, and Tubercle. Chronic Suppuration. Prevention and Treatment of Chronic Inflammation.

Chronic inflammation is a term frequently made use of; but I am not acquainted with any work in our language which may serve to point out the pathological considerations which it involves. On this account, though the subject is perhaps too obscure for investigation in an elementary work, I have thought it advisable to offer a few remarks concerning it ; rather, indeed, with the idea of attracting the attention, than of satisfying the inquiries of the student.

Chronic inflammation occurs frequently, and in almost every variety of structure : in the lungs, where it lays the foundation of consumption ; in the brain, liver, spleen, and kidney. All the serous and mucous membranes of the body are subject to it ; and in many cases this proves a most formidable affection, as in chronic dysentery and catarrhus senilis. The substance of muscle, and the different species of fibrous membrane, appear to be the seat of chronic inflammation in some forms of rheumatism. The skin is of all textures the least liable to chronic inflammation, unless, indeed, with some pathologists, we place in this class lepra, psoriasis and other varieties of chronic cutaneous disease. The same affection falls also within the observation of the surgeon. Gleet, inflammation of the prostrate gland, scrofulous enlargements of absorbent glands, chronic ophthalmia, and ozæna (or the chronic inflammation and ulceration of the Schneiderian membrane,) may be taken as instances.

Chronic inflammation is sometimes a primary, and at other times a secondary affection, that is to say, it succeeds acute inflammation ; and this is the most common form in which it appears, witness gleet and dysentery. In other cases it begins almost imperceptibly, and its advances are slow, often exceedingly insidious, being unaccompanied by any symptoms which could betray, even to the experienced practitioner, the existence of such a disease. Nowhere is this better exemplified than in some forms of chronic peritonæal inflammation ; but the same thing has been observed also in cases of chronic inflammation of the membranes of the brain, and even of the heart itself. In these instances, not only are there wanting all local symptoms of inflammatory action, but there are not even any constitutional symptoms ; at least none of sufficient importance to attract attention. This, however, is rare ; and chronic inflammation, both primary and secondary, exhibits for the most part local and constitutional symptoms, less indeed in degree, but the same in kind, with those which accompany acute inflammation. These vary of course, with the part affected. Sometimes, as in chronic laryngitis, there are local symptoms, but no sensible affection of the constitution. (When the general system is implicated, the symptoms are usually those of fever.) The pulse is quickened ; there is a white tongue, thirst, and some degree of restlessness. Occasionally, however, in a state of chronic inflammation, the tongue is clean, there is no thirst, but the pulse is feeble and languid, the extremities are cold, and the slightest exertion occasions fatigue, general uneasiness, and pain across the loins. All these symptoms mark a state, not of fever, but of atony and debility. The term *asthenia* has been applied with much propriety, by some pathologists, to express this state of the general system. Many of the protracted cases of bronchial inflammation, particularly those which occur in old people, exhibit, in the greatest perfection, the characters of *asthenic inflammation.*

The causes of *primary* chronic inflammation are involved in great obscurity. There is reason to suspect that cold has sometimes induced it ; or the long continuance of some mechanical irritation, as in the case of chronic inflammation of the brain, from spicula of bone ; but it is seldom that we can attribute the disease to so obvious a cause. A scrofulous habit of body appears to favour the disposition to chronic inflammation, but it often occurs where it would be mere hypothesis to attribute it even to that obscure source.

The nature of that action of vessels in which chronic inflammation consists, has been long an object of research. By some, it has
been defined to be that state of increased action of vessels, which
is neither so far subdued as to tend to resolution, nor so violent as
to form abscess ; but this goes only a little way in explaining the
difficulty. From the appearance of the eye in some cases of chronic ophthalmia, and from the effects of the *juvantia* and *lædentia* in
this and many other instances of chronic inflammation, it would
seem probable that a *relaxation* of vessels prevails, rather than any
increase of their action. It must be confessed, however, that this
object of inquiry is obscure ; and perhaps the truth, if it could be
obtained, of no practical application. In France, a doctrine obtains, that chronic inflammation has its seat in two distinct orders
of vessels, *sanguiferous* and *lymphatica capillaries ;* but as this piece
of pathology has never been received in this country, it will not be
necessary to inquire into its merits.

The effects of chronic inflammation vary with the texture of the
part affected. A simple thickening of structure is a common appearance, both in serous, mucous, and cellular membranes. Sometimes the thickening assumes the form which has been called *tuberculated accretion.* At other times the part inflamed is converted
into cartilage and bone. Instances of ossific deposition taking place
in consequence of chronic inflammation occur in chronic laryngitis,
chronic pleurisy, and chronic pericarditis. A further effect of
chronic inflammation (confined however to serous membranes) is
the extensive union of opposite surfaces. *Scirrhus* is generally accounted the effect of chronic inflammation in a glandular organ.

The origin of *tumours* in different structures, is a subject that has
excited much attention among pathologists. In many cases it is
presumed that their growth is referable to the same action of vessels by which all parts of the body are formed ; but in other cases,
there is reason to believe that they may have had their origin in a
state of chronic inflammation of vessels. Closely allied to tumours
are *tubercles ;* but the views which are entertained by pathologists
of the origin and nature of tubercle, will come better under discussion hereafter, when treating of pulmonary consumption.

The last effect of chronic inflammation which I shall notice is
suppuration, and it is one of those which we have most frequent
occasion to witness in practice. The fact of the formation of purulent matter in cysts and other structures, without any evidences of

previous inflammation, was well known to John Hunter, who had particular views of his own regarding it. But they are very nnsat. isfactory ; and until further light is thrown upon the subject, it may not be improper to consider these collections of matter as the re. sult of chronic inflammation.

To some, the subjects which have now been discussed may ap. pear too indefinite and obscure to be legitimate objects of investiga. tion, particularly in an elementary work. To this I would reply, in the energetic language of Bichat,* " that in explaining the ani. mal œconomy, it is doing much to indicate analogies ; to show the uniformity of an unknown phenomenon with another about which all the world are agreed." " In every branch of science," adds this author, " it would be well if the principle was thoroughly appreciated—that nature, greedy of her means, is prodigal of re. sults ; that a small number of causes everywhere preside over a multitude of effects, and that the greater part of those about which we are doubtful, are referable to the same principles with others which appear to us evident."

The treatment of chronic inflammation is very little understood. It is often said, that parts which have been much weakened, es. pecially by large bleeding during the acute stage, are liable after. wards to fall into the state of chronic inflammation. The remark however is not of general application, and this form of disease is oftener attributable to a neglect of those vigorous measures which would have cut short the acute stage of inflammation at its com. mencement. Chronic inflammation is almost as much out of the control of medicine as acute inflammation is under it. Nature sometimes works a cure ; but in many cases, more particularly of primary chronic inflammation, nothing is found effectual in check. ing the disease. The general system of treatment must depend up. on the state of the constitution. Four plans of treatment have been advised, and each has been found serviceable under different cir. cumstances.

1. Where fever is present, blood-letting, purging, and saline me. dicines, with a low diet, are to be recommended.

2. Where the pulse is feeble, and there is a decided loss of tone in the system, myrrh, benzoin, the balsam of copaiba, steel, and bark, are unquestionably useful.

* Traite des Membranes, page 189.

3. Where the disease is purely local, it is best treated by leeches, blisters, and issues, upon the principle of counter-irritation.

4. Where these means fail, an *alterative* plan of treatment may be resorted to. This is done under the idea of giving a new action to the vessels. Upon this principle, mercury is employed in the treatment of chronic hepatitis, alkalies in the scrofulous inflammation of absorbent glands, and sarsaparilla and guiacum in chronic rheumatism.

CHAP. IV.

PHRENITIS AND HYDROCEPHALUS.

Acute Idiopathic Phrenitis of Adults. Chronic Phrenitis. Symptomatic Phrenitis. Delirium Tremens. Its Symptoms, Nature, and Treatment. First Notices of Hydrocephalus, or Infantile Phrenitis. Its several Stages described. Variety in the Symptoms. Duration of the Disease. Prognosis. Diagnosis. Appearances on Dissection. Pathology. Treatment of Hydrocephalus. Remarks on the Chronic and Congenital Hydrocephalus.

PHRENITIS, or acute idiopathic inflammation of the brain or its membranes, is a disease so singularly modified in its principal features by the circumstance of age, as to require that it should be considered separately as it occurs in adults and in children. The distinction between *phrenzy* and *water in the head* is acknowledged by sound pathology as well as by the world at large ; but the former teaches that the two diseases run into each other by insensible degrees, and that the generic term phrenitis is strictly applicable to both. The former is an acute, the latter a subacute inflammation.*

The acute idiopathic inflammation of the brain in adults first engages our attention. This formidable disease is characterized by the following symptoms : violent inflammatory fever, redness of the eyes and face, intolerance of light and sound, great head-ache, with extreme restlessness, and, above all, early and fierce delirium. A very peculiar disposition to *self-injury* may be remarked in the progress of this disease. The patient obstinately shuts his teeth, and refuses both sustenance and medicine. If a penknife or razor be at hand, he frequently, and often too successfully, attempts his own life. Acute phrenitis, as it occurs idiopathically in hot cli-

* See Appendix ; Note L.

mates, has frequently been traced to excessive fatigue, under exposure to the rays of a vertical sun. In this country it is occasionally observed originating in anxiety of mind, or in a plethoric
habit of body from the inordinate use of spirituous liquor. Genuine phrenitic inflammation occurs too as a consequence of erysipelas of the face, and of small-pox ; but upon the whole, it is much
more commonly the result of fractures of the cranium and other
violent external injuries ; and comes therefore more within the
province of the surgeon than of the physician.

The acute phrenitis of adults is a disease of great danger, and it
may commence in any of the textures within the cranium. Some
pathologists have recently attempted to distinguish, by the peculiar
train of symptoms during life, the structure principally implicated,
but I believe without sufficient grounds. Various morbid appearances have been noticed after death, depending for the most part
on the character of the affected structure, of which the following
are the most important. When the dura mater is inflamed, effusion of coagulable lymph sometimes takes place, and adhesions
form. At other times, pus is found covering a portion of the membrane; or the membrane itself is eroded by ulceration ; but this
latter occurrence is by no means frequent. Inflammation of the
pia mater, when it runs high, generally proceeds to suppuration :
—that of the arachnoid membrane to thickening of its structure,
and serous effusion. Inflammation of the *substance of the brain*
seldom extends over any large portion of that viscus. Its usual
termination is in abscess.*

The treatment of genuine phrenitic inflammation is to be conducted on the common principles ; but the measures of depletion
must be prompt and vigorous, proportioned to the violence of the
symptoms, and the importance of the organ attacked. Twenty
ounces of blood should be taken from the arm in a full stream, and
repeated as circumstances may require ; or the temporal artery
may be opened, which in this violent disorder is occasionally very
serviceable. Purging by jalap and calomel (R No. 8,) or by the
mixture R No. 14, is to be steadily pursued. The head should be
shaved, and kept cool by ice, cold water, or the lotion, R No 109.

---

* The reader should not fail to consult the splendid work of Dr. Hooper,
entitled "The Morbid Anatomy of the Human Brain." The effects of
phrenitic inflammation are there exquisitely delineated in a series of coloured engravings.

The strictest quiet is to be enjoined and the patient closely and un. interruptedly watched.

Chronic inflammation of the brain and its membranes is a state of disease by no means uncommon. It seems to occur, in some cases, as a consequence of falls and blows on the head ; but in most instances, its origin is altogether inscrutable. It generally terminates in abscess. The symptoms which it occasion are sin. gularly diversified, and the skill of the experienced practitioner is often baffled in attempts to determine its existence. Death is usu. ally preceded by a short period of coma. Could the nature of the disease be ascertained during life, a seton in the neck and re. gular purging would afford the only legitimate hope of relief.

I have already spoken of the tendency of common fever, both in this country, and still more in warm climates, to implicate the brain, and give rise to all the symptoms of phrenitic inflammation. Whether these depend on *true* inflammation, or are attributable to a mere state of *congestion* in the vessels and sinuses of the head, is a matter of no great practical importance ; but the occurrence of such symptoms demands the serious attention, and their man. agement the utmost skill of the practitioner.

There is a very singular affection of the brain and nervous sys. tem called DELIRIUM TREMENS, which deserves notice in this place, from the risk which exists of confounding it with true phrenitis. It has for its pathognomonic symptoms, delirium (sometimes fierce, but more generally restrainable,) delusions of sight, trembling of the hands or whole frame, and complete sleeplessness. Fever is here seldom strongly developed, and the pulse wants the character of true inflammation. A like combination of symptoms, with the addition of damp perspirations, sometimes occurs in the latter sta. ges of fever, and I have witnessed it as a sequel or metastasis of acute rheumatism. Under all circumstances, delirium tremens in. dicates extreme danger. It arises in a very large proportion of cases from the excessive use of ardent spirits ; but a few instan. ces have been traced to other sources, such as the poison of lead, the habitual use of opium, and strong metal emotion. It appears to have for its proximate cause a peculiarly excited state of the

nervous system ; but the occurrence of such symptoms in cases of
extreme inanition would lead to the belief that exhaustion of nervous power expresses perhaps more accurately its intimate nature.
Delirium tremens usually runs its course in about four or five days.
It sometimes terminates in a fatal epileptic fit. It is universally admitted that this complaint does not admit of depletion by blood-letting. Much mischief indeed has followed its employment. Leeches
however are occasionally useful, and sometimes in its early stage
indispensable. The principal aim of the physician should be to
calm and support the nervous system, and if possible to procure
sleep. Opium answers all these indications, and must be given in
full and frequently repeated doses. Where the complaint can be
traced distinctly to the excessive use of ardent spirits, the accustomed stimulus must not be too rapidly withdrawn. Wine or brandy, in moderate quantities, should be administered. Æther, ammonia, camphor, and hyoscyamus, have also been found beneficial.
It is unnecessary to add, that moderate purging should also be directed, for in so disordered state of the nervous system, the secretions can scarcely fail to be greatly vitiated.*

Children are very subject to an affection of the brain, commonly
known by the name of hydrocephalus. Different opinions have
been entertained of the nature of this complaint. By Dr. Cullen
it was called apoplexia hydrocephalica. Some have viewed it as
more nearly allied to the class of dropsies ; but modern pathologists incline to the belief that it is a subacute inflammation of the
membranes of the brain, and therefore, in strict nosological language, the *phrenitis hydrocephalica* or *infantilis.* The disease,
though very common, was not described with any degree of accuracy until about ninety years ago, by Mr. Paisley, in vol. iii, Ed.
Med. Essays. In 1768 it was made the subject of an essay by
Dr. Whytt. In 1808 a very complete description of the disease
appeared from the pen of Dr. Cheyne. Dr. Monro has recently
described it with great accuracy in the first volume of his Morbid
Anotomy of the Brain.

Hydrocephalus prevails chiefly among children from the third to
the sixth year of life. It has been noticed, indeed, as early as the
second year, and as late as the fourteenth. After that period it is
seldom met with. From the circumstance of its occurring for the

* See Appendix ; Note M.

most part in children, the symptoms of the disease do not always
admit of being very accurately ascertained. This contributes, with
some other circumstances which will hereafter be noticed to render the diagnosis more difficult in this disease than in any other to
which the human body is subject. Hydrocephalus may, for the
purposes of instruction, be considered as exhibiting four stages or
sets of symptoms; but the distinction must be viewed as a very
arbitrary one; and it should be thoroughly understood, that, in many cases, the symptoms of different stages will be found blended
together, or one or more of them altogether wanting.

1. The symptoms which characterize the first, or premonitory
stage of hydrocephalus, are those of common *infantile fever* such
as often accompany the state of dentition, or a foul stomach, or a
disordered state of the bowels, more especially when complicated
with the presence of worms. The pulse is quick, the skin hot, the
sleep disturbed, the tongue white; there is some degree of nausea
and vomiting, with thirst, restlessness, and loss of appetite. The
child droops. The fauces being very dry, he picks the nose so as
often to make it bleed. The body wastes, and the skin is flabby.
The symptoms have irregular exacerbations and remissions; so
that this state of disease is generally known by the name of *infantile remittent fever.* An exacerbation usually takes place towards
evening.

2. The second set of hydrocephalic symptoms are those which
more unequivocally direct attention to the head as the seat of disease. They are, head-ache, sometimes diffused, sometimes refered to a particular spot; impatience of light and noise; a flushed
countenance; præternatural redness of the conjunctiva; contracted pupil; tossing of the arms to the head, and occasional screaming or shrieking without any obvious cause. With these are joined
the common symptoms of infantile fever, and they denote what pathologists consider the state of acute inflammatory action of the
vessels of the brain.

3. The train of symptoms which characterize the third stage of
the disease are of a different kind. The pulse, before quick, becomes slow, intermitting, or irregular. The pupils are permanently
dilated, and cease to contract on the approach of light. There is
strabismus, or squinting. Instead of being restless, and tossing
about his arms, the child falls into a state of stupor, and is insensible to things and persons around him. The screaming fits occur

20

more frequently, and there is an almost constant moaning. The child will often vomit on being brought into the erect posture. Any sudden exertion brings on a fit of convulsion, in which the child dies. These symptoms are supposed to mark that water is now poured out by the vessels of the brain, particularly by those of the arachnoid membrane and choroid plexus.

4. If the child survives this stage, it is occasionally found that after a time the pulse again rises, so as to beat 150 or more in a minute, and is withal small and feeble. The child lies perfectly insensible, and takes no nourishment from actual inability to swallow. The stools and urine pass involuntarily. The face is pale; the tongue dry and brown. Subsultus tendinum, convulsions, or partial paralysis (as of the levator palpebræ) occur; occasionally one side becomes perfectly paralytic. Severe pustular opthalmia is sometimes witnessed. The immediate approach of death is often preceded by gangrenous spots, or ecchymoses, appearing particularly about the neck, hips, or tips of the ears. This combination of symptoms I have several times seen to occur where the child, during the previous stage, had been kept in a state of perfect quietude.

I have already alluded to the great variety which exists in the symptoms of hydrocephalus, and above all, in the order in which they appear; but of some of these it will be proper to take more particular notice. The first stage is sometimes wanting, the attack being *sudden*, and perhaps the first evidence of the disease a strong convulsion fit. In many instances the pulse never becomes slow. In a still larger proportion of cases the disease never exhibits that remarkable change from the slow to the *rapid* pulse, which characterizes the fourth stage. Occasionally there is neither permanent contraction nor dilatation of the pupil, but throughout the *whole* course of the disease an irregularity in the contractions of the iris may be noticed. The pupil dilates on the approach of the candle, and contracts as it recedes. In a few cases I have seen children continue sensible to the last moment. Other, and even more singular varieties in the symptoms of hpdrocephalus will be found recorded in the writings of authors.* It is certainly worthy of remark, considering the universality of *delirium* as a symptom of

---

* See Monro on Hydrocephalus, page 96.

phrenitis in the adult, that aberration of intellect can scarcely be said to occur in this, or indeed in any of the diseases of early life.

The duration of hydrocephalus is liable to almost as much variation as the symptoms which characterize it. It has been known to prove fatal in a week. Some cases run on even as far as two months, but these are comparatively rare. The average duration of the complaint may be stated to be three weeks. The general opinion of the world has sufficiently stamped the *prognosis*. Dr. Whytt did not save more than one out of twenty cases. Many practitioners of great experience have seen only two or three instances of favourable termination, when the symptoms were so strongly marked as to preclude all possibility of being deceived as to the nature of the complaint. It must be confessed that the *diagnosis* is difficult, yet I am satisfied that many cases of genuine hydrocephalus have been recovered by judicious treatment, which (on that very account perhaps) were considered to be only disordered states of the primæ viæ. I have witnessed one case of recovery after the occurrence of complete hemiplegia.

To determine what the diseases are, with which hydrocephalus is liable to be confounded, is an object of some importance. 1. The first is common or typhus fever. The only manner of guarding against this source of fallacy is by hearing steadily in mind, that idiopathic fever is not common in young subjects, and that hydrocephalus is. Unless the evidence therefore be very unequivocal (as where the disease can be *distinctly* traced to contagion,) the symptoms should always be attributed to hydrocephalus, and not to typhus.

2. The second source of difficulty in the diagnosis, arises from the *early* symptoms of hydrocephalus being in every respect the same with those which accompany abdominal irritation; but chiefly from the important pathological principle, that several abdominal diseases, particularly those of children, are liable in their progress to affect the brain and nervous system, and to produce symptoms resembling those of the *latter* stages of hydrocephalus. The exact nature of these abdominal affections has been a frequent subject of dispute. By some it is supposed that derangements in the *hepatic* system have a strong tendency to produce hydrocephalic symptoms; but I do not believe that the liver is more, if even so much concerned in this as the the stomach and intestinal tract. A mere functional disturbance of these organs gives rise to remitting fever,

head-ache, and vomiting. The presence of worms creates a degree of irritation that in the most striking manner counterfeits hydrocephalus. But of all the states of abdominal disease which are
liable to be mistaken for it, by far the most important is inflammation and ulceration of the mucous coat of the small intestines, particularly the ileum. In its latter stages, I have seen this disease
attended in children with coma, dilated pupil, and screaming, constituting a secondary affection of the brain and nervous system.

3. With reference to the diagnosis of hydrocephalus, it must
further be observed, that in children the latter stages of what appears to be *pneumonia* are sometimes attended with coma and
screaming,—the early symptoms, that is to say, having been difficult breathing, a hard pulse, and cough. These cases are extremely deceiving. On dissection the thoracic viscera often appear healthy, while the ventricles of the brain are perhaps loaded with serum. The circumstance is well deserving of notice, as, without
some explanation, the practitioner might be exposed to the opprobrium of having misunderstood the case.

Dissections in hydrocephalus exhibit the ventricles more or less
distended with fluid. The quantity varies much, and can never be anticipated from the violence of the preceding symptoms.
From one to six or eight ounces are generally found. The effused
fluid does not coagulate on the application of heat, like the serum
of the blood, or many other dropsical fluids. It has never happened to me to see any flakes of lymph floating in it. Where the disease occurs at an early period of life, the quantity of effusion has
sometimes been such as to cause a tumour on the anterior fonta-
nelle. In a case recorded by Dr. Baillie, the ossa parietalia were
separated to a considerable extent, after being to all appearance
firmly closed.* Tumours, probably of a scrofulous kind, have been
also met with, of different sizes, situate either in the substance of
the brain or cerebellum, or attached to the membranes. It has
often occurred, that where hydrocephalic symptoms have been the
most strongly marked, no morbid appearances have been discovered in the brain on dissection. In these cases it is generally supposed, that the disease has proved fatal during the first stage ; but in
a certain proportion of them, organic disease sufficient to account

* Medical Transactions of the College of Physicians, vol. iv. p. t.

for death might. possibly be found in some other part of the body, were the dissection fully prosecuted.

We have stated, that hydrocephalus is one of the forms of phrenitic inflammation ; but it must be admitted that such a view of the disease is not perfectly satisfactory. This may be gathered from the very rare appearance of flakes of lymph, or of suppuration in the brain, as consequences of hydrocephalus ; and from the great mortality which attends the disease, in spite of the vigorous measures of depletion which are so constantly practised, and which would not fail to relieve inflammatory affections in other parts. In what circumstances hydrocephalus differs from common phrenitis has never been accurately explained. It is commonly stated, that the first stage of hydrocephalus is one purely of increased excitement of vessels, and that serum is not effused until the pupils are dilated, or strabismus, or the slow pulse come on. This piece of pathology has always appeared to me to be doubtful. I am inclined to think, that the vessels of the brain throw out an undue proportion of water even from the very first, and that the symptoms of *compression* which mark the advanced stages of the disease are owing to the *accumulation* of water in the ventricles, rather than to incipient effusion.

The only predisposing cause of hydrocephalus that is known, is the scrofulous diathesis. Its occurrence in scrofulous families, its alternation with other forms of scrofulous disease, its connection with scrofulous deposits in the brain, and other textures of the body, form the strong grounds on which this opinion is supported. Its most common exciting causes are, teething ; cold ; suppressions of tinea capitis, or of scrofulous runnings behind the ears ; injuries to the head ; and previous diseases, especially measles, scarlatina, and hooping cough. We are authorized in laying it down as a general rule, that in all the febrile disorders of children, there is a *tendency* to that form of phrenitic inflammation which terminates in serous effusion. In the treatment of infantile diseases this principle must be steadily kept in view, as it is *practically* of much more consequence than any attempt to discriminate them from hydrocephalus by fine and arbitrary distinctions. It is unquestionable, that the disease has arisen in many cases without the slighest assignable cause.

The object of treatment in hydrocephalus is to diminish that general inflammatory excitement, and that flow of blood to the head, which exist during its early stages; and afterwards to promote, if possible, the absorption of the effused fluid. In what we have call-ed the first or premonitory stage, reliance is to be placed on purga-tive medicines, particularly rhubarb and calomel, or the powder of scammony and calomel (R No. 10) in doses sufficient to ensure a full action on the bowels. When the symptoms of phrenitic inflam-mation, or as some would rather say, of cerebral excitement, deve-lop themselves, the jugular vein must be opened, or a vein in the arm, and from four to six ounces of blood taken away. I have open-ed the temporal artery under these circumstances with the best ef-feet. Of the indispensable necessity of blood-letting in hydroce-phalus, I can hardly express myself too strongly.* Much of the danger commonly imputed to this disease may be referred to the neglect of this necessary evacuation. If bleeding in the jugular vein, or arm, should unfortunately be found impracticable, or consi-dered decidedly inadvisable, leeches or cupping may be substituted, and their operation assisted by purging with calomel and jalap, or the strong aperient mixture (R No. 14,) and by the application of cold to the head. In a few instances I have had recourse to the cold affusion. The child may further be directed to take every three hours a saline draught, with antimonial wine and the tinc-ture of digitalis, as in the formula No. 38.

When the symptoms lead to the notion that water is effused, bleeding is for the most part ineffectual, and even sometimes abso-lutely prejudicial. It ought not however to be forgotten, that the symptoms of effusion are equivocal, and that an inflammatory con-dition of the cerebral vessels does not always subside, even when effusion has actually taken place. Blisters should now be applied, either to the crown of the head, or to the arm, or better perhaps to the back of the neck. At an earlier period of the disease, they ap-pear rather to increase irritation. At all times considerable cau-tion is requisite in applying blisters to children. Their skins are generally very delicate and irritable, and in feverish states of the body (when the skin is *hot* and *dry*) they occasionally produce very high local inflammation, ending in sloughing or gangrene, or such a degree of nervous irritation, as terminates the life of the child

---

* Some excellent observations on blood-letting, as applicable to the dis-eases of infantile life, man be found in Dr. Clarke's Commentaries on the Diseases of Children, chap. vi, pages 148—160.

by a convulsive fit. Occasional purgatives and the exhibition of
digitalis may be continued, with a view of directing the fluids upon
the bowels or the kidney. Under the idea of stimulating the absorbents, mercury is nearly always resorted to. Calomel, in large
and frequent doses, is recommended by some even from the very
first, but the propriety of this practice is very questionable. Mercurial inunction is preferred by others; and towards the latter stages
of the disease, this method of treatment has certainly proved effectual in some cases. The medicine frequently shows its influence
upon the system, by affecting the bowels. Salivation is not easily
excited in children, but it sometimes occurs, and has even occasioned considerable inconvenience.

It remains for me to notice the chronic form of hydrocephalus,
or that which is accompanied by enlargement of the skull.* Sometimes this disease is congenital, but more usually it begins during
the first month. In consequence of the bones of the cranium giving way, the usual symptoms of compression do not come on. The
size which the head attains in this disease is often enormous †. On
dissection, the brain appears flattened out, but it will be found to
weigh about as much as a healthy brain would have done at the
same age. In the progress of the disease, the functions of the body
generally are very little, often not at all impaired till a short time
before death. It is almost incredible how little the powers of the
mind are affected by this disorder. Dr. Monro states, that in no
instance seen by him could it be said that the intellect was deranged. In one remarkable case, of twenty-six years duration, in which
the head measured 44 inches in circumference, the patient displayed a very affectionate disposition towards his parents, entered into
the amusements of his brothers and sisters, and enjoyed a tolerably retentive memory. Attempts have been made to afford relief
to this apparently hopeless state of disease by tapping, and a case,
successful for a time, is recorded in the Medico-Chirurgical Trans-

* This complaint has been frequently, but very improperly, termed *hydrocephalus externus.*

† I made the following measurements of the head of a child eleven months
old, who died of chronic hydrocephalus under my care, December 28, 1818.
—Greatest circumference of the head 23 inches,—smaller circumference
22 1-4 inches; distance of the parietal bones from each other, 7 inches.
Four pints of fluid were contained within the brain.

actions (vol. ix, page 354).   More recent observations have shown, that the risk from this operation is great, and that it is not general. ly to be recommended.   Bandaging of the head has been tried, but without material benefit.   The complaint does not necessarily prove fatal at an early age, a few cases being on record of its con. tinuance to an advanced period of life.*

* See Appendix ; Note N.

OPHTHALMIA.

Structures primarily affected. Inflammation of the Conjunctiva. Mild and Purulent. Consequences of Purulent Ophthalmia. Causes of this Disease. Peculiarities of Scrofulous Ophthalmia. Of Syphilitic Iritis. Principles of the Treatment of Common Ophthalmia. Of Scrofulous and Variolous Ophthalmia.

THE attention of medical authors has been strongly directed to the subject of ophthalmia during the last twenty years, chiefly in consequence of the general introduction into the army of the purulent or Egyptian ophthalmia. This happened in the year 1800; previous to which time, neither the seat of the disease, nor the precise character of its consequences, had been described with any degree of accuracy. The circumstances that render the study of this disease so difficult, are the varieties of structure which we meet with in the complicated organ of vision, where membranes, cartilages, humours, ducts, glands, and hairs, are all intimately connected together. It will not be necessary however here, to enter with any degree of minuteness into the consideration of ophthalmia, because it has latterly been almost wholly taken out of the bands of the physician. Still the outlines at least of the pathology of ophthalmia should be understood by every student of physic; and further, a brief notice of them will be necessary to complete our view of the inflammatory affections of the body.

Inflammation may begin in almost every one of the structures of which the eye is composed; but the principal primary seats of ophthalmia are, the tunica conjunctiva, the sclerotica, the iris, and the meibomian glands. The phenomena of the disease are remarkably modified by diversities of exciting cause, more so perhaps in this than in any other instance which could be brought forward.

21

This principle therefore it will be necessary to bear in mind, in the short sketch which will be offered of the symptoms and progress of the disease. The structure most frequently affected is the conjunctiva, in function resembling a mucous membrane, though in appearance more nearly allied to those of the serous class. The inflammation of this membrane is characterized in mild cases, and where the disease arises from common causes, by pain, intolerance of light, a sensation of sand in the eye, head-ache, redness of the eye, and an *increased flow of tears*. The general febrile symptoms are slight, or perhaps altogether wanting. The disease gradually goes off without leaving any permanent bad effects.

In the severer forms of ophthalmia, the invasion is often sudden, the progress of the disease rapid, and its result disorganization of all or some of the structures necessary to vision. Besides the symptoms already enumerated, there occur in this form of ophthalmia, swelling of the eyelids, and secretion of purulent matter by the inflamed membrane, often in enormous quantity, and from a very early period of the disease. The conjunctiva quickly loses all traces of transparency, and exhibits instead, a mass of spongy red granulations, in which the transparent cornea may sometimes be observed as at the bottom of a well. This inflammatory thickening of the membrane, from the increase of its vessels, is called *chemosis*. The other symptoms are in a proportionate degree of violence. The head-ache is excruciating. The smallest ray of light gives intense pain. The febrile symptoms which accompany this state of disease run high, and are for the most part aggravated towards evening.

This is the disease known by the name of the purulent or Egyptian ophthalmia. Its further progress depends in a great degree upon the measures of treatment which may be adopted in its early stage. If these are judicious, the symptoms begin to yield about the third day, and in the course of some weeks the eye is restored to its natural state. But if the disease be unusually violent, or its early stages neglected, disorganization of the eye follows to a greater or less extent.

Sometimes the inflammation spreads to such a degree, that every part of the ball of the eye becomes involved in one uniform mass of suppuration, and the eye is totally lost. This however is rare. The disorganization is generally confined to one or other of its different structures. The inflammation, for instance, spreads from the conjunctiva covering the sclerotic coat, to that more delicate part of the membrane which extends over the cornea, and the consequence is either opacity or thickening of the cornea occasioning total or partial blindness ; or open ulceration of the cornea, a state of disease attended with a remarkable degree of pain ;—or lastly, *interstitial* ulceration of the cornea. This last affection is correctly speaking, ulceration of the proper membrane of the cornea, the delicate layer of conjunctiva which covers it remaining entire. This kind of ulcerated cornea occurs often in debilitated states of the system, and is accompanied by a deficiency, or total absence, of that action in the vessels which is necessary to repair the loss of substance. It is therefore often relieved by bark, and other tonic medicines, and by stimulant applications to the eye itself.

Pustular ophthalmia, as this is called, sometimes spreads to the deep-seated membranes. The iris in particular is frequently so affected, and the consequences are various. Lymph or pus may be effused into the anterior chamber of the eye. If pus is effused to any extent, the cornea is pushed forward, presenting the appearance called hypopion, or poached eye ; or it may be ruptured and the iris protruded, constituting that painful and nearly incurable condition called *staphyloma*. Another effect of the inflammation spreading inwards is, that the iris contracts adhesions, particularly with the capsule of the crystalline lens, and with the posterior layer of the cornea, whereby the motions of that membrane are lost, and blindness, to a greater or less degree, produced.

Occasionally it happens that the *eye-lids* continue to suffer, either with, or without permanent disorganization of the eye itself. The internal surface of the eye-lids for instance, remains red and granular ; and this in its turn renews the inflammation of the conjunctiva covering the ball of the eye, and leads perhaps to opacity of the cornea. At other times the cartilaginous edges of the eye-lids are the parts affected, and the eye-lids are either everted, forming the disease called *ectropion*, or the tarsi are turned inwards upon the ball of the eye, constituting the *entropion*. Both these states of disease of the palpebræ are tedious, and often difficult to manage. They require surgical operation. The only other consequence of acute ophthalmia which it is necessary to allude to here, is that state of *chronic* inflammation of the conjunctiva which is frequently left, especially in weak and scrofulous habits.

Before proceeding to notice the other varieties of ophthalmia, it may be proper to inquire into the causes of that common form of it, whose principal symptoms and consequences have been now detailed.

Mechanical and chemical irritations, such as acrid fumes, a drop of spirit getting into the eye, an eye-lash turned inward, walking against a very strong wind, or too long exercise of the eye, are frequent causes of ophthalmia. In no part of the world is it a more common disease than in Egypt, and several causes have been assigned for its prevalence in that country. The fact appears to be, that a great many circumstances, each of them sufficient to produce ophthalmia, are there combined; such as great heat succeeded by heavy dews; bright light; a burning wind from the desert, and innumerable particles of fine sand everywhere floating through the air.

But besides these causes of ophthalmia, which may be supposed to operate upon the eye *directly*, there are many, which act through the medium of the general system. Cold may be mentioned as one of the most frequent. Bile and sordes in the stomach and bowels have also occasioned ophthalmia. The purulent ophthalmia of infants has been attributed by some to this source. Iutemperance leads to a chronic state of inflammation of the eye. The presence of fever in the body, or the operation of the exanthematous poisons, have brought on ophthalmia, as we judge from its so frequently accompanying small-pox, measles, catarrh, and hydrocephalus. In many cases ophthalmia must be regarded merely as the evidence of an inflammatory or very highly excited state of the vessels of the brain. It frequently accompanies the secondary fever of small-pox. As it often happens that inflammation of one eye is succeeded by a corresponding affection of the other, sympathy of the eyes has been justly regarded as an exciting cause of the disease. *Habit* may be looked upon in the same light. It is well ascertained, that a soldier who has once suffered from a severe attack of ophthalmia, is liable to have it renewed by very slight causes, such as a night-guard or a debauch. No doubt can be entertained, that among the exciting causes of ophthalmia *contagion* deserves to be noticed. This has been disputed, but not by those whose opportunities of observing the disease have been upon an extensive scale. The experience of the army fully warrants this principle of pathology.

One of the most remarkable of all the exciting causes of ophthalmia still remains to be mentioned :—the repulsion of gonorrhœa or metastasis from the urethra to the eye. The occurrence is rare but it is sufficiently ascertained. Some have attempted to explain the phenomenon by supposing that there is a direct application of the gonorrhœal matter to the eye ; but this is altogether an unsat-isfactory hypothesis. Ophthalmia from repelled gonorrhœa is al-ways a violent disease, resembling in every respect the worst forms of Egyptian ophthalmia. While the eye continues to be inflamed, the discharge from the urethra generally ceases. The circumstan-ces which tend to produce this metastasis, or translation of the dis-ease, have never been explained, though they are probably within our reach.

Such are the most important of the causes of common inflam-mation of the eye ; and we have next to notice those which do not merely operate as exciting causes, but which have a further effect in giving a peculiar *character* to the disease. Of these the most important are scrofula and syphilis.

When ophthalmia occurs in a scrofulous habit of body, the parts most usually attacked are the conjunctiva, the tarsi, and the mei-bomian glands.* The disease is very common in young children from the time they are weaned, and is often the first indication of the presence of the scrofulous diathesis. Scrofulous ophthalmia occurs both in the acute and chronic from. The appearance of the eye in either is very characteristic. The disease is attended with a high degree of impatience of light, and a profuse secretion of tears, greatly exceeding what might have been expected from the corresponding severity of other symptoms. It is accompanied by a copious secretion from the glands of the tarsi of a thick matter, which during sleep agglutinates the eye-lids. Besides those con-sequences which it has in common with some other species of oph-thalmia, the scrofulous inflammation of the eye is often followed by ulceration of the cartilaginous edges of the palpebræ, which under bad management may continue to harass the patient for a number of years. It must be remembered, however, that this chronic in-flammation of the tarsi (the *ophthalmia tarsi* of Dr. Cullen), though very frequently, yet is not always dependent upon the scrofulous disposition.

---

* For a very clear and practical detail of the symptoms and treatment of scrofulous ophthalmia, see Jeffrey's " *Cases in Surgery*," London, 1820.

The venereal poison is occasionally the cause of inflammation of the conjunctiva, but for the most part, venereal ophthalmia assumes the form of inflammation of the iris. In this disease there is increased sensibility of the eye, with pain in the eye-ball, without the usual redness of the conjunctiva. The fine hair-like vessels of the iris may be observed injected with red blood, or small specks of blood may be seen extravasated upon that membrane. In a more advanced stage of the disease, the fibres of the iris are occasionally agglutinated. The edge that looks inwards appears thickened and immovable. A layer of lymph, or a globule of pus, may be seen upon it; or it is found adhering to the cornea or capsule of the lens. The latter stages of *iritis* are attended with severe pain, aggravated towards night.

Such are the appearances of venereal ophthalmia. The power of calomel over this state of disease is admitted to be very great; and it must therefore be considered a very singular circumstance in the history of iritis, that it has sometimes been *brought on* by calomel. This idea at least is entertained by some, but by others the correctness of the opinion has been called in question.

The treatment of ophthalmia involves too many surgical details to be entered upon with any minuteness here. During its early stages and before any disorganization of structure has taken place, its treatment must be conducted on the general principles which have been already explained. In the purulent and pustular forms of ophthalmia, the depleting system must be early resorted to, and vigorously pursued. Bleeding at the arm (in some cases opening the temporal artery) local blood-letting, especially by cupping-glasses applied to the temples, active purging, blistering, and nauseant doses of emetic tartar, are to form the groundwork of the treatment. Warm narcotic fomentations to the eye, assiduously applied, are of considerable use. In milder cases, leeches, purgatives, and cold lotions, will be sufficient. When the disease has assumed a chronic character, some applications of a stimulant kind, as the diluted citrine ointment, alum lotions, or the vinous solution of opium, are eminently serviceable. When the disease has advanced to such a point that any of the structures within the orbit are injured, the case becomes purely surgical.

Scrofulous and venereal ophthalmia require a treatment adapted to the particular circumstances of the exciting cause. In iritis from the syphilitic virus, mercury, as I have stated, is indispensable. In scrofulous ophthalmia an antiphlogistic plan of treatment must be judiciously combined with the administration of such medicines, and the observance of such a regimen, as are found useful in counter-acting the scrofulous disposition. A grain of calomel should be given every other night. The collyrium (R No. 115,) should be employed during the day ; and the ung. zinci applied to the edges of the eyelids every night. In severe cases change of air will be found indispensable.

The variolous ophthalmia is perhaps of all the varieties of this complaint the most uncontrollable. It commences, for the most part, about the eighth or ninth day of the eruption, when the scab-bing process is about to take place.) It is a *pustular* inflammation, often associated with violent diffuse inflammation of the integuments in some part, which runs on to sloughing or gangrene, or with ex-tensive cutaneous ulceration and hæmorrhage. This condition of the surface precludes in a great measure the employment of active measures for the relief of the eye, and the consequence is either total destruction of that organ, or such disorganization as leads to eventual blindness. Bleeding from the arm, leeches to the temples, and active cathartics, afford the only effectual means of relief. Mercury is here useless, and local applications of a stimulant kind improper.

, *Symptoms of Catarrh. Its Causes and Consequences. Peculiarities of the Epidemic or Contagious Catarrh. Treatment of Catarrh. Symptoms of Cynanche Tonsillaris. Its Causes, Terminations, and Treatment. Symptoms, Causes. and Consequences of Cynanche Parotidœa.*

CATARRH is the inflammation of the Schneiderian membrane. Dr. Cullen united it with inflammation of the mucous membrane lining the bronchia, but separated it from the other phlegmasiæ, on the plea of a peculiarity in the mode of its termination. On several ac-counts it is advisable to deviate from both these points of arrange-ment. Catarrh is characterised by a sense of fulness in the nose, of weight or fulness in the head, with an altered state of the secre-tion of the part, and more or less general fever. At first, the se-cretion from the membrane is altogether checked. The nose is stuffed and dry. After a time a thin acrid fluid is secreted, which gradually increases in quantity, becomes opaque, and alters in co-lour, until at length it is restored to its healthy condition. The in-flammation generally extends to the mucous membranes in the neighbourhood ; and hence redness and watering of the eyes, hoarseness, a sense of rawness in the windpipe, cough, and often a degree of oppression about the chest, with difficulty of breathing, accompany the other symptoms.

This disease, if properly attended to, seldom lasts long, but by neglect it is protracted, and not unfrequently leads to severe bron-chial inflammation, or to pneumonia—in scrofulous habits to affec-tions of the larynx, hæmoptysis, and phthisis. In some persons there is a very strong disposition to catarrh, and this is one of the marks of a scrofulous constitution. The only exciting causes of common catarrh are cold, and changes of weather ; but there is a

influenza

very curious variety of this disease, which arises apparently from contagion, and is well known under the name of *the influenza.* From the earliest records of the world epidemic catarrhs have been noticed. In the last century fifteen are distinctly described, the most remarkable of which was that of 1782. The chief peculiari. ties of the contagious epidemic catarrh are, that its attack is for the most part very sudden, and accompanied with an uncommon degree of languor and debility. This usually continues through the whole course of the disease, and even sometimes after the other symptoms have declined. It runs its course in three or four days. It is attended with a more urgent head-ache, and with more disorder of the stomach than occur in common catarrh. But se. vere as it sometimes is, the influenza is not a disease of danger. The bills of mortality seldom indicate any notable increase in the proportion of deaths during the existence of such an epidemic. El. derly persons are those who chiefly suffer by it, from the copious effusion of a viscid secretion into the air-passages.

On every occasion when an influenza has prevailed, the question has been agitated, whether it spreads by contagion and personal intercourse, or arises from some peculiar state of the atmosphere. Each of these opinions has found its supporters ; but a third class of pathologists hold a middle course, and while they admit the doc. trine of a particular contagion, maintain that it is conveyed by the air. Upon comparing the evidence which has been collected toge-. ther, with the view of elucidating this point, it is impossible, I think, not to perceive that the phenomena are best explained upon the principle, that the disease is propagated by contagion and person- *contagious* al intercourse. The difficulties which lie in the way of this ex- planation are obviated by the supposition of some *peculiarities* in the contagion of catarrh. There is every reason to believe, that the sphere of contagious influence differs in different diseases. That of small-pox has been shown by Dr. Haygarth to be very limited. Now, in the present instance, it is probable that the con- tagion is of a very diffusible nature—that the contagious effluvia will float to a considerable distance from the infected individual. It appears further, that its latent period is very short, perhaps not exceeding a few hours. On these principles we may account, in a manner sufficiently satisfactory, for the anomllies which the his- *a* tory of influenza presents. The circumstance of its travelling from the most distant parts of the world, and resisting in its progress the

22

extremes of European heat and cold, is conclusive as to its being something more than a common catarrh, produced by variations of atmospheric temperature.

Treatment Catarrh is seldom a disease of sufficient importance to become an object of medical treatment. In many cases it may be left with perfect safety to nature, when a spontaneous perspiration will commonly relieve the symptoms. If it prove somewhat more severe, the patient should keep within doors, abstain from animal food, take a dose of salts, and promote diaphoresis by the pediluvium and mild diluent drinks. To alleviate the cough, if it prove urgent, recourse may be had to a mucilaginous mixture, or an oily emulsion, as in the forms Nos. 57, 58, and 59. The hoarseness and sensation of rawness in the trachea are often lessened by the use of Mudge's inhaler. If there is considerable oppression about the chest, with difficult expectoration, and fever, antiphlogistic measures of more activity must be resorted to, proportioned to the violence of the symptoms, such as will hereafter be mentioned when treating of thoracic inflammation.

The epidemic catarrh is generally, but not invariably, more severe than the common form of the disease. The same general system of treatment is to be recommended also here. It appears of importance to promote diaphoresis and expectoration, by the employment, first, of antimonials, and afterwards of preparations of squill. Gentle aperients, and opiates at night are advisable. On account of the debility which usually accompanies the latter stages of this disease, bark and cordials are often necessary at that period.

CYNANCHE TONSILLARIS is the inflammation of the mucous membrane of the fauces, affecting especially the tonsils, and from thence spreading, so as to occupy, in many cases, the palate, uvula, pharynx, and membrane lining the back part of the nose. It is readily distinguished by the redness and swelling of the internal fauces, by the difficulty of deglutition, and the accompanying fever. When the inflammation runs high, the swelling of the tonsils is sometimes so great as to impede deglutition altogether, and patients have suffered severely, under such circumstances, from hunger and thirst. It sometimes extends to the orifice of the Eustachian tube, and pro-

duces deafness. Food or drink attempted to be swallowed are
sometimes returned by the nose, and this is a sure sign of very severe inflammation. In many cases, the tongue cannot be protruded without occasioning considerable pain. It is seldom that the
breathing is affected.

The febrile symptoms which accompany cynanche tonsillaris are
often urgent, and almost at all times severer than could have been
anticipated from the extent of local disease, or the importance of
the organ attacked. The pulse is often as high as 120, and the
tongue covered with a thick coat of fur. Much febrile debility attends this disease, particularly where the inflammation, in its appearance and progress, has the characters of erysipelas, more
than of phlegmon. The duration of the disease is very various.
Under common circumstances it will subside by resolution in the
course of a few days ; but occasionally, a great degree of debility
continues, and the convalescence is protracted for many weeks.

1. Cynanche tonsillaris frequently terminates, when the inflammation is active, by suppuration in one or both tonsils. The rapidity with which pus sometimes forms in the loose texture of these
organs is very remarkable, but occasionally six or seven days
elapse before the inflamed and highly stretched membrane gives
way spontaneously. The matter of the abscess is fœtid and nau-
seons. The bursting of it is always followed by a great and in-
stantaneous relief.

2. When the inflammation, instead of being of a vivid red colour, has an aspect inclining to purple, we consider that it partakes
of the nature of erysipelas, and it will then generally be found to
terminate by superficial vesicles and ulcers, of a white or grey colour, similar in their nature to *aphthæ*. These often create a great
deal of alarm from their resemblance to the sloughs of cynanche
maligna, but they commonly go off in a few days, and are productive of no other inconvenience.

3. In some cases, the inflammation will neither advance nor re-
cede ; and I have in vain attempted to determine upon what this
depends. It is most common in persons of a scrofulous habit of
body, and who from their aspect might be considered as predisposed to phthisis pulmonalis. After the lapse of a fortnight or three
weeks, the disease will in such cases commonly give way, but occasionally a permanent enlargement of the tonsil remains. This,
I think, chiefly occurs in delicate young women.

Cynanche tonsillaris is a disease of little or no danger, scarcely any fatal cases of it being on record. It is rendered severe by neglect ; and danger may sometimes be apprehended from the tonsils pressing on the glottis. Its immediate exciting cause is, in all cases, exposure to cold, as from getting wet feet, or from sitting in a partial current of air, particularly if the body be previously overheated. It affects chiefly the young, and those of plethoric habit. It occurs especially in the spring and winter seasons, and in cold and variable climates. Habit increases the disposition to the disease, so that some persons scarcely ever pass twelve months without experiencing an attack of it, and in them it is induced by very slight causes. This affection occurs symptomatic of scarlatina, and small-pox, and it sometimes attends measles, lichen, catarrh, and croup. It is occasioned also by the poison of mercury and the venereal virus; but in all these cases there will be found sufficient in the aspect of the disease, or the concomitant symptoms, to prevent ambiguity in the diagnosis.

An antiphlogistic system of treatment is required in cynanche tonsillaris, but venesection is seldom, if ever, necessary. Leeches to the external fauces have been recommended, and are frequently very serviceable. If the inflammation runs high, the tonsils, or more properly the velum pendulum palati, may be scarified, and a little blood so obtained affords very effectual relief. In slighter cases, it will be sufficient to rub the throat with some rubefacient liniment, as the *linimentum ammoniæ*; and to direct the frequent use of a repellant gargle, as of the infusion of roses with a due proportion of tincture of capsicum (R No. 106.) In all cases, a saline purgative, as an ounce of the sulphate of magnesia, is advisable ; but if much fever be present, the patient should be confined to bed, and the saline draughts (R Nos. 39 and 40) administered. If suppuration is likely to take place, it may be promoted by the employment of mild emollient gargles, as of the dec. hord. compos. of the London Pharmacopœia. An emetic is sometimes directed with perfect safety, with the view of promoting the bursting of the abscess. The decoction of bark may be employed as a gargle when there are superficial ulcerations or specks, but taken internally it will be found to aggravate the febrile symptoms. As long, therefore, as the pulse remains frequent, with thirst and restlessness, saline draughts only should be given. When the fever

subsides, the decoction of bark and acid (R No. 68) may be administered with advantage.

When the disease is disposed to be stationary, a blister to the
fauces, or better to the upper part of the sternum, or behind the
ears, will prove useful. In the state of chronic enlargement of the
tonsil, little can be done by internal medicine ; and gargles, even
of the most powerful kind, are generally quite ineffectual. The
disease sometimes yields in the most unexpected manner, probably
in consequence of some change taking place in the constitution,
the nature of which is altogether inscrutable. Some have recommended the removal of the part, either by the knife, or by ligature,
when the disease has lasted a considerable time. In many cases
this may be done with great propriety ; but as a general rule it
should not be resorted to, unless the breathing be impeded, or
cough or some other serious inconvenience be produced.

_____

CYNANCHE PAROTIDŒA, or the mumps, is the inflammation of
the parotid gland, interesting chiefly in a pathological point of view.

It begins by symptoms of fever, soon followed by swelling of the
gland, appearing as a tumour at the corner of the jaw, and gradu-
ly extending over the face and neck. The swelling continues to
increase till the fourth day, and then usually goes off by resolution.
The disease chiefly attacks children. It is often epidemic, and
manifestly contagious. Occasionlly however it attacks adults, occurs *sporadically*, and is attributable to cold. In a few cases it has
been known to terminate by suppuration.

The most curious circumstance connected with the history of
the mumps, is its tendency to affect the testicle by metastasis, and
this most remarkably when it occurs in adults. The testicle swells
as the inflammation of the parotid gland subsides ; but this secondary affection seldom lasts long, or proves troublesome. In a considerable number of cases, a further translation has taken place to
the brain, and symptoms of genuine phrenitis have supervened.*

* See a very instructive history of an epidemic mumps that prevailed on
board his Majesty's ship Ardent, in November 1807, by Mr. Noble—Ed.
Med. and Surg. Journal, July 1808.

It does not appear that either of these metastases can be prevent.
ed by medical treatment, or that they are relieved by any attempts
to bring back the inflammation to its original seat.   They must be
treated in every respect as idiopathic inflammations of the testicle
and brain.

Setting aside this consideration, the mumps can scarcely be said
to require medical assistance.   A saline purgative, warm fomenta.
tions, and confinement to the house, are all that it appears neces.
sary to insist upon.

CHAP. VII.

Laryngeal Inflammation. Symptoms of Acute Laryngitis. Its Causes and Treatment. Symptoms and Progress of Chronic Laryngitis. Symptomatic Affections of the Larynx. Treatment of Chronic Laryngitis. Of Croup. Its Symptoms and Progress. Of the Disposition to Spasm in Croup. Of the spurious or Spasmodic Croup. Appearances on Dissection. Causes of this Disease, predisposing and occasional. Treatment of Inflammatory Croup. Of spasmodic Croup. Of Bronchial polypus, or Chronic Croup.

THE inflammatory affections of the wind-pipe, though comparatively rare, are yet diseases of great importance ; for this organ is essential to life, and the smallest disturbance of its function is sufficient to put life in danger. Inflammation of the larynx and trachea may co-exist, but they oftener occur independent of each other; and as their pathology is in many respects different, we shall consider them as distinct diseases. The larynx is subject both to acute and chronic inflammation, and these will require separate consideration.

Acute laryngitis is a very uncommon disease, and, until lately, appears to have been overlooked by authors. The fullest, and I believe I may add the original account of the disease is by Dr. Baillie[*] in 1809, whose observations comprise almost every thing hitherto known concerning it. Since the appearance of Dr. Baillie's paper many well marked cases of the same affection have been published by Dr. Farre, Dr. Arnold, and others. It is characterized by fever, pain referred to the larynx, difficulty of breathing

[*] Vide "Transactions of a Society for the Improvement of Medical and Chirurgical Knowledge," vol. iii, page 275. A very distinct case of acute laryngitis, with dissection, had previously been detailed by Mr. Mayd. See Med. Communications, vol. ii, page 479. 1799.

and of swallowing, hoarseness, or complete loss of voice, and spasmodic exacerbations of all the symptoms, creating a sense of suffocation which is urgent in the extreme. In some cases the pain is increased by pressure upon the thyroid cartilage. The disease is attended by the perpetual hawking, or spitting up of a tough gelatinous mucus. If the epiglottis partake of the inflammation, which it often does, any attempt to pull the tongue forward will be attended with pain. In the course of the disease, the cellular membrane, in the neighbourhood of the larynx has been observed to take on inflammatory action, from which has resulted hardness and fulness of the throat externally. In mild cases deglutition is but little impeded; but in most of the severe cases on record, the attempt to swallow fluids is followed by a violent spasm, sickness, and vomiting, and the fluid itself is sometimes forcibly ejected by the nose. The usual duration of the disease is four days. It is one of the most urgent danger.

On dissection, the inner membrane of the larynx is found red and thickened, or œdematous. Pus is frequently met with in the sacculi laryngis; and sometimes, though not often, there is an effusion of coagulable lymph upon the membrane, as in croup. Acute laryngitis has only been known to arise from cold. It occurs chiefly in persons turned of forty, and Dr. Baillie suspects that a disposition to it is given by previous attacks of cynanche tonsillaris. As far as my observation extends, it occurs chiefly in languid and exhausted habits, and is *preceded* by a long period of debility, and mental anxiety. It seems to prevail mostly in the months of March and April. The diagnosis from cynanche tonsillaris is sufficiently obvious. From cynanche trachealis, it is distinguished by the want of that peculiar sound of the breathing which we shall presently speak of, and by the period of life at which it occurs.

The treatment of the disease is to be regulated by the view which has been taken of its pathology. A very prompt and vigorous practice can alone offer any prospect of successful termination. Large bleedings are required; and at the onset, they should be pushed so as to produce fainting. Leeches may be applied to the throat when the violence of the symptoms has been subdued; and a brisk cathartic given as soon as the power of deglutition has been in some degree restored. Any attempt however to give medicines internally while deglutition is dreaded, will aggravate the sufferings, without lessening the dangers of the patient. The bowels should at first be

opened by means of emollient glysters. The evident tendency to
spasmodic exacerbation in this disease renders it probable that opium may be advantageously given, when the proper evacuations have
been premised. As a last resource some have recommended tracheotomy ; but, upon the whole, considering the disadvantageous
circumstances under which the operation must here be performed,
it can scarcely be thought advisable.*

Chronic inflammation of the larynx is far from being so rare as
the acute form of the affection. It usually begins by pricking pains
in the larynx, some degree of fever, cough, and difficulty of breathing. The most striking symptom of the disease, when fully formed,
is the long inspiration which occurs in consequence of the constriction of the glottis. The breathing is attended too with a peculiar
noise, not unlike that which characterizes croup. To these symptoms are usually added, a copious but difficult expectoration of ropy
mucus, a peculiar hoarseness or huskiness of voice, and often some
degree of pain of the chest. The disease is attended by a slow, or
hectic fever. The pulse is never full or strong, but always very
frequent. The skin is hot, the tongue cherry red and dry, and the
bowels costive. As the disease advances, respiration becomes more
and more difficult, and is aggravated in paroxysms, during which
the face often becomes livid. The patient at length dies from suffocation. The duration of the disease is various, extending from
three to twelve months.

On dissection, ulceration is found within the larynx, generally
in the sacculi laryngis ; and along with this there is commonly
some degree of thickening of the surrounding parts, and in a great
majority of cases, ossification : spicula of bone, that is to say, are
to be felt within the ulcerated cavity. This phenomenon is not peculiar to ulcerated states of the larynx. I have observed it in a variety of cases of internal ulceration. Upon what pathological principle this connection of ulceration with ossification depends, has
never, as far as I know, been hitherto explained.

The repeated application of leeches to the throat affords the best
prospect of relieving this very dangerous disease. Vomiting is allowed by all to be very prejudicial, as it creates much pain. Any
expectorant medicines which may be given, therefore, should be of
the mildest kind. Alterative courses of calomel, cicuta, and opium, are usually recommended, with the decoction of sarsaparilla,

* See Appendix ; Note O.

and a milk diet. Blisters may be tried. Bronchotomy has been performed in several cases, in some of which it has proved partially, and in a few permanently beneficial.

Permanent hoarseness, unattended by pain, fever, expectoration, or any other mark of disease, is far from being uncommon. It appears to consist in a thickening of the membrane lining the larynx. This, and probably all states of chronic inflammation and ulceration of the larynx, are symptomatic of some constitutional affection, generally of scrofula, and a diseased state of the larynx is frequently complicated with true tubercular phthisis, constituting that variety of the disorder termed *phthisis laryngea.* I have seen it orginate also in a constitution worn down by syphilis and mercury. In the progress of consumption, particularly towards its latter stages, it is not unusual to find a violent pain come on, referred to the larynx, and attended with hoarseness. From the violence of the pain, it might be supposed owing to inflammation; but leeches and blisters are of no service, and it generally goes off in four or five days. It is probably a sympathetic pain connected, perhaps, with the recurrent nerve. Dr. Cheyne, in his pathology of the larynx and bronchia, speaks of an affection, in every respect similar to that which we have called chronic laryngitis happening as a consequence of measles. It prevails chiefly among children of scrofulous families, and proves very fatal.

CROUP.

Croup, or the acute inflammation of the mucous membrane of the trachea, was not described with any degree of clearness by the ancient authors. The first regular history of it is to be found in the letters of Martin Ghisi, 1749. Dr. Home, of Edinburgh, made it known to the practitioners of this country by his "Enquiry into the Croup," published in 1765. For the fullest account of the disease which has since appeared, we are indebted to Dr. Cheyne.* †

* The Pathology of the Membrane of the Larynx and Bronchia. Edin. 1809,

† See Appendix; Note P.

Lymph

Croup is characterised by inflammatory fever, a sonorous inspiration of a very peculiar character, and difficult respiration, aggra-
ted in paroxysms. It prevails chiefly from the first to the third
year of life ; and though occasionally met with as late as the tenth
or twelfth year, it is yet clear that the tendency to it diminishes in
a remarkable manner as life advances. The almost complete immunity from genuine croup enjoyed by adults, is perhaps referable
to some alteration which the mucous membrane of the trachea undergoes about the age of puberty. It is not to be understood however that in advanced life inflammation never affects the trachea,
but merely that the symptoms of such a disease are not then distinguishable from the more common varieties of *pneumonia*.

The true symptoms of croup are often preceded by those of
common catarrh, and sometimes by ulcerated sore throat. Occasionally, however, they show themselves from the very first, coming on towards the evening, or perhaps during the night. The child
wakes with an unusual cough ; and the inspirations, particularly
those which immediately follow the cough, are long, and attended
with that crowing noise, which is the most striking characteristic
of the disease. Feverish symptoms succeed, and often run high.
The pulse is frequent and hard, with thirst and extreme restlessness. The natural functions, as well as those of the brain, are not
always disturbed to a corresponding degree. I have seen a child
taking food and running about, while the disease was making rapid
advances. If it proceed unchecked, all the symptoms are quickly
aggravated. Respiration becomes more laborious, the cough troublesome, and the expectoration difficult, until the child dies, either
suddenly in a paroxysm of dyspnœa, or more gradually by *suffocation*. The usual duration of the disease, when violent, and unin- *time*
fluenced by medical treatment, is about thirty-six or forty hours.
Its danger is such, that if the alarming symptoms are not moderated during the first twelve hours, it generally proves fatal. If, by
the efforts of nature or art, the child recovers what has been called *Second*
the *second stage*, the convalescence is always tedious, and is at- *Stage*
tended by the expectoration of portions of a membrane, whose origin and nature will presently be noticed. In a milder form of the
disease, where the difficulty of breathing is not so urgent at the
commencement, the cough about the second day becomes loose
and the skin moist, the fever abates and the voice gradually recovers its natural tone.

One of the most important considerations in the history of croup, *tendency to exacerbation an argument for spasmodic character of disease* is the disposition which it shows to occasional *exacerbations* of all the symptoms. This tendency to spasm is apparent in all the diseases which affect the air passages, whether arising from inflammation or not. It is observable in laryngitis, acute and chronic bronchitis, hooping-cough, and asthma. It is no less manifest in croup; and some have contended that these exacerbations mark the true nature of the disease, and point it out as one of a *spasmodic*, rather than of an inflammatory nature. Such an opinion is countenanced by the well-ascertained fact, that children are occasionally affected by a kind of *croupy* inspiration, apparently the result of spasm of the muscles about the glottis, which abates and recurs, without producing in the intervals any unpleasant effects. To such *spasmodic croup* a disease, the term spasmodic or *spurious* croup has been applied. It is frequently accompanied by partial, and sometimes by general convulsions, or other marks of cerebral irritation.* It is reasonable to presume these cases depend principally upon the high degree of irritability in the child's system; but they have for their exciting causes, painful dentition, a foul state of the stomach, or accumulations in the bowels. The diagnosis of this, the spurious, from the true inflammatory croup has excited much attention. It is however not always easy, nor am I inclined to attach any great degree of pathological or practical importance to it : first, because there is reason to suspect that the one may degenerate into the other ; and secondly, because the chief danger in croup arises from neglecting the disease in its early stage.

false membrane   Examination of the trachea, in those who die of croup, has made us acquainted with a very peculiar morbid appearance ; viz. an adventitious membrane, or tube of coagulable lymph, which is thrown out by the inflamed vessels of the trachea, and in a great measure blocks up the passage. It arises a little below the larynx, and extends, in many cases, to the bifurcation of the bronchia. A semi-purulent fluid is commonly found in the trachea at the same time, and occasionally tracesare also met with of pulmonic inflammation. Frequent as is the appearance of such a præternatural membrane in those who die of croup, it is by no means to be considered as a constant or necessary part of the disease. Its formation is often indicated by the manner in which the child breathes—throwing the head back, so as to put the trachea upon the stretch.

* Consult Dr. Clarke's " Commentaries on the Diseases of Children." chap. iv, page 87.

The most usual exciting cause of croup is cold, and particularly exposure to a damp atmosphere. It prevails, therefore, chiefly in winter and spring, and is more common in the cold and temperate climates than between the tropics. Children who have once had an attack of croup, are liable to have it renewed on the application of very slight causes. A common catarrh will, in such constitutions, be often attended by croupy symptoms, until the thirteenth or fourteenth year of life. Second attacks of croup are seldom so violent as the first, but they always require the utmost caution on the part of the practitioner. Pathologists have almost invariably agreed in stating that the croup is not contagious. Some cases, however, which have lately fallen under my care, incline me to believe, that this opinion has been adopted without due consideration; and in a disease so violent and fatal as croup, it is highly important that this question should meet with attention. It is acknowledged by Dr. Cheyne, that in those cases which are attended, at the commencement, by a sloughy state of the fauces, a suspicion of contagion may be entertained; but he suggests that these are cases of cynanche maligna, upon which croupy symptoms supervene. Such an explanation of the circumstance is certainly plausible, but without attempting to determine whether it be pathologically correct, I feel myself bound to act upon the principle, that croup, in its worst or most malignant form, is capable of being communicated by *contagion.**

With a view to treatment, croup has been divided into two stages; the first being that of inflammatory action, the second being distinguished by the formation of that præternatural membrane, which we have already described. During the former, the chief reliance is to be placed on general and local bleeding, the warm bath, blisters, an emetic, and occasional purgatives. If these means fail to give relief in the first period of the disease, the object is then to promote expectoration, to relieve the disposition to spasm which so generaly prevails at that time, and to support the strength of the system, which will commonly be found to have suffered from the previous measures of depletion. For these purposes, recourse may be had to preparations of squill, camphor, æther, digitalis, and opium, and to various medicines of the tonic and cordial kind. Some add to this an occasional emetic, the exhibition of small doses

* This question is considered, and various cases cited, illustrating the facts, in the Lond. Med. and Physical Journal for Oct. 1825, and Jan. 1826.

of calomel, and, as a last resource, bronchotomy.   To this sketch of the general plan of treatment in croup, I shall subjoin a few prac. tical suggestions.

ipecac.   A vomit of ipecacuanha, administered at the very outset of the disease, appears in some instances to have checked it altogether. The continued exhibition of emetics, with the view of removing the mucus or lymph, which may be collected in the trachea, is a prae. tice which cannot be recommended.   Some authors have noticed, that there is difficulty in exciting vomiting in this disease, but this I have never experienced.   In a few cases, on the contrary, I have found vomiting a very troublesome symptom.   The great nicety in

Blood-letting   the treatment of croup consists in the management of the general and local blood-letting.   Children do not bear the evacuation of blood like adults; and in this disease it has appeared to me to in. crease, in some instances, the disposition to spasm about the glottis. The relief, however, afforded to the breathing, by taking away a few ounces of blood from the jugular vein, in a full stream, is al. ways great and immediate, and should never be neglected in the early periods of the disease.   If the symptoms recur, and the pulse continues hard, it may be repeated a second time, but a few leech. es to the throat will often supersede the necessity of further deple. tion from the system.   The draught (R No. 38) may be given every two hours, preceded by the purgative powder (R. No. 10.)

calomel   The exhibition of calomel in small, but frequently repeated doses (as from one to five grains every two hours) has been strongly re. commended by some practitioners, even from the commencement of the disease ; but my own experience would incline me to say, that the advantages of this practice have been rated much too high.

Blisters   ly.   The propriety of applying large blisters to the throat, has also appeared to me very questionable.   Experience, as well as theory, induce me to think, that the irritation produced by blisters may sometimes extend to the inflamed membrane, and aggravate the symptoms of the disease.   The warm bath frequently affords great

Bath   relief to the breathing, and may be directed at night, or even twice during the day.   When the measures of depletion have been car. ried as far as the strength of the constitution admits, recourse must

digitalis   be had to such medicines as allay irritation and promote expecto. ration.   The tincture of digitalis may be exhibited in small doses ; and to the draught containing it may be added a proportion of oxy.

squills   mel of squills, and of the compound tincture of camphor (as in R No. 88.)   Laudanum, or the spt. æther. sulphur. may be substitu.

Laudanum

ted. The operation of bronchotomy has been suggested, but in croup I believe it to be altogether inadmissible.

The complaint which I have described under the title of _spas. modic croup_ is one of comparatively little danger, and will generally be found to yield to a gentle emetic, followed by a dose of calomel and rhubarb. It certainly is dependent in many instances upon a disordered condition of the primæ viæ. In urgent cases, threatening fits, leeches should be applied to the temples. When the croupy inspiration recurs at intervals for a considerable length of time, assafœtida may be given with advantage. During the period of dentition, the free scarification of the gums should never be, omitted.

There is a very rare disease affecting adults, called _bronchial polypus_, which is believed to be dependent upon chronic inflammation of the mucous membrane of the windpipe and bronchia. It is characterized by catarrhal symptoms, wheezing, and the expectoration of portions of a membrane which must evidently have lined those parts. Such _polypi_, as they have been called, are sometimes solid, but more commonly tubular. The fit of coughing which displaces them is often alarmingly violent. The disease has been known to last many years,*

* The writers on it are Dr. Warren, in Coll. Trans. vol. i, p 407 ; and Dr. Cheyne, in Edinburgh Med. and Surg. Journal, vol. iv, p. 441.

Pleurisy, Bronchitis & PNEUMONIA.

ACUTE inflammation occurring in any of the structures within the thorax, is what is understood by the term PNEUMONIA, the different species of which, as detailed by nosologists, have always had a reference to the particular structures which are the seat of disease. The principal of these are the pleura, the mucous membrane of the bronchia, and that continuation of it which lines the air-cells of the lungs, the proper cellular structure of the lungs, and the pericardium. In the present chapter, I shall confine my attention to the acute inflammation of the three first of these textures, and shall subsequently treat of the sub-acute and chronic forms of bronchial inflammation, of phthisis pulmonalis, or chronic inflammation of the substance of the lungs, and of the acute and chronic pericarditis.

Thoracic inflammation, in all its various forms, is characterized by the combination of the four following symptoms,—fever, pain of the side, difficult breathing, and cough; which constitute, therefore, the definition of pneumonia. But each of these symptoms is variously modified by circumstances; of which the most important is the structure, primarily or most essentially implicated. The pleura being that, the inflammation of which exhibits most perfectly the characters of the genus, I begin by describing the symptoms of *pleurisy.*

1. An acute pain of the side, highly aggravated on full inspira-

tion, is the leading characteristic of this disease. The respiration is short and hurried, and is generally performed with most difficul-ty when lying on the side affected. A hard and short cough is al-most always present; and, as it aggravates the pain, is stifled as much as possible by the patient. At first it is commonly *dry*, that is to say, without expectoration. The accompanying fever is ur-gent. The pulse is frequent, strong, and *hard*. The tongue is loaded with a thick fur. Thirst, restlessness, a hot skin, and a scanty and high-coloured state of the urine may be noticed. The concurrence of these symptoms precludes all possibility of ambi-guity as to the nature of the disease, or the requisite means of re-lief. When blood is drawn from the arm, it will be found *cupped* and buffy. In some cases, inflammatory action is confined, through-out the whole course of the disease, strictly to the pleura. In oth-ers it implicates, to a greater or less degree, the contiguous por-tions of the substance of the lungs.

2. When the mucous membrane lining the larger branches of the bronchia is affected by acute inflammation, that is to say, in *acute bronchitis*, the following is the character of the symptoms. It may be right first to mention, that this form of thoracic inflam-mation is less frequent than the preceding, though on the whole more dangerous. The most urgent symptoms is a sense of *tight-ness* or constriction about the chest, referred generally to the pit of the stomach, but sometimes very unequivocally to the precise seat of the disease. Respiration is hurried, and accompanied by a wheezing in the throat, although the thorax can perhaps be expan-ded to its full extent. There is cough, which from the first is at-tended with some degree of expectoration. The general febrile symptoms are very severe. The pulse is frequent, but it often wants that fulness and hardness which characterise pleurisy. Not unfrequently it is intermitting. There is always observable a re-markable expression of *anxiety* in the countenance, generally with paleness. The functions of the brain are here more disturbed than in the common cases of thoracic inflammation. In the progress of this disease, authors have noticed, that occasionally, at a partic-ular period, the constitutional symptoms are suddenly converted from those of high inflammatory action into such as indicate ex-treme debility, or exhaustion.

3. The *substance* of the lungs is also the seat of acute inflamma-tion, and the term *peripneumony* is usually applied to this form of thoracic inflammation. In some of these cases, the inflammation

24

occupies the ramifications of the *mucous* membrane, but the proper cellular texture of the lungs (or parenchyma) is probably in others the primary structure affected. The student however need not perplex himself by attempts to establish a diagnosis between peripneumony and acute bronchitis. It is rather in deference to commonly received opinion, than from a conviction of their real differences, that I am induced to treat of them separately.

The usual symptoms of peripneumony are, an obtuse pain, sometimes referred to the side, but more usually to the sternum, or epigastrium, and occasionally to the back or shoulder; impeded breathing, which is often particularly difficult in the recumbent posture; a moist cough; and fever, the character of which, however, is subject to great variety. Sometimes there is so little constitutional disturbance, so little febrile oppression, that the disease makes rapid advances before its nature is suspected. Sometimes the pulse is hard, but much more commonly it is oppressed, labouring, and full. Peripneumony is often attended by a puffiness of the features, lividity of the lips and under the eyes, eruptions about the lips, and occasionally head-ache; symptoms obviously referable to the difficulty experienced in the transmission of blood through the lungs.

It is certainly of importance to be aware of the minute differences in the *symptoms* of pneumonic inflammation; but to detail them would serve only to distract the attention from those great features of it now enumerated, which the student should keep steadily in view. The variety in the *progress* of the disease demands a more extended notice. The insidious manner in which it sometimes makes its approach, is the first point which should be urged, so directly opposed as it is to the *sudden* attack experienced in other cases. It is well worthy of remark, that a degree of inflammatory action may, and often does exist in the lungs for many weeks, without producing any serious disorganization in their structure. At other times, the continuance of inflammation, even for a few days, lays the foundation of extensive and irremediable mischief. Notwithstanding, however, the importance of the organ attacked, the prognosis in pneumonia is not unfavourable. There is no form of inflammatory affection which is so completely under the control of the physician as this. Resolution, therefore is its most frequent termination; but it is to be observed, that in all the forms of bronchial inflammation, and in a large proportion also of the most genuine cases of pleurisy, the subsidence of inflammation is attended

by an increased secretion from the mucous membrane of the bronchia.

1. This important principle points out the necessity of attending
accurately, during the whole course of the disease, to the *state of
the expectoration*; by which, no less than by the variations in the
four leading symptoms already stated, is the progress of the inflammation to be judged of, and the treatment regulated. A copious
and easy expectoration of mucus marks the decline of the disease.
Nor is the prognosis less favourable, if the sputa be tinged with
blood. A cream-like deposition in the urine, and a copious warm
perspiration, are equally evidences of the subsidence of inflammatory action. Under certain circumstances, however, the secretion
from the mucous membrane of the bronchia may be so profuse, as
to exhaust the patient by the quantity of the discharge, or by the
necessary efforts for its expulsion.

2. Allied, in some degree, to the termination by mucous expectoration, is that by serous effusion into the air-cells. So far, at
least, it is allied, that we presume this effusion takes place from the
vessels of the inflamed membrane ; but in a practical point of view,
they differ most essentially. Mucous expectoration is always desirable. Serous effusion is almost uniformly fatal. The effused
fluid is serum, or, more strictly, water ; and it takes place, not so
much when the disease has a tendency to *resolve* as during the
height of inflammatory action. It has been supposed that the disposition to *serous effusion* is sometimes given, or increased, by the
too liberal employment of the lancet in the prior stages of the disease ; but I have more commonly found it to occur where no treatment whatever had been adopted. The rapidity with which it
takes place is a circumstance deserving of notice. The symptoms
which attend it are, a livid appearance of the whole countenance,
and a sudden sinking of the pulse, with urgent dyspnœa. It is, I
believe, peculiar to peripneumony, and those diseases which have
supervening peripneumony, and it proves fatal by suffocation.

3. Every form of pneumonia occasionally terminates by suppuration, which may be either diffused or circumscribed. When the
disease is violent, the constitution much enfeebled, and the pleura
the chief seat of disorder, pus is frequently thrown out by the inflamed membrane without ulceration, and is found after death floating loose in the cavity of the thorax, constituting *empyema*. Acute
bronchitis in like manner sometimes terminates by a profuse secretion of true purulent matter from the vessels of the inflamed mem-

brane. These states of disease are usually fatal. Pleurisy and peripneumony on the other hand occasionally terminate by the formation of one or more abscesses, which in this situation are called
vomicæ. The symptoms of vomica are, a frequent and full pulse, the
continuance of dyspnœa, a sensation of weight, or fulness in a particular part of the chest, and after a certain time (three weeks or a
month) hectic fever and purulent expectoration.   The danger attending vomica will be proportioned to the strength of the constitution and the size of abscess. In a strong habit of body even a large
vomica will occasionally heal, but in a debilitated subject no reasonable hope of recovery can be entertained.   The matter expectorated is often exceedingly fœtid, a circumstance which will assist
in the diagnosis of simple vomica from tubercular consumption.
Gangrene (or rather sloughy abscess) of the lungs has been described by Laennec, and others. The occurrence is rare, and never
very distinctly characterized during life.

4. Pleurisy is frequently followed by *adhesions* of the opposite
surfaces of the pleura to each other.   It is remarkable, that this
takes place without being productive, as far as can be judged, of
any particular inconvenience to the breathing. In some cases serum
is effused with or without coagulable lymph, and the result is *hydrothorax.*

5. Coagulable lymph is sometimes thrown out by the vessels of
the proper cellular texture of the lungs, giving rise to what has
been called *hepatization,* or hardening of the lungs, a state in which
they are impervious to air, and of course incapable of performing
their functions.   The state of condensed or hepatized lung is not
uncommon.   When simple, that is, uncombined with tubercle, it
principally occurs in persons of strong fibre and plethoric habit,
giving rise to the following combination of symptoms :—difficult
breathing, cough, giddiness, and permanently loaded tongue, without emaciation or œdema. It may continue for a considerable time.
At length, however, acute inflammation supervenes, speedily proving fatal ; or the symptoms gradually merge in those of common
consumption. (Polypous concretions in the heart and great blood-
vessels are usually met with in persons thus carried off,) marking
the *entonic* character of the preceding inflammation.

6. It remains to be noticed, that occasionally, and more especially in the peripneumony of children, no morbid appearance is
discoverable after death, except perhaps a slight engorgement
of a portion of the lungs with blood. This renders it probable,

that, independent of effusion and consequent suffocation, pneumonia may prove fatal through the mere violence of inflammatory action. This principle in pathology will hereafter be more fully illustrated.

Pneumonia is, perhaps, the only inflammatory affection which occurs with equal frequency at every period of life, and under every variety of habit, circumstance, and situation. Its most common exciting cause is cold, and alterations of atmospheric temperature. It often supervenes on other diseases ; such as measles, small-pox, catarrh, hooping cough, and occasionally rheumatism and gout. The disposition to pneumonia is much increased by long-continued exercise of the lungs in speaking, by severe exercise of the body generally, and by its having before occurred. It is a frequent effect of that habitual indulgence in spirituous liquors, so common in the lower orders of this country. It prevails chiefly in the winter and spring seasons, like every other form of thoracic disease.

The principles of treatment in pneumonia are sufficiently simple ; but the *extent* to which evacuation should be carried, having a due regard to the period of the disease, the nature of the prevailing epidemic, the age and circumstances of the patient, and the urgency of the symptoms, must be regulated by a habit of discrimination, that can be acquired only by clinical observation. In the acquisition of this knowledge, so essential to the safety of the patient, the student may perhaps be assisted by a few considerations which it shall be my object now to lay before him.

1. In bleeding from the arm we possess a power of controlling pneumonic inflammation, the efficacy of which has been acknowledged in all ages, and is obvious, indeed, to the most superficial observer ; nor is it difficult to account for this, when we reflect that the morbid action occupies the branches of the pulmonary artery, with which the veins of the body generally are physiologically associated. Beneficial as bleeding is, much must of course depend on the period of the disease at which it is first practised, on the manner in which it is performed, the quantity drawn, and the frequency of its repetition. Above all, in estimating the probable advantage of blood-letting in any particular case, the natural strength of the constitution is to be looked to. Weakly habits will not bear the extent of blood-letting which is necessary to subdue a severe attack. Old persons and infants have not the power of regenerating blood so quickly as adults. Physicians have been struck, at all times, with the effect produced by taking the blood from a *large orifice*, in this and other urgent cases of local inflammation ; and it

(margin handwriting: Quantity of blood)

certainly cannot be too strongly urged as an indispensable point in practice. The orifice should be such as to allow a pound of blood to flow in five, or at furthest in six minutes. The quantity to be taken at one time cannot be defined with any degree of accuracy. A pound of blood may be looked upon as a proper *average* for an adult. As a general rule it may be stated, that some effect ought to be produced on the *system*, before the orifice is closed; either faintishness, or sickness, or diminution of pain, or of the strength of arterial contraction.

2. In all cases of pneumonia of the least severity, bleeding from the system must be repeated, and the principal circumstances by which the frequency of its repetition is to be regulated, are the state of the symptoms, and the appearance of the blood drawn. Blood-letting is better borne in pleurisy than where the mucous membrane of the bronchia is the chief seat of disease; and as expectoration of mucus is one of the means by which all inflammation within the chest is relieved, venesection, on several accounts must be practised with great caution when that symptom occurs. When suppuration has commenced, copious bleedings are inadmissible, but small bleedings may then often be resorted to, with the happiest effect. Although the presence or absence of buff is not to decide our practice as to future bleeding, still, when present, it may often materially *assist* us in our judgment. If the blood, besides being buffy, be cupped, and *fringed* at the edges, we need have little hesitation in repeating the evacuation. Should the blood appear with a flat surface of buff, and the coagulum be loose, further bleeding may indeed be still necessary, but it must be practised with very great caution. In the pneumonia of infants, and occasionally with adults also, leeches and cupping may be substituted for bleeding at the arm; but the circumstances warranting this are very few.*

3. Moderate purging, by castor oil, or the neutral salts, is a useful auxiliary in the treatment of pneumonia; but the advantages of purging are, upon the whole, much less obvious in thoracic diseases, than in those of the head or abdominal cavity. Any attempt to overcome decided thoracic inflammation by severe purging will always prove ineffectual, and often prejudicial.† Refrigerant medicines, as nitre (R No. 37,) may be employed with great propriety. A free expectoration being, as we have said, the means which na-

* See Appendix ; Note Q.   † See Appendix ; Note R.

ture most commonly adopts for carrying off inflammation within the chest, it might be supposed that expectorant medicines would prove useful ; but the reliance to be placed upon them is very small. Antimony and ipecacuanha are the only ones of this class which can be recommended. The oxymel of squills (R No. 86) is useful, but should be delayed till the inflammatory symptoms have in some degree subsided. Opium is quite inadmissible during the active stages of pneumonic inflammation. Even in the more advanced periods of the disease, it must be given with extreme caution, on account of its tendency to check expectoration. Some practitioners are disposed to place considerable reliance on the combination of opium with calomel. It will be found however a very inefficient substitute for blood-letting, and it is too active a medicine to be employed as a mere auxiliary.

4. Blisters are unquestionably of the greatest importance in the treatment of pneumonia, but they should not be applied while the pulse is hard, and the blood appears cupped. It is not until the tone of the system has been lowered by venesection, that their good effects will become apparent.

5. If the inflammation has terminated in suppuration, besides the small bleedings already recommended when the difficulty of breathing becomes particularly urgent, advantage will be derived from the continued exhibition of the tincture of digitalis. The strength of the patient must now be supported by a light, nutritious diet, but wine is to be avoided. The operation of *paracentesis thoracis* is probably advisable in certain cases, both of vomica and empyema ; but the observations of authors on this piece of practice are very scanty, and my experience does not enable me to supply the deficiency.

6. The hepatized state of lung is be combated by external irritants, such as the ointment of tartarized antimony (R No 114,) or the antimonial ambrocation No. 110, by repeated blisters and issues, low diet, occasional aperients, and lastly by mercurial alteratives and diuretics, such as the pill (R No. 105.)

CHAP. IX.

SUBACUTE AND CHRONIC BRONCHITIS.

Prevalence and general Character of Bronchial Inflammation. Its subdivisions. Subacute Bronchitis, or Peripneumonia Notha. Of Chronic Bronchial Inflammation. Connection of Bronchitis with Abdominal Disease. Of Dropsy consequent upon Chronic Bronchitis. Morbid Appearances. Treatment of Bronchial Inflammation by Antiphlogistic Measures. Stimulants. Opiates. Expectorants. Blisters.

THE most frequent of all the diseases of cold climates is subacute and chronic inflammation of the mucous membrane of the bronchia, commonly known by the name of *winter cough*; and it cannot therefore but be considered a matter of great surprise, that the pathology of this disease should have been so long overlooked. By all the ancient writers, and by modern authors, up to a very late period, the disease was noticed, indeed, under the vague and unscientific denominations of tussis, catarrhus senilis, rheuma catarrhale, and bastard peripneumony; but their ideas concerning it were very confused and unsatisfactory. The nature of the peripneumonia notha of Sydenham, in particular, was a theme of endless controversy.

Dr. Badham, in 1808, first wrote expressly on inflammation of the mucous membrane of the bronchia, and gave to it the appropriate name of bronchitis. His views concerning this affection are very clear and just, and his work deserves to be noticed, as a pathological essay of the highest merit. The attention of the author was, perhaps, too exclusively directed to that severe but rare disease, which we have already alluded to under the title of *acute bronchitis* His deficiencies, however, have been, in a great measure, supplied by the industry of later writers, among whom Dr. Hastings, of Worcester,* deserves particular mention; and the pa-

---

* A Treatise on Inflammation of the Mucous Membrane of the Lungs, by Charles Hastings, M. D. London, 1820.

thology of the mucous membrane of the bronchia therefore, though far from being complete, may now be considered as having attained some degree of precision.

The general character of chronic bronchial inflammation is drawn from the symptoms of cough and mucous expectoration ; but dyspnœa, attended with wheezing, is nearly always present also, and with it may be observed a tendency to spasmodic exacerbation of all the symptoms. It is obvious, therefore, how closely allied are the symptoms of bronchitis to those of croup and peripneumony. To some, perhaps, it may not appear necessary to draw very minute distinctions between the inflammations of different portions of the same membrane,—still less to proceed to a subdivision of the cases of bronchial inflammation ; but it it will not, I am persuaded, be looked upon in this light by the practical physician. He will keep in view the extreme frequency of these affections ; he will acknowledge the necessity of variation in his mode of treatment, and be sensible of the utility of regulating that treatment by some sort of pathological principle. I shall offer no apology therefore for attempting to discriminate the different forms of chronic bronchial inflammation which we meet with in practice, or even for pushing this division beyond the limits which Dr. Badham and others have hitherto assigned it. It is unnecessary to premise, that these distinctions are arbitrary and made solely with a view to practice. A gradation may be traced in nature, from the most acute form of bronchitis, which attacks suddenly, and proves fatal, perhaps in a week, to that the origin of which is imperceptible to the patient, and which he carries about him for a long series of years.

Three great divisions of chronic bronchitis might be made, having a reference to the state of the accompanying constitutional symptoms. Sometimes fever is present, to a greater or less degree ; sometimes the constitution is wholly unaffected ; and at other times, lastly, it is in the state of *asthenia* ; but a more extended view of the subject will be requisite for the purposes of practice.

1. There is a species of bronchitis which is attended with considerable febrile derangement of the system, and which runs its course in about three weeks, or a month, generally so severe as to confine the patient to bed for a part of the time. This I would distinguish by the name of *subacute* bronchitis. It is the peripneumonia notha of Sydenham, who has admirably described its symptoms and treatment. To those who have once suffered by it, it is apt to recur

25

every year, and commonly about the same season. It is attended by
the expectoration of puriform mucus, and respiration is performed
with a wheezing noise.   Occasionally, the cough occurs in paroxysms of great violence, terminating by the vomiting of food ; and
the disease then so closely resembles the hooping-cough, that, for
a time, it is with difficulty distinguished from it ; but the diseases
are very distinct in their origin, termination, and treatment. Subacute bronchitis is to be treated on the common principles applicable
to all inflammatory diseases.   It requires venesection two or three
times, to the extent of ten ounces each time, and with intervals of
two or three days, and is much benefited by saline and antimonial
medicines.

2. This disease, if neglected in its early stages, sometimes terminates in ulceration of the mucous membrane of the bronchia, the
principal symptom characterizing which is the expectoration of a
purulent matter, of a *greenish* colour and smooth appearance. This,
with attention to the preceding symptoms, will assist in distinguishing the disease from phthisis pulmonalis, where the matter expectorated usually assumes the form of globules of a white, or straw
colour. The pulse here is frequent and often full, while, at the same
time, great debility prevails. The patient can generally take a full
inspiration, which is scarcely ever possible in an advanced stage of
consumption, as will hereafter be more fully noticed.   Ulceration
of the bronchia occurs only in persons advanced in life. It is a disease of great danger, but still, occasionally subdued.   The ulcers
are found upon dissection to be always superficial, and generally
small.   This disease will be assisted by a moderate exhibition of
tonics, as myrrh ; but upon any urgent aggravation of the symptoms, blood must be taken from the 'arm to the extent of four or
six ounces.

3. These cases are very rare, however, when compared with
those which I would designate by the name of *common chronic* bronchitis, and which constitute the great bulk of all the cases of chronic or *winter* cough. The symptoms of most importance in a pathological view are, the frequent pulse and the slightly furred tongue
which attend it, pointing out that the constitution is in a state
of febrile excitement.   There is great variety in the other symptoms, but a few of the leading points may be worthy of notice.
When pain is complained of, it is generally refered to the head, or
the iliac region, referable, I believe, to the injury done to the bowels by the mere violence of the cough.   A deep inspiration will al-

most always be followed by a fit of coughing, but it will seldom cause or aggravate pain. The difficulty of breathing is often very trifling when the patient is sitting quiet, but it is highly increased by any exertion of walking, more particularly by going up stairs, or ascending a hill. After such an effort the patient appears gasping for breath, and ready to faint from weakness. He can sometimes lie on both sides, but the horizontal posture generally increases dyspnœa; and consequently, in the severer forms and latter stages of the disease, he passes both his days and his nights in a great chair.

The cough, in common chronic bronchitis, occurs in fits, lasting several minutes; and these, in a vast proportion of cases, happen in the morning when waking, or on going to bed at night. The irritability of the membrane is obviously increased in this disease; and exposure of the skin to the cold air proves, by sympathy, a source of irritation. In like manner, a change of weather, or the inhalation of smoke or vapours, or the taking in of food, brings on a fit of coughing. The matter expectorated varies very much in appearance, but still more in *quantity*. Sometimes it is thick and ropy, sometimes thin and frothy, and occasionally in such enormous quantity as to excite astonishment. I have seen three pints of a thin mucus brought up in twenty-four hours, and that without any other very urgent symptom. Some attention, with a view to practice, is to be paid, as to whether the expectoration be easy or difficult.

Coldness of the lower extremities is generally complained of, as was long ago noticed by Hoffman. The patient becomes weak, and makes great complaints of the languor and lassitude which oppress him. As the disease advances he loses flesh, and a disposition to phthisis is often suspected. However difficult or needless it may be to establish an accurate diagnosis between the acute forms of bronchitis and peripneumony that between chronic peripneumony (or consumption) and the subacute and chronic bronchitis is both important and attainable, but it cannot be clearly explained until the symptoms and progress of the former disease have been under discussion. Besides the symptoms of febrile excitement already mentioned, it will commonly be found, that in the early stages of all severe bronchial affections, and in the latter periods of slighter ones, the functions of the stomach and bowels are impaired. There is loss of appetite, a weak digestion, flatulence, an unpleasant taste in the mouth in the morning, and costiveness. The duration of this form of bronchial inflammation is very various. It

has very little tendency to wear itself out, and, if suffered to run its
own course, continues often during the whole winter, and yields
only to the change of season. It is not a disease of danger, until
by frequent recurrence it has worn down the system.

4. There is a peculiar form of bronchial inflammation unattended
by any symptoms of disordered constitution. The patient, on first
waking, is attacked with a severe and loud fit of coughing, which
continues to harass him for half an hour after rising. It recurs occasionally during the day. It is attended with little or no expectoration, and appears to consist chiefly in an *increased irritability* of
the membrane. But that it is closely allied to a state of inflammation
is probable from this, that the affection can always be traced to
cold. It is not permanently benefited by any plan of treatment
which I have been able to devise, except change of air. The hy-
drocyanic acid, given in doses of three drops twice a day in lac-
amygdalæ, has occasionally proved useful.

5. Bronchial inflammation is sometimes attended, particularly
in old people, with those marks of loss of tone in the system which
pathologists have generalized under the term *asthenia.* This form
of the affection has long been known by the name of *catarrhus senilis.* It is marked by profuse expectoration, a feeble and languid
pulse, a disposition to sleep, and extreme weakness of the limbs.
It proves fatal to many old people—it is usually said, by suffocation, but this is doubtful; for in the latter stages of bronchial inflammation of the true asthenic character, the effusion of mucus
in some measure ceases, and the patient dies from *exhaustion*, often
very unexpectedly. This form of chronic bronchitis is sometimes
met with at an earlier period of life. Women who have suckled
their children too long are occasionally the subjects of it. It proves
particularly tedious and severe in such persons as have led irregular lives, and indulged freely in spirituous liquors; but in them it is
generally associated with *hepatization,* or some other form of disorganization of the substance of the lungs.

Chronic bronchitis is, certainly, for the most part, a primary disease, and attributable to cold and moisture. I have observed that
foggy weather is very apt to bring it on. But it frequently also
supervenes upon other diseases, both of an acute and chronic kind;
such as the febrile eruptions, chronic cutaneous affections, and
diseases of the abdomen. The connection of bronchitis with disordered conditions of the abdominal viscera has long been known.
Worms have been observed to create cough. Dyspepsia, and dis-

eases of the liver, are often attended by the common symptoms of
chronic bronchitis. In some cases this connection may be accidental; but in many, it is, I believe, strictly *sympathetic* ;—that is to
say, the disease of the bronchia has not its origin in cold, and can
be relieved only by relieving the abdominal affection. The precise
nature of this relation between the viscera of the thorax and abdomen, it is, perhaps, impossible to ascertain exactly ; but it
should be borne in mind, that it is to a certain degree mutual ; and
therefore it becomes often a matter of great difficulty to determine,
in complicated cases, whether the system of treatment should be
directed, in the first instance, to the relief of the thoracic or of the
abdominal derangements.

Among the symptoms which supervene on chronic bronchitis,
œdema of the feet and legs deserves particularly to be noticed.
Dr. Hastings seems inclined to attribute this dropsical effusion directly to inflammation of the mucous membrane,* but general pathology would rather induce us to suppose, that some mechanical impediment exists in such a case to the free passage of blood through
the lungs, whereby the right ventricle of the heart is gorged or distended, and the whole venous system disturbed in its function.

The morbid appearances presented by the mucous membrane of
the bronchia, after being long subject to chronic inflammation do
not appear to throw much light on the *ratio symptomatum*, or to direct us in any degree to the proper treatment of the disease. The
membrane appears discoloured ; sometimes of a vivid red colour,
sometimes inclining more to purple. Its structure is often thickened, and not unfrequently the surface of it is pulpy. Mucus is generally found, to a considerable extent, filling the bronchia and air-
cells.

The general principles of treatment in subacute and chronic
bronchitis have never been very accurately laid down by authors.
It must be regulated by reference partly to the constitutional, and
partly to the thoracic symptoms. In the subacute forms of the disease, antiphlogistic measures of greater or less activity are always
to be resorted to. When the cough occurs in paroxysms of extraordinary length or violence, or when there is a tensive pain of the
forehead, or of the iliac region, blood must be taken from the arm.
In very severe cases, a repetition of small blood-lettings is neces-

* Hastings on " Inflammation of the Mucous Membrane of the Lungs,"
chap. v.

sary to overcome the disease. In cases of less urgency, it will be
sufficient to direct saline draughts, with twenty drops of tincture of
hyoscyamus, and ten of antimonial or ipecacuanha wine. The bowels should never be suffered to become costive.   It was a favourite maxim with the old physicians, that it is only in stomach (or
sympathetic) coughs that purgatives are beneficial, and that the
true pectoral coughs are more relieved by diuretics.   This is true
to a certain extent, but occasional purging by the draught No. 21
will nevertheless be found very beneficial.

Where the system is much debilitated, the tongue clean, and no
thirst present, advantage will be derived from the exhibition of ammoniacum (R No. 94,) myrrh, and acids. In this state of the system, narcotics, more especially opium, are not only useful, but oft-
en quite indispensable. They allay that irritation of the membrane
which would otherwise prevent the patient from getting sleep. They
are best given in a full dose at night.   Where the irritability of
the membrane is very great, with little constitutional disturbance,
demulcent mixtures (R Nos. 57, 58, 59.) with the addition of a proper proportion of the vinegar or tincture of squill, will be found very
serviceable.   I have derived much advantage from the formula No-
95 ; but the indiscriminate employment of those medicines which
have been called *expectorant*, in cases of chronic bronchial inflammation, cannot be defended on any principle, theoretical or empirical.

Combinations of expectorant with anodyne medicines are famil-
arly known under the name of *cough pills*, and almost every praetitioner has his favourite formula.   That which in my hands has
proved very serviceable, is R No. 87. One pill may be taken twice
or thrice a day.   Most of these formulæ contain a proportion of
calomel, and its employment in small doses undoubtedly contributes
to relieve the breathing in obstinate cases of chronic bronchitis.
It will be found indeed, in all cases of dyspnœa unattended by corresponding fever or cough, that the exhibition of three or four
grains of calomel in a pill affords very effectual relief. Five grains
of Plummer's pill taken at bed-time is sufficient in slighter cases.
When the tone of the stomach is impaired by the long continuance of the disease, bitters are of considerable service, and may be
advantageously united with the narcotic and expectorant medicines
already recommended, as in R No. 92. Coughing is an act in which
the diaphragm is mainly concerned, and hence it is that a gentle
stimulus to the stomach so often aids expectoration.

Blisters are useful in almost every form of winter cough, when applied judiciously. The symptoms, which in an especial manner call for their employment, are a cold skin, a languid circulation, and an oppression in the breathing. An uniform moderate temperature, warm clothing, and a light diet, are quite indispensable. If the disease prove very óbstinate, a change of air should be directed ; for it may then be considered as kept up, in some measure, by habit. Warm weather has a very striking influence in many cases of obstinate chronic bronchitis ; and therefore when the disease has recurred several times, and is brought on by slight vicissitudes of temperature, it may even be proper to recommend removal to a warmer and steadier climate.

CHAP. X.

General Pathology of Consumption. *Morbid Conditions giving rise to consumptive Symptoms. Of Tubercular Phthisis in detail. Origin and Nature of Pulmonary Tubercle. Its Connection with Scrofula. Progress of the Symptoms in Consumption. Phthisis Incipiens, and Confirmata. Characters of Hectic Fever. Diagnosis. Prognosis. Principles of treatment in the incipient, and in the confirmed Stage of Consumption.*

CHRONIC inflammation of the *substance* of the lungs is so uniformly connected with wasting of the body, as to have obtained for itself the distinguishing appellation of *consumption*, or *decline*. Its amazing prevalence, and almost uniform mortality, entitle it to the fullest attention; but independent of this, it is a subject which involes many curious pathological speculations. Consumption is a febrile disease, but the character of the accompanying fever differs from any thing we have yet examined. It is the chronic inflammation of a cellular, structure, but that structure had previously been diseased. It occurs, for the most part, in that peculiar habit of body (the *scrofulous*) which is characterized by a delicate organization of blood vessels; and it exhibits therefore, in all its stages a strong disposition to *hæmorrhage*.

Cough with expectoration, difficult breathing, and wasting, are the *leading* symptoms of consumption; and pathology would bear us out in applying the term at all times to such a combination of symptoms. But physicians have generally agreed in restricting it to those cases where the symptoms arise from *ulceration of disorganized lungs*, the principal disorganizations being hepatized induration, and tubercle. There are other morbid conditions of the respiratory organs however which may, and frequently do, give rise to all the symptoms of genuine consumption. They are, first, chronic inflammation and ulceration of the larynx, trachea, and bronchia; secondly, chronic inflammation of the pleura; and thirdly, vomica, the sequel of acute inflammation in lungs previously *sound*. The second of these forms of thoracic disease is rare, and hardly distinguishable during life. The others have been already treated of, and they are only referred to in this place, that the student may have before him, in one view, a sketch of the general pathology of consumptive diseases.

Of the two principal forms of consumption, *viz.* ulceration of *hepatized* lungs, and ulceration of *tuberculated* lungs, it is unnecessary that I should treat separately. They give rise to nearly the same train of symptoms, they are equally dangerous, and they are not unfrequently found to co-exist.* Of the former it is sufficient to say, that it is the occasional consequence of pneumonic inflammation and repeated catarrhs in any habits, but more especially in persons indulging freely in the use of ardent spirits. It may occur therefore at all ages, but is most common in the middle period of life :—*viz.* between the ages of thirty and fifty.

The great and peculiar feature of phthisis pulmonalis is its connection with *tubercle of the lungs;* and before the phenomena of the disease, the diagnosis, or prognosis, can be properly understood, the nature of tubercle must be explained.†

Tubercles are rounded, firm, white bodies, varying from the size of a pin's head to that of a garden pea, frequently found interspersed through the whole substance of the lungs, but most usually met with in its upper and posterior parts. Frequently they occur in clusters. In their earliest state they are solid, and of cartilaginous hardness. No blood-vessels can be traced in them even by a microscope, and the finest injection does not penetrate them. They are situate not in the air cells, but in the proper cellular texture of the lungs, and are without any cyst.

Even in this state, tubercles create a degree of impediment to

* Dr. Willan remarked, in 1797, that of the cases of consumption occurring in London, not more than *one-fourth* arose from the slow and successive suppuration of tubercles in scrofulous constitutions; but this is probably underrating the proportion of tubercular phthisis; for of thirty-five consecutive cases of consumption, examined at St. George's Hospital, eight were of pure hepatization, twenty-two of pure tubercular disorganization, and five were mixed cases.

† On this subject consult Dr. Stark's Works, 4to. 1788 (or Medical Communications, vol. i. page 359;) Dr. Baillie's Morbid Anatomy, and the works of Laennec.

the breathing, by occupying a considerable space in the body of the lungs. They prevent the free transmission of blood through that vascular organ, and occasion, therefore, a rupture of some of the smaller vessels, and consequent spitting of blood, when by any cause the impetus of the blood, is increased. But these are only a small part of the evils which result from the presence of tuber. cles. Though no blood-vessels can be traced in them, they are susceptible of inflammation, the effect of which is to convert the tubercle into a white capsule containing pus ; or when a cluster of tubercles inflame together, to form an abscess of considerable size. The internal surface of the bronchia communicating with this abscess appears red and inflamed. The contiguous portions of the substance of the lungs are differently affected in different cases. Sometimes their texture is unaltered, but more commonly it is rendered red, solid, and impervious to air. The smaller blood. vessels are commonly destroyed ; and the larger, before they reach the abscess, are wholly, or partially, filled with a kind of fibrous substance, by which severe hæmorrhagy is prevented, even though a great extent of lung be injured. It is imagined, that upon an average, three-fourths of the substance of the lungs are rendered unfit for respiration in the progress of consumption, before the pa. tient sinks.

Tubercles have been occasionally found in the lungs of children at a very early age, but they are not commonly met with until a short time before the completion of the growth of the body. In a few cases they appear to have been formed at a very *advanced* pe. riod of life. They are at all times morbid growths ; and it it cer. tainly an important object to determine, if possible, the manner in which their formation takes place, and the circumstances which give occasion to it. On these questions, however, pathologists are much divided. Some maintain, that tubercles are deposited by a peculiar action of vessels, altogether distinct from inflammation, that their formation is unattended by the usual accompaniments of inflammatory action, and that in fact inflammation is the couse. quence rather than the cause of tubercle. Others contend that tubercles (more especially as they occur in the lungs) are simply the result of a low degree of common inflammation ; and this opin. ion is corroborated, first, by finding them associated with the other more acknowledged *effects* of inflammation, and secondly, by ob. serving that when occurring singly, their appearance has been preceded by the ordinary symptoms of catarrh or peripneumony.* The question in dispute is one of the most difficult in general pathology, and it will probably long remain open to discussion. All parties however are agreed in the important fact of the intimate connection of tubercle in the lungs with the *scrofulous* diathesis. This appears in the occurrence of phthisis in scrofulous families, and in persons who exhibit other marks of the scrofulous disposition. It is illustrated also by the analogy which subsists between the progress of inflammation in a tubercle, and in a *gland* affected by scrofula. In both it is of the same *chronic* kind, tending to the formation of the same sort of thick curdly pus. It is brought on in both by the same causes, and relieved by the same means.

The symptoms of tubercular consumption are next to be explained, and they are sufficiently uniform to admit of a precise detail.

A sense of tightness across the chest and of internal heat, with a slight tickling cough, are among the first symptoms that mark the approach of a decline. The patient is languid, and has the feeling of slight pains in some part of the chest, when he ascends a flight of stairs, or takes any considerable exercise. The pulse will commonly be found, even in this early period of the disease, somewhat accelerated. These symptoms however, being very slight, are often overlooked, both by the patient and his friends, until the occurrence of *hæmoptysis*, which may be said to characterize the first stage of phthisis pulmonalis, with as much certainty as purulent expectoration does the second. The spitting of blood recurs at irregular times and in variable quantities. By degrees, the cough becomes more and more troublesome. A fixed pain in some part of the thorax, or about the pit of the stomach, is now complained of. Respiration is hurried, and the patient unable to expand the chest, even in the slightest degree. There is difficulty in lying on one or other side, or sometimes on the back ; and, at length, the nature of the disease is put beyond doubt by the occurrence of *purulent expectoration* and *hectic fever*.

The expectoration of a thick pus, generally in the form of globular lumps, of a straw colour, occasionally tinged with blood, and always more or less mixed with mucus, is indeed the peculiar feature of this disease ; but perhaps too much stress has been laid upon the necessity of distinguishing in pulmonic diseases between

* On this subject, see Dr. Alison on " The Pathology of Scrofulous Diseases," in the Transactions of the Med. Chir. Society of Edinburgh, vol. i.

the different *kinds* of expectorated matter. An extensive observation of disease will show, that its appearance varies extremely, not
only in different individuals, but even in the same individual on
different days, and different times of the day, and that its qualities
may alter, without materially altering the danger, still less the nature of the disease.

Hectic fever (the other diagnostic mark of confirmed phthisis) is
the fever of irritation and weakness. It is commonly attendant on
extensive and protracted ulceration, because this is one of the most
common ways in which that irritation throughout the body, and that
degree of constitutional weakness is kept up, which is necessary to
its development. But genuine hectic sometimes occurs without any
ulceration, as in delicate women who suckle their infants too long,
in children of weak habits, and in adult men after confluent small-
pox, or in the latter stages of diabetes. Under all circumstances
it presents very nearly the same characters. It is a *remitting* fever,
having its exacerbation between five and six o'clock in the afternoon,
at which time rigors occur, lasting about an hour, and succeeded
by an increase in the quickness of the pulse, the heat of skin, the
thirst, general uneasiness, and restlessness. About ten o'clock at
night the sweating begins, which is the natural crisis of the hectic
paroxysm. The patient then gets some sleep, but the sweating for
the most part continues ; and when he wakes in the morning he
finds himself bathed in perspiration. It is a remarkable circumstance, that this disposition to sweating is sometimes local, being
confined, for instance, to the head and neck, or to the inferior extremities. These are the *colliquative* or weakening night-sweats,
which afford so striking a characteristic of hectic fever.

The pulse in this form of fever is always very quick, generally
averaging 120, but frequently it will be found for weeks together
as high as 144. The skin is hot, but not in proportion to this extraordinary rapidity of the pulse. The vessels of the adnata lose whatever redness they may have had in health, and the eye becomes of
a leaden or pearly hue. The countenance is pale in the morning;
but towards evening, when the febrile exacerbation occurs, the
cheeks exhibit that circumscribed redness, known by the name of
the *hectic flush*. The urine, from the very first, is high coloured,
and deposits, on cooling, that copious branny red sediment upon
which the older pathologists laid so much stress.

Under common circumstances, the functions of the stomach are
but little impaired. The appetite may even continue good. There

is not much thirst, except towards night, or what results from the medicines taken ; and the bowels are at first unaffected. Yet with all this, emaciation takes place, and frequently proceeds rapidly, and to an extreme degree. This is first observable in the face, which becomes thin and long, and the eyes appear sunk in their orbits. Closely connected with the emaciation, is the loss of muscular power, which also proceeds to a great extent, and is often the earliest prominent symptom of this peculiar affection of the system.

A circumstance well deserving of attention in the phenomena of hectic fever, as pointing out a striking difference between it and idiopathic fever, is the little disturbance which takes place in the functions of the brain. Head-ache does not always occur during the periods of exacerbation, and it is seldom present at other times. Delirium is very rare, except perhaps for a few hours before the patient's death. Even this is not constantly observed, for in many instances the senses remain perfect even to the last gasp of breath which is drawn. A degree of languor generally prevails, but in a large proportion of cases the mental faculties continue quite unimpaired throughout the disease. I have sometimes even thought, that a præternatural vigour of mind was perceptible while the body was suffering under the most exquisite form of hectic. One exception must be made, applicable at least to that which attends consumption. On the prospect of his own recovery, the judgment of the phthisical patient is nearly always erroneous. The most obvious indications of danger are over-looked ; and, full of hope, he is busied only in the anticipation of approaching convalescence.

The only other peculiarity of hectic fever which I have to notice, is the tendency which exists, in its latter stages, to an affection of the mucous membrane of the ileum. This is indicated by colliquative diarrhœa, the occasional appearance of blood in the motions, and a præternatural redness and *tenderness* of the tongue, followed in most cases by the appearance of aphthæ in the mouth. On dissection, especially if such symptoms have been present for any length of time, inflammation and ulceration of the ileum of a peculiar character are met with, but not so constantly as to warrant the belief, that in all cases these symptoms depend on an *inflammatory* state of the intestines. Sometimes the bowels are merely irritable.

Such are the characters of hectic fever ; and as they are always

most strikingly displayed in the progress of tubercular consumption, they will seldom fail, in conjunction with the local symptoms
already enumerated, to afford evidence sufficiently decisive of the
nature of the disease. There are some symptoms however, which
occasionally occur in the progress of consumption, which require
a separate notice. I may first mention, that it is not uncommon to
have in the course of the disease an accession of acute pleurisy,
or of inflammation of the peritonæal surface of the liver. Further,
as phthisis frequently supervenes on other diseases, its symptoms
are somtimes so complicated with those of the primary disorder,
that much discrimination is required in forming a judgment as to
the true nature of the case. In many instances the symptoms of
such diseases correspond very closely with those of phthisis ; and
this applies more especially to certain morbid states of the larynx
and trachea, and to some obscure affections of the heart and great
vessels. I have already alluded to the hoarseness which attends
consumption, and to that sympathetic affection of the larynx which
is so frequent in its latter stages.

Dropsy, particularly of the cellular membrane, is by no means
uncommon in this disease. Œdema of the feet and ancles is sufficiently decisive of it, but it frequently extends also to the legs and
thighs. This has commonly been attributed to *debility*, to that same
relaxation of the capillaries to which we are in the habit of aseri-
bing colliquative perspirations. But this theory is doubtful, because
in many cases, where an equal, or even a greater degree of muscular weakness prevails, there is no appearance of dropsical effusion.
I should presume it is simply referable to some unusual difficulty
experienced in the transmission of blood through the lungs.

The diagnosis of genuine (or tubercular) consumption from that
state of thoracic disorder which we have called *vomica*, where no
pre-existing disease of the lungs modifies the phenomena, and also
from chronic inflammation of the *bronchia*, is a matter, often of great
consequence, but as often of very considerable difficulty. Indeed,
it baffles in many cases the skill of the most experienced physician.
It is to be effected principally by a knowledge of the constitution
of the patient and of his family predispositions ; but much too may
be learned by a close attenion to the *progress* of the symptoms, and
the order of their succession. A careful examination of the thorax should never be omitted. The degree to which the ribs can
be elevated should first be ascertained, and percussion may then
be practised on the different parts of the chest in succession. The

clearness or dullness of the sound emitted affords an obvious and very useful test of the degree to which consolidation of the lungs has gone. Dr. Laennec of Paris was further of opinion, that a *va-riety* of sounds issued from the chest in diseases both of the heart and lungs, sufficiently permanent and characteristic to afford as-sistance in diagnosis. To distinguish these he invented an instru-ment called the stethoscope, the utility of which however is great-ly lessened from the very long practice and the nice habit of dis-crimination which its employment is generally admitted to demand.*

It is unnecessary to treat formally of the *prognosis* in consump-tion. The common observation of the world has sufficiently stamp-ed its character as the most destructive disease in this island,† and in its confirmed stage, almost hopeless. The duration of the complaint however it is scarcely possible to define with any degree of accuracy ; for a galloping and a lingering consumption are al-most equally frequent. M. Bayle speaking of the usual duration of phthisis, informs us, that out of 200 cases, 104 died within nine months. In many instances there are threatenings of the disease for several winters before the symptoms assume any degree of ur-gency. They are often checked by the return of mild weather, but perhaps even in a still more remarkable manner, by pregnancy. The months of December and January are observed to be particu-larly fatal to phthisical patients. Sometimes they die from extreme weakness, exhausted by the discharge of pus, and the colliquative perspiration and purging ; at other times more suddenly, suffocated by the accumulation of pus in the bronchia, which they are unable to expectorate ; and in some rare cases, quite unexpectedly, by the rupture of a large blood-vessel in the lungs, the consequence of ul-ceration.‡

It is melancholy to reflect how very little this disease is under the control of medicine ; and before I can enter upon the consid-eration of the principles which are to guide us in its treatment, I

* The reader who desires further information concerning the stethoscope may consult Dr. Forbes's translation of Laennec's works. He will there also find useful and most accurate descriptions of the different varieties of thoracic disease, and of the morbid appearances which they present.

† The deaths throughout England by consumption are calculated at one in five, and amount therefore annually to about 55,000. They constitute one fourth of the deaths in London, according to the bills of mortality.

‡ See Appendix; Note S.

must record the failure of every plan for its effectual cure, which
human ingenuity has yet devised.

The first principle which it appears of importance to inculcate is,
that in phthisis active measures cannot be pursued; and that this
must be compensated by a strict attention to a number of lesser
circumstances, which in many other diseases may be neglected
without detriment to the patient. We are to bear in mind, that
consumption, though an inflammatory affection, is principally characterized by its occurring in a *scrofulous*, which is commonly a
weak habit of body, and in an organ loaded with tubercles, the inflammation of which runs rapidly to suppuration. The chief objects
of consideration, therefore, are, how these tubercles may either
be absorbed, or kept in a quiescent state; in what respect their
treatment when inflamed, differs from that of common pneumonia;
and how the constitution may be best supported in the protracted
suppuration to which their inflammation leads. In the treatment of
phthisis much nicety is required. On the one hand, we have to
combat the actual presence of inflammation; and to bear in mind,
on the other, the danger of exhausting the constitution.

The question has been frequently agitated, whether tubercles
can be absorbed, and by what medicines that desirable object can
be effected. Emetics have been recommended by some, the muriate of baryta by others; but though there is every reason to believe, that tubercles have in some cases dispersed, yet this effect
appears to be as completely out of our control, as the manner of
their formation is beyond our knowledge. All that can reasonably
be expected from medicine, is to keep them in a quiescent state;
and this is to be done by a strict attention to diet, air, exercise, and
by avoiding all those causes which we shall notice hereafter, as
likely to bring on hæmorrhagy of the lungs.

The diet of a person who has shown a disposition to phthisis,
should be nourishing, and calculated to afford strength to the system, without creating a disposition to febrile excitement. For this
purpose, farinaceous preparations of all kinds with milk should be
recommended. Animal broths, with fish and a proportion of plainly
dressed meat may also be allowed; but all highly seasoned dishes,
and food which is difficult of digestion, and fermented and spirituous liquors are to be strictly prohibited. Nothing appears more
likely to correspond in every respect with this *indication of cure*,
than the breathing a free and pure air; and its advantages in consumptive cases are generally acknowledged. The air of a large

town, loaded as it is with smoke and effluvia, has long been considered hurtful. The patient should be sent therefore to the country; and, if possible, a situation selected, which is sheltered from
cold bleak winds, and where the soil is gravelly.

To those whose circumstances will admit of it, we should advise the removal to a warm climate. Consumption, though far from
being uncommon in the southern countries of Europe, is, upon the
whole, less frequent there than in cold climates; but between the
tropics it is a disease nearly unknown. This consideration, were
it not for the danger of the endemics of those countries, would induce us to prefer the Bermudas, or even the West India Islands,
as a residence for consumptive patients. But even in the South
of Europe, particularly the climate of Naples, holds out many advantages; and a timely removal thither, with regularity of living,
may be recommended to those who are *threatened* with consumption, with a fair prospect of overcoming the tendency to the disease.*

With the enjoyment of a free and pure air, moderate exercise
should also be advised. A sedentary mode of life, and close application to study, or business, have frequently proved the exciting
cause of the disease; partly, perhaps, by the bent position in which
the thorax is so long kept, but principally from the want of that due
exercise which is essential to the preservation of the health and
strength of the body. With the view of affording, at the same
time, both exercise to the body and relaxation to the mind, a jour-
ney during the summer months is particularly useful.

When hæmoptysis has occurred, and when the symptoms warrant the belief that inflammatory action is going on in the lungs,
measures of more activity must be pursued. Bleeding from the
arm has been recommended as a means of putting an *immediate*
check to the progress of the disease; but this is too often a vain
hope; and blood-letting must, therefore, at all times be resorted to
with caution, and a due consideration of the habit of body in which
consumption occurs. Where the pulse is hard and contracted, and
the pain and cough urgent, blood must of course be drawn from
the arm, as in pneumonia, and repeated according to the strength

* This point, and the utter hopelessness of success from the removal to a
warm climate in the advanced stages of consumption, have been urged upon the attention of practitioners with much force, by Dr. H. W. Carter.
See " *Remarks upon the Effects of a Warm Climate in Pulmonary Consumption and some other Diseases.*" Medical Transactions, vol. vi. 1820.

of the habit, and severity of the symptoms. At any period of the disease, if pleuritic symptoms supervene, with a loaded state of the tongue, blood may be abstracted ; and commonly a few ounces taken from the arm will be preferable to the application of leeches.

Blisters afford great relief to the cough and tightness across the chest, and they may be repeatedly applied with great advantage through the whole course of the disease. I have never seen sufficient benefit derived from issues and setons to warrant me in recommending them. Active purging is inadmissible, but an occasional dose of castor oil, or of rhubarb, will be found very useful. Mild diaphoretic and expectorant medicines may be exhibited frequently through the day. Attention to the state of the skin, indeed, is very necessary in this disease, as in every other in which the lungs are implicated. An uniform temperature of the body should be promoted by warm clothing. In some cases it may be necessary during the whole winter, to confine the patient to apartments which are of a regulated temperature.

In consumptive complaints digitalis is universally employed. That its powers have been extravagantly over-rated, I cannot doubt ; but it appears in some cases to quiet the cough, and to be an useful narcotic. In this view I am inclined to think it preferable to conium, and even sometimes to opium. I have never observed any good effect to follow from pushing the dose of this medicine to such an extent as materially to affect the pulse.

In the confirmed stages of consumption, it is necessary to support the strength of the system by tonics ; and the mistura ferri composita, in doses proportioned to the state of the system, is, perhaps, under all circumstances, the best form of tonic which can be recommended. In some cases, however, it seems to increase the febrile excitement, and to aggravate the cough and dyspnœa. The sulfate of quinine may then be substituted, as in R No. 73.

Attention must chiefly be directed, in the latter periods of the disease, to the relief of urgent symptoms. The night sweats, which so greatly harass and weaken the patient, are in some degree checked by full doses of æther taken at bed-time. Cough may be alleviated by demulcents ; diarrhœa by chalk, catechu, and aromatics. Both these objects will be promoted, with the additional advantage of procuring sleep, by the last resource of medical art, opium, and this valuable medicine should be freely given, increasing the dose regularly, so as to ensure to the patient the full benefits which it is capable of affording. Six grains of Dover's powder, with three of extract of hyoscyamus, made into two pills, may at first be given every night at bed time.   Laudanum, or the liquor opii sedativus, may be administered at a later period, in combination with almond emulsion, chalk mixture, infusion of catechu, or with æther, sub-carbonate of ammonia, and camphor julep, according as cough, looseness, or languor predominate : injections of thin starch with laudanum (R No. 107,) will be required when the diarrhœa is particularly harassing.

CHAP. XI.

PERICARDITIS.

Pathology of the Heart. Inflammation of its investing Membrane. When first noticed. Symptoms of Acute Pericarditis. Prognosis. Diagnosis. Morbid Appearances. Causes. Metastasis of Acute Rheumatism. Treatment of Acute Pericarditis. Symptoms and Treatment of Chronic Pericarditis.

THERE is scarcely a subject in the whole range of medical literature, which opens so extensive and important a field of investigation as the pathology of the heart. It has excited the attention of physicians from the earliest times ; and in the elaborate dissèrtations of Morgagni concerning the morbid anatomy of the heart,* we see that every advantage had been taken of one means of arriving at a knowledge of this interesting branch of science. In the attempts, however, which were made to connect the diseased appearances of the heart, found after death, with the symptoms which occurred during life, the older pathologists unquestionably failed ; and it has been reserved for our own times to infuse some portion of accuracy into this part of the inquiry. Much, however, still remains to be done ; and though the difficulty of the subject must universally be admitted, still it does not appear to be, like some of the obscure and controverted points in the science of medicine, beyond the pale of legitimate investigation. These remarks apply equally to the acute and chronic disease, to which the heart and its investing membrane are subject. The latter are very numerous, and constitute the different species of angina pectoris, to which our attention will hereafter be directed. The acute diseases of these parts will form the subject of the present chapter.

There is every reason to believe, that when the heart is inflam-

* Morgagni de Causis et Sedibus Morborum per Anatomen indagatis, lib. ii, epist. 16 and 27.

ed, the primary seat of disease is the pericardium. In one or two cases, indeed, the substance of the heart has been found inflamed, without a corresponding affection of the investing membrane ; but the occurrence is so rare, that it will be sufficient in this place to have thus alluded to it. Inflammation commencing in the pericardium is, on the other hand, by no means unfrequent ; and though it occasionally dips down a little way into the substance of the heart, still the character of the disease is the inflammation of a serous membrane, and the disease itself, therefore, is correctly denominated PERICARDITIS. Such a form of thoracic inflammation was acknowledged by many of the old nosologists ; but their notions regarding it were very confused, and the most important circumstance in its pathology was altogether overlooked ; I mean, its connection with acute rheumatism. The honour of this discovery is due to Dr. David Pitcairn, who first noticed the fact in 1788 ; and upon the strength of whose authority it was mentioned by Dr. Baillie in 1797. The first distinct account, however, which appeared in this country, of the disease, since called *rheumatism of the heart*, was from the pen of Sir D. Dundas.* Pericarditis is a primary as well as a secondary disease ; but the symptoms by which both forms of the affection are characterized are so similar, that it is unnecessary to separate their consideration.

Inflammation of the pericardium is ushered in, and accompanied in its course, by the usual febrile symptoms. The *local* symptoms are in some measure the same with those of the common forms of pneumonia ; but such as peculiarly point out that the pericardium is the seat of disease, are the following. There is pain referred to the region of the heart, or more properly to the *scrobiculus cordis*, sometimes pungent as in pleurisy, but often described as a suffocating weight, extending to the right side. The patient complains of a violent *palpitation*, and the motions of the heart are often perceptible at a considerable distance. A strong pulsation of the carotid arteries, attended with noise of the ears and giddiness, is not an unfrequent symptom. The manner of the patient's breathing is to be attended to, as occasionally affording evidence of the exact seat of disease. It is often by catches, or starts ; and the chest can generally be filled, though gradually. Dyspnœa is an urgent symptom, much aggravated by motion or exertion of any kind, so as to occasion an apprehension, on the part of the patient

* Medico-Chirurgical Transactions, vol. i, page 37. London, 1809,

of immediate death. There is usually present, also, a short, dry, but incessant cough, aggravating the other symptoms, and fie. quently excited by pressure on the epigastrium. The pulse, which is always very frequent, bounds against the finger with a haish jar- ring feel, at first regularly, but as the disease advances, irregularly both in point of force and frequency. The tongue is white, and the skin often bathed in sweat, as in acute rheumatism.

Unless some degree of relief is obtained, the countenance be. comes livid, the eye glassy, and the patient sinks. Should the ur- gent symptoms only be palliated, the disease degenerates into the state of chronic pericarditis, the symptoms of which will presently be enumerated. Under more favourable circumstances, the pa- tient gradually recovers ; but, upon the whole, the prognosis is un- favourable as to ultimate and complete recovery. A quick pulse, and occasional palpitation, will always be found to remain behind, with a strong tendency to relapse ; the recurrence of the disease being, if possible, still more dangerous than the primary attack.

The diagnosis of pleurisy and pericarditis is often a matter of difficulty, although apparently there are sufficient symptoms already detailed, to distinguish these diseases under every possible circum- stance. The appearance of the countenance may sometimes be resorted to, in aid of the other symptoms. Common inflammation of the lungs frequently proceeds to a great extent, without a cor- responding change of countenance ; but in pericarditis there oc- curs, from the very earliest periods, a peculiarly anxious expres- sion of the features, commonly with paleness. This symptom, however, fails as a diagnostic mark between this disease and acute bronchitis, which has often, I believe, been mistaken for it ; but the error is fortunately of no practical importance.

On dissection of those who die of acute pericarditis, the mem- brane appears externally denser, and more opaque than natural, and numerous vessels are seen ramifying on its surface. On cut- ting into the sac of the pericardium, it is found gorged with serum, in which shreds of coagulable lymph are floating. Recent lymph will be found also covering the surfaces of the membrane ; and in some places the heart and pericardium will, perhaps, be seen to ad- here. The muscular structure of the heart in contact with the pe- ricardium becomes much more crowded with vessels than in its natural state ; and sometimes extravasated blood, or globules of pus, may be found dispersed through it. Along with these appearances, others are often noticed, denoting the extension of the in-flammation to the diaphragm, pleura, or substance of the lungs.

Cold, and the metastasis of acute rheumatism, are the only known exciting causes of acute pericarditis. One instance of the disease, with which I am acquainted, was obviously owing to the patient having slept on a pavement, during a frosty night, while in a state of intoxication. Another I traced as distincly to travelling on the outside of a coach during a cold and rainy night. But it is unquestionable, that the extension or metastasis of acute rheuma-tism is by far the most common cause of inflammation of the heart. The circumstances which lead to this have never been very accu-rately investigated. In some instances, but by no means generally, the affection of the joints is relieved when inflammation attacks the heart. On the other hand, it has been found, that a fresh acces-sion of inflammation has sometimes come upon the joints, during the existence of active pericarditis. All periods of life are liable to inflammation of the heart, but it chiefly prevails between the ages of fourteen and thirty. Both sexes are in like manner its subjects, but I think it is most common among females. Persons of a broad chest and plethoric habit of body, appear to be those most particularly predisposed to it.

The treatment of acute pericarditis, supposing the disease to be ascertained with perfect accuracy, will not differ, in any material point, from that proper to be pursued in other cases of thoracic in-flammation. Venesection must be promptly had recourse to, and pushed to a very considerable extent. Depletion is, for the most part, borne well in the early stages, and the blood is always highly cupped and buffy. Some degree of caution may be necessary when there is any considerable *intermission* in the pulse ; but this symp-tom is by no means to deter us from the vigorous employment of the lancet, should it be called for by others of an unequivocal char-acter. Considerable benefit is often experienced in this disease from local blood-letting ; and it has the advantage of being applica-ble, when the state of the system is unfavourable to further deple-tion from the arm. Fomentations in the first stages, and blisters at a somewhat more advanced period of the complaint, are exceed-ingly useful.

Purgative, saline, and antimonial medicines are to be freely ex-hibited. The combination of five grains of calomel with as many of antimonial powder, is well adapted for those cases in which venesection is ill borne. Some benefit is experienced from giving small doses of mercury, in combination with other antiphlogistic measures. For this purpose the pill (R No. 16) may be recommended. Digitalis is of some use ; but care must taken not to push its exhibition so far as to affect the pulse, and interfere with those symptoms by which we are to judge of the necessity of further evacuation. Opium, if advisable at all, should be given at night, in combination with ipecacuanha. Thus exhibited, it sometimes relieves the tickling cough, which is very harassing to the patient, and procures for him a few hours rest.

It has been already observed, that there is a state of *chronic pericarditis* ; and we are next to inquire into the symptoms, progress, and treatment of this affection. Some differences of opinion have been entertained regarding the precise state of disease to which this term should be applied ; and here I would, in the first place, give a caution to the student as to the degree of importance which, in the present state of our knowledge, is to be attached to the distinctions among the chronic diseases of the heart, which pathologists have attempted to establish. It is seldom that they are observed to exist separately ; and consequently their diagnostic symptoms have never been ascertained with that precision, which would warrant the expectation of their becoming applicable to practice. This observation will hereafter be illustrated when treating of angina pectoris, and the other structural diseases of the heart ; but it is applicable also to the case of chronic inflammation of the pericardium.

Without wishing to deny altogether the pathological importance of that distinction between simple dilatation of the heart, and chronic inflammation of its investing membrane, which Mr. Burns has been at pains to inculcate,* I would apply the term chronic pericarditis to that state of the heart which is very often left by acute inflammation of the membrane, and found after death to be connected with adhesion of the heart to the pericardium. Such a

---

* See " Observations on some of the most frequent and important Diseases of the Heart." Edin. 1809, page 53.

state of the heart is frequently accompanied by more or less enlargement of that organ ; and it has been noticed that this is in
the area of its cavities, rather than in the thickness of its muscular
parietes.   Complete adhesions of the heart to the pericardium
have occasionally been found, without any previous symptoms of
acute inflammation ; nay, sometimes, I believe, without any evideuces of disease at all.   It appears that habit will, in many cases
reconcile the heart to a degree of restraint in its action, which at
first may have been almost insupportable to it.   When the adhesions are partial and long, Dr. Baillie is of opinion that little or no
inconvenience may be felt ; but when close, and extending over
the whole surface of the heart, very considerable disturbance is
generally produced,—so much indeed as sometimes to prove fatal.

The symptoms of chronic pericarditis are not always, it must be
confessed, well defined ; and many, even of those which are considered of most importance, are occasionally present in hysteria
and dyspepsia ; but still, in a great majority of cases, the diagnostic symptoms are sufficiently apparent.   They are, a constant
sense of oppression about the region of the heart, often, but incor-
rectly, termed *palpitation* ; pain, sometimes in the situation of the
heart, but more commonly referred to some distant part ; pulsation
in the epigastrium ; and dispnœa, aggravated by the slightest exertion of the body, or any strong emotion of mind.   To a person
so affected, the climbing a pair of stairs, or the ascent of a hill, are
insurmountable obstacles.   At night the patient is disturbed by
dreams of headlong precipices and rushing waters, of quick pur-
suit and impossible escape.   The pulse is full, strong, and jarring,
and the whole frame appears to vibrate with the systole, and dias-
tole of the heart.   In the worst cases dropsy succeeds.

The duration of the disease is very various.   While it sometimes
proves fatal in a few weeks, or months, it is occasionally protracted even for years, and medicine has certainly considerable power
in controlling this very formidable affection.   It is satisfactory to
know, that such symptoms as I have now detailed, have been in
some instances completely subdued.

The following plan of treatment has been found efficacious, and
is consonant to general principles.   It consists in keeping down
the action of the heart by occasional purgatives, and a very light
diet ; in avoiding all severe exercise, and restraining, as far as possible, those emotions of mind which tend to hurry the circulation.

28

A drain should be established in the neighbourhood of the heart, by means of a seton, which should be kept open for at least six weeks. Small doses of digitalis and calomel, in combination with extract of cicuta (as in R No. 54,) have had a well-marked effect in moderating the pulse, and diminishing that general irritability of the frame, which a chronic state of disease in the heart commonly induces. When from cold, or any other accidental cause, the symptoms become unusually severe, blood must be taken from the arm to the extent of eight ounces.

CHAP. XII.

In the abdomen, a variety of structures are met with, all of course subject to inflammation. These it will be necessary briefly to notice, before the several kinds and characters of abdominal inflammation can be justly appreciated. There is, in the first place, the peritonæum, the most extensive serous membrane of the body, lining the viscera and the muscular parietes of the abdomen. Whatever portion of it be primarily attacked, the general characters of the inflammation remain the same, receiving only some slight addition or modification from the structure and functions of the subjacent viscus. It is to Bichat we are indebted for our present notions of the general nature and modifications of peritonæal inflammation. They had formerly been confounded with diseases, commencing in the organs invested by this membrane. Bichat first pointed out, as an important principle both in pathology and practice, that a morbid state of the peritonæum was compatible with, and frequently attended by a healthy state of the parts which it covers. This principle had been partially known before, but never distinctly avowed, or thoroughly investigated.

The second of the structures within the abdomen, is the parenchyma of the solid viscera ; and the third is the mucous membrane of the intestinal canal. The inflammatory affections of each of these parts will require a separate consideration.

The peritonæum is subject to two kinds of inflammation, the

acute and chronic, very distinct from each other in their character
and progress.   The acute form of peritonæal inflammation is that
to which my attention will first be directed.*

This disease begins with rigors, a quickened pulse, and other
marks of fever.   From the commencement it is usually attended
with its characteristic symptom—pain of the abdomen, increased
on pressure ; but it will 'occasionally be observed, that pain of the
back is chiefly complained of for the first four-and-twenty hours.
In some cases, the invasion of the disease is sudden, and the pain
becomes in a short time almost intolerable.   In others, the advance
of the disease is more gradual, and the pain is felt only on pressure.   At first, it is commonly confined to one spot, more partien-
larly to the navel, but by degrees it extends over the whole abdomen.   With very few exceptions, indeed, the pain of peritonæal
inflammation is constant.   The pulse is about a hundred in a minute,
varying however very much in character, but for the most part contracted, and hard, or wiry.   There is great thirst, and the tongue
is covered with a cream-coloured mucus.   The abdomen is swelled and tense.   The patient lies on his back and frequently complains even of the weight of the bed-clothes.   Peritonæal inflammation may exist with every possible state of the evacuations.   If severe, and suffered to proceed, it usually proves fatal between the
seventh and tenth day ; the countenance collapsing, the pulse becoming very indistinct, and the extremities cold.

On dissection, the peritonæum generally, or in some of its parts,
will be found minutely injected with blood, the convolutions of the
bowels loosely glued together, and serum (in which flakes of lymph
may be observed floating,) or sometimes pure pus, in considerable
quantity, effused into the cavity of the abdomen.   Ulceration of the
peritonæum has been met with, but it is a rare appearance.   The
intestines are occasionally distended with air, constituting tympa-
nitis.

Such is the general character of peritonæal inflammation, whether the omentum, or the mesentery, or the surfaces of the different
solid and membranous viscera, or that portion of it which lines the
muscular parietes of the abdomen, be the chief seat of disease.   Its
symptoms are in some respects modified by the structure and func-

---

* In this and the two following chapters, I have derived the greatest assistance from Dr. Pemberton's " Practical Treatise on various Diseases of
the Abdominal Viscera."   London, 1806.—This useful work should be in
the hands of every student.

tions of the subjacent viscus ; and these modifications have been assumed by all nosologists, as the ground-work of a subdivision of this affection into several species. It is certainly a curious circumstance, considering the tendency to spread, which the inflammation of membranes, both serous and mucous, generally exhibits, that peritonæal inflammation should sometimes be so completely confined to one portion of its extent, that these nosological distinctions become applicable in practice. The particular symptoms which characterize inflammation of the capsule of the liver, will be best explained when the corresponding affection of the parenchyma of that organ comes under review. For the present, therefore, I confine my attention to the symptoms of Gastritis and Enteritis. The inflammation of the omentum, mesentery, and peritonæal coverings of the spleen, pancreas, uterus, and bladder, offer no phenomena of any particular interest.

GASTRITIS is a very rare disorder ; and the few cases of it on record are primary inflammations of the mucous, and not of the peritonæal coat of the stomach. The symptoms usually attributed to inflammation of the peritonæal coat of the stomach, are an acute pain, and sense of burning heat in the epigastrium, vomiting, increased by the mildest ingesta, extreme debility, a remarkable anxiety of countenance, and delirium.

Inflammation of the paritonæal coat of the intestines, or ENTERITIS, is, on the other hand, the most frequent of all the forms of peritonæal inflammation ; and it is also the most dangerous, and the most rapid in its progress. It has been known to prove fatal in four days. Besides the symptoms already enumerated as characterizing peritonæal inflammation generally, enteritis is distinguished by great prostration of strength, restlessness, a continual tossing of the arms, nausea and vomiting, an expression of great anxiety in the countenance, and *costiveness.* This last symptom, though not constantly, is yet so generally met with in cases where the peritonæal surface of the bowels is *primarily* affected, that it may be looked upon as one of the diagnostic marks of the disease. Where peritonæal inflammation however occurs in the course of typhoid or other fevers, diarrhœa is generally observed to prevail. In enteritis, the pulse is often very obscure, but generally quick, hard, and incompressible. The tongue is white, with a streak of brown fur down the middle. The pain, which is usually referred to the navel, is aggravated occasionally in paroxysms, probably from spasmodic contractions of the muscular coat of the bowels. In the

worst cases, delirium comes on about the sixth or seventh day (seldom earlier) and death speedily follows.

The extreme feebleness of the pulse, the coldness of the extremities, sunk features, hiccup, and other marks of failure of the powers of life, which occur in the last stage of enteritis, are often said
to denote that gangrene has taken place; but in a great number of
instances, these symptoms occur without the slightest trace of gangrene being discoverable on dissection. Sufficient cause of death is
to be found in the *extent* and *violence* of inflammatory action. When
gangrenous spots do appear, it is supposed by some pathologists
that the inflammation has spread to the muscular structure of the
intestines.

Acute peritonæal inflammation occurs to all ages,* and at all
seasons of the year.   Cold combined with moisture, is presumed
to be its most common exciting cause ; but enteritis has not unfrequently been brought on by causes applied more directly to the
membrane itself; such as a full meal of high-seasoned food, intemperance, and accumulation of hardened fæces.   It has been often
aggravated, perhaps even actually induced, by strong, and especially *spirituous* cathartics.   In some instances it has been owing
to causes which no prudence could avert ; such as intus-susceptio,
morbid elongations of the mesentery and omentum strangulating a
portion of intestine, and a wound of the bowel in the operation of
tapping.   There is a particular species of peritonæal inflammation,
which occurs to women after child-birth, and is generally known
under the name of *puerperal fever.*   Whether the local disease be
primary or secondary, is still a matter of doubt ; but there is every
reason to believe that the affection, whatever be its nature, is contagious, and communicable by the clothes of the practitioner.
Though sometimes fatal, it is seldom so severe, or so rapid in its
progress, as common peritonitis.

The only diseases with which I have ever seen peritonæal inflammation liable to be confounded are, colic, and affections of the
kidney, probably from calculus.   In regard to colic, it must be
borne in mind, that peritonitis has, in some cases, succeeded violent attacks of the colic ; and the possibility of this conversion
should never be lost sight of while engaged in establishing the diagnosis.   Colic is distinguished from peritonæal inflammation by

* A distinct case of peritonæal inflammation, occurring in an infant a
week old, and proving fatal on the fifth day, is recorded by Dr. Garthshore.
Med. Communications, vol. ii. page 44.

the absence of fever, by the pain occurring in paroxysms, with occasional intervals of complete ease, and by its being alleviated,
rather than increased, on pressure. With respect to afiections of
the kidney, I have seen them attended with severe and constant
pain of the whole abdomen, costiveness, nausea, and vomiting ; but
the pulse was slow in these cases, and pressure on the belly did not
aggravate the pain.

The general prognosis in peritonæal inflammation, particularly
in enteritis, is, upon the whole, unfavourable. The disease, it is
true, is very much under our control at first ; but if neglected, even
for twenty-four hours, the mischief is sometimes irremediable.
The sequelæ of the disease too are very formidable—agglutination
of the bowels, dropsy, and a tendency to relapse. The particular
prognosis is to be regulated almost entirely by the *extent* of pain.
When the boundaries of the inflamed portion of membrane can be
ascertained, judicious measures will probably save the patient. In
weakened habits, when the *whole surface* of the membrane is affected, recovery is almost hopeless. To have procured a free passage of the bowels is, of course, a favourable symptom ; but it is
very far indeed from being decisive as to the subsidence of inflammatory action.

When the disease is once ascertained, the treatment is sufficiently simple. Purgative medicines are not to be given at first, while
active inflammation is going on ; but blood is to be taken from the
arm to the extent of at least sixteen ounces ; and if the pain on
pressure continue unabated, this should be repeated in six or eight
hours, before any attempts are made to open the bowels by medicine. In very urgent cases, it is advisable to place the patient in
a warm bath, and in that situation to open a vein. The abstraction of a quantity of blood is thus rendered not only more effectual, but more *certain*. It was long ago observed, that the blood does
not always appear buffy in the early stages of enteritis. No reliance therefore can be placed on this symptom. Nor is the practitioner to be deterred by the marks of *oppression*, or apparent exhaustion, which often occur in the outset of the disease. The
pulse commonly rises as the system is freed from the load which
oppresses it. In addition to bleeding at the arm, or sometimes as a
substitute for it, particularly where the seat of pain is limited, or
when the strength of the patient is likely to fail, ten or twelve
leeches may be applied to the abdomen. They sometimes give
great and immediate relief. A blister should not be applied until a

later period of the disease. The practice of applying a blister, in all cases of local pain, without due regard to its cause, cannot be defended. In peritonæal inflammation it is particularly hurtful, as it takes away our best guide in the adminstration of other remedies. Warm fomentations are greatly preferable in an early stage of the disease, and should be applied diligently on any return of pain.

Inflammatory action must mainly be subdued by the measures now alluded to. Internal medicines however are not to be neglect. ed, and mild laxatives, in small and frequently repeated doses, are the most useful. Castor oil and Epsom salts (R No. 27 and 29) or the infusion of senna and tamarinds of the Edin. Pharm. (R No. 24,) may be mentioned as well adapted to the circumstances of this disease. If the stomach is very irritable, and rejects medicine in the fluid form, small doses of calomel, in union with the extract of hyoscyamus, will sometimes be retained, and prove useful. Frequent emollient glysters are very serviceable, and should never be neglected. Effervescent draughts may also be tried. A tobacco injection has been mentioned as affording some chance of relief, but it cannot be recommended.

Chronic inflammation of the peritonæum is not unfrequent, and there is very considerable uniformity in the symptoms and progress of the disease. Its advances are very insidious. Occasional pricking pains over the abdomen, with a quickened pulse, and coated tongue, give the first evidence of disease. The pain, or *tightness*, of which the patient complains, is occasionally aggravated in paroxysms of geat violence. This tendency to periodical exacerbation in the pain, is an important index of chronic peritonæal inflammation. The pulse remains steadily above 100, and is often full. During the early stages of the disease, the patient continues his ordinary occupations, but complains always of an increase of pain or soreness across the abdomen, from fatigue. There is thirst, and want of sleep and appetite. As the disease advances, the features appear sharp and contracted, and the countenance pale, sallow, or doughy. The tongue is either of a bright red colour, or covered with a thick mucus. The taking of food creates much uneasiness, particularly a sense of weight in the abdomen. There

is no considerable tension in common cases, but a degree of hardness in the viscera may often be distinctly traced. Costiveness
usually prevails, and increases very considerably the distresses of
the patient. I have seen this go on to perfect *ileus* (stercoraceous
vomiting). Great emaciation and debility succeed, and the patient
ultimately dies hectic, and exhausted. The duration of the disease
varies from three or four to twelve months. It is full of danger.
I have seen but one case recover where the symptoms were strongly marked. Relapses are to be dreaded, even though a diminution
of the pulse, and of pain, should indicate a degree of improvement.

On dissection, the peritonæum appears discoloured, and often
thickened to a great extent. Tuberculated accretions of different
forms are found attached to it, sometimes appearing like bunches
of grapes. The convolutions of the intestines are matted together, and often form with the liver, omentum, and other viscera,
a mass, in which it is scarcely possible to distinguish one part from
another. In many cases there is an effusion of dropsical fluid, and
occasionally of purulent matter, with or without ulceration of the
peritonæal membrane. The subjacent viscera are sometimes perfectly healthy.

The disease for which chronic peritonitis is most liable to be
mistaken is ascites, or ovarial dropsy (an accidental, and by no
means frequent symptom, being looked upon as the primary disease). Several persons have been tapped for this complaint. A
few pints of water are perhaps discharged, but without affording
any relief to the sufferings of the patient.

The causes of this affection are involved in great obscurity. I
have seen it occur as a consequence of common fever; but it is
doubtful, if that hardness of the abdomen, which is occasionally
met with in convalescence from typhus, and recovered from, is
really attributable to chronic peritonæal inflammation. All ages
are subject to this disease. In children it is by no means uncommon, and it constitutes one of the forms of *marasmus*, as I shall
hereafter more fully point out. It appears to be connected at that
period of life with the scrofulous diathesis; and I have noticed, as
a peculiarity of the disease when so occurring, that erosions take
place of the peritonæal and mucous coats of the intestines, by
which a quantity of matter, which had been formed by the diseased peritonæum, finds its way into the intestine, and is discharged

29

by stool. This form of the affection I have ventured to call the scrofulous inflammation of the peritonæum.*

The method of treatment in chronic peritonitis is very little un-derstood, but the following plan offers the best prospect of success. Topical bleeding, to the extent of six ounces, may be directed twice in the week, while the sensation of pricking pain continues. Some-times I have found it necessary to bleed from the arm. Without free alvine evacuations, the distress becomes quite insupporta-ble; but large quantities of purgative medicines, which are some-times given, under the idea that the disease consists only in fœcu-lent accumulations, are decidedly prejudicial. Some gentle mer-curial preparations, and blisters may be tried. In one case, I thought benefit was derived from digitalis. A light diet of milk and vegetables should be strictly enforced. Opium is often indis-pensable in the latter stages of the disease.

* See Medico-Chirurgical Transactions, vol. xi, page 258.

Liability of this membrane to inflammation, both Acute and Chronic. Aphthous Diarrhœa of Children. Inflammation of the Mucous Membrane of the Stomach in Adults. Of the Mucous Membrane of the small Intestines in Adults. Of Dysentery. Its Causes. Symptoms. Morbid Appearances. Treatment. Symptoms and Treatment of Chronic Dysentery.

THE pathology of the mucous membrane of the alimentary canal is a subject of great extent and importance, but it has rot yet been investigated with all the accuracy which it deserves. While some parts of it are well understood, others are involved in a degree of obscurity which it will require a long course of observation to clear up. One of the most obvious of its general principles, is the great, liability of the membrane to inflammation. Such an affection occurs both in an acute and chronic form,—as idiopathic, and as supervening on other diseases,—in adults, and inchildren. There appears to be a peculiar tenderness and susceptibility of inflammation in this membrane during the first years of life, and this points out the great importance of regulating the diet of children with the most scrupulous care.

The mucous membrane of the intestinal canal, as has been remarked by Dr. Baillie,* is more disposed to become *ulcerated* than any other membrane of similar function in the body. It is difficult to assign a satisfactory reason for this; but it probably depends on some minute difference of structure. There is a good deal of resemblance, observes this author, between the structure of the inner membrane of the trachea, and that of the urethra, and their secretions likewise are not very different. The inner membrane

* Morbid Anatomy. 5th edit. page 169.

of the intestines, however, has a structure and secretion peculiar to itself.

As a general principle it may be stated, that inflammation occurring in any one part of the mucous membrane of the alimentary canal, is apt to spread to others. Thus it is, that when we observe apthæ in the mouth, we may expect, on dissection, to find ulceration of the ileum. But it is to be observed, also, that the appearances of inflammation are in some cases confined to one portion of its extent. It is not uncommon, for instance, to find ulceration of the ileum terminating by a distinct line at the valve of the colon, and the mucous membrane of the large intestines altogether free from disease. I shall now describe, very briefly, the symptoms and progress of the inflammation of the mucous membrane of the intestines, as it occurs at different periods of life, and in different parts of the membrane, but without pretending to fix, with any degree of accuracy, the precise portion of it occupied by the disease.

APHTHA.

Infants are subject to an inflammatory affection of the mucous membrane of the alimentary canal, general classed as a species of diarrhœa, but known also by name of aphtha, or *the thrush*, from a symptom which attends it in one of its stages. It chiefly occurs between the fourth and eighth month, and among such as are fed wholly or partially upon spoon-meat. There is reason to believe, that it is always connected with an improper diet. It is characterized by vomiting, fœtid eructations, and pain, apparently referred to the epigastrium; tormina, diarrhœa, and some degree of tenderness of the belly on pressure. The stools are green, and slimy, or tinged with blood. Frequently they are ejected with great force. As soon as any food is taken into the stomach, the child has a motion, giving the appearance as if it passed immediately through the bowels. As the disease advances, the tongue becomes red; the mouth is covered with aphthæ, and the verge of the anus appears inflamed. The brain also becomes affected, illustrating that important pathological principle which I had occasion to allude to, when treating of the diagnosis of hydrocephalus. The child is frequently drowsy, before the aphthæ appear. This symp-

tom is vulgarly called sleeping for the thrush. Coma is occasionally observed to come on towards the termination of the complaint.
The infant rapidly emaciates.

This disease is a true inflammation of the mucous membrane of
the bowels. On dissection there appear, in various parts of the
inner surface of the intestines, particularly the ileum, irregular
patches of inflammation, slightly elevated above the surrounding
parts, and often covered with minute vesicles and ulcers.* It often proves fatal in a short time, and requires therefore, great attention in its early stages. The treatment should be begun by an
emetic, consisting of four grains of ipecacuanha. Small doses of
castor oil, or of rhubarb and magnesia, should then be given frequently, while the urgent symptoms continue. Mucilaginous and
anodyne injections may be thrown up, with the view of sheathing
the lower parts of the inflamed membrane. A warm bath is frequently serviceable. Great attention should be paid to the diet of
the child, which must consist altogether of milk, or of the lightest
farinaceous preparations.

An affection, very similar to the proceeding, is met with in children from the period of weaning, as late as the fourth or fifth year
of life, and even later. It is attributable, I believe in most cases,
to an improper course of diet ; very often to a diet composed of a
larger proportion of animal food, than the stomach, at that age, is
capable of digesting. It\is of a more chronic nature than the *aphthous diarrhœa* of infants at the breast. It frequently goes on to
complete emaciation, and it constitutes, in fact one of the forms of
the atrophia of children,—a disease which has received the various names of tabes mesenterica, marasmus, and infantile remitting fever.

On dissection, in these cases, the mucous membrane of the bowels is found extensively ulcerated, and the mesenteric glands more
or less enlarged ; but this last appearance is probably dependent on
the former. Whether there is a disease of the mesenteric glands,
primary, and independent of disease in the intestines, and how far
it may be looked upon as a frequent occurrence, are points in pathology which do not appear to have been hitherto very accurately
investigated.

---

* Vide Dr. Abercrombie, on the Pathology of the Intestinal Canal. Ed.
Med. and Surg. Journal, 'July 1820, page 326. A valuable paper, from
which I have derived much useful information.

The mucous membrane of the *stomach* is liable to be affected by inflammation, in consequence of acrid matters swallowed. It has been supposed, that arsenic proves fatal by bringing on inflammation of the stomach; but Mr. Brodie has shown the incorrectness of this as a general proposition. In some cases, indeed, there can be little doubt, that after a certain time, inflammation of the mucous membrane of the stomach does come on in consequence of arsenic, and the case published by Dr. Roget* may be brought forward as an instance; but even here the symptoms of high nervous irritation predominated greatly over those of the local inflammation. Dr. Baillie states,† that on dissection, an extreme degree of redness then appears in the inner membrane of the stomach. Portions of it are sometimes destroyed, and occasionally a thin layer of coagulable lymph is thrown out. Such appearances however cannot be relied on as proofs of poisoning.

Inflammation of the mucous membrane of the small intestines occurs in *adults*, both as an idiopathic affection, and as symptomatic of other diseases,—in an *acute* as well as chronic form. The symptoms by which it is characterized are not always very distinct; and hence it is, that the disease, though by no means uncommon, has hitherto remained without any appropriate designation from nosological writers.‡

It is attended with a diffused soreness over the whole abdomen, rather than with pain. This is sometimes increased on pressure, but never to the extent that prevails in peritonæal inflammation. There is no considerable tension in the belly. The pulse is quick, with thirst, *languor*, and considerable febrile oppression. By these symptoms we distinguish *inflammation* of the mucous membrane of the bowels, from that state of *irritation* of the membrane, which exists in common cases of diarrhœa; but it must never be forgotten, that the two states of disease are closely allied, and, in fact, run into each other by insensible degrees. The tongue is *red, and smooth*, and eruptions take place about the lips. Vomiting is fre-

* Medico-Chirurgical Transactions, vol. ii, 1811.
† Morbid Anatomy, page 147.
‡ It has sometimes been called the intestinal catarrh. *Enteritis Mucosa* is perhaps its legitimate denomination.

quently noticed, with loss of appetite, indigestion, and irregularity in the alvine evacuations. Diarrhœa is almost uniformly present ; the stools are slimy, and tinged with blood. In severe cases, pure blood is occasionally passed in considerable quantity. An increased secretion of mucus from the intestines constitutes one of the principal features of the disease. It must be confessed, however, .that in the appearance of the evacuations there is considerable diversity. In some instances inflammation exists to a considerable extent, while the motions differ but slightly from those of common diarrhœa. Nothing perhaps more strikingly distinguishes this complaint than that degree of morbid irritability of the whole intestin. al canal, by which food, even of the lightest kind, or a little cold water taken into the stomach, stimulates the rectum to immediate contraction.

The disease is always tedious, but not commonly fatal. It occasionally proves so, with or without supervening peritonæal inflammation, or it passes into a chronic state, in which the patient at length sinks exhausted. The chronic form of the affection is marked by pain of the abdomen, diarrhœa alternating with costiveness, increasing weakness and emaciation, hectic fever, and a tongue præternaturally red, or aphthous. It is certainly a curious circumstance, that the appetite, in this state of disease, often continues good.

The appearances, on dissection, vary very much with the degree of violence in the inflammatory action, or what is nearly the same thing, with the period of disease at which death takes place. Sometimes we observe only an increased redness of the whole membrane ; at other times, irregular patches of inflammatiom may be traced, elevated sensibly above the sound parts. The lower end of the ileum has been long observed to be the most common situation of these morbid appearances. Ulcers are frequently met with there, of an oval shape, having elevated edges. Sometimes a considerable extent of the inner membrane of the intestine is seen completely stripped from the mucular coat, or hanging attached to it in tattered shreds. In a few cases the ulceration perforates the peritonæal coat, and a portion of the contents of the intestines passes into the general cavity of the abdomen, producing inflammation that speedily proves fatal. Inflammation of the intestine, sometimes, although rarely, advances to mortification.

The causes of this affection of the internal membrane of the bowels are not very well understood. A disposition seems to be

given to it by irregular habits of life, and one attack certainly favours a recurrence of the complaint. It prevails at times epidemically. I have seen it in its idiopathic form, arising from accidental exposure to cold and moisture, but it is much more commonly
witnessed as supervening on other diseases. It appears in the progress of continued fever, consumption, and all diseases attended
with hectic, and it is one of the most frequent sequelæ of measles.
It would seem, indeed, as if inflammation and ulceration of this
structure readily took place, whenever the system was in the state,
either of very high, or very long protracted inflammatory excitement.

If the disease comes under treatment in an early stage, great
advantage will be derived from taking away ten or twelve ounces
of blood from the arm. This I have several times seen to give an
immediate check to the disease. At a later period, leeches prove
an excellent substitute. Active purging is carefully to be avoided.
Small doses of castor oil (R No. 27,) or the sulphate of magnesia
with a few drops of tinctura opii (R No. 31,) will occasionally be
found useful ; but in the irritable condition of the bowels that then
prevails, soothing, anodyne, and demulcent medicines (R Nos. 49
and 58,) are much preferable. Starch injections with laudanum
may be recommended where the tenesmus is very troublesome.
When the feverish symptoms subside, and the diarrhœa lessens, a
gentle tonic will be useful ; and after giving trial to a great variety, I
have found none answer the purpose so well as myrrh, four grains
of which may be added to the draught R No. 68. Particular attention should be paid to the diet of the patient, which should be of
the lightest kind. All fermented liquors, and at first, broths also
should be strictly prohibited.

When the disease has assumed a chronic form, with extensive
ulceration, the treatment is very precarious. Astringents and bitters, with laudanum, are indispensable with the view of checking
the diarrhœa, but the astringent tinctures should carefully be avoided. Catechu appears to me to be less irritating than any of those
to which I have given trial. A pill consisting of one grain of calomel with the extr. hyoscyami (R No. 55,) may be administered at
night with considerable advantage. Change of air may be advised, and a milk diet. Under this treatment I have seen very many
unfavourable cases gradually recover.

DYSENTERY is a disease closely allied in its symptoms to that which was last under examination ; and though it would probably be going too far to say, that in cases of mild dysentery there is always inflammatory action of the vessels of the mucous membrane of the intestines, yet in severe cases of the disease, this certainly happens ; and there can be no great error in considering dysentery as at all times arising from, or strongly tending to, such a state. This view of the *proximate cause* of the disease is borne out by a consideration of its remote causes, of its symptoms, and of the efficacy of a treatment similar to that which is adopted in other inflammatory affections. Dissection also leads to the same conclusion ; for ulceration and mortification are here commonly met with, as in the inflammations of other parts. We presume that in dysentery the principal seat of disease is the inner membrane of the *great* intestines, for morbid appearances chiefly present themselves in that part of the alimentary canal.

Dysentery is peculiarly the disease of warm climates and seasons. Between the tropics it often rages with a degree of violence, of which no adequate idea can be formed, from instances of the complaint witnessed in this country. A sudden check to perspiration is perhaps the most common of its exciting causes. The night dews of hot countries are therefore particularly to be guarded against ; but excessive fatigue and long exposure to the direct rays of the sun appear in some cases to have brought it on. Some stress has been laid upon irregularity of diet (such as eating abundantly of ripe fruit,) as tending to dysentery, but its influence has probably been over-rated. That contagion has occasionally operated as a cause of this disease, in camps and on board slave ships, cannot, I presume, be questioned ; but neither in this country nor in tropical climates is dysentery contagious under common circumstances.

The characteristic symptoms of dysentery are griping pains of the bowels, and a frequent desire to go to stool, the evacuations being watery, mucous, or bloody, and without any admixture of natural fæces. The patient perpetually complains of a *load* in the intestines, which he endeavours to throw off by violent efforts of straining, and though he feels them to be ineffectual, he is unable to resist them. Small lumps called *scybala* are sometimes passed, but their appearance is not uniform, nor of any particular importance.

This state of disease in the alimentary canal is always accompanied by fever ; in many cases of a highly inflammatory character

30

The pulse is very frequent; the mouth and fauces dry and clam-my. The tongue is covered with a dark fur in the centre; or, when much bile is secreted, with a yellow fur at its posterior part; or it is red and polished. In severe cases the stomach becomes very irritable, the mildest fluids being rejected, while an unceasing thirst prevails; or that state of sympathetic irritation in the whole tract of the alimentary canal takes place, by which *tormina* and *tenesmus* immediately succeed the swallowing of the blandest li-quids.

The nervous system suffers also severely. Nothing appears to weaken the body so much as dysenteric purging. In very bad cases, hiccup, cramps of the gastrocnemii, and strangury occur; and great exhaustion of power is evinced in the staggering or giddiness, and even syncope, which take place when the patient is brought into the erect posture. The duration of the disease is subject to great variety. The acute dysentery of hot climates sometimes proves fatal in a few days; but in a practical point of view it is more im-portant to bear in mind the disposition of the disease to assume a *chronic* form.

In very severe and protracted dysenteries, dissection exhibits the inner membrane of the great intestines thickened, and formed into small irregular tubercles of a white or yellowish colour, with thick-ening of the peritonæal and muscular coats. In some instances, patches of the membrane have been observed in a state of high inflammation. Occasionally it is found abraded or extensively ul-cerated. This appearance has been seen to extend to the small in-testines. In tropical dysenteries the colon has sometimes been found decidedly in a state of mortification; and fæces have even escaped through the mortified gut into the cavity of the abdomen. With these, which are the true dysenteric appearances, marks of peritonæal inflammation are not unfrequently united.

The treatment of dysentery is to be regulated by a consideration, first of the tendency to inflammation which exists in the mucous membrane of the intestines; secondly, of that apparently spasmo-dic contraction of the muscular fibres in contact with the diseased membrane, by which the fæces are retained; and lastly, of that morbid increase of irritability in the whole extent of the alimentary canal, which prevails in this as well as other affections of its mu-cous membrane.

If the pain be constant and severe, and the pulse strong, or cor-dy, blood should be taken from the arm, particularly in a case

which comes early under treatment. But the employment of *pur.*
gatives constitutes the most important part of the cure of dysentery.
They must be steadily persisted in, until *fæcal* evacuations have
been produced, and that sensation of load in the bowels completely
removed, which leads to the effort of straining. Then, *and not
until then*, may the practitioner desist from the free use of his ca.
thartics. Almost every kind of purgative medicine has been tried,
and at different times recommended. Provided a due effect be pro.
duced, it does not appear to be of much consequence which of them
is selected ; but the liquid *form* is generally to be preferred. A
pill of six grains of calomel, followed immediately by an ounce of
the sulphate of magnesia, will commonly be found to answer well.
In some cases, the oleum ricini may be preferable. If the stomach
rejects these medicines, some other form of cathartic (R No. 5 or
13) is to be chosen ; the opium being added with the view of allay.
ing irritation. Purgative enemata are found insufficient to overcome
the disease. An ointment containing opium applied to the anus
after every loose motion will greatly relieve the smarting which
the acrid secretions of the bowels produce. *

When proper fæcal evacuations have been procured, it will generally be proper to continue the same medicines in smaller doses
(R No. 15 and 31) ; and if after that, pain and diarrhæa continue,
anodyne draughts (R No. 48,) and mucilaginous anodyne injections (R No. 107) will be found very useful. The pulv. ipec. comp.
either in the dose of fifteen grains at bed time, or of six grains every six hours, is well adapted to this state of the disease. It promotes perspiration, a proper attention to which is very requisite du.
ring the whole course of the complaint. The effect of this medicine will be materially aided by the warm bath. In hot climates,
the exhibition of mercury, pushed so as to produce salivation, has
been recommended as an effectual method of putting a check to
the advances of dysentery.† The testimonies in favour of this practice are certainly very strong ; at the same time we have no reason
to believe that a vigorous and well.regulated employment of the
means already recommended, is less efficacious in hot climates
than we find it in our own.

Chronic Dysentery is the sequel of the acute stage. It is some-

* See Appendix ; Note T.

† See a Paper by Dr. Fergusson, in the Medico-Chirurgical Transactions,
vol. ii, page 182.

times connected with structural derangement, particularly ulceration of the mucous membrane of the colon ; but at other times it appears to be only a continuance of that diseased action previously established. In the former case purulent matter may sometimes be detected in the motions ; but, for the most part, the local symptoms will only differ in the degree of their violence from those of the acute stage. This is a very dangerous form of disease. When the membrane is *extensively* ulcerated, extreme weakness and emaciation follow, and the patient is at length worn out by the inccssant discharge which is kept up. It is surprising however to observe how long he will sometimes linger under circumstances apparently hopeless. In such a state, the slightest irregularity of diet, or regimen, aggravates the symptoms. Ulceration of the intestines has been supposed to heal with difficulty under all circumstances ; but it is obvious that the healing process will go on most favourably, when a light, unirritating, and easily digested food is taken. A gentle action should be kept up also in the bowels, so as to prevent accumulation and distension. Hence we may see the propriety of directing an occasional dose of rhubarb and calomel (R No. 12), or of castor oil, when there is any considerable degree of griping pain.

When the circulation is languid, and the constitution much weakened, it is reasonable to suppose that the local action of ulcers will also be weak and indolent, and likely to be improved by such medieines as promote digestion, and give *tone* to the system.* This conclusion is supported by experience. Benefit has been derived, in many cases of chronic dysentery attended with ulceration, from the exhibition of a decoction of bark, myrrh, the aromatic confection, balsam of copaiva, and other stimulant and tonic drugs (R Nos. 63, 71, 78.) When the evacuations are copious, but unattended with pain, and probably kept up by an irritable state of the membrane, astringents, absorbents, and opiates (R No. 100) may be required ; but in every case their effects are to be carefully watched, and omitted altogether, if they bring on tormina. Lime water taken freely has an excellent effect, particularly where there is nausea with acidity. The sulphate of copper, in the dose of two grains twice or thrice a day, has been found a useful astringent in

---

* Consult Bampfield's Practical Treatise on Tropical Dysentery, which contains a very full and judicious exposition of the varieties of the chronic form of the disease, and of the principles of its treatment,

chronic dysentery. It not unfrequently happens that the patient gradually recovers his strength, appetite, and flesh, during a moderate state of diarrhœa. In some instances it is found, that small doses of mercury (either in the form of hydr. cum creta, pil. hydr. or calomel) in combination with ipecacuanha, contribute to an improved appearance of the secretions of the intestines. The complication of dysentery with chronic hepatitis, which is occasionally met with, will be an additional motive for the exhibition of mercurial alteratives.

Such are the principles upon which the treatment of chronic dysentery is to be conducted. They should be well understood, because an injudicious practice may do much harm, though the best regulated may prove ineffectual.

Acute Inflammation of the Peritonœal covering of the Liver. Diagnosis. Inflammation of the Substance of the Liver. Terminations of this Disease. Of Hepatic Abscess. Causes of Acute Hepatitis. Treatment. Of Chronic Hepatitis. Its Causes, Symptoms, and Treatment. Torpor of the Liver. Diagnosis of Hepatalgia.

THE peritonæum forming the capsule of the liver is liable to acute inflammation; and it is the common form of hepatitis which we have occasion to observe in this country. The *substance* of the liver is also the seat of inflammation, both acute and chronic. This disease too is occasionally met with here, but both are infinitely more frequent in hot climates, where hepatitis may justly be considered as *endemic*.

The peculiar symptoms which denote that the peritonæal surface of the liver is the seat of inflammation are, pain in the right hypochondrium, shooting to the back and shoulder, generally very acute, permanent, and increased on pressure; a white and dry tongue, hurried respiration, cough, and difficulty of lying on the eft side. Jaundice occasionally occurs, and more particularly, it has been supposed, where the membrane covering the concave surface of the liver is affected; but it is not to be considered as a necessary concomitant of the disease. The bowels are sometimes constipated. At other times, diarrhœa is present. Indeed inflamed liver and dysentery frequently coexist in the same patient.

Some stress has been laid on *cough*, as a symptom of acute hepatitis, because it is likely to create difficulty in distinguishing this disease from inflammation within the chest. It is sometimes loose, but more commonly dry, and appears in many cases to be owing to the spreading of inflammation from the surface of the liver to the diaphragm. A full inspiration does not always produce *cough*, though it increases *pain*; and very generally this symptom does

not appear till the second or third day of the disease. In this manner, and by the increase of pain from pressure, we are commonly
able to distinguish acute hepatitis from pneumonia. The diagnosis
between inflammation of the liver, and spasm of the gall ducts from
the passage of a biliary calculus, will come under consideration
hereafter, when the symptoms of jaundice are explained.

Whether the hepatitis of warm climates begins in the membrane
or parenchyma of the liver, is of little moment ; for it is abundantly obvious, that in a large proportion of cases, the latter structure
becomes quickly, and to a great extent, involved in the disease.
The symptoms which characterise acute inflammation of the substance of the liver, are in most respects the same with those of its
peritonæal surface ; but in addition to them, some degree of swelling is generally to be felt externally ; the pain is more obtuse than
when the membrane is affected ; jaundice takes place ; the urine is
of a deep saffron colour ; the tongue is covered with a white, or
sometimes a yellowish fur ; the pulse is frequent and hard ; the skin
hot and dry ; and commonly there is nausea and vomiting, not probably from inflammation, but extreme irritability of the stomach.

In hot climates, the inflammation of the substance of the liver
often advances with great rapidity, so that in a short time suppuration takes place ; and it has been observed that an abscess forms
in the liver as rapidly where the local pain is trifling as where it is
intense.*   In cases of hepatitis, originating in this country, abscess
of the liver must certainly be viewed as an uncommon occurrence.
That suppuration will take place, may be inferred from the pulse
continuing full and frequent, and the pain urgent, with *rigors.*
When abscess has actually formed, there will be a sense of weight
in the part, with *throbbing* pains, occasional flushings of the countenance, night perspirations, and other marks of hectic fever.

The further progress of the disease is subject to great variety.
Hepatic abscess frequently proves fatal without any escape of its
contents, but at other times the matter works its way out by one
or other of the four following modes.   Adhesions sometimes form
between the liver and the parietes of the abdomen ; the tumour becomes more and more prominent ; and the matter is discharged by

* Dr. Clark, of Dominica, relates a case (Duncan's Medical Commentaries, vol. xiv,) where suppuration began on the fifth day of the disease,
and on the twenty-ninth the abscess burst; almost the whole substance of
the right lobe of the liver being destroyed.

an external opening. The usual situation of such a tumour is between the third and fourth false ribs. Sometimes, where such adhesions have not formed, and the walls of the abscess are thin, the
matter bursts into the cavity of the abdomen, bringing on peritonæal inflammation, which quickly proves fatal. Occasionally the
matter of the abscess finds its way by ulceration into the colon or
stomach ; and patients have recovered where there was reason to
believe that such an event had occurred. Lastly, it is by no means
uncommon for abscess of the liver to form a communication with
the cavity of the thorax by erosion of the diaphragm. Pus will then
be discharged (generally along with bile) by the bronchia, giving
rise to the very curious symptoms of *bilious expectoration* ; but the
patient seldom recovers. The abscesses formed by an inflammation of the liver are often of enormous size, capable of holding several quarts of matter. Very frequently *hydatids* are found accompanying them, and they add greatly to the danger of the disease.
The pathology of these morbid productions is very little understood. They have been found in all the great cavities of the body,
but more frequently attached to the liver than in any other situa-
ion. Under any circumstances, abscess of the liver is a dangerous
state of disease. It is only where the abscess is small, that recovery can, with any degree of confidence, be anticipated.

The causes of acute hepatitis are the same with those of inflammation generally ; but a very strong predisposition to it is given by
hot climates, and a long course of full living with indulgence in
spirituous liquors. Heat appears to have some peculiar and inexplicable influence upon the liver. To this principle only can we
attribute the frequency of hepatic complications with the intermittent and continued fevers of warm countries, the occurrence of
cholera and other bilious affections in this country during the summer and autumn months, and the general prevalence of hepatitis in
tropical regions.

It has been remarked, that the liver in warm climates seems to
be the seat of disease nearly in the same proportion that the lungs
are in Great Britian. Many of those who suffer from acute and
chronic hepatitis in this country have had the foundation of the disease laid by residence in a hot climate. The predisposition to liver disease which is given by high living and spirituous liquors,
though less interesting in a pathological view, is practically of far
more importance ; and it is applicable not only to acute inflammation of the liver, but to every form of chronic derangement of the

hepatic system, whether occurring in hot or cold climates. It must not however be forgotten in practice that genuine acute inflammation of the liver is occasionally met with in this country, where no suspicion of high living can be entertained ; in delicate chlorotic young women for instance, and in the latter stages of phthisis pulmonalis.

The treatment of hepatitis when it occurs in cold or temperate climates, and when it may be considered as confined altogether, or nearly so, to the investing membrane of the liver, is to be conducted on the principles which were laid down in the last chapter, as applicable to peritonæal inflammation generally. Bleeding from the arm, and locally by leeches or cupping, with fomentations and blisters, are principally to be relied on ; but the employment of saline purgatives (R Nos. 20 and 29) is also of very essential benefit. A purgative draught (R No. 21,) with a few grains of calomel, may even be ordered immediately after the first bleeding. Purging appears to be a means of diminishing inflammatory action, very well calculated for diseases of the liver. Pathologists have imagined that the peculiar distribution of the blood in the venous system of the abdomen may in some measure account for this. By increasing the secretions of the intestinal canal, it has been supposed, with some appearance of reason, that congestion of blood in the vena portarum, and consequent distension of the liver, may be, to a certain degree, lessened or prevented.

It has long been observed, that the blood which is drawn in inflammation of the liver, exhibits the very remarkable appearance of *greenish buff*; and different ideas, none of which however are very satisfactory, have been entertained regarding the cause of this phenomenon. The great danger of suppuration in the hepatitis of hot climates makes it necessary to be prompt in the employment of venesection. The same consideration induces some to employ *mercury* on the first attack. The propriety of this practice in hot climates cannot properly be judged of by experience acquired here, but theory and analogy seem equally opposed to it. When the febrile symptoms abate, however, recourse should undoubtedly be had to this remedy, in the manner which will presently be noticed. It is seldom that mercury is absolutely requisite in the acute hepatitis of this country ; but under proper management, it may be resorted to even here, in the latter stages of the disease, with some prospect of shortening the convalescence.

In the hepatitis of hot countries, the vigorous employment of the

31

lancet and of active mercurial purgatives (Nos. 5 and 8) can alone ensure a fortunate termination. The deceitful remissions which sometimes occur in the progress of the cure must not throw the practitioner off his guard, but on the first return of pain, the same remedies must be again resorted to.

The term CHRONIC HEPATITIS is not confined strictly to that state of slow inflammation of the liver which is attended by fever, and which terminates like other inflammations in suppuration, though such a disease exists, and is by no means uncommon ; but it is extended in common language so as to include different chronic affections of the liver, which may or may not have their origin in inflammation. It does not appear necessary, with a view, to practice, to attempt any minute distinctions between the different chronic diseases of the liver, although, in a pathological point of view, it must certainly be considered a matter of some interest. Were it even possible to ascertain during life the symptoms by which they could be distinguished from each other, it does not appear that we could as yet, apply our knowledge to the discrimination of remedies. The appearances which the liver presents in cases of chronic hepatitis are, simple enlargement without alteration of structure, enlargement with increased hardness, or præternatural softness and flaccidity of its substance, a small and contracted state of the gland, an unhealthy mottled aspect of its peritonæal coat, an ash-coloured hue of its substance, abscesses, and lastly, various kinds of tubercle. Of all the modifications of chronic disease of the liver, the most important is tubercle.*

The symptoms of chronic hepatitis are various, but at the same time in many cases so obscure, that while persons have been suspected of it, whose livers were perfectly sound, others have died, in whom the disease had remained unsuspected during life. The characteristic symptoms of the disease are, a sense of weight, or a dull numb pain in the right side or back, pain at the point of the shoulder, or a sense of heaviness or weariness in the right arm, a sallow countenance, and yellow tinge of the conjunctiva. In some

* This portion of the Morbid Anatomy of the Liver has been examined by Dr. Farre with great attention, in a work expressly dedicated to that subject.

cases, the enlarged liver can be distinctly felt under the finger. The pulse varies in point of frequency, but is feeble and often in-termitting ; the tongue is permanently loaded, and the appetite impaired. The urine frequently deposits a pink sediment. Venous hæmorrhages take place from the stomach and intestines, referable probably to the difficulty which the blood finds in passing through the vena portæ. For the same reason the external veins of the ab-domen appear swollen. Pimples break out on the nose and fore-head, and the face acquires a bloated appearance. Extreme lan-gnor, dejection of spirits, and sleepiness are often noticed. Dys-pepsia and atrophy are also prominent symptoms.

The observations already made on the causes of acute hepatitis apply equally to this form of the affection. It is sometimes the the *result* of acute inflammation, but it sometimes also precedes that state of disease. Enlargements of the liver have been the consequence of long continued intermittents. Chronic hepatitis may last a long time ; but in most cases it sooner or later ends in u ᴉsy, which proves fatal. The prognosis therefore should always be ᴉarded, particularly in elderly subjects. The probability of succt ᴉ in the treatment of the disease will depend partly on the state oɪ the constitution, and partly on the extent of morbid altera-tion which the *structure* of the liver has undergone.*

The means of relief are comprised in a course of regular mode-rate purging ; gentle doses of mercury pushed so as to affect the system ; the occasional exhibition of bitters and acids, especially the nitric acid ; with a light diet, and abstinence from all fermented and distilled liquors. Dr. Pemberton speaks highly of the efficacy of the extract of taraxacum (R No. 76.) Removal to a cold climate is often found indispensable in the chronic affections of the liver which occur to residents in the East and West Indies.

The chief reliance, as far as medicine extends, is of course to be placed on purging and mercurials. The natural purging waters, as those of Cheltenham, are well adapted to this complaint ; but the Seidlitz, Epsom, or Rochelle salts, in doses so regulated as to keep up a gentle but constant action on the bowels, are, probably, equal-ly effectual. Calomel or the blue pill may be given in small doses

* For the fullest information concerning hepatitis, and for numerous splen-did delineations of hepatic disorganizations, especially abscess, the reader is referred to Mr. Annesley's great work, entitled, " Researches into the causes, nature, and treatment of the Diseases of India," 4to. 1827.

at night, but it commonly answers better to direct a scruple or half a drachm of the strong mercurial ointment to be rubbed on the side every night, till the mouth be touched. This effect should be kept up, though cautiously, for several weeks. If feverish symptoms appear, or are aggravated under the use of this remedy, it should be immediately relinquished. The nitro-muriatic foot-bath has been found useful.

In torpid states of the liver especially such as are connected with dram drinking, and where there is reason to believe that a vitiated secretion of viscid bile is taking place, some benefit is derived from alterative doses of mercury combined with the steady use of bitter and warm purgatives. The pill (R No. 15) taken every night is well adapted for this purpose ; and the mixture (R No. 23,) composed of senna, gentian, an aromatic, and an alkali, may be directed in the dose of an ounce twice a day. The compound decoction of aloes (R No. 32,) affords another combination very useful in such cases.

There is an affection of the side, frequent in young women, called *hepatalgia*, which has been by many conceived to depend on some low or chronic kind of inflammation in the vessels of the liver. Indeed such cases are often designated as those of chronic hepatitis. There is a well-marked distinction however between these two diseases ; and as the former is one of the most genuine *chronic* disorders which come under the physician's care, I shall delay further notice of it, until the subject of jaundice has been discussed.

CHAP. XV.

Symptoms of Acute Rheumatism. Disposition to Metastasis. Causes. Seat of Rheumatism. Of the Rheumatic Inflammation of Synovial Membrane, or Arthritis. Principles of Treatment in Acute Rheumatism. Of Chronic Rheumatism. Varieties in the Symptoms of this Disease. Causes. Remarks on the Mode of Treatment applicable in the several varieties of Chronic Rheumatism. Peculiarities of Sciatica.

RHEUMATISM is an affection of the extremities and external coverings of the human body, occupying the muscular, tendinous, and fibrous textures, and characterized by pain, stiffness, and swelling of a joint, with or without fever according to the violence of the disorder. In common life, a threefold distinction is made *viz.* into the true rheumatism, the rheumatic gout, and the rheumatic fever. The two latter alone merit the title of *inflammations,* but there is obviously a close analogy in the pathology of all these affections. In their symptoms and mode of treatment however sufficient difference exists to entitle them to separate examination. It is certainly a curious circumstance, considering the frequency of this complaint, that there should still be so much obscurity in regard to several of the fundamental doctrines connected with rheumatic inflammation. This may be partly explained, perhaps, from its being a disease of so little danger, as never to have received any elucidation from the labours of the morbid anatomist.

We shall begin by the consideration of the highest grade of rheumatism, the rheumatic fever of the world, the acute rheumatism of nosologists, a painful and severe disease thus characterized. It is ushered in by a sudden attack of rigors, followed by the usual symptoms of pyrexia, and is particularly distinguished by the great pain and swelling which affect one or more joints, coupled with an utter inability to move them, and very commonly with considerable redness. The affected joints are acutely tender to the touch. The pains are aggravated towards night, and for the most part, at all times, from external heat. The swelling, except in certain cases hereafter to be specified, does not take the form of the joint, but is diffused over the cellular membrane in its neighbourhood. Several joints are commonly affected at the same time, but one of the most singular phenomena of rheumatic inflammation is the strong tendency which it exhibits to *shift its situation* : to abate in one or two joints, often very suddenly, and to become as suddenly violent in another, and a distant part.

The accompanying fever presents several important peculiarities. The pulse seldom exceeds 100 or 110 in the minute; but instead of the hardness which characterizes inflammatory fever, it is full, soft, and as it were *round*. The skin, instead of being hot, harsh, and dry, is commonly in a state of profuse perspiration ; and a remarkable acid odour of its secretion may be noticed. The tongue is always deeply loaded. The papillæ appear elongated, and covered with a thick and abundant mucus. The functions of the brain are in a peculiar manner exempt. Head-ache is seldom present in any form of rheumatic inflammation, acute or chronic ; and delirium is almost unknown. There is a great thirst, but rarely any nausea, or vomiting. The bowels are costive, though easily made to move. There is a sallowness in the aspect, and a peculiar expression of the countenance, sufficiently distinct from that of common febrile anxiety.

Different as are the local and constitutional symptoms from those of other phlegmasiæ, the terminations of rheumatic inflammation are no less peculiar. The local inflammation may run high, but it never proceeds to suppuration. It is seldom, indeed, that any permanent injury is done to the joint ; for if effusions of a transparent gelatinous fluid into, or around the sheaths of tendons and the capsular ligaments, take place, they are commonly absorbed in a short time. The most important consideration in this view of the subject is the disposition which exists, in a state of acute rheumatism, to an affection of some internal organ by *metastasis*, or rather by an extension of inflammation ; for it is not often that the joints are relieved when this event takes place. The organ chiefly liable to be so affected is the heart, and it is from this occurrence alone that any danger in the progress of the disease is to be apprehended. The symptoms that result are those of common thoracic inflammation ; the tendency to which, therefore, constitutes an important object of attention in the treatment of acute rheumatism.

It has already been remarked that the circumstances which lead to this extension of rheumatic inflammation to an internal organ have never yet been accurately investigated.

No disease is more liable to relapse on slight occasions than acute rheumatism. Going out a little too early in the open air, too much exercise of a particular joint, or an excess in diet, have frequently brought it back in all its former violence. Acute rheumatism is characterized also by a tendency to recurrence after a long interval. Those who have once suffered from an attack of the disease should therefore be particularly careful to avoid what we shall point out as its exciting causes, or to obviate them by proper attention to clothing. Rheumatism is certainly the most tedious of all the acute inflammations. In many cases it appears to run a defined course, which does not admit of being shortened by any process of treatment, and in a certain length of time to wear itself out. This is seldom less than a month, or longer than six weeks. That the acute sometimes terminates in a state of chronic rheumatism cannot be doubted ; but, instead of being a frequent occurrence, as is often imagined, this is in fact rare ; though the recovery from genuine acute rheumatism is tedious, it is usually perfect.

Children are very seldom the subjects of acute rheumatism. It most commonly occurs from the age of puberty to the thirtieth or thirty-fifth year of life, and chiefly affects those of sanguine temperament, robust form, and plethoric habit of body. It prevails principally in the months of December and January, and least frequently in August and September. Cold, with moisture, particularly where long applied, is certainly the most common, and perhaps it might be added its only exciting cause. Hence it is that we find it attributed, in a large proportion of cases, to sleeping in damp beds, living within damp walls, sitting in damp clothes, or working in damp situations.

Very little is known regarding the precise seat of inflammation in acute rheumatism. It appears to be situated primarily in capsular ligaments, tendinous sheaths, and aponeurotic expansions ; but the cellular membrane around the joints probably partakes of inflammation in the active form of the complaint. In this, perhaps, consists the principal local distinction between acute and chronic rheumatism. In some instances of disease, not usually distinguished by the physician from those of common rheumatism, though known to the world by the name of the *rheumatic gout*, the swelling will be found to take the exact form of the joint, or of a bursa in its neighbourhood ; and the affection is then simply *inflammation of synovial membrane.* By some pathologists it is imagined that such a disease is altogether distinct from rheumatism, and the term *arthritis* has been applied to it. It occurs both with or without fever. It appears to differ from rheumatism in its causes, progress, and treatment, as well as in its symptoms. It has been traced, for instance, to repelled gonorrhœa. It is frequently confined to a single joint, as the knee, or the elbow, and then commonly falls under the cognizance of the surgeon. It exhibits less tendency to shift its situation from one joint to another, and is more under the control of local remedies, than genuine, or as it may be called, *diffuse* rheumatism. As this subject however is very obscure, but still more, as it has not yet received those illustrations which may probably throw considerable light upon the nature of the affection, I simply state the circumstances, without venturing an opinion on the pathological principles which they involve. Blisters are very serviceable in these synovial or bursal forms of rheumatism, and they may be applied as soon as the acute pain attending the first stage has subsided.

If an opinion were formed from the various, and even opposite modes of treatment which have been recommended in the common acute rheumatism, not upon theoretical grounds, but after ample and successful experience, it might rationally be supposed, that the disease occurs in the most opposite states of the system ; but this opinion is not borne out by the observation of symptoms. I believe the better conclusion to be, that acute rheumatism is at all times a tedious, and rarely a dangerous disease ; that a large proportion of cases would recover with very slight care ; and that, in many, medical treatment is of little further service than as obviating the tendency to internal inflammation. It cannot, I think, be doubted, with regard to the power of *cutting short* the disease, that a considerable difference exists between rheumatism and common inflammation.

Three plans of treatment have been advised in the acute rheumatism. 1. The usual antiphlogistic system, consisting of bloodletting, purgatives, saline and antimonial medicines. 2. Opium and calomel. 3. Bark.

1. The authority of Sydenham is in favour of the first; and though it is impossible to call in question the very remarkable efficacy of opium, or of opium in combination with calomel, in many

cases of this disease, yet the plan of treatment which that judicious physician employed, will be found, upon the whole, the most gen. erally efficacious. The important distinction to be kept in view between the practice in acute rheumatism and that in other inflam. matory affections is, that while in the latter, a continuance of the same symptoms calls for a repetition of the same evacuation, it does not do so in the former. To subdue rheumatic inflammation by the lancet alone (even if possible) would be to weaken the system unnecessarily ; for it is to be remembered, that, in this disease, the inflammation is not in an organ essential to life. Sixteen ounces of blood may at first be taken from the arm; and repeated two days afterwards, if the pain continues urgent. The blood will al. ways be found highly cupped, and buffy. The further treatment of the disease may commonly be entrusted to purgatives, antimo- ny, and nitre ; but venesection must again be had recourse to, if internal inflammation supervenes. The purgative draught (R No. 22,) containing the powder of colchicum, will be found very effec. tual ; and when the febrile symptoms have somewhat abated, ad· vantage is derived from the exhibition of the vinum colchici (R No. 44 ;) but it is in the subacute and chronic forms of rheumatism that the efficacy of this medicine is best displayed.

2. The power of opium, and of calomel in combination with opi- um, in repressing acute rheumatic inflammation, is unquestionably very great ; and, under certain circumstances, it may be allowable to resort to them. It will seldom be found that calomel, even in large doses, affects the salivary glands, while the body is suffering under acute rheumatism.

3. Bark was introduced as a remedy in acute rheumatism, with the highest encomiums, by Dr. George Fordyce, and Dr. Hay· garth ; but as far as my observation extends, it has not answered the expectations which might have been formed of it from the tes- timony of these authors. It has appeared to me to be of use only in the latter periods of the disease, when considerable pain and stiffness of the joints are frequently found to exist, but with a *natu-ral* state of the pulse and tongue.

In the true acute rheumatism local applications to the affected joints are of little service ;—or rather, in most cases, of no service at all. This remark applies equally to fomentations, cold lotions, rubefacient liniments, and blisters. Not so, however, is it with re- gard to diet. In acute rheumatism, the functions of the stomach are often little impaired ; but a free indulgence of the appetite pro·

32

tracts the complaint, frustrates the effects of other remedies, and
has certainly contributed to give to rheumatism that character of
tediousness, which makes it the opprobrium of physic. Broths and
jellies, animal food in every shape, as well as wine and porter, are
to be prohibited ; and a cool, spare, vegetable diet strictly enforced.

———————

CHRONIC RHEUMATISM is of constant occurrence, and this circumstance alone is sufficient to point out that it is not often the sequel of the acute form of the disease. It is characterized by pain
of the joints aggravated on motion, stiffness of the joints, thickening of the several structures in their vicinity, or increased effusion
into the synovial bags. It is readily distinguished from the acute
rheumatism by the want of inflammatory fever, and of redness in
the affected part. To this kind of affection the term *rheumatism*
is, in common language, specially appropriated.

1. Three species of chronic rheumatism may be distinguished.
The first is that which is connected with a state of febrile excitement in the system, and which would be more correctly designated
by the term *subacute rheumatism*. It is known by the pains occasionally shifting their situation suddenly, as in the acute form of the
disease, and by their being increased by warmth, and especially,
at night, by the warmth of the bed. The frequent occurrence of
œdema along with the affection of the joints, may serve to distinguish this from the other species of the disease. Those joints which
are surrounded by a large mass of muscular substance, and which
are the most constantly exerted, are especially liable to it, such as
the hip, and joints of the lumbar vertebræ. This state of chronic
rheumatism is accompanied with a white tongue, thirst, a quickened pulse, and a costive state of the bowels.

2. The second species of chronic rheumatism is marked, not by
any degree of excitement in the system, but by the absence of constitutional symptoms. Here it is not unreasonable to believe, that
there may be a loss of tone in the vessels of the affected part. It
is not so common as the preceding species, but it sometimes follows
it. Stiffness of the joint is here the prominent symptom. *Pain*, in
this form of the complaint, is often not at all felt except on motion,
or on occasion of changes in the heat or moisture of the atmosphere. It is relieved rather than increased by the warmth of bed.
The pain and stiffness do not shift from joint to joint. Spontaneous

coldness of the limb, and even a degree of paralytic torpor, are of. ten complained of by the patient. The pulse is seldom quick, or the tongue white.

3. The third species of chronic rheumatism is attended with perma. nent derangement in the structure of the joint; and it is that form of disease which has been ably described by Dr. Haygarth, under the title of Nodosity of the joints. The ends of the bones, the pe. riosteum, and ligaments become thickened; and nodes form upon them, often to such an extent as to distort the joint in the most un. sightly manner. This form of rheumatism chiefly affects the fin. gers, but I have seen it also in the knees and ancles. It is princi. pally met with in women, after they have passed the period of menstruation. It is attended with pain of the joint, particularly severe at night.

The usual causes of chronic rheumatism are exposure to cold and moisture, or to partial currents of air; local injuries, such as strains and bruises; and it is also one of the common effects of the syphilitic poison, and of mercury. The structures affected in chronic rheumatism are those called by Bichat *fibrous*;—*viz.* the periosteum in every part of its extent, the tendons and tendinous sheaths of muscles, the ligaments around the joints, the investing membranes of the nerves and of the teeth, and not unfrequently the substance of muscle itself. The sclerotic coat of the eye, which has a dense structure of an analogous kind, is subject also to a spe. cies of *rheumatic* inflammation. To distinguish this affection is by no means easy; nor is this the only instance in which chronic rheumatism has given occasion to difficulties in diagnosis. Lum. bago has been mistaken for nephralgia or lumbar abscess; rheu. matism of the intercostal muscles for pleurisy; and sciatica for ul. ceration within the cavity of the acetabulum.

No general rules of much importance can be laid down for the guidance of the student in the treatment of chronic rheumatism. Some attention must be paid to the state of the constitution, as di. rected in page 172; and perhaps more can be done in that way, to. wards the relief of the complaint, than is generally supposed; but the remedies, both internal and external, must be varied according to their effects, and the particular circumstances of each case. In. stead, however, of a bare enumeration of the remedies that have been tried, and occasionally found useful in chronic rheumatism, it may be advisable to attempt, at least, to point out a few principles that may prove of general application.

1. In some of the forms of sub-acute rheumatism, particularly lumbago and sciatica, the local abstraction of blood by cupping will be productive of great benefit. Where the pains are very severe, it may even be necessary to take blood from the arm, which in this state of disease will always be found cupped and buffy. Leeches are well adapted to those cases of chronic rheumatism, where there is pain and swelling of a joint from distension of the synovial membrane. Dr. Haygarth recommends their application where an enlargement of the extremities of the bones has taken place.

2. The cure of chronic rheumatism may occasionally be effected by promoting diaphoresis. This mode of treatment is adapted to those cases where there exists some degree of febrile excitement, where the pains are of recent date, and shift from one joint to another. The warm bath may be directed twice in the week (provided the pulse be perfectly free from all activity,) and the diaphoretic draught (R No. 45,) consisting of the liquor amm. acet. and small doses of Dover's powder, given repeatedly during the day. It is unnecessary to add, that neither in this, nor in any other form of chronic rheumatism, can any thing be hoped for without proper attention to clothing, and above all, the use of flannel as an under dress.

3. In the same description of cases which are benefited by diaphoretics, the vinum colchici may be had recourse to with great advantage. Where there is any considerable degree of effusion, either within the capsular ligaments or the bursæ, or where the cellular membrane in the neighbourhood of the joint is œdematous, I think that I have seen the colchicum particularly useful. The form of draught (No. 46,) may be recommended. Occasional purging (twice or even three times in the week) by senna in union with salts, or with the powder of colchicum (R Nos. 21 and 22,) should never be omitted. I have seldom experienced much benefit in this complaint from the exhibition of antimony.

4. Where great torpor and debility of the general system prevails, stimulant and tonic medicines of different kinds have been administered with advantage, the principal of which are gum guaiacum and the volatile alkali, or their combination, the volatile tincture of guaiacum, the oil of turpentine, the balsam of Peru, and mezereon. Bark, both in the form of decoction and powder, unquestionably possesses considerable power over certain forms of chronic rheumatism attended with general torpor : and arsenic has proved successful, even when the *structures* about the joints had

become partially disorganized. The good effects of all these remedies will be considerably aided by the diligent use of stimulating embrocations (such as the compound camphor or soap liniment,) friction alone appearing to be a powerful means of exciting the languid action of the vessels. The formula No. 112 is strongly recommended by Dr. Bardsley. In all cases of chronic rheumatism of long standing, permanent stiffness of the joint is chiefly to be dreaded, to which nothing contributes so much as neglect of the due exercise of the joint. To this, therefore, patients should always be encouraged, as a matter of great consequence with a view to their ultimate recovery.

5. Mercury, pushed so as to affect the mouth, is very effectual in the cure of rheumatic affections of a chronic nature. It appears to operate as a general *stimulant*. The best mode of administration is five grains of the blue pill taken night and morning. In many of these cases it has been supposed, that a syphilitic taint may have existed in the constitution and kept up the disease ; but very frequently, there is no foundation for such a suspicion. Where rheumatic pains can be traced to cold while the system was under the influence of mercury, decoctions of sarsaparilla, guaiacum, and the elm bark, the powder of sarsaparilla in doses of two drachms three times a day, with other vegetable alteratives, may be tried with a reasonable prospect of advantage.

6. No one remedy, perhaps, is of such general application in the treatment of chronic rheumatism as local warm bathing. In that severe form of the disease which has been called nodosity of the joints, scarcely any thing else can be relied on to soothe pain and relax the rigid fibres. The efficacy of the waters of Bath and Buxton, even in very obstinate cases, is generally acknowledged. They are applicable, however, only in that species of rheumatism which is unattended by inflammatory excitement.

7. In all cases of chronic rheumatism, *pain* is, if possible to be relieved ; and, generally, opium will be found the only effectual resource. Ten, or even fifteen grains of Dover's powders should be given every night at bed-time. Opium taken at night in conjunction with calomel, is particularly serviceable when the pulse and tongue give evidence of general vascular excitement. Where opium disagrees with the system, the extracts of conium or hyoscyamus may be substituted (R No. 55). The costiveness which all narcotics occasion is to be carefully obviated by some aperient taken the following morning (R Nos. 15 and 32.)

There appears to be something peculiar in the pathology of that variety of rheumatism termed SCIATICA. It is conjectured, that in this disease there is a degree of inflammation present either in the substance or in the cellular envelope of the great sciatic nerve. It is attended with excruciating pain, extending down the thigh, particularly urgent about two or three o'clock in the morning. It occurs chiefly in persons of robust habit; and it is, in almost all cases, extremely tedious. The neuralgic affection called ischias nervosum, closely resembles it in many of its features. Cupping, blistering, and active mercurial purgatives long and steadily continued, are required for its cure; with opium, in doses proportioned to the severity of the pain. In obstinate cases, an issue should be directed. The application of the *moxa* has occasionally given relief, and as a last resource, is certainly worthy of a trial.

LUMBAGO is the rheumatism of the lumbar vertebræ, or rather of the large masses of mucular substance attached to them, and serving for the support of the body. It is distinguished from nephritis by the aggravation of pain on stooping. It is a less violent form of ailment than the preceding, and yields, for the most part to strong, stimulating embrocations (R No. 112,) active aperients (R No 21,) and Dover's powder, in full doses, taken at bed-time.

Rheumatism of the thoracic parietes is called PLEURODYNE, or bastard pleurisy. It is to be distinguished from true pleurisy by the character of the pulse, and the absence of constitutional derangement. It is a very transient form of rheumatism, best combated by the warm bath, and frictions with soap liniment and laudanum.

ɔi

OF THE GOUT.

*Its Pathological Connection with Rheumatism. Division into acute and
Chronic Gout. Symptoms of acute Gout. Of Chronic or Irregular Gout.
Predisposition to Gout. Exciting causes of Acute Gout. Proximate
Cause of Gout. Principles of the Treatment of Gout.*

GOUT is a disease, which, though possessed of many peculiar characters, is yet intimately associated, in a pathological view, with
rheumatism. It is scarcely, indeed, two hundred years since they
were first accurately distinguished.* But though the diagnosis is
very important, and has contributed essentially to the elucidation
of this branch of pathology, still it must not be forgotten, that a
close affinity subsists between these diseases, that they run into
each other by insensible degrees, and that the term *rheumatic gout*,
so frequently employed in common life, is at the same time strictly scientific. The general features of resemblance between gout
and rheumatism may be traced in the identity of the structures
which are attacked, in the similarity of the terminations of the
two diseases, and in their mutual tendency to affect some internal
organ by metastasis. The leading points of difference are to be
found in the joints principally affected, in the progress of the symptoms, in the *predisposing*, and lastly, in the *exciting* causes. All
these are well expressed in Dr. Cullen's excellent definition of
gout. It may fairly indeed, be admitted, that no subject in the
whole extent of medical science has been investigated with such
attention as the gout; and by no one certainly has that investigation been prosecuted with so much success as by Dr. Cullen.

Gout, in its regular form, is a genuine inflammatory affection of

* The term *rheumatism* was first employed, and the disease separated
from the *arthritis* of old authors, by Ballonius, in his Treatise " De Rheu-
matismo et Pleuritide dorsali." 1642.

the fibrous membranes, running a defined course, and attended by
the common symptoms of inflammatory fever.   This is the regular
or acute species of the disease.   In a large proportion of cases,
its attack is confined to a single joint, and that one, the first of the
great toe.   But as in other inflammatory affections, there is here
also a chronic form of the complaint, called in common language
the *irregular* gout ; and to this a third variety may be added, which
occasionally supervenes upon both the other species,—I mean the
retrocedent gout, where a metastasis takes place to some internal
organ, giving rise to symptoms either of visceral congestion or of
inflammation.

An attack of acute gout sometimes comes on suddenly, without
any warning, but for the most part it is preceded for two or three
days by symptoms indicating general disturbance of the system.
The principle of these are lassitude with depression of spirits, coldness of the feet and legs, numbness, with a sense of pricking or itching in the lower extremities, cramps of the muscles of the legs, an
irritable state of the bladder, but chiefly a great degree of disturbance in the functions of the stomach.   There are present also,
symptoms of fever ; such as disturbed sleep, scanty and high-coloured urine, cough with expectoration of mucus, and a costive
state of the bowels.   The attack of local inflammation commonly
takes place about two or three o'clock in the morning, with more or
less shivering, succeeded by the common symptoms of pyrexia, and
aways almost with intense pain of the joint.   In a few hours the joint
becomes swelled and red, and very painful to the touch.   The feverish symptoms continue for three or four days, generally exhibiting
the usual exacerbation towards evening.   The redness and swelling then gradually abate ; and as the disease wears off, it leaves
the patient, not as in a common fever, weak and debilitated, but
enjoying better appetite and better spirits, than he had experienced
for some time before.

But this is only a *paroxysm* of gout.   The disposition to recur,
frequently too at regular intervals, constitutes another, and a most
important feature of the disease.   By degrees these intervals become shorter, and the paroxysms themselves more severe ; and
while the constitution falls more and more under the influence of
the disease, it makes corresponding encroachments in respect of the
parts which it attacks.   At first, it confines itself to a single joint
of one foot ; by degrees it affects several joints, and both feet, either together, or in succession ; and at length its ravages extend to

every joint of the body. When it has subsisted for a certain time, a saline matter is thrown out by the inflamed vessels, and deposited upon the periosteum, the ligaments of the joints, the cellular mem-brane around them, the bursæ mucosæ, and even in some cases be-tween the cutis and cuticle.* This accumulates after repeated pa-roxysms, so as to obstruct, during the intervals of health, the mo-tions of the joint, and, when fresh inflammation supervenes, to ag-gravate very considerably the sufferings of the patient. It is some-times effused in such quantity as to occasion concretions of a large size, tedious ulcerations about the joint, or even complete anchylo-sis. The matter has been found, by analysis, to consist of the urate of soda. For this discovery we are indebted to Dr. Wollas-ton.†

In the chronic or irregular gout, the symptoms do not follow that defined course which is witnessed in the acute species of the dis-ease. The appearances of external inflammation are slighter, but there is equal or even more œdema, and always so much weakness of the neighbouring muscles, that the motion of the joint is great-ly impaired. Sometimes it leaves the joint first attacked, and fixes on some distant part; or, after harassing the patient by affecting different joints in succession, returns to that in which it was origin-ally seated. With these local symptoms are conjoined a variety of others, indicating general constitutional disturbance, such as feel-ings of languor and dejection, cramps in different parts of the bo-dy, particularly distressing at night, palpitation, costiveness, heart-burn, a chronic cough, and in the worst cases, wasting, and that general depravation of the whole habit which is commonly called *cachexia*.

The retrocedent gout is that form of the disease, where, during the existence of the more usual symptoms, some internal organ be-comes affected. The stomach, intestines, heart, and brain have at different times been observed to be the seat of retrocedent gout. Some differences of opinion exist as to the precise nature of the affection in cases of this kind. The symptoms, in many instances, warrant the suspicion of *inflammation* ; but it is doubtful if this holds good, when the stomach or the brain are attacked.

There are several very important considerations connected with the causes of gout, predisposing and occasional ; and among them

* Vide " Moore on Gouty Concretions or Chalkstones." Med. and Chir. Transactions, vol. i, page 112.
† Philosophical Transactions, 1797.

the first in point of pathological interest is the influence of *heredi-tary predisposition*. This principle is now for the first time brought under consideration, but it is one of extensive application, and will hereafter be adduced to illustrate the pathology of some of the most important diseases of the body, such as hæmoptysis, scrofula, epilepsy, mania, and asthma. It may be stated as a general prin-ciple, that such an hereditary predisposition as we have supposed to exist, both with regard to these diseases and to gout, may be assisted by different circumstances, or it may be so far counteract-ed by others, as that it never shall exert during life any influence in the production of disease. Persons too, without hereditary dis-position, may *acquire* the gout, or any other of the complaints as-sociated in this respect with it; so that, as a doctrine in pathology, it must be received with limitations; but it is not on that account the less certain or important. Hereditary predisposition is greater or less, according as it is on the side of both parents, or of one only. Attempts have been made to estimate the proportion which the ca-ses of acquired gout bear to those where an hereditary tendency can be traced; but the calculations that have hitherto appeared are far from being satisfactory.

Gout chiefly prevails among men. This is not to be ascribed to any peculiar exemption which the female sex enjoys from gout, but to a difference in those habits of life which contribute to the devel-opment of the disease. Where the gout appears in women, an he-reditary predisposition to it will probably be met with, both on the father's and the mother's side. A gross and corpulent habit of body, with fulness of the veins, and a relaxed or loose state of the solids, is observed to give a tendency to gout. The same remark, however may certainly be extended to acute rheumatism. The ex-emption of youth from gout is a striking character of the disease, as was long since urged by Hippocrates. Dr. Heberden,[*] whose experience in gout was probably more extensive than that of any physician who ever lived, never saw an instance of the disease be-fore puberty. It seldom, indeed, appears before the age of thirty-five.

But of all the circumstances which give a tendency to gout, next after a hereditary predisposition, the most important are, full living, and especially the free use of animal food,—an habitual indulgence in wine,—and inactivity of body. The gout, therefore, is almost

---

[*] Commentarii de Morbis, page 33.

wholly unknown among persons employed in constant bodily labour, and chiefly supported upon vegetable aliment. It has been
attempted, by several writers, to estimate the relative degree of
importance which should be attached to each of these three predisposing causes of the disease, and pathologists generally attribute to
the free use of *wine* the principal share in the production of gout.
Van Swieten states, that the gout was unknown in Holland till wine
was substituted for beer. This doctrine, however, admits of some
doubt. The disease occurs frequently in certain classes of persons
in this country, where an indulgence in animal food and inactivity
of body can alone operate. I am inclined to think, therefore, that
these, if they have not a superior, have at least an equal share in
the production of gout in the upper ranks of life. They all concur
in producing that plethoric state of the body, on which the predisposition to gout appears mainly to depend.

The exciting causes of the gout, or those which more immediately bring on a paroxysm, are such as in a plethoric habit of body
induce a state of weakness, or irritability. Of these the most common are indigestion, produced either by the quantity or quality of
the aliment ; intemperance, particularly in the use of *acescent* wines
such as champaign and claret ; excess in venereal pleasures ; intense application to study, with night watching ; mental anxiety ;
excessive evacuations ; cold, especially when applied to the lower
extremities ; severe exercise, so as to occasion fatigue ; sprains
and contusions, and lastly, very sudden changes in the manner of
living, not only from a low to a full diet, but what is important also in practice, from a full to a very spare diet.

The *proximate* cause of gout has been studiously investigated by
almost every writer on the disease. The favourite doctrine has
been that gout depends upon a certain morbific matter, always
present in the body, which thrown out upon the joints, or other
parts, produces the several phenomena of the disease. By some,
even of the latest writers on gout, this theory has been supported,
and the morbific matter has been pronounced to be an *acid.* Many
ingenious arguments have been brought forward in its favour, but
the doctrines of the *humoral* pathology have fallen into oblivion,
and in this instance, at least, scarcely merit revival. With respect
to the analogy between gout and gravel, sufficient evidence has
been adduced to render it probable that a pathological connection
really subsists between these diseases ; but its precise nature is not
ascertained.

A regular fit of the gout is so far from being a disease of danger, that it is considered by many as the precursor of health and strength. It would be, perhaps, fortunate for gouty persons if there were less foundation for this opinion ; for, under such an impression, a system is too often pursued, which, in the first instance, rivets the disease in the constitution, and ends by undermining it.   The principles of treatment in gout are different from those which obtain in other in-flammatory affections.   The paroxysm of local inflammation, not being attended with danger, may be to a considerable degree disre-garded ; while the efforts of the practitioner, should be steadily ex-erted during the intervals of the paroxysms, to prevent their recur-rence, by a due attention to the predisposing and exciting causes.

In a paroxysm of acute gout, the antiphlogistic regimen is to be enforced, the bowels are to be kept open by cooling laxatives (R No. 22,) and saline draughts may be given at proper intervals. The efficacy of colchicum, in checking the first approach of a fit of the gout, and moderating its violence when it has come on, is es-tablished by very ample observation.   For this purpose, either a drachm of the vinum colchici ; or a proportionate dose of the *Eau Medicinale,* may be given at once, or the draughts (Nos. 44 and 46,) at proper intervals.   It is seldom that general measures of greater activity than these are called for.   With regard to local treatment, experience has fully proved that patience and flannel may safely be trusted to.   Leeches and linseed meal poultices are occasion-ally requisite.   Cooling lotions sometimes afford relief ; but there are instances in which any application of cold to the affected joint aggravates pain, and increases the tendency to metastasis.

Cases of chronic or irregular gout are to be treated according to the symptoms which may arise ; but no attempts should be made, by the liberal use of wine, or by local irritants, to bring on the acute state of the disease.   A light diet and regular moderate exercise, with laxatives, absorbents, and the occasional use of bitters, so as to improve the tone of the system, and regulate the functions of the stomach and bowels, will be requisite in this form of the complaint. Where an internal organ is attacked, constituting the retrocedent species of gout, the treatment is to be conducted upon the same principles as are applicable in a corresponding idiopathic affection of the part.

In the intervals of the paroxysms, the great objects of attention are *diet* and *exercise.*   There is high authority for saying, that the gout may be entirely prevented by constant bodily exercise and a low diet ; and this, not only where an hereditary predisposition exists, but even where that disposition has already manifested itself by paroxysms of the disease. To ensure, however, the success of these measures, care must be taken to avoid the *exciting* causes formerly enumerated.

It has always been an object of interest to discover some medicine that might obviate the necessity of any restraint upon the diet or regimen of the patient ; and at different times remedies have been extolled for the *effectual* prevention of the gout. The principal of these are certain combinations of bitters, and various forms of alkaline medicines ; but though they may have succeeded, for a time, in warding off a fit, they are incapable of effecting any such change in the constitution as may altogether prevent the recurrence of the disease.

ERYSIPELAS.

Symptoms of the Idiopathic Erysipelas. Its tendency to affect some internal Organ. Causes of idiopathic Erysipelas, predisposing and occasional. Question of its Origin from Contagion. Principles of treatment in the Idiopathic Erysipelas. Of the external Treatment proper in this Disease.

HAVING already offered an opinion regarding the general pathology of erysipelatous inflammation,—having attempted, that is to say, to point out its seat, its relation to phlegmon, and the peculiarities which distinguish it, I have now to detail the symptoms, causes, and principles of treatment of that idiopathic ailment to which the term ERYSIPELAS has been considered more peculiarly to apply. The general character of this disease corresponds perfectly with that form of the affection which is familiar to surgeons, as arising from burns and scalds; and as the frequent consequence of wounds, punctures, operations, compound fractures, and the application of poisons, or acrid matters, to the skin. Many of the observations, therefore, which I shall have to offer on the *idiopathic* erysipelas, apply equally to the other forms in which this species of inflammation appears; but it will be more consonant to the general design of this work, to confine my attention to that form of the complaint which falls more exclusively under the cognizance of the physician.

The idiopathic erysipelas may commence on any part of the skin, but the face and legs are most usually affected. It is ushered in by febrile symptoms of considerable severity, which continue through the whole course of the disease. The pulse is always frequent, and commonly full and hard. The functions of the brain are much disturbed, and drowsiness, or confusion of the head, amounting in some cases to delirium, accompanies the hot stage.

On the second, or, at furthest, on the third morning from the attack of rigor, redness and swelling appear on some part of the skin,
very frequently on one side of the nose, spreading rapidly to the
rest of the face, or extending over the scalp, neck, and shoulders.
There is a distressing sense of heat and tingling in the inflamed
surface. The whole face becomes turgid, and upon the second or
third day from the appearance of inflammation, the eye-lids are
commonly closed. In some instances the disease goes off simply
by desquamation of the cuticle, but more usually, after a certain
time, blisters arise of different sizes, containing a thin yellowish or
transparent serum, which speedily burst, and leave the skin, in that
part, of a livid colour. In some places purulent matter forms, and
this is very frequently observed to happen in the loose cellular membrane of the eyelids. A disposition to œdematous effusion is not
uncommon, and under certain circumstances erysipelas verges to
gangrene; but this is rarely observed, except where it occurs as a
consequence of severe injuries.

The duration of the disease is liable to considerable variation.
In young persons it commonly terminates in six or seven days; but
in those more advanced in life, it is often protracted to the twelfth
day, or even later. The febrile symptoms do not always cease
with the subsidence of external inflammation. In the progress of
the disease, and especially towards its latter stages, they assume,
in many cases, a well-marked *typhoid* character; and great debility always characterizes the period of convalescence.

The tendency in erysipelas to spread to some internal organ, is
a circumstance in the history of the disease of the utmost importance. It is the great source of *danger* in idiopathic erysipelas,
and it regulates, in no inconsiderable degree, the treatment. Pleurisy or severe bronchial inflammation have been observed in some
cases; but the brain is the organ chiefly liable to be affected.
There appears, indeed, to be some peculiar and hitherto unexplained conection between erysipelatous inflammation and disease of
the brain. The symptoms are those of phrenitic inflammation;
and some of the purest specimens of phrenitis met with in this
country are attributable to this cause. In certain cases, the inflammation of the skin abates when the affection of the brain supervenes; in others, the internal and external inflammation proceed together.

The causes of idiopathic erysipelas are not well understood.
There is, in some persons, a strong disposition to this kind of in-

flammation ; and in them it is brought on by very trifling causes. Such a disposition appears, in some families, to be hereditary ; and it may possibly depend on a peculiar organization of the skin.　To the latter circumstance we may, perhaps, refer the greater prevalence of the disease among females.　It is certainly a very remarkable fact, that while the erysipelas *sometimes* attacks the robust and plethoric, it is, upon the whole, much more commonly met with among those who have been debilitated, either by previous disease, or long residence in a hot climate, or unwholesome diet, or bad air.　It may occur at any age.　There is a species of erysipelas which attacks new-born infants, particularly in lying-in-hospitals and workhouses ;* but it is chiefly the disease of adult life, and of old age.

The discussions regarding the contagiousness of erysipelas, have been as keen as on every other occasion in which the doctrine of contagion is involved.　Dr. Wells † has collected several examples of the communication of erysipelas by contagion in private families ; and in my own practice this fact has been most strikingly exemplified.　In hospitals, it is well ascertained that it frequently spreads by contagion, particularly where there is a defective or *ill-regulated* system of ventilation.　Admitting this, I think at the same time it cannot be questioned, that erysipelas prevails at at some seasons, and under certain circumstances of the air, more than at others.　What the peculiar conditions of the atmosphere are, which dispose to erysipelatous inflammation, have not been determined.　The occasional cause to which *idiopathic* erysipelas is commonly attributed is cold applied when the body is overheated ; but intemperance, and exposure to strong heat, have been also considered as giving rise to it.　In many cases no exciting cause of any kind can be traced, and it is strictly a *spontaneous* disease.

The treatment of erysipelas has proved a fertile theme of controversy.　It has been supposed, that the common principles applicable to other inflammatory diseases are inapplicable here ; but the supporters of this opinion do not seem to have taken into consideration the variety of causes from which erysipelas originates, and the almost infinitely varied circumstances of situation, age, and constitution, under which it appears.　Keeping these in view,

---

* See Dr. Garthshore, in Medical Communications, vol. ii, page 28.

† Transactions of a Society for the Improvement of Med. and Chir. Knowledge, vol. ii, art. 13.

it does not appear that any important difference of principle is to be established between the treatment of erysipelatous and of common phlegmonous inflammation.

1. The acute idiopathic erysipelas of the face, occurring out of an hospital, to a stout plethoric young man, is to be treated like any other inflammatory affection. Blood is to be taken from the arm, to the extent of sixteen ounces, and repeated if necessary. It is very seldom, if ever, that more than two bleedings are required. Local depletion by leeches, and still better by free incisions, are often of essential service in erysipelas of the extremities. Purgative medicines are to be given at the same time.' The period of convalescence will be shortened by bark and cordials.

2. If erysipelas occurs under circumstances less decisive of the inflammatory nature of the accompanying fever, the chief reliance should be placed on the exhibition of purgatives, especially calomel, jalap, and senna. The saline aperients, too, frequently exhibit a very remarkable influence over this species of inflammation.

3. When erysipelas occurs to aged people, and in debilitated habits; when it originates decidedly from contagion; when it happens in an hospital, to persons suffering under, or recovering from, a tedious illness; when it is attended by a feeble pulse, a brown tongue, and a disposition to gangrene, the system is to be supported (perhaps even from the very first) by bark aromatics, the volatile alkali, and wine. The draught (R No 71) may be recommended under these circumstances. With this plan, the occasional exhibition of a purgative may be united with the best effect, and a preference may then be given to castor oil.

4. When phrenitic inflammation occurs as a consequence of erysipelas, it is to be treated by venesection, blisters, and purgatives, not regulated by any consideration of the *cause*, but merely by the state of the pulse, and character of the accompanying fever.

5. Different external applications have been proposed in erysipelas, such as cold lotions, warm and spirituous fomentations, and dry powders. Their influence upon the disease does not appear to be very great; and, therefore, that one should be selected which best relieves the heat and uneasy sensation which the patient experiences. The cold spirituous lotion (R No. 109) will commonly be found to answer this purpose. It is certainly preferable to the application of dry powders, which irritate and heat the skin, and in this way often prove prejudicial. In many cases, however, of idio-

34

pathic erysipelas, it will be found advisable to refrain altogether from local applications. When there is a tendency to gangrene, stimulating lotions containing camphor prove serviceable, by supporting the tone of the vessels.

* See Appendix; Note U.

CHAP. I.

Character of the Order of Hæmorrhagies. Degree of Importance to be attached to the Doctrine of Hæmorrhagy. Hæmorrhagies general or local. Active or passive. Of Anæmia. Hæmorrhagy connected with Plethora, local Congestion, and weakness of the Coats of Vessels. Causes of Hæmorrhagy, predisposing and occasional. General Principles of Treatment in the Diseases of this Order.

THE diseases comprised in the order of hæmorrhages are, in every point of view, much less interesting than the inflammations. They are of less frequent occurrence, and seldom met with in an idiopathic form. Indeed, it is only by a stretch of nosological refinement that they can be considered in the light of a distinct order of diseases. The rupture of a blood-vessel is not necessarily connected with a train of other symptoms, and is therefore itself rather an accident or a *symptom*, than a state of disease. While engaged in the investigation of the phlegmasiæ, we were content to refer the phenomena to the presence of *inflammation*. In the class of hœmorrhagies, we must always look to something beyond, and endeavour to determine upon what ulterior cause the rupture of the vessel depends.

The general doctrine of hæmorrhagy has, nevertheless, always excited attention in the schools of physic ; and much learning has unquestionably been shown in investigating the principles which it involves. Dr. Cullen's dissertation on this subject must be considered as a remarkable specimen of acute pathological research ; but these discussions, not having the same influence on practice with some of those which have been already before us, do not require the same attention from the student, and will therefore be only briefly alluded to in this place. Without venturing upon those abstruse theoretical speculations concerning hæmorrhagy, in which some authors have indulged, it may, however, not be altogether uninteresting to notice the principal points which have been thought of importance ; and this more particularly, as it will afford an opportunity of exhibiting, in a connected view, several diseases included in this order, the particular consideration of which will be taken up in future parts of the work. Although there may not prove to be many points of analogy among them, it will not be the less useful to notice the principal circumstances in which they differ, and above all, the various, and even opposite states of the system in which they occur.

1. Hæmorrhagies may be divided, in the first place according as they are general or local. A general disposition to hæmorrhagy is not common ; but it occurs in scurvy, and in a disease of a very singular kind, known by the name of the *hæmorrhœa petechialis*. The pathology of this affection is but little understood. Different speculations have been thrown out concerning it, which will hereafter come under our notice, when considering the class of chronic constitutional diseases ; but for the present, it may be sufficient to state, that it appears to be wholly different from scurvy, that it has some obscure connection with disease within the thorax, and that it is occasionally to be treated by antiphlogistic measures. A general disposition to hæmorrhagy occurs also in many acute diseases, more particularly in different forms of inflammatory and typhoid fever.

Local hæmorrhages may be arranged according as they happen in one or other of the three great cavities or divisions of the body. Hæmorrhagy from the vessels of the head occurs either as *epistaxis*, or as *apoplexy*; diseases which have, in some cases, an important pathological connection. Hæmorrhagy from the thorax is denominated *hæmoptysis*. Hæmorrhagy from the abdominal cavity assumes the several forms of *hæmatemesis, melæna, hæmorrhois, hæ-maturia*, and *menorrhagia*. Two or more of these forms of local hæmorrhagy are occasionally present at the same time, or occur *vicariously* to each other, illustrating strongly the importance of the general doctrine of hæmorrhagy. They show that hæmorrhages, even the most partial, or apparently accidental (such as that

which sometimes follows the extraction of a tooth,) are yet connected with a morbid condition of the *whole* arterial system, which
is unable to preserve its surface unbroken.

2. From the situation assigned to hæmorrhagic diseases in most
systems of nosology, symptoms of *fever* might be expected; but
one of the most important considerations in the general doctrine of
hæmorrhagy, is the frequency of its occurrence without any evidence of febrile excitement existing in the system. In some cases, hæmorrhagy is preceded by rigors; and during the flow of
blood the pulse is frequent, full or even hard, the skin is hot, and
there is thirst and restlessness. At other times, hæmorrhagy exists
with a state of general constitutional debility, and arises from causes that obviously weaken the tone of the system; as is well exemplified in some of the cases of menorrhagia. These facts have
long been known; and they have given rise to one of the oldest
pathological distinctions among hæmorrhagies; *viz.* into the *active*
and the *passive*.

3. All hæmorrhagies when long continued are apt to induce a
very alarming state of constitutional weakness. The blood degenerates into a state of morbid tenuity. It is rather bloody serum
than blood. Even in the heart itself but little crassamentum will
be found. This condition of the fluids is generally known by the
name of *anæmia*, and it perhaps sometimes exists independent of
hæmorrhagy. Its symptoms are a pale and bloodless countenance,
great weakness, disposition to syncope, loss of appetite, indigestion, swelled legs, and a pulse, weak, tremulous, and intermitting.
It is most commonly witnessed in women suffering under cancer
uteri, and its attendant hæmorrhagy.

4. In estimating the circumstances which may lead to the accidental rupture of a vessel in an internal part, there are three
which chiefly merit attention. The first of these is the quantity
of blood in the body; the second is the force of the heart's action
(these two constituting the impetus, or *momentum* of the blood;)
and the third is the strength of the coats of the containing vessel,
depending principally on the *original* constitution or structure of
the body. By one or other of these considerations, we may explain the manner in which different circumstances act as the predisposing or occasional causes of hæmorrhagy, and the *modus operandi* of the remedies which are resorted to for its relief or removal.

1. Plethora, or præternatural fulness of the blood-vessels, is a

state of the body, the reality of which is established by ample, as
well as the most simple evidence. It is the common consequence of
full living, and of a sedentary life ; and it proves a frequent source
of disease.   A man too full of blood becomes heavy and languid.
A state of over-distension in vessels gives a disposition to increased action in them; hence it is, that whatever leads to *general plethora* is so frequently found to be a predisposing cause of inflammation, and of hæmorrhage, and even of fever.   It will be remembered, however, that a state of plethora, is by no means essential
to hæmorrhage, which is compatible even with a state of morbid
tenuity of the blood.

2. The mere force of the heart's action has something to do
with the occurrence of hæmorrhagy; for heat, and violent exercise of the whole body, as in running, are among the most frequent
of its exciting causes ; and they can only act by hurrying the circulation.   The idea entertained by old pathologists of a *spurious*
plethora has been long abandoned.   But the more necessary circumstance to be kept in view, is the connection of hæmorrhagy
with the state of partially increased action of vessels, or irregular
determination of blood ; or, as it is now more commonly called, *local
congestion*.   This has always been recognised as a principle in pathology of the highest importance ; and it is undoubtedly the most
generally applicable of any which have been established in the
whole extent of pathological science.   We have seen it influencing the phenomena and treatment of every form of idiopathic fever.   It is the very basis of all reasoning on the subject of inflammatory action ; and we shall subsequently find it to extend to many of the most important chronic diseases of the body.   In what
manner this local determination of blood is brought about,—how
it is that the heart, which appears calculated to supply blood equally to all parts of the body, should distribute it unequally, are questions which the inquiries of physiologists have not, hitherto, enabled us to decide.   The fact itself, however, is well ascertained ;
and it strongly illustrates the great principle, which, though generally professed, has yet been too frequently lost sight of—that the
doctrines of hydraulics are but distantly applicable to those of the
circulation of the blood.*

* See a very ingenious Essay by Mr. Charles Bell, entitled, " On the
Forces which circulate the Blood, being an Examination of the Difference
between the Motions of Fluids in living and dead Vessels." London, 1819.

With this doctrine of local congestion, that of hæmorrhagy is closely connected, as will hereafter be illustrated in several ways; by the phenomena, for instance, of epistaxis and apoplexy; by the effect of posture in favouring different forms of hæmorrhagy; and by the fact, that exercise of the lungs in singing, or loud or long speaking, will occasion a fit of hæmoptysis. We have already seen, that the state of hæmorrhagy is sometimes dependent on that of *inflammation*) as in the instance of dysentery and pneumonia; and there is reason to believe, that, in some other cases, the same pathological connection may subsist, although it be less apparent. The general analogy between these states of disease may be fur-ther traced in the similarity of their predisposing and exciting cau-ses, in the effects of the *juvantia* and *lædentia*, and in the appear-ance of the blood drawn. In almost all cases of hæmorrhagy at-tended with symptoms of constitutional excitement,—that is to say, (in all states of active hæmorrhagy, the blood drawn will appear buffy and cupped.) This phenomenon was considered by Dr. Cul-len of such frequent occurrence, as to merit notice in his definition of the order.

By some pathologists it has been conjectured, that the evolution of organs at different periods of life is one cause of those partial congestions of blood which take place in the body, and which, by over-distending a particular set of vessels, dispose them to rupture. (It has generally been observed, that epistaxis is the hæmorrhagy of childhood; hæmoptysis, of the age of puberty; and that the ab-dominal hæmorrhagies occur in the more advanced periods of life.) It is possible, that *many* circumstances contribute to this peculiari-ty in the phenomena of the hæmorrhagies; but the theory which ascribes it to partial plethora from the evolution of organs has prob-ably some foundation in nature.

The third general condition of the body which was noticed as tending to hæmorrhagy, is (a weakened state of the coats of the blood-vessels.) This usually depends on original formation, and is not unfrequently hereditary. In some constitutions the arterial system appears to be peculiarly weak and lax; and it has been conjectured, that this often occurs of a scrofulous diathesis. In these habits it is reasonable to suppose, that the blood-vessels will give way from the application of causes which would have no such effect in a different habit of body. An idea is entertained by some pathologists, that mere *laxity* of the coats of vessels, independent of actual *rupture*, is sufficient to cause the effusion of blood. That

the colouring particles of the blood may *exude* along with the secretions of the part in certain relaxed conditions of a membrane is
probable ; but it is questionable how far this corresponds with genuine hæmorrhagy.

Hæmorrhagy may take place both from veins and from arteries ;
and frequent attempts have been made to explain what circumstances determine the one or the other of these events. It is generally admitted that arterial hæmorrhage is most frequent in early
life, and venous hæmorrhage at an advanced age. This circumstance is believed to depend upon certain differences in the *relative density* of the coats of arteries and veins at different periods of
life. The portion of the *venous* system most liable to hæmorrhagy
is the vena portæ. This vessel appears to differ in structure, as
it certainly does in distribution, and probably in function, from the
other veins of the body, and to partake closely of the nature of an
artery. We presume, that in hæmatemesis, and in certain cases
of abdominal hæmorrhage, the rupture takes place in some of the
branches of the vena portææ. Whenever there is a disposition to
hæmorrhagy, ether venous or arterial, it is reasonable to expect
that the vessels will give way in that part where they are least supported by integuments, or surrounding muscular or ligamentous
substance. Hence we may perceive, why hæmorrhages are so
much more frequent from the lungs, and the vessels of the Schneiderian membrane, than from any other part of the body.

4. The general principles of treatment in hæmorrhagy must be
varied to meet the varying circumstances under which it occurs.
A very eroneous idea once prevailed in the schools, that hæmorrhagies were salutary efforts of nature, and that they were to be
encouraged rather than checked. This originated, in part, from
the temporary relief which the patient experiences from the discharge of blood ; but the reasoning by which the doctrine is supported is vague, and the practice to which it leads, at least in the
great majority of cases, dangerous. We may not always have it
in our power to check hæmorrhagy, but we should at least attempt it.

The principal objects of treatment in cases of internal hæmorrhagy are four ;—to diminish plethora, where it can be rendered
probable that it exists ; to lessen the *vis a tergo*, or the force of the
heart's action ; to induce the formation of a coagulum about the
ends of the ruptured vessel ; and lastly, to bring on contraction of
the muscular fibres of the vessel, and of the parts in its vicinity.

Treatment

Upon one or otherof these principles may be explained the mode of action of each of those means, which have been found useful in the treatment of internal hæmorrhagy. They are, blood-letting, digitalis, purgatives, cold, the exhibition of astringents (such as alum, the superacetate of lead, and the mineral acids ;) and lastly, opiates and tonics. Some degree of doubt prevails as to the propriety of administering opium in a state of hæmorrhagy, and certainly it is not adapted to every form of the disease. It is chiefly indicated where the hæmorrhagy is of the *passive* kind ; and where it appears to come on from a *habit*, which the system has acquired, of relieving itself at particular times. This disposition in hæmorrhagy arising from internal causes, to recur after certain intervals, and often at stated periods, is a very curious, but, at the same time, one of the most general and best established of the principles which regulate its phenomena.

The application of this principle to the treatment of hæmorrhagy, and the adaptation of the different means which have been enumerated, to the several circumstances under which hæmorrhagy occurs, will become objects of inquiry in future chapters.*

* Epistaxis, and hæmoptysis, being the only species of hæmorrhagy attended, in common cases, with *pyrexia*, and the consideration of which does not involve that of chronic local disease, can alone be considered with propriety in this part of the work.

CHAP. II.

Symptoms of Epistaxis. Periods of Life at which it occurs. Exciting Causes. Epistaxis symptomatic of other Diseases. Treatment of Epistaxis, internal and external.

THE vessels that ramify upon the Schneiderian membrane are very numerous, and from their forming a net work, which is covered only by thin and delicate integuments, easily ruptured. The flow of blood from them, when it does not happen from accidental causes, is usually preceded by symptoms marking a determination to the head, such as throbbing of the carotid and temporal arteries, head-ache, flushing of the cheeks, giddiness, and a sense of weight, or fulness, in the nose; or by such as indicate a general state of increased action throughout the whole arterial system, as a quickened pulse, restlessness, disturbed dreams, thirst, diminished secretion of urine, and costiveness. The blood commonly flows from one nostril only; but often in quantity that may reasonably occasion considerable anxiety. Nor is it the occurrence of a single fit of hæmorrhagy which is alone to be considered; in almost all cases, it recurs for several weeks at certain intervals, and often tends very materially to weaken the body.

Epistaxis (for so this hæmorrhagy is called) happens equally to both sexes; and it may occur at all periods of life, but is chiefly observed to prevail among young persons advancing to puberty. In this case it may be considered as one of the evidences of that irregular distribution of blood, which characterizes the period of puberty, and which so strikingly manifests itself in the irritable constitution of the female. This principle in pathology will hereafter form the groundwork of our reasoning concerning the symptoms of *amenorrhœa*. The frequency of epistaxis at this period of life is very remarkable; and there can be no question, that if it be not excessive, it is productive of no particular inconvenience ;—in some constitutions it may even serve to diminish plethora. If it recurs, however, with great frequency, and is very copious, it becomes an object of serious attention. It is then commonly said to mark a state of arterial plethora. This is doubtful. It much more obviously points out a state of weakness in the original structure of the vessels of the body. It was an observation of Hippocrates, that persons subject while young to severe and obstinate bleedings at the nose, easily fall into dangerous diseases of the chest ; more especially peripneumonies, hæmoptysis, and consumption.

Hæmorrhage from the nose occasionally occurs in the middle periods of life ; but it becomes (common towards the decline of life,) when it probably depends upon the same causes which lead to apoplexy and palsy.

Among the exciting causes of epistaxis, pathologists have enumerated both heat and cold, and in different ways both may contribute to the occurrence of the hæmorrhagy. It frequently comes on without the slightest apparent cause, but is obviously attributable in other cases to exertions of the body, such as running, coughing, or blowing the nose. Particular postures favour it, as stooping, or lying with the head low. On this account, persons liable to epistaxis are frequently attacked by it on first waking. Epistaxis is occasionally to be traced to the suppression of some usual evacuation, especially in young women to the suppression of the menses. Under such circumstances, it has sometimes afforded relief to other symptoms.

Hæmorrhagy from the nose is a symptom of different diseases ; and as such, not less deserving of attention than when it occurs in an idiopathic form. It is met with in some of the severest cases of inflammatory fever, in low typhus, in the small-pox, and in several chronic diseases, as hooping-cough, and scurvy. After what was stated in the last chapter, it will be obvious, that in each of these cases, the occurrence of the hæmorrhagy is attributable to different causes. In conjunction with other symptoms, epistaxis always affords an important index of the *state* of the system, and proves an useful guide in practice. It is a very old and just remark, that hæmorrhagy from the nose accompanies some forms of abdominal disease, particularly obstructions of the spleen. The obscurity in which the functions of that organ are involved, would alone prove an insurmountable obstacle to any attempt at an explanation of the phenomenon.

Idiopathic epistaxis, when it occurs in *young* persons, and not in an excessive quantity, is scarcely an object of medical treatmen'. A light diet, with an occasional dose of salts, however will certainly be advisable. In severer cases, cold is to be applied to the head and back. Purging, regular exercise, early rising, and a diet strictly antiphlogistic, are then to be recommended. The tincture of digitalis in union with the sulphuric acid and infusion of roses, will also be found very useful. When epistaxis occurs in the middle or more advanced periods of life, it is often excessive, and is asse-ciated with plethora, and high vascular excitement. It then fre-quently becomes necessary to use very active means. Blood must be taken from the arm even till the patient faints. The nostrils are to be plugged up, both anteriorly and posteriorly, by dossils of lint dipped in an astringent solution, such as the liquor aluminis com-positus. The bowels are to be kept freely open, for a considerable time, by the mixture (R No. 14,) and a very spare vegetable diet rigidly enforced.

CHAP. III.

HÆMORRHAGY FROM THE LUNGS.

Circumstances under which Hæmoptysis chiefly occurs. Pre disposing Causes. Exciting Causes. Prognosis. Connection of Hæmoptysis with Tubercular Phthisis. Principles of Treatment.

THE discharge of blood from the lungs is usually accompanied by symptoms denoting determination to that organ, amounting in some cases, perhaps, to actual inflammation. There is a sense of fulness, heat, weight, tightness, or oppression about the chest, increased on full inspiration, some uneasiness in breathing, and a short tickling cough. Symptoms of fever are also present, such as shiverings, pains in the back and loins, a flushed countenance, lassitude, costiveness, a dry skin, and a hard pulse; but these are subject to great variety. I have seen the pulse, for instance, feeble and indistinct, so as to be hardly perceptible. The spitting up of blood is commonly preceded by a degree of irritation felt about the larynx, and a saltish taste perceived in the mouth. The quantity of blood brought up is very various. A slight tinge of the expectoration is sufficient to characterize the disease, as it marks the hæmorrhagic tendency, and may quickly be followed by a gush of blood. Again, it is sometimes so profuse as to occasion alarm for the immediate safety of the patient. It commonly recurs for several days together, and is often renewed upon very slight exertions. The blood is of a florid colour and frothy.

To distinguish this disease from hæmatemesis, or vomiting of blood is often more difficult than might be anticipated, owing to the occurrence of vomiting during the discharge of blood from the lungs; but in ordinary cases, an attention to the preceding symptoms, to the appearance of the blood, and to the general habit of body, will be sufficient to establish the diagnosis.

1. The most important considerations connected with hæmoptysis are those which relate to its predisposing and exciting causes; for by these we are to form our judgment of the probable termina-

tion of the disease, and be in a great measure guided in our method of treatment. Of the former, however, one only can be considered as under our control, and that one, the least frequent of
the whole :—I mean, _plethora_ of the system generally. The simple rupture of a blood-vessel in the lungs, from fulness of blood
and increased action, either within the chest, or throughout the
body, independent of any peculiarity of structure, has sometimes
been observed, but it is unquestionably a rare occurrence ; and this
must surely be a matter of surprise, when we reflect how numerous and how large the blood-vessels of the lungs are, and by what
a very delicate membrane they are covered and supported. Under
such circumstances, however, hæmorrhagy may occur from the
lungs, as from the vessels of the Schneiderian membrane. By rest
and low diet, the ruptured vessel would soon heal, without any further bad consequence.

2. The second predisposing cause of hæmoptysis, is the _scrofu-_
lous diathesis, or that habit which is marked, among other peculiarities, by a general delicacy of structure throughout the body—light
and thin hair, a smooth and soft skin, a lax muscular fibre and slender form. Of this delicacy of structure the blood-vessels appear
to partake ; and consequently a disposition to _hæmorrhagy_ becomes
also a character of scrofula. That it should particularly appear
in the lungs, might be conjectured from what has just been stated ;
but a further disposition in such a habit of body to this form of
bæmorrhagy is given by _tubercle_, the connection of which with
scrofula has been already noticed. It is necessary however to
add, that weakness of the vessels of the lungs, disposing them to
rupture, is often met with independent of scrofula. Hence it happens that some persons spit blood from any cause that weakens the
body generally.

3. The third circumstance giving a predisposition to hæmoptysis
is _period of life_. It rarely happens to children under the age of
twelve years, and is not frequent after that of five-and-thirty. It
chiefly prevails between the ages of fifteen and twenty-five. Pathologists have attempted in several ways to explain this circumstance. It has been said to depend upon the growth of the thorax
continuing, after other parts of the body have been fully evolved,
manifested by the increased width which the chest acquires at that
period of life. Dr. Cullen has imputed it, in part at least, to a
want of due balance between the aortic and pulmonary systems,
which must chiefly be felt at that age, when the former has arrived

at its utmost extension and resistance. To whatever cause it is to be ascribed, there can be no question as to the general correctness of the position, that this particular period of life gives a remarkable predisposition to hæmorrhagy from the lungs.

4. The fourth predisposing cause of hæmoptysis is _mal-forma-tion of the chest_, which obviously acts by preventing the due expansion of the lungs. Persons who have suffered in early life from rickets, to such an extent as to affect the spine or ribs, are very liable at another age to hæmoptysis. The scrofulous habit of body is characterized by prominent shoulders, and a narrow chest; and this is one, among other reasons, why the scrofulous diathesis is so frequently accompanied by a tendency to hæmoptysis, upon all occasions which impel the blood with any degree of increased impetus upon the vessels of the lungs,—in other words, upon the application of the _exciting_ causes. These are very numerous, some acting more immediately upon the lungs, and some indirectly through the medium of the general system.

Among the exciting causes of hæmoptysis, which act directly upon the weak blood-vessels, the most important are external injuries; violent exercise of the whole body, as in running, or wrestling; or of the lungs in particular, as in loud or long speaking, playing on wind instruments, or glass blowing. Those which act indirectly are full living, and particularly the free use of wine; alternations of atmospheric temperature, and, as some allege, of atmospheric pressure; sudden exposure to cold after being overheated; the suppression of usual evacuations; and apparently in some cases the amputation of a limb.

The _prognosis_ in hæmoptysis is to be regulated by the following considerations. As far as it is idiopathic, and as the mere effusion of blood is concerned, it is certainly favourable. Dr. Heberden, in the course of a long life, saw only one case of death from the excessive loss of blood. In a large proportion of cases, however, hæmorrhagy from the lungs is but a symptomatic affection; and the prognosis, therefore, merges in that of _consumption_. The connexion that subsists between these two diseases, hæmoptysis and tubercular phthisis, is in a practical point of view of the highest importance. The subject was formerly noticed when treating of consumption, but I have hitherto delayed mention of it, because it was desirable that the student should view pulmonary hæmorrhage somewhat abstractedly in the first instance, and afterwards as forming one in that series of symptoms which constitutes phthisis pulmonalis.

Treatment

As the prognosis in hæmoptysis is intimately connected with that of consumption, so also is the prevention and treatment of the disease. All that I shall now attempt, therefore, is to point out, in a few words, the method of treatment which is to be recommended with the view of checking the *immediate* effusion of blood.

While the blood is actually flowing, little can be done further than to admit cool air, and to avoid every kind of exertion, more particularly speaking. Ice, or ice-cold acidulated drinks, may be freely administered, and the diluted sulphuric acid, in the dose of thirty or forty drops every six hours. In some few cases, it becomes necessary to open a vein in the arm while the patient is expectorating blood. This however may generally be deferred for a few hours, when feverish symptoms supervene. The pulse becomes full and hard, the skin hot, and there is a sense of oppression about the chest. The blood will generally be found buffy. A saline purgative is then to be given, and cold acidulated drinks persevered in. The necessity of a second bleeding will be judged of by the state of the pulse, the habit of body, and, the appearance of the blood first drawn ; but unless the symptoms are urgent, it will commonly be advisable to trust, from this period, to nitre, sulphuric acid in the infusion of roses (R No. 99,) and tincture of digitalis. If the patient be threatened with a return of the hæmorrhage, ten or twelve leeches should be applied to the chest ; and if necessary, recourse had to alum (R No. 97) and the super-acetate of lead (R No. 98.) The bowels are to be kept open by saline purgatives. A light vegetable diet is to be directed, and by degrees some gentle exercise should be taken. Where a fixed pain is complained of, and the smallness of the pulse forbids bleeding, a blister may be applied. With the view of relieving the cough, a linctus of oxymel, or the mucilaginous mixture (No. 55,) containing a proportion of the syrup of poppies, may be taken frequently during the day.

Occasionally, a different plan of treatment should be adopted. When the spitting of blood takes place in warm and relaxing weather, when the pulse is weak, and the ordinary evidences of febrile excitement wanting, we may reasonably presume that the rupture of the blood-vessel has been owing to relaxation and debility. Under such circumstances, leeches and active aperients are carefully to be avoided. The patient is to be directed to take one or two glasses of port wine daily, and every six hours a draught composed of ten drachms of decoction of bark, with twenty minims of elixir of vitriol.

PART II.

CHRONIC DISEASES.

PRELIMINARY REMARKS.

THE term chronic disease has been employed by physicians in a double signification, which, though sufficiently intelligible to those who have had opportunities of seeing disease extensively, may, without previous explanation, become the source of some embarrassment to the student. In the perusal of the preceding pages, this may perhaps have been experienced; but it is now more particularly necessary to clear up any such difficulties, as chronic diseases are henceforth to be the sole objects of investigation.

The term *acute*, in medical language, is in strictness applied to such diseases as run a short and defined course : - *chronic* to such as are lingering, and of uncertain duration ; but, in common discourse, acute and chronic are frequently taken in the sense of *febrile* and *apyrexial*, because febrile diseases, for the most part, run through their stages rapidly, while such as are unattended by fever are usually of long duration. There is sufficient foundation in nature for both these pathological principles to entitle the physician to employ the terms in such a sense ; but is necessary to apprise the student, that they are by no means of universal application. The history which has been given of consumption, of chronic rheumatism, and of chronic peritonitis, will be sufficient to show, that diseases attended with a certain degree or kind of fever are sometimes tedious in their progress, and irregular in their periods and symptoms, In the present division of the work, it will be shown that the converse of this proposition holds equally true, and that diseases, unattended by fever, are sometimes rapid in their progress, and uniform in their symptoms. Apoplexy and hydrophobia may be taken as examples. These must be viewed, however, as *exceptions* to a

general rule ; or rather as facts supporting the opinion formerly ur·
ged (Introduction, page 2,) that the nature of the subject renders
fruitless any attempt to give a *perfect* idea of diseases by considering them separately and piecemeal,—that is to say, as exclusively
general or local, external or internal, acute or chronic.*

The general character of chronic diseases may be viewed as the
reverse of that which distinguishes diseases of an acute kind.
Throughout the latter a considerable similarity of pathology will
have been observed to prevail. There is a remarkable uniformity
also in their symptoms and periods. They run their course in a
short time—often in a defined time. In all of them may be traced
a disposition to terminate in the recovery of health. Medicine ex·
erts over the greater number of them a very obvious power; and
the principles of their treatment may, in most instances, be consid·
ered as tolerably well ascertained.

Chronic diseases, on the other hand, are very tedious : some of
them may even be present in one shape or another during the
whole course of life. In their progress they are very irregular.
The protæan forms which they assume not only perplex the prac·
titioner, but present difficulties almost insurmountable to the author
who would accurately describe them. Though not commonly, or
necessarily, accompanied by fever, yet feverish symptoms may
arise in all of them, at any period of their course. Much obscurity
pervades their pathology. The reasonings concerning some of
them do not readily assimilate with the views entertained of other
disorders. Lastly, the principles of treatment in chronic diseases
are neither uniform nor well understood. In many instances they
are wholly unknown ; but were they even better ascertained, it is
doubtful how far the physician could avail himself of such knowl·

---

* The ancients called those diseases acute, which being seated chiefly in.
and attended with a rapid ebullition of, the fluids, run their course quickly.
On the other hand, they called such diseases chronic, as proceed from a vi·
tiated condition of the solids of the body, or from preternatural grossness of
the fluids, on which account they either move very slowly towards concoc·
tion, or else never reach it.—*See Baglivi de Praxi Medica, lib. ii, cap. 1.*

edge. In the cure of chronic diseases, indeed, as Baglivi observes, neither fortune nor art avail him much. It is seldom that he observes in them any disposition to terminate spontaneously in the recovery of health; and they are unquestionably much less under the control of medicines than acute disorders.

Although this may be the general character of the class of diseases which form the subject of the present division of the work, it is not on that account to be supposed that they are less worthy than others of attentive examination. The practical physician will find abundant occasion for the exercise of his skill, if not in the cure, at least in the relief of these complaints; and to the pathologist, chronic diseases are an endless subject of curious investigation. Their history and pathological relations, indeed, involve some of the most abstruse and recondite points in medical literature. To lay open and explain these, as far as the author's knowledge extends, and the state of the science admits, will be a principal object with him in the present volume. Where he fails in throwing light on the difficulties which he may encounter, it will at least afford him satisfaction to have suggested fit subjects for the inquiries of those who may come more qualified for the task.

CLASS I.

CHRONIC DISEASES OF THE ENCEPHALON.

CHAP. I.

CHARACTER, GENERAL PATHOLOGY, AND CONNECTION OF THE
CHRONIC DISEASES OF THE ENCEPHALON.

*Of Neurosis, or disturbed Function of the nervous System, independent of
Fever. Diseases arranged under this Head. Their chief Characters.
Coma. Convulsion. Mental Aberration. States of the Brain in these
Diseases. Chronic Inflammation. Congestion. Imperfect Supply of
Blood. Affection of the Brain and Nerves independent of the circulat-
ing System. Pressure. Other Points of connection among the Chronic
Diseases of the Encephalon. Their Conversion into each other. General
Principles of their Treatment.*

THERE are not, perhaps, in the whole circle of medical science,
any diseases offering so many interesting points of research to the
speculative physician, as those which derive their character from
disturbance of function in the brain and nervous system, independent of the presence of fever. They may be associated together
as the diseases of *primary neurosis*, and they constitute a series,
which it cannot but be useful to examine in the first instance in a
general manner. It will be found that they have a common character, and many points of mutual connection. To explain these
will not only be the means of preventing hereafter much needless
repetition, but it will serve to impress upon the student the importance of those pathological relations among diseases, which serve
equally to improve and to facilitate practice.

The diseases comprised in this series are, apoplexy, palsy, epilepsy, mania, chorea, tetanus, hydrophobia, neuralgia; to which
may be added, syncope, asphyxia, and hypochondriasis. Though
deriving their character principally from a morbid condition of the

nervous system, they are all more or less connected with disturbed function in other parts. The four last mentioned, however, are so intimately connected with disorder in other organs, that in the present chapter I shall merely keep them before me, with a view to some points in their general pathology, reserving their separate consideration to future parts of the volume.

Physiology teaches, that among the several functions of the brain and nerves, of which some are well, and others only imperfectly ascertained, the principal are, sensation, voluntary motion, and the manifestation of the mind. It is natural to expect, that from disturbance in them the chief characters of the *neuroses* should be derived; and accordingly we find that Coma, Convulsion, and Mental Aberration, are the three great classes to which we may refer the symptoms of these diseases.

1. Coma consists in the loss of sensation, thought, and *voluntary* motion. In this state of disease, however, the organs of involuntary motion preserve their functions, and consequently it is by the continuance of the pulse and of the breathing, that we distinguish between coma and the states of syncope and asphyxia. But though in this manner we are enabled to mark the diagnosis between coma and the *disordered* conditions of body with which it is liable to be confounded, there are two states, consistent with health, from which it cannot be distinguished by such a criterion ; I mean the states of *sleep* and of *intoxication*. In all cases of suspected coma, it is necessary for the safety of the patient and the credit of the practitioner, that this point should receive attention. If duly kept in view, there is no great probability of any error occurring ; for it is inattention to the circumstance, and not any difficulty in deciding upon it when once suggested, from which mistakes have originated. Coma is distinguished from sleep by the impossibility of rousing the patient by shaking, noise, or otherwise. The smell of the breath will, for the most part, be sufficient to characterize the state of intoxication ; but in extreme cases there will always be difficulty, for actual coma may possibly have supervened. At all times attention should be paid to the circumstances which *preceded* the attack ; for by this means not only will ambiguity be prevented, but the physician will obtain such an insight into the causes of the disease and the habits of the patient, as will assist materially in directing his practice.

The abolition of sense and voluntary motion then constitutes perfect coma ; and it is the distinguishing feature of apoplexy, the first disease which will be noticed in the present series. It remains to state, that the loss of these functions is not always complete. Partial deprivations, both of sensation, thought, and voluntary motion, occur in the chronic diseases of the brain, and afford many of the most prominent symptoms of such disorders. Of this kind are preternatural drowsiness, or lethargy, paralysis of particular muscles, indistinctness of vision, amaurosis. They are all referable, however, to the general head of coma.

2. The second set of symptoms occurring in the chronic disease of the encephalon, may be classed together under the head of convulsion, or spasm. The state of convulsion is commonly defined to be that wherein the *voluntary* muscles of the body are excited into action by powers independent of the will. It is not, however, peculiar to those muscles. Not unfrequently those of involuntary motion are similarly affected, the diaphragm for instance, and smaller muscles of inspiration, as in asthma, or the muscular coat of the stomach or intestines, as observed in colic. It would appear indeed as if no particular fibres were exempt from spasmodic contraction, excepting those of the heart.

Of the voluntary muscles of the body it has been remarked, that those which are most immediately under the influence of the will, and most frequently employed, are those principally affected in convulsive disorders ; and the same observation will be found applicable to paralytic affections. Of this kind are the muscles of the eyes, eyelids, face, arms, and legs. Spasms of these muscles are observed in chorea, hysteria, and all the lighter forms of nervous affection ; while spasms of the muscles of the neck, back and belly, occur in tetanus, hydrophobia, epilepsy, and indicate a severer kind, or more aggravated *degree* of disease.

Convulsions have been divided into two kinds—the permanent, and that which alternates with relaxation ; in other words, the *tonic* and *clonic*. Tetantus affords an instance of the one, hysteria of the other. The distinction is of little consequence, unless coupled with the pathological principle, that the tonic or *tetanic* spasm is a disease of infinitely more importance than the *common* or clonic spasm. The former arises from causes over which we have little or no control, and is, at all times, a state of the utmost danger ; while the latter (to which the term *convulsion* is more especially supposed to apply) is frequently little more than the evidence of a peculiarly irritable disposition in the nervous system, which may exist, even to a great extent and for a long time, without exciting any uneasiness for the ultimate safety of the patient. In all reasonings indeed concerning a disease accompanied with clonic or common spasm, it is necessary to look to the original constitution and temperament of the individual. There exists in some persons an *irritable* habit of body, a disposition in the system to be excited on slight occasions, and consequently, a more than ordinary tendency to *spasm*. This manifests itself even when any function of the body becomes, from *accidental* circumstances, disturbed. Such a habit of body has been denominated by some physiologists the nervous *temperament*. It is characteristic of the infantile period of life and of the female sex. The distinction between this *irritable habit of body* and the *morbid state of convulsion*, though sufficiently apparent in common cases, is yet on many occasions a matter of considerable difficulty. In point of fact they will be found to run into each other by insensible degrees, constituting, as we shall afterwards show, one of the many interesting features in the pathology of epilepsy.

Independent of those convulsive actions of the whole body to which the term *fits* is popularly applied, there are a variety of *partial* convulsions, referable to this general head, which occur as evidences of chronic disease within the brain. Of this kind are, permanent contraction of the iris, irregular contractions of the muscles of the eye, constituting *squinting*, and the convulsions of the pterygoid muscles, commonly called *grinding of the teeth*.

3. The symptoms by which chronic disease of the brain manifests itself, may be referred, in the third place, to the head of *Vesania*, or mental aberration. Of this disordered condition of the brain, physicians have noticed many varieties. It may be either temporary or permanent; in other words, it may assume the form of delirium or mania. It may be either general or partial; that is to say, the powers of thought may be completely lost, as in the case of *idiotcy*; or some one faculty of the mind may be disturbed, while others remain perfect, or only partially impaired. Sometimes for instance, the imagination labours under a strong and unconquerable delusion, while the memory is perhaps still enjoyed in full perfection. This constitutes the highest grade of mental aberration, and is the characteristic feature of *mania*. At other times the memory fails, while the powers of perception are still uninjured. This is a frequent consequence of severe injuries of the head, and of paralytic seizures. It is a very common attendant also on

37

that morbid change in the structure of the brain, which gradually takes place in the latter periods of advanced life.

Aberrations of mind, lastly, vary in their character and intensity. Sometimes they are attended with fierce excitement, violent aversion, and a disposition to commit acts of violence on themselves or those around them. At other times the delusion of mind is accompanied with a sense, hardly less formidable, of melancholy and settled despondency. To the lighter shades of this disordered condition of the mind, physicians have commonly applied the term *hypochondriacism*. Occasionally, we find maniacal aberration coupled with a perfect tranquillity and self-content.

After noticing the general character of the diseases usually called *nervous*, I proceed to inquire into the opinions commonly entertained regarding their pathology and proximate cause. And here it is to be remarked, in the first place, how manifestly a large proportion of such cases are connected with, and therefore probably dependant upon, certain disordered states of the *circulating* system. That this principle is not of universal application, I shall presently have occasion to show; but, in the mean time, it will be right to point out what those derangements of the circulating system are, which are so closely interwoven in the pathology of nervous diseases.

1. The first of these is *chronic inflammation* of the substance of the brain, or of its meninges. That this is the true *proximate cause* of many cases of chronic disease of the encephalon, is abundantly proved by the appearances found on dissection; which are, depositions of coagulable lymph upon the surface of the brain, thickening of one or more of the membranes, and suppuration. These *unquestionable* marks of inflammatory action, are however, but rarely met with, in comparison with two others, frequently adduced as evidences of the same state of disease;—I mean increased vascularity within the cranium, and serous effusion between the membranes, or within the ventricles. These appearances are very common in different diseases, but in none are they so generally met with as in chronic affections of the nervous system. There are few instances, indeed, of any morbid change of structure in the brain existing without them. Pathologists have differed, however, in their estimate of the importance to be attached to them, especially to that of serous effusion. The general opinion appears to be, that though it cannot be assumed as a proof of the existence of actual inflammation within the brain, it must yet be allowed to

denote a degree of morbid *excitement* of the vessels of the brain, not far removed from inflammatory action.

2. The second of the morbid conditions of the circulating system, connected with nervous disease, is *simple congestion* of blood in the blood-vessels. This may arise either from an extraordinary flow of blood into the arteries of the brain, or from the difficulty experienced in the return of blood to the heart. The peculiar structure of the large venous trunks of the brain is calculated to lead, under certain circumstances, to *stagnation*, or, as is now more commonly called, *venous congestion* in the head. That such a state of the circulating system in the encephalon does occasionally exist, there cannot, I presume, be a doubt ; but it may be fairly questioned how far we are able to judge of its existence, with any degree of accuracy, by examination made after death. It is at least sufficiently ascertained, that that fulness in the vessels of the brain, so often found upon dissection, and supposed to denote *congestion*, depends in a great degree on the position in which the body had lain previous to examination.

3. The third of those states of disease to which our attention must be paid in this inquiry, is *hæmorrhagy*. The rupture of a blood-vessel within the brain acknowledges many of the laws which affect other hæmorrhages ; but the want of outlet for the effused fluid, the peculiar delicacy of the structure of the brain, the importance of its functions, and above, all, the remarkable effects of pressure upon its substance, give to the *hæmorrhagia cerebri* an interest far superior to what belongs to any other form of hæmorrhagic disease. The symptoms produced by effusion of blood within the brain, are, with few exceptions, those of apoplexy ; and the nature and varieties of cerebral hæmorrhagy will accordingly constitute the most important feature in the pathology of that disease.

4. The fourth morbid condition of the circulating system observed in certain diseases of the nervous kind, is *an imperfect supply of blood*. The brain, like every other organ of the body, is dependent for the due exercise of its functions on the circulation. It can neither perform them properly when the supply of blood is too great, nor when it is defective. Syncope is the usual result of a want of due supply of blood to the brain ; but convulsions occasionally arise from the same cause, as is well exemplified in the instance of puerperal hæmorrhage. It is not often that we have to apply this principle in the pathology of nervous diseases ; but in a

general view of the subject, such as we are now taking, it would have been improper to omit it.

5. In like manner, it becomes necessary to notice a fifth state of the circulating system which is occasionally present in nervous diseases ;—I mean the supply of blood _imperfectly oxygenated_, and therefore unfit for supporting the functions of the nervous system. This principle, it is true, like the last, is very limited in its application ; but it enters into the pathology of apoplexy, and is the foundation of many of our reasonings concerning asphyxia.

I have already remarked, that there are conditions of cerebral disease, independent, as far as we can judge, of the circulating system.

1. The first of these is simple compression. This may arise either from a coagulum of blood, a soft tumour, a bony excrescence, a depressed portion of the skull, or the presence of some foreign body. The effects of pressure vary extremely, according as it takes place _suddenly_ or gradually. In most instances, as already observed the symptoms occasioned by pressure on the brain partake of the _comatose_, or apoplectic character ; but instances are upon record, particularly in the case of gradual pressure, where such a state has been followed by symptoms, not of insensibility, but of high nervous excitement—by mania and convulsions.

2. There still remains to be stated one principle of very general application in the pathology of nervous disorders. Hitherto we have had some cognizable cause for the symptoms—the effusion of blood, inflammation, or the pressure of a tumour. But it is further to be remembered, that there exists an affection of the brain and nerves equally independent of pressure, and of all disturbance in the circulation within the encephalon. The best illustration of this principle is afforded by the phænomena of the narcotic poisons, where coma and convulsion are produced by means, which obviously act on the sentient extremities of the nerves, and which, we may fairly presume, deprive the nervous substance of its _mobility_, or its power of receiving or communicating impressions. Such a pathological principle is necessarily obscure, from the very nature of the functions concerned, but it will be found an indispensable one on many occasions ; as, for instance, in any attempt at explaining the pathology of tetanus and hydrophobia, or in elucidating those varieties of epilepsy and chorea which depend upon the sympathy of the brain with some distant organ. The principle being once established, there remains no longer any difficulty in under-

standing why, in a great variety of cases of chronic disease of the brain, no morbid appearances of any kind are found upon dissection. This interesting fact, indeed, has been denied by some, and explained away by others; but it is too frequent and too obvious to be thus disposed of. The student in medicine may here receive an important lesson. He may learn from this, that the causes of *death* are often as obscure as the sources of life and health; and that morbid anatomy, with all its acknowledged advantages, may, if pursued too exclusively, injure rather than assist the conclusions of the pathologist.

The observations now offered on the character and general pathology of nervous diseases, will tend to point out the very intimate connection subsisting among them. The same thing will be further illustrated by a view of their predisposing and exciting causes, by a consideration of their mutual conversion, and, lastly, by a survey of the principles of treatment applicable to the greater number of them. But before adverting to these topics, I would wish (without, however, going into any detail on the subject) to notice the attempts which have been made to connect particular symptoms observed during life with certain appearances found after death;—— in other words, to establish *minute diagnosis* among the morbid affections of the several structures contained in the encephalon. Pathologists, more especially those of recent times, have been at pains to distinguish inflammation of the arachnoid, from a similar affection of the other membranes;—extravasation into the ventricles, from extravasation with laceration of the substance of the brain;— disease of the anterior, from disease of the posterior lobes of the brain;—injury of the brain, from injury of the medulla oblongata. It would be presumptuous to say, that attempts of this kind are altogether nugatory; but it cannot be denied, that hitherto very little success has attended them, that the rules laid down by authors are subject to such numerous exceptions as to interfere greatly with their application in practice; and lastly, that no reasonable hope exists of deriving from them, even if considerably improved any portion of practical advantage.

It is of more importance to trace the *analogies* among the chronic diseases of the encephalon than their minute shades of difference; and we shall be assisted in this, in the first place, by considering the similarity, and even, in many cases, the identity of their predisposing and exciting causes. Mania, for instance, and epilepsy, are hereditary. The exciting causes of epilepsy are for

tbe most part those also of apoplexy and palsy.   Chorea, hysteria
and many varieties of epilepsy have a common origin in a disordered state of the stomach and bowels.   But in no way is the connection among these diseases so strikingly displayed as in the circumstance of their mutual conversion, and in their manner of running into each other by insensible degrees.   I have already alluded to this in the case of hysteria and epilepsy ; but it is equally
well marked with regard to palsy and apoplexy, syncope, and convulsion, convulsion and mania, mania and apoplexy.   One individual of a family has had epilepsy, while others have been deranged.
Epileptics commonly die with comatose symptoms.   Neuralgic affections are not unfrequently succeeded by amaurosis, or by apoplexy.   Instances of this important principle in pathology need not
be multiplied, as they must be familiar to all who have enjoyed any
share of general practice.

It remains only that, I notice the principles of treatment applicable to the greater number of the diseases which are now under
consideration ; and it will be found, that the pathological analogies
subsisting among them are strikingly confirmed by the effects of
the *juvantia* and *lædentia*.   The depleting and lowering system
adapted to the particular circumstances of each patient, and the
peculiarities of each disease, is that upon which the physician
places his chief reliance ; and it is, with some few exceptions, of
powerful efficacy in all of them, whether exhibiting the character
of coma, of convulsion, or of mental aberration.   This is the great
principle kept in view, whether we employ bleeding, purging, leeches, cupping, local cold, blisters, issues, and setons ; or content
ourselves with remedial means of a less formal though not less useful character, such as a cooling spare diet, regular exercise, or a
course of aperient mineral waters.   By these means, early, steadily,
and judiciously applied, we may often do a great deal towards the
relief, or permanent cure, of the chronic diseases of the brain ;
while without them, and depending upon stimulants and antispasmodics, our expectations will be but too often baffled.

Premonitory Symptoms. Varieties in the Apoplectic Seizure. Appearances presented during the Apoplectic Fit. Prognosis. Appearances on Dissection. Predisposition to Apoplexy. Exciting causes. Speculations concerning its proximate Cause. Subdivision of Apoplexies. Treatment to be pursued during the Fit. Prophylaxis.

In the last chapter, I had occasion to explain the sense in which physicians employ the term coma ; and I then stated, that apoplexy is a disease of which coma constitutes the leading feature. Coma, or the abolition of the functions of the brain and nerves, may be the consequence of external injuries, or it may occur without any obvious assignable cause. In the former case, it is an object of attention to the surgeon, and is often remediable by surgical operation. In the latter case, it falls under the cognizance of the physician, and is by him denominated spontaneous coma, or apoplexy.

It is very seldom that this dreadful visitation is experienced without the occurrence of symptoms to warn the patient of its probable approach. There are a few instances, indeed, of any kind of severe disease occurring without some premonitory symptoms ; but they are not often so unequivocal as those which indicate the apoplectic tendency. With a view to practice, such symptoms are of infinitely more importance than those of the fit itself ; and they accordingly require the most serious attention from the physician. For the sake of perspicuity, they may be arranged according as they affect the head generally, the external senses, the internal senses, or the organs of voluntary motion.

To the first class belong pain of the head (generally a dull pain, with a sense of weight, but occasionally a more acute pain, accompanied with the feeling of the head being bound round by a cord or wire ;)—giddiness, particularly on stooping, or any attempt to

turn the head quickly round ;—throbbing of the temporal arteries.
To the second class belong transient deafness, ringing in the ears,
epistaxis, obscurity or irregularity of vision, transient blindness.—
To the third, stupor, drowsiness, incoherent talking, a state resembling intoxication, disturbed sleep, failure of the memory, loss of
temper.—To the fourth, twisting of the mouth, falling of the eyelid, numbness and weakness of a finger, dragging of the leg, stam-
mering. After experiencing, for a longer or shorter time, one or
more of these warnings, the patient falls into the apoplectic fit ;
and Dr. Abercrombie has well described the several ways in which
this takes place.*

1. In the most usual form of apoplectic seizure, the patient falls
down *suddenly*, deprived of sense and motion, and lies like a person in a deep sleep. He neither hears nor sees, nor feels. Unconscious of every thing around him, he is alike insensible to the
exertions of his medical attendants, and the anxieties of his friends.
The suddenness of the attack is that feature of the disorder which
most immediately impresses itself upon the notice of observers ;
and being so very general, the disease has from this circumstance
in all ages received its name.

2. The second form of apoplectic seizure commences by a sudden attack of violent pain of the head, accompanied with paleness
of the face, sickness at stomach, vomiting, and transient loss of
recollection. The patient, in some instances, falls down in a state
resembling syncope, but recovers in a few minutes, and is able to
walk. After a few hours, however, the head-ache continuing, he
becomes oppressed, and *gradually* sinks into perfect coma.

3. The third form of apoplectic seizure begins with a sudden
attack of *palsy* of one side, with loss of speech, which after the
lapse of some hours passes gradually into apoplexy.

In whichever way the apoplectic fit commences, there are certain appearances presented during its continuance, which merit attention. The pulse, at first, is commonly small and irregular ; but
as the system recovers from the shock, the pulse becomes full and
strong, and is generally slower than natural. Respiration is much
embarrassed, being always slow, and occasionally irregular. In
all the severer degrees of the disease, this laborious breathing is
accompanied by *stertor* ; and a frequent appearance is that of foam,
or frothy saliva, excreted from the mouth, and blown away from

* Edinburgh Medical and Surgical Journal, vol. xiv, p. 554.

the lips with considerable force. This latter symptom has always been looked upon as indicative of the greatest danger.

The skin is commonly warm, and bathed in a copious perspiration. In the worst cases of the disease, a cold clammy sweat has been observed. The face is generally pale ; the cornea dull and glassy ; and the pupils permanently dilated. The teeth are closely clenched ; and the power of swallowing, though seldom wholly lost, is for the most part so much impeded, as to oppose the most serious obstacles to the administration of remedies. The bowels are torpid, as is usual in all cases of cerebral oppression, and they resist the action even of powerful cathartics. If blood is drawn from the arm, the coagulum is commonly firm ; and Sir Gilbert Blane states that it is in most instances buffy.

The duration of the apoplectic fit varies from two or three hours to as many days. Thirty hours may be called the average duration of those cases which have fallen under my own observation. Instances, indeed, are on record of *sudden death* from apoplexy ; but in many of these there are grounds to suspect, that the immediate cause was to be found in some affection of the heart, or large vessels in its neighbourhood, rather than in injury to the brain. Genuine apoplexy, commencing in the manner I have descibed, and attended with all the symptoms just enumerated, almost always ends fatally. When a recovery, either perfect, temporary, or partial, takes place, it will usually be found that some of the more decided evidences of perfect coma have been wanting : the patient has given evidence of feeling when his limb is grasped, or the lancet used ; the pupil has obeyed in a certain degree the stimulus of light ; the mouth has not been firmly closed, nor the power of swallowing wholly lost ; there has been no stertor, or foaming at the mouth ; nor were the premonitory symptoms strongly marked. Under such circumstances our prognosis may be somewhat more favourable ; though it should even then be guarded by the reflection, that if recovery does take place, it is seldom complete. An incurable palsy may remain ; or the memory wholly or partially fail ; or an imbecility of mind, approaching to mania, may be left. But besides this, in every case where a decided apoplectic fit has been experienced, a relapse is to be dreaded ; and recovery from a second attack, though sometimes witnessed, is yet a rare event.

The opportunities which the fatality of this disease has afforded to the physician for prosecuting his researches into its nature and seat, have not been lost ; and we have accordingly a most extended

38

morbid appearances

record of the appearances found on dissection in apoplectic cases. Their variety is very great, and must be fully appreciated before any attempt can be made to explain the pathology of the disease.* Extravasation of blood in some part of the encephalon, is by far the most common appearance, and is that which is generally to be anticipated. Such extravasation may take place between the membranes of the brain, on its surface, about its basis, within its ventricles, or in the midst of its substance. The quantity of fluid effused is as various as its situation ; and the violence of the symptoms is found to bear a reference partly to the *quantity*, and partly to the particular *seat* of extravasation. An extensive effusion of blood is equally to be dreaded wherever it takes place ; but slight effusion is generally stated, and probably with justice, to be more dangerous in certain situations than in others. (It is believed, for instance, to be much more alarming, and attended with more formidable symptoms, when occurring on the medulla oblongata, than in the anterior lobes of the brain.)

The next most usual appearance in those who die of apoplexy, is the effusion of serum, either upon the surface of the brain, or within the ventricles. In some cases we meet with turgescence of the smaller vessels, or of the great sinuses of the brain, but without effusion either of blood or serum.

These are the common appearances presented on examination of those who die of apoplexy ; and, considering their frequency, it is undoubtedly a surprising circumstance, that every now and then, after the most unequivocal symptoms, the head presents, on dissection, nothing morbid or uncommon. Some pathologists explain this by supposing, that effusion or disorganization may have taken place, but in a degree so minute as to escape observation. Others imagine, that more decided appearances may have existed, but were overlooked in the hurry of examination. A third class maintain, that there may be morbid phænomena present during life, which disappear prior to dissection ; while others avow their persuasion, that in some other part of the body (the thorax, for instance, or spinal marrow,) the cause of death existed, and might by judicious examination have been detected. These arguments may have

---

* The student who desires further information on this subject, or on that of apoplexy generally, may consult with the greatest advantage the first volume of Dr. Cooke's " Treatise on Nervous Diseases," where, besides much useful original matter, he will find references to all the best authorities.

weight in particular cases, but their *general* tendency is disproved by an extended survey of the chronic derangements of the brain and nervous system.

The predisposition to apoplexy has attracted much attention from medical authors, and many contradictory opinions have been brought forward concerning it.

1. The tendency to apoplexy is given, in the first place, by certain *conformations of body*. The apoplectic *make* has been remarked, indeed, in all ages. A large head, a short thick neck, a florid complexion, broad shoulders, short stature, with a tendency to corpulency, are the prominent features of the apoplectic figure. Nevertheless, apoplexy is sometimes met with in spare subjects with pale countenance. Peculiarity in the formation of body being often hereditary, a tendency to the disease may naturally be expected to prevail in particular families ; but independent of this, there may exist a *constitutional* tendency to disease of the head, the knowledge of which will materially assist in forming a right judgment on the origin and probable tendency of particular symptoms.

2. The predisposition to apoplexy is connected, in the second place, with a certain *period of life*. Hippocrates said, that apoplexies were chiefly generated between the fortieth and sixtieth year ; and Cullen further remarks, that as life advances, the tendency to this disease increases. There is no doubt that in early life it is rarely met with ; but it is far from being uncommon between the twentieth and thirtieth year. By many pathologists it has been held, that the greater liability to the disease at an advanced period of life, is owing to an ossified or otherwise diseased state of the coats of the cerebral arteries ; which is stated to be then of frequent occurrence. It is supposed to give increased facility to extravasation within the encephalon, just as the same morbid structure in other parts is imagined to lead to aneurism. There is, probably, some foundation for this opinion, though it may have been pushed too far by certain of its supporters. While we are ready to acknowledge, then, that the rupture of a blood-vessel within the brain may sometimes be connected with a diseased state of the coats of the arteries, we must not, on the other hand, forget, that, in probably a *larger* proportion of cases, it is merely the result of a *morbid action* of vessels, analogous to that which takes place in hæmoptysis.

3. A predisposition to apoplexy is further given by such *habits of life* as tend to produce plethora generally, to drive the blood in

more then ordinary quantity upon the vessels of the brain, or to
prevent its free return to the heart.   Hence it is, that full living,
habitual intoxication, sedentary pursuits, too great indulgence in
sleep, intense and long-continued thought, have always been accused of leading to apoplexy.

The principal *exciting* causes of apoplexy, are the distension of
the stomach by a full meal, the immoderate use of wine or spirits,
straining to evacuate a costive stool, violent exercise, very long or
loud speaking, severe fits of coughing, tumours on the neck, stooping, the recumbent posture, and, lastly, violent passions of the mind.
It is a singular circumstance, that both heat and cold, when in an
extreme degree, may occasion apoplexy.   The coup de soleil of hot
climates has been considered, on good authority, to be of the nature of apoplexy.   The improper use of the warm bath has, under
my own observation, brought on complete and fatal apoplexy.   On
the other hand, excessive cold produces a torpor and sleepiness,
apparently of the comatose kind.   This was strikingly exemplified
in the celebrated adventure of Dr. Solander and Sir Joseph Banks
on the mountains near the Straits of Magellan.   The disposition to
sleep is almost irresistible ; but, in the emphatic language of Dr.
Solander, whoever indulges it, " wakes no more."

It belongs to this place to remark, that an apoplectic attack is
not uncommon in the progress of other diseases.   It occasionally
occurs in fevers, small-pox, rheumatism, gout, and hooping-cough :
and it is a still more frequent consequence of organic diseases of
the heart, more particularly of such as are attended with a bound-
ing pulse, and in their course become complicated with dropsy.

I am unwilling to place in the catalogue of the exciting causes
of apoplexy, certain others which have been mentioned by authors ;
because the very circumstance of naming them as such, involves the
difficult question of the nature of the affection which they produce.
To this class belong opium, tobacco, and the other narcotics ; the
carbonic acid, and other irrespirable gases ; catain poisonous vegetable matters (as the upas antiar, and woorara) ; and lastly, lightning.   The consideration of their effects and of their mode of action will be reserved for discussion in the chapter on asphyxia.

In the remarks now offered, I have attempted, as much as possible, to confine myself to facts, and to avoid all allusion to the variety
of opinions which have been entertained respecting the proximate
cause of apoplexy, and consequently respecting the division of the
disease into different species.   These topics, however, must be ac-

knowledged to be of no small importance; and it will be my endeavour to lay before the student such a view of them, as may assist him in unravelling the difficulties in which this portion of medical science is involved.

It has been the great object of pathological writers to discover
some one morbid condition of the brain which is present in every
case of apoplexy, some have stated this to be *effusion*. Others have
generalized further, and considered *pressure* as the real efficient
cause of the apoplectic phenomena. A third class of pathologists
have held, with Dr. Abercrombie that irregular or *interrupted circulation* is the general principle applicable in all cases of apoplexy.

Each of these opinions has been supported by ingenious arguments ; and that in particular which attributes the disease to *pressure* on the cerebral mass or its appendages, is undoubtedly applicable to a very large proportion of cases. The proof of its appli-
cability as a proximate cause *in all cases*, is however, even in this
instance, highly defective. Extravasation of blood is the most usual source of that pressure which occasions apoplexy ; yet extravasated blood has been on several occasions found in the brain, without any comatose symptoms having existed during life. The same
thing is even still better ascertained with regard to serous effusion
and sanguine congestion, which are presumed to be the next most
usual sources of pressure in apoplectic cases. These facts, taken
in connection with those which substantiate the frequent occurrence
of apoplexy without leaving any cognizable traces of disease after
death, appear to warrant the opinion, that the *single* principle so
long sought for by pathologists does not exist ; and that, in point
of fact, the apoplectic state is the result of different morbid conditions of the system.

These speculative notions concerning the proximate cause of apoplexy have not been confined to the closet of the pathologist ; they
have given occasion to the subdivision of apoplexies into different
species, important, it is said, in practice, as leading to diversities
of treatment. By many of the distinguished systematic writers in
medicine, great stress was laid on the division of apoplexies into
sanguineous and *serous*, and the doctrine continues, in a certain degree, to influence the notions and practice of modern physicians.
Certain symptoms have been described as peculiar to the serous
apoplexy, and plans of treatment have been recommended, adapted
only to that species of the disease. These conclusions, however,
are neither borne out by facts, nor rendered probable by patholo-

gical reasoning. The distinctive characters described by authors,
are seldom met with so strongly characterized as to warrant an
opinion concerning the exact nature of the case. Even where they
have been the most distinctly marked, the appearances on dissection have frequently disappointed the expectations of the practitioner. Pathological reasoning would incline us still further to distrust such distinctions, as it would tend to show that the effusion of
blood and that of serum depend here, as in many other cases upon
the same general cause. As far, then, as they simply express a
fact discovered after death, the term *serous* and *sanguineous* may
be admitted ; but they can never with propriety be employed during life, under the impression of establishing more accurate diagnosis, or of facilitating practice.

If these objections apply to the old division of apoplexies into
sanguineous and serous, there are others no less forcible, which
may be urged against the modern distinctions of *meningeal* and *cerebral*, or of simple apoplexy, and of apoplexy complicated with
paralysis. But these have never been formally acknowledged by
any writers in this country ; and no practical benefit that I am
aware of, would result from their adoption, were it even ascertained, that there was a foundation for them in nature. I have, therefore, deemed it unnecessary to enlarge on the subject in a purely
elementary work.

The doctrines here laid down are now to be applied to an illustration of the principles and details of treatment proper in apoplectic
cases. From the remarks just offered on the distinctions of apoplexies, we may, in the first place, deduce, one very important
rule, *viz.* that all cases of apoplexy are to be treated on the same
general principles ; and that though the details must necessarily
be varied, according to the age and constitution of the patient, the
severity of the disease, or other accidental circumstances there is
no class of apoplectic affections which requires a *distinct* system
of management.

In the actual paroxysm of apoplexy, the patient should be moved into a spacious apartment, and cool air freely admitted around
him. His head should be raised ; ligatures of all kinds, especially
about the neck, should be loosened ; and the legs and feet may
with propriety be placed in warm water. A strong disease, however, as Aretæus observed, requires a powerful remedy, and blood-
letting has at all times been resorted to as holding out the best
prospect. Many objections have been urged against it ; but it still

continues, and must for ever continue to be employed. In the most
aggravated form of the disease, indeed, neither bleeding nor any
other remedial means can reasonably be expected to effect a cure;
but there are no grounds for believing, that, with common caution,
the danger of the patient is *increased* by it. No one certainly
would venture to advise repeated and indiscriminate abstraction of
blood, without reference to its effects, or to any of those rules by
which we regulate the application of the lancet in other cases.
This would be a blameable empiricism; but at the same time the
student should feel, that blood-letting is the only effectual remedy
in apoplexy, and he should not be discouraged from it by any theoretical notions. The observations of Dr. Fothergill, and others
who have opposed the employment of blood-letting, tend rather to
establish the dangerous nature of the disease than the impropriety of the practice. We cannot it is true, remove by this means
blood which has been actually extravasated; but we may prevent
further effusion, and lessen general compression. In slighter cases, we may relieve the excitement and tension of the vessels
within the head, and possibly prevent effusion altogether.

On the first attack, therefore blood should be drawn from the
arm to the extent of one or two pounds; and this should be repeated in four or five hours afterwards, unless very unequivocal symptoms of amendment have appeared. The propriety of pursuing
the evacuation further, must be determined by the peculiar circumstances of the case. It ought to be known, that from six to
eight pounds of blood have been taken from a person, by no means
robust, before the disease began to yield. On the other hand (as
Dr. Latham has well observed, in commenting on the propriety of
bood-letting in cases of sudden seizure,*) attention must always be
paid to the *constitution* of the patient; and it must be borne in mind,
that a practice highly proper in persons of corpulent habit, firm
muscles, and florid complexion, would probably be detrimental in
emaciated subjects, with flaccid muscles, cold extremities, and a
small thready pulse.

The advantages of opening the temporal artery or jugular vein,
in preference to bleeding from the arm, have often been insisted
on, but apparently without sufficient reason. It is enough that the
evacuation be made in a full stream, and carried to such an extent
as to affect the system. Cupping from the nape of the neck is a

* Transactions of the London College of Physicians vol. vi, p. 248.

powerful means of relieving tension within the craneum, and as an auxilliary, may be resorted to in apoplectic cases with a fair pros- peet of advantage. In some constitutions, it may even supply the place of general blood-letting.

Every exertion is to be made to exhibit purgative medicines; but the clenching of the teeth and the paralytic state of the organs of deglutition often render this a matter of extreme difficulty. Croton oil, in the dose of two or three drops, is well deserving of a trial. Some calomel may be laid upon the tongue, and a strong infusion of senna with jalap given by teaspoonfuls, until a full effect has been procured. The operation of these medicines may be promoted by sharp purgative glysters.

Cold applications to the head have been found advantageous in some instances, and are certainly preferable to blisters. These are the only powerful means of *generally acknowledged* efficacy, which we possess in the treatment of apoplexy. The exhibition of *emet- ics* has, indeed, been extolled by some as highly useful, and even as superior to blood-letting; but the practice has never been gen- erally followed ; and there is no small difficulty in understanding how it could be carried into effect in those severe cases, to which it is considered as particularly applicable. In the instance of an apo- plectic seizure immediately succeeding a full meal, an emetic might perhaps be advisable ; but even under such circumstances, it would be improper to rely upon it to the exclusion of other remedies.

Apoplexy being so very fatal a disease, it is incumbent on the physician, in all cases where he has reason to suspect a predispo- sitiou to it, to employ steadily such *prophylactic* measures as are cal- culated to avert the danger. A cool spare diet, abstinence from all fermented or spirituous liquors, regular exercise, abridging the usu- al number of hours allotted to sleep, keeping an open body, and, in some instances, establishing a drain by means of an issue, or seton, are those on which his chief reliance ought to be placed. A blister to the shaved scalp will be found decidedly efficacious. Dr. Cheyne[*] speaks highly of the powers of antimonial powder in constitutions predisposed to this form of sanguine conjestion and effusion.

When giddiness, fulness of the face, hæmorrhagy from the nose, or throbbing of the arteries of the head are present, blood must be taken either from the arm, or from the nape of the neck by cup- ping, according to the degree in which the general system parti- cipates in the disturbance.

[*] Dublin Hospital Reports, vol. 1, page 315.

Relation of Palsy to Apoplexy. Distinctions among Paralytic Affections. Cerebral Palsies. Hemiplegia. Appearances on Dissection. Paraplegia. Partial Palsies depending on Disease of the Encephalon. Palsy independent of any Affection of the Brain. Palsy from Cold. From Lead. Treatment of Hemiplegia and of Paraplegia—of Amaurosis— and of saturnine Palsy. Of the shaking Palsy.

MEDICAL authors have almost uniformly agreed in uniting the consideration of apoplexy and palsy ; and there can be no question but that these diseases are, in many of their great pathological features, very closely associated. There are points, however, in which they as widely differ ; and it will conduce to a clearer understanding of what is known regarding the nature and varieties of palsy, if it is treated as a distinct affection. A vast number of very intricate questions are involved in the consideration of palsy. To all the difficulties connected with the pathology of apoplexy, are added many peculiar to itself. These it will be my endeavour to point out to the notice of the student ; but I shall not consider it incumbent upon me to examine into the merits of the different speculations to which they have given rise.

A superficial survey of the phænomena of palsy would lead to a distinction among the cases of this disease, into such as are connected with a morbid state of the encephalon, and such as, being *to all appearance* independent of any affection of the brain, originate, we may fairly presume, in some condition of the nervous filaments themselves, by which they are rendered incapable of receiving or transmitting impressions. The former, being infinitely the most common, will in the first instance require attention.

The most perfect form of cerebral palsy is *hemiplegia;* in which the affection extends over the whole of one side of the body, from the head to the foot. Sometimes it takes the form of *paraplegia*,

39

or palsy of the lower extremities ; and, in some rarer instances, the affection is confined to the loss of function in a particular nerve. Each of these varieties of cerebral palsy will require separate investigation.

1. Hemiplegia, to which form of the disease the term *palsy* is in common language appropriated, has generally been considered as a minor degree of apoplexy. The attack of it is sometimes unexpected, but more commonly it is preceded for several days, or even weeks, by one or more of those symptoms formerly described as the forerunners of apoplexy ; such as giddiness, drowsiness, numbness, dimness of sight, failure of the powers of mind, forgetfulness, transient delirium, or indistinctness of articulation. For the most part, the paralytic seizure is sudden ; but occasionally the approaches of the disease are made more slowly ;—a finger, a hand, or an arm, the muscles of the tongue, of the mouth, or of the eyelids' being first affected, and the paralytic state gradually extending to distant parts. It is a common observation, that hemiplegia is, in most instances, preceded by a genuine fit of apoplexy ; but this opinion will hardly be borne out by facts ; and it is, *a priori*, rendered improbable by a comparison of the frequency of palsy, with the rarity and acknowledged fatality of apoplexy. It is true, that the patient, on occasion of the paralytic *stroke*, is often observed to labour under more or less of temporary coma, but the apoplectic paroxysm is hardly ever complete. It will be found in practice, that palsy is much more commonly the *precursor*, than the *consequence* of apoplexy.

It is often been remarked, as a very singular circumstance, that in hemiplegia, as well as in other varieties of palsy, the power of sensation should remain perfect, while that of voluntary motion is wholly lost. This curious fact has perplexed physiologists in all ages, and various theories have been offered in explanation of it. Even in the present improved state of our knowledge, however, regarding the functions of the brain and nerves, these must be considered as hypothetical. Cases, indeed, have undoubtedly occurred, wherein sensation was impaired, as well as the power of voluntary motion ; nor are there wanting instances of the total loss of sensation ; or of the loss of sensation on one side, with that of motion on the other. These latter cases, however, under the most favourable supposition, are so rare as hardly to merit notice. So far from there being *commonly* a loss of feeling attendant on palsy, it is not unusual to observe sensation morbidly increased. A disa-

greeable feeling of creeping, for instance, is occasionally complained of ; rheumatic and nervous pains affect the limb ; and blisters
and phlegmons occasion the usual degree of inconvenience.

The temperature of the paralytic limb, as far as my own observation extends, is commonly preserved ; though to the patient's
feelings it may sometimes appear hotter, sometimes colder than
natural. On this subject also, a considerable diversity of opinion
has prevailed. Mr. Earle* has found reason to believe, that paralytic limbs are of a much lower temperature than natural ; that
they are incapable of supporting any fixed temperature ; that they
are peculiarly liable to partake of the heat of surrounding media ;
and cannot, without injury, sustain a degree of warmth, which to
a healthy limb would prove in no degree prejudicial.

I have commonly observed, that the pulse in the paralytic limb
is weaker than that of the sound one. The mouth in hemiplegia is
always distorted, and a peculiar expression of countenance is giv-
en by the torpor of one side of the face. The saliva, in many cases, dribbles away ; and the tongue, when protruded, is turned to
one side. The speech is indistinct, and considerable difficulty is
often experienced in swallowing liquids. Severe pains of the limbs
or of the head are occasionally noticed. After the disease has subsisted for a certain length of time, the muscles, apparently from
want of use, shrink and waste, and become flaccid. Sometimes a
degree of œdema supervenes, with a tendency to gangrene, especially on blistered surfaces.

In hemiplegia, the vital and natural functions are but little, if at
all impaired. The bowels indeed are sometimes torpid ; but there
is no reason to believe, that the loss of nervous power extends, in
common cases, to any of the internal organs. It is a curious circumstance too, that the senses are in general but little affected.
The phænomena of hemiplegia, in fact, as Dr. Yelloly has remarked,† are principally confined to such parts as derive their nerves
from the medulla oblongata and spinal marrow, and in this we may
trace an important distinction between palsy and apoplexy.

The mental faculties almost always suffer. Sooner or later the
intellect is weakened, the memory more or less impaired, and even
the passions are sensibly affected. A mind once vigorous, firm, or
placid, becomes, after a severe paralytic attack, weak, timid, ca-

* Medico-Chirurgical Transactions, vol. vii, page 179.
† Medical-Chirurgical Transactions, vol. vii, p. 214.

pricious, and fretful. To these general rules there may be found, however, I am well aware, many exceptions.

Instances are on record of *perfect* recovery from the attack of hemiplegia, but they are extremely rare. Sometimes, as I have already mentioned, the paralytic seizure is only the precursor to a complete fit of apoplexy, which commonly proves fatal in a few days. The more usual progress of the disease, however, is characterized by a slow but gradual and imperfect amendment, continuing for two or three months, until the patient, with some support, is able to walk about, dragging along the paralytic limb.

After remaining in this helpless condition for some years, and frequently suffering from attacks of pain of the head or giddiness, he either dies of an attack of apoplexy, or of some new disease. In a severer form of the affection, the patient never makes any advances at all towards recovery. For many weeks or months he is confined to his bed, and at length gradually falls into a state of lethargy, or coma, in which he dies.

The opinions already delivered, regarding the proximate cause and general pathology of apoplexy, apply also, in a great degree, to hemiplegia, as will be rendered evident by a notice of the appearances usually found on dissection of those who either actually die of palsy, or who during life had experienced one or more paralytic attacks.

In those cases of paralysis which pass quickly into apoplexy, the common apoplectic appearances are met with ; in most instances, extravasations of blood ; but occasionally serous effusion into the ventricles. In the more chronic forms of palsy, there is no appearance so common as discoloration, or some other diseased state of the corpora striata ; but various other organic læsions of the brain and its membranes have been also observed. Of this kind are—encysted suppuration, induration of a part of the brain, flaccidity and softness of a portion of its substance, effusions of serum in various parts and in various quantities, tumours, and lastly, clots of blood imbedded in the substance of the brain, or sometimes only cavities, in which it is presumed that such clots had formerly existed. The latter set of appearances have lately given rise to considerable discussion. It has been supposed that blood extravasated during the apoplectic or paralytic fit may in time become absorbed ; and that in proportion to the degree of this absorption, will be the more or less perfect recovery of the patient. These conclusions, however, appear to have been hastily drawn, for they are not borne out by more recent observation.

Much importance has always been attached to the singular cir-cumstance of the morbid appearances presented by the brain hav-ing their seat in the side opposite to that of the paralytic affection. The fact was noticed in the writings of Hippocrates, Galen, and Aretæus, and its correctness is sanctioned by many modern au-thorities more especially by the accurate observations of Morgag-ni and Dr. Baillie. Although exceptions to it have unquestionably been met with (notwithstanding the positive assertions to the con-trary of some late French pathologists,) it must be acknowledged as a phænomenon of very general occurrence ; and from the earliest times attempts have been made to account for it. The notion of a decussation of nervous fibres was originally entertained by Aretæ-us, and applied by him in explanation of the fact. The subject has since been often brought under discussion, but by no one in so ela-borate a manner as by Dr. Yelloly, in the first volume of the Me-dico-Chirurgical Transactions.* The principle of *decussation* seems to be generally admitted, but the difficulty consists in determining its seat ; some placing it in the corpus callosum, others in the tu-berculum annulare, the medulla oblongata, or the medulla spina-lis. Pathologists have supported their respective opinions by much ingenious argument ; but in the estimation of Dr. Yelloly, the pre-ponderance is considerably in favour of that which makes the tu-berculum annulare the seat of decussation.

It is not always that traces of morbid structure are discovera-ble in those who have suffered during life from hemiplegia ; but this circumstance does not militate against the notion of an iden-tity in the pathology of hemiplegia and apoplexy. Such an opin-ion, moreover, is corroborated by the identity of their predisposing and exciting causes ; and, upon the whole, were it required to state in a few words the relation of these diseases to each other, it might be urged, that there *are* points of distinction between them, yet too obscure to be defined with accuracy ; and that in common prac-tice, they may be safely viewed as modifications of each other.

2. Paraplegia, or palsy of the lower half of the body, though far less frequent than hemiplegia, ranks next in importance to it. The loss of nervous power is here entirely confined to the pelvis and lower extremities. This affection sometimes arises, as will

* Page 105, et. seq.

hereafter be mentioned, from local causes injuring the spinal marrow ; but it is as a disease depending upon some morbid state of the cerebral system, that I am now to consider it. Dr. Baillie is, I believe, the first who fully established the important pathological principle which I am now to illustrate, and to his paper I am indebted for the following outline of this variety of palsy.*

Cerebral paraplegia occurs chiefly in the middle or more advanced periods of life, and is more frequent in men than women. The approach of the disease is never sudden : at first there is only a sense of numbness, with a stiffness or awkwardness of motion in the lower limbs ; but by degrees the patient is unable to walk without support. As the disease advances, the urine passes off, at first in a feeble stream, at length involuntarily. The bowels are costive, but from loss of power over the sphincters, the motions frequently pass unrestrained by the will. Patients in this complaint may live for a long time ; but at the end of some years they usually die with their constitutions entirely exhausted. In a few instances recovery takes place.

The connection of these symptoms with disease of the brain has been in some cases proved by dissection ; and in others it has been rendered almost equally certain by the general symptoms of cerebral disease present at the same time. Dr. Baillie has seen paraplegia accompanied by giddiness, drowsiness, impaired vision, paralytic dropping of an eyelid, defect of the memory, loss of mental energy, and lastly, numbness and weakness of one or both of the upper extremities. These circumstances afford strong evidence that·the cause of the disease exists within the cavity of the skull, and that it consists in some mode of pressure upon the brain.

3. There are a variety of cases in which the loss of nervous power is confined to a particular organ, or muscle, or set of muscles ; and yet from the manner in which the affection begins, from the symptoms which attend it, and the course which it afterwards runs, it is obvious to the pathologist that the source of the mischief must be sought for in the great centre of the nervous system. Innumerable degrees of paralytic affection may be observed in practice, from the torpor and weakness of a single finger, up to complete apoplexy, in which sense and motion perish throughout the

* Vide Transactions of the College of Physicians of London, vol. vi, p. 16 ; and London Medical and Physical Journal for May 1827, vol, lvii, page 392.

whole body. To enumerate these different partial palsies would be unnecessary ; it is sufficient to say, that among the most fre-quent will be found amaurosis, or palsy of the optic nerve, palsy of the muscles of one side of the face, palsy affecting only the muscles of deglutition, or the neck of the bladder, and palsy of an arm, a hand or a finger. It is wholly beyond our power to compre-hend how it happens that a cause, operating upon the brain gen-erally, should produce effects so partial and at such a distance from the actual seat of disease.

The difficulties which we have to encounter in any inquiry into the pathology of paralysis, are greatly increased when the investi-gation is extended to those cases of general and partial palsy, which are, to all appearance, totally unconnected with any derange-ment of structure or function in the encephalon. That such cases do occur is unquestionable ; and it must be left to future inquirers to determine in what manner these apparent inconsistencies are to be reconciled.

In the year 1820, I had an opportunity of seeing an instance of general palsy of the kind now alluded to, the history of which is fully detailed in the London Medical Repository.* The disease ran a very singular course, terminating, after the lapse of above eight months, in the complete recovery of health. During the whole of this long period there did not occur one symptom which could warrant me in looking to the brain as the source of the disor-der. The vital and natural functions were also undisturbed, nor was there any evidence of disease within the theca vertebralis. It is obvious, therefore, that this affection was, in its pathology, totally distinct from the ordinary forms of paralysis. A case very similar in its leading symptoms, but different in its termination, is record-ed by Dr. Powell† in a paper containing many important patholo-gical views of palsy. He brings forward this case among others, in support of the opinion, that certain paralytic affections, both par-tial and general, originate in a peculiar condition of the *nerves alone ;* that they are independent of any morbid affection of the blood-vessels of the head ; and that they are produced in many in-stances by cold, and in some by sympathy with particular states of the stomach, or other distant local irritations. The nervous fibril-læ are here rendered incapable of transmitting impressions, either to or from the cranium.

* Vol xvi, p, 265, October 1821.
† College Transactions, vol. v, p. 105.

There was a reasonable presumption, that in the case just detail-ed *cold* was the exciting cause, and the opinion is strengthened by a consideration of the frequency with which cold operates as the cause of paralytic affections of a more partial kind. The muscles of the face, of the arm, and of the foot, have often been found par-alysed by exposure to cold, more especially when conjoined with moisture. Various instances of the kind might be quoted from the writings both of ancient and modern authors.* The union of palsy and rheumatism is a frequent occurrence in the lower ranks of life, and is therefore familiar to those who are in the habit of attending workhouses and parochial infirmaries.

There are many other causes of partial palsy, however, besides cold. Paraplegia depends, in a variety of cases, upon a diseased state of the spine, produced by mechanical injuries. The scrofu-lous incurvation of the spine, to which infants and children are lia-ble, is attended also in its progress by paraplegic symptoms. Par-tial palsy originates, in some instances, from long-continued exer-cise of particular muscles, or violence done to them. There is rea-son to believe, that occasionally it is connected with inflammation of the substance of the nerve, or of its covering. There is a fourth class of partial palsies, which apparently depend upon some irrita-tion in the bowels.

By far the most common, however, of all the causes of partial palsy, is the poison of lead, which appears to exert some peculiarly noxious power over the nerves of the fore-arm and hand. Innu-merable instances of the deleterious effects of lead, in the several shapes of colic, palsy, and epilepsy, are met with among plumbers, painters, and workers in lead-mines, manufacturers of white lead, and others whose occupation exposes them to the influence of this metal.† It is certainly a curious circumstance, that some constitu-tions should be so much more easily affected by the poison of lead than others. There are persons, who, in a very short time, suffer severely from it in their general health, while others receive no injury, though exposed to its influence during a long series of years. The remarkable effect of lead however now adverted to, and called in common language the *dropped hand*, is infinitely more common

* Consult Dr. Cooke's excellent work on " The History and Method of Cure of the various Species of Palsy," pp. 64 and 95.

† For a full account of the peculiarities of the paralysis saturnina, I must refer to Clutterbuck, " On the Poison of Lead."

among painters than in any other class of persons engaged in lead-works, and it is probable therefore that the constant exercise of the fore-arm in painting has some influence in producing this peculiar symptom.

Palsy is a complaint, which, from very early times, has been considered almost incurable ; nor have the labours of modern phy-sicians succeeded in removing this opprobrium from medical sci-ence. It is sufficient to mark the numbers of paralytic persons in our streets, to form an idea of the inutility of medical practice in this disease.

The close analogy existing between the pathology of apoplexy and that of palsy, has led to the employment of blood-letting, both general and topical, in every variety of palsy, but more especially in hemiplegia ; and very decided benefit has been occasionally de-rived from this practice. It is obviously best adapted for those cases which are attended with evidences of general plethora, or of strongly marked determination to the head. The evacuation of blood, by cupping from the nape of the neck, is *generally* to be pre-ferred to bleeding from the arm ; but it is quite impossible to lay down rules for the administration of this remedy, considering how much must always depend upon the particular constitution and hab-its of the patient.

All authors agree as to the benefit which may be reasonably ex-pected from cathartic medicines. Jalap, scammony, and the more stimulating purgatives, are to be preferred ; and their combination with calomel affords a powerful means of relieving tension and con-gestion within the head. Emetics have found many advocates upon the continent ; but the partial advantages derived from them do not appear to counterbalance the inconveniences which they necessa-rily occasion. Blisters to the nape of the neck have afforded con-siderable relief, but I think I have seen more benefit derived from them when applied to the shaved scalp.

These observations apply to the treatment of hemiplegia in its early state. The system of treatment must of course be different, when the disease has subsisted for any length of time, and when all traces of affection of the head have ceased. Medicines of a stimulating quality have then been administered, with the view of rousing the torpor of the nervous power. Externally, physicians have had recourse to frictions, blisters, issues and setons, sina-pisms, embrocations of various kinds, warm bathing, electricity, and galvanism. The waters of Bath and Buxton enjoy a conside-

40

rable reputation for efficacy in paralytic cases. Internally, tonic medicines of different kinds have been commonly directed, more especially aromatics, the sub-carbonate of ammonia, the heating gums, chalybeates, bitters, and plants containing an acrid essential oil, such as mustard and horseradish. The formulæ, Nos. 60, 62, and 77, may be tried ; but the prospect of advantage from them is not great.

Besides these, medicines of a narcotic quality have been at different times recommended in the cure of palsy ; more particularly the nux vomica, the arnica montana, and the rhus toxicodendron. That these drugs produce some very remarkable effects upon the nervous system, cannot be questioned. They will frequently occasion twitchings and convulsive motions, and a sense of tingling or pricking in the paralytic limbs ; but these effects are, in many cases, rather painful than useful to the patient. Some instances are recorded of apparent benefit from them ; but upon the whole, they cannot be trusted to, and there is always some danger of their proving injurious to the general health.

The treatment of cerebral paraplegia is to be conducted on the same general principles. Dr. Baillie states, that though no plan of treatment has proved very successful, yet that he has employed with advantage, cupping, blisters, a seton in the nape of the neck, purgative medicines (consisting of the compound extract of colocynth, jalap, and the neutral salts,) and an alterative course of mercurial preparations. The same author further states that in a few instances he has seen benefit from frictions to the lower limbs, continued for an hour twice a day, and in one case advantage was derived from electric sparks. He is disposed also to think favourably of tepid bathing, both in fresh and sea water.

In the management of the different varieties of *partial* palsy, the physician must be guided by the pathological views recently adverted to. Some do not appear to demand any remedial treatment, while others are as decidedly benefited by the judicious administration of medical and surgical aid. It would be unnecessary to go into any detail on this subject ; but in consideration of the frequent occurrence of amaurosis and of saturnine palsy, as objects of attention to the physician, I shall make a few remarks on the treatment particularly applicable in these cases.

AMAUROSIS, or palsy of the optic nerve, generally comes on gradually, being preceded by the appearance of motes or small bodies seen floating in the air, or of a mist or network like black lace spread before the eye. It has for its remote causes exposure to intense heat or light, employment of the eye in very delicate pur. suits, irregularity of the digestive organs, strong mental emotions, and irregular habits of life. In some cases it is connected with an inflammatory or congestive state of the vessels of the brain, and is found associated with other forms of nervous disease. An here. ditary predisposition to amaurosis has been noticed in several fa. milies.

Very ample evidence has been brought forward by Dr. Vetch* and others, of the benefit to be derived from general blood-letting in amaurosis. Carried to the extent of producing syncope, it has proved, in many cases, the surest means of combating that conges. tive state of the deep-seated vessels of the eye, upon which the paralytic affection of the nerve appears mainly to depend. The necessity of this evacuation, however, is not to be judged of by the usual symptoms of ophthalmic inflammation. Its effects are to be assisted by the application of leeches, by purgatives and blisters. Mr. Travers, in the treatmet of amaurosis, recommends in the first instance the employment of medicines calculated to regulate the functions of the digestive organs, and subsequently, such general tonics as the system can bear. Emetics have been much employ. ed by continental physicians.

The origin of SATURNINE PALSY has been already adverted to. Its cure is always tedious and often precarious. Mercury has been strongly recommended by Dr. Clutterbuck, who relates several ca. ses in which its good effects were evident. From my own ob. servations, however, I should be inclined to form a very different estimate of its efficacy ; and in its stead to recommend for gene. ral adoption the plan which I have known so successfully pursued in the hospital at Bath, viz. the application of blisters to the wrist ; a warm bath twice in the week ; warm pumping on the affected joint ; occasional aperients, and the use of the battledore splint, as advised by Dr. Pemberton. The drinking of the Bath waters may perhaps contribute to improve the general health ; but I am per. suaded that the only effectual system of treatment consists in the

* Practical Treatise on Disorders of the Eyes, by John Vetch, M. D. London, 1820.

steady and long-continued employments of *local* stimuli. On the Continent the warm sulphureous waters of Barege and Aix-la Chapelle are highly extolled.

A few lines may be devoted to the consideration of that nervous affection which has been called skaking palsy, the *paralysis agitans* of some nosologists. In this disease the muscles of one or both the superior extremities are in a state of continual tremor. By degrees the trembling extends to one or both legs, and the patient walks with increasing difficulty. The body is bent forward. Articulation is indistinct, mastication troublesome, and at length the saliva dribbles from the mouth. As the muscular weakness increases, the agitation of the body becomes more and more vehement, continuing even during sleep. Delirium, drowsiness, and other marks of exhaustion, precede the fatal event. The complaint often lasts for many years, without impairing in any degree the mental faculties. Such a condition of nervous disorder is peculiar to persons advanced in life. Nothing is known regarding its remote causes. It is conceived to depend on some morbid state of the medulla oblongata and upper portions of the spinal marrow, the exact nature of which has never been ascertained, but it may reasonably be ascribed to the mere alteration which time produces on the cerebral textures. Medicine appears to exert no influence whatever on this disease. Blisters to the nape of the neck with aperients, are indicated, but they have been tried and found as ineffectual as the class of tonics. Upon the occurrence of giddiness, however, or any unusual aggravation of the ordinary symptoms, cupping glasses may be applied to the neck with a fair prospect of advantage.*

* Vide Parkinson's " Essay on the Shaking Palsy." London, 1817.

CHAP. IV.

EPILEPSY.

Nosological Distinctions. Phænomena of the Epileptic Paroxysm. Varieties. Natural Progress of the Disease. Prognosis. Predisposition. Dependence of Epilepsy on derangement of the natural Functions. Stomach and Bowels. Uterus. On some primary morbid Condition of the Encephalon—functional—structural. Practice during the Paroxysm. Principles of Treatment during the interval. Agency of antispasmodic Medicines.

MANY circumstances conspire to give an interest to epilepsy : the great frequency of the disease, the class of persons among whom it chiefly prevails, the alarming character of its symptoms, the obscurity in which its pathology is involved, and the difficulties, which from the earliest times, have been experienced in the relief of it. No other disease has ever procured for itself so large a share of popular attention. In remote times it was universally attributed to the immediate agency of evil spirits, and viewed with a kind of reverential awe, which obtained for it the name of *morbus sacer.** Among the Romans the forum broke up when an epileptic was seized with a paroxysm of his disease.

Although the characters of epilepsy are thus sufficiently distinct to have attracted in all ages the notice of the world, considerable difficulty has been found in contriving a definition of it which may include every form of the complaint ; and not less, perhaps, in establishing the precise nosological distinction between it and the

---

* To the physician, nothing certainly can be more instructive than observing, that of the sick who were brought to our Saviour to be healed, the greater number were paralytics, and those who were possessed of " unclean spirits." While he learns from this how unchanged are the features of these diseases, he cannot, on the other hand, fail to appreciate, in all its force, the mighty miracle of their cure.

other varieties of convulsive disease. This may chiefly be traced to the want of a proper understanding of the true meaning of *disease*, in opposition to the *symptoms* by which it is characterized. Convulsion is a symptom, and not a disease ; though many nosologists have so termed it. Epilepsy, on the other hand, is strictly a disease, consisting of a succession of paroxysms of *convulsion*. To complete the definition, nosologists have added the clause, *with insensibility*, and by this they distinguish epilepsy from hysteria.

The *species* of epilepsy which have been described by authors are mere technical expositions of its various exciting causes. Like many other affections, it is both idiopathic and symptomatic ; but the phenomena of the epileptic paroxysm are, in both cases, the same. I shall first describe the usual appearances, and then notice the most important of those varieties which have been recorded.

The epileptic fit for the most part occurs suddenly. The patient falls to the ground ; and the disease has hence received the appropriate name of the *falling sickness*. When the complaint is fully established, it is usual for the patient to experience certain warnings of the approach of a fit, which though lasting only a few seconds, enable him to make some preparations for it. The most frequent of these warning symptoms are head-ache, giddiness, dimness of sight, or flashes of light passing before the eyes, ringing in the ears, and coldness of the extremities. Some persons are apprized of the approach of the fit by the appearance of particular spectres ; but the most common of all epileptic warnings is that singular sensation of tremor, or coldness, or numbness, which has been called the *aura epileptica*. It begins at the extremity of a limb and gradually ascends to the head, when the paroxysm of coma and convulsion ensues.

During the fit the convulsive agitations of the body are violent. The eyes are fixed and reverted and the pupils permanently contracted ; the teeth gnash against each other ; the tongue is thrust forward, and often severely bitten, and there is foaming at the mouth; the breathing is irregular and laborious, and the pulse for the most part small and contracted. Complete insensibility prevails. The fit varies in duration, from a few minutes to a quarter or even half an hour. In some cases it has lasted even longer. On its cessation the patient remains for some time motionless, insensible, and apparently in a profound sleep. From this he recovers by degrees, but without any recollection of the circumstances of the fit. It leaves him weak and exhausted, and for the rest of the

day he generally complains of a degree of stupor and sense of oppression in the head. In many cases this has amounted to actual
mania, continuing for two or three days.

The periods of recurrence of the fits are too various to admit of
being stated with any degree of accuracy. When the disease first
develops itself, the intervals are long, perhaps two or three months.
As it becomes more firmly rooted in the system, the fits recur with
a corresponding frequency, until at length the patient hardly passes a day without one. It is important, however, to bear in mind,
that genuine epilepsy never occurs oftener than this; and therefore, when a person has more than one fit in the day, we may reasonably conclude that the disease is of an *hysterical* nature.

Epileptic fits occur at all hours; but much more commonly during the night than in the day; sometimes on first going to sleep;
but more usually, as far as my own observations extend, on waking in the morning. It is reasonable to conclude that there is
some peculiarity in the state of the brain during sleep, which is
highly favourable to the development of the epileptic paroxysm.

The varieties in the phænomena of the epileptic fit are very interesting; and they have induced Dr. Prichard (from whose valuable work I have derived great assistance in the present and succeeding chapters) to found upon them a three-fold division of the
disease.* The first, or common form, is that which I have just
described; characterized by insensibility, and general convulsions,
or *struggling* of the whole body. The second is the *tetanoid* epilepsy distinguished by the loss of sense and consciousness, with
tonic spasm or *rigidity* of the muscles. There is the same *suddenness*
of the seizure in this as in former species; and though the attacks
are very different in their aspect they are manifestly allied in their
nature. The third form of epilepsy is marked by fits of insensibility, with perfect *relaxation* of the muscular system. Dr. Prichard
distinguishes this by the term *epileptic leipothymia*. It bears a close
resemblance to the apoplectic state; but its recurrence in paroxysms, and the whole tenour of the disease prove it to be connected
pathologically with epilepsy. To these may be added a fourth and
still more singular variety, to which authors have given the name
of *catalepsy*. The reality of such a state of disease has frequently
been called in question, but without sufficient reason. One instance

* Treatise on the Diseases of the Nervous System, by Dr. Prichard, London, 1822, vol. 1, p. 87.

of it has fallen under my own observation.   The affection consists
of paroxysms of reverie, in which the patient remains unconscious
of external impressions, and incapable of voluntary motion, though
retaining the position in which he was first seized.   The fit seldom
lasts more than a few minutes, and leaves no traces of itself in the
memory.   The disease has in several instances passed into common epilepsy.

It has been noticed by authors, that some degree of consciousness is occasionally preserved in the genuine epileptic paroxysm ;
but such an occurrence is very rare, and seldom permanent, proving only a prelude to the total abolition of sense.   In a few cases
the recovery from the fit has been as sudden as the seizure ; nor
are the succeeding head-ache and stupor observed invariably.

Such are the more common modifications of the epileptic paroxysm.   In whichever way the disease manifests itself, it goes on to
produce other and more serious injury to the constitution.   In the
first place, the mental faculties become gradually and permanently
more and more impaired ; the memory fails, and a state of mind
closely verging on idiotism is at length brought on.   In almost all
epileptics a vacant expression of countenance is observable, which
once seen cannot easily be forgotten.   Yet here, too, we may incidentally mark the endless variety in the phænomena of disease.
It has happened that a person, subject in youth to epilepsy, has
risen in maturer years to the highest honours of a state, and been
celebrated for political and literary talents.

Epilepsy, when once thoroughly rooted in the habit, will generally be found to bring on, sooner or later, some other form of encephalic disease—hydrocephalus, mania, apoplexy, or palsy.   The
complication of epilepsy with mania is at once the most frequent
and the most formidable.   Of one of these, in most instances, the
epileptic patient dies ; but it is not to be overlooked, that epilepsy
sometimes terminates, in the third place, fatally and suddenly,
without inducing any secondary affection.   This, though seldom
witnessed among adults, is not uncommon in the epilepsy of children ; and assuredly it cannot be a matter of surprise ; it can only
lead us to reflect, how wonderful must be the structure of that delicate system, which can resist, in ordinary cases, the repeated attacks of so dreadful a disease, and how little pathology can assist
us in unravelling such a mystery.

On the morbid appearances observed in those who die of epilepsy, I have nothing to state of any importance.   A turgid condition

of vessels, both in the membranes and substance of the brain, has been noticed in some cases, with or without effusion of serum. Tumours, exostoses, and abscesses, have been discovered in others : but in none has dissection thrown any light on the peculiarities which distinguish the convulsive from the other varieties of encephalic disease.

In offering a few remarks on the predisposition to epilepsy, I have first to notice, that it is obviously an *hereditary* disease in many instances. In others, the parents and relatives of the patient may not, it is true, suffer from actual epilepsy, but they will often be found affected by other maladies of the same class, such as palsy, connate idiotism, or mania. The intimate connection subsisting among the different forms of nervous disease will enable us still to trace, in these circumstances, the principle of hereditary predisposition.

Epilepsy undoubtedly prevails, for the most part, in what has been termed the *nervous* habit or temperament of body. Dr. Cullen designated this peculiar condition of the frame by the term *mobility of constitution*, and it entered deeply into all his speculations concerning epilepsy. It is that state wherein impressions, both on the mind and body, produce more than their usually corresponding effects,—in which hope elates, and fear depresses, and wine excites, more than could reasonably be anticipated. To this circumstance alone are we warranted in attributing the well-established fact, that epilepsy is mainly the disease of early life. It was a maxim of Hippocrates that epilepsy never *originates* after the twentieth year. There are exceptions to the rule, but the remark amply proves the extent and accuracy of his researches.

Epilepsy is generally considered as equally frequent in both sexes. My own observations would lead me to believe, that it is considerably more prevalent among females than males ; and the fact, if correct, may be attributed partly to the greater *mobility* of habit in the female sex, and partly to the peculiar character of the *exciting* causes of the disease. These constitute, in fact, the most interesting points in the pathology of epilepsy, and they well merit a detailed investigation. I may begin by noticing the connection of epilepsy with a deranged state of the natural functions, constituting the *epilepsia occasionalis* of Dr. Cullen ; and then proceed to show how it depends, in other cases, upon some primary morbid condition of the encephalon. This latter variety of the disease Dr. Cullen has designated by the title of *epilepsia cerebralis*.

1. The symptomatic or *occasional* epilepsy is of two kinds ;—
41

the enteric, or that which is connected with disturbance of function in some portion of the alimentary canal ; and the hysteric, or that which has its origin in disturbed functions of the uterus. Speaking generally, we may say, that the first is peculiar to children under the age of fourteen; and the second to women between the ages of fourteen and twenty.

The first source of that irritation in the alimentary tract which leads to epilepsy, is painful dentition. It is a fruitful cause of the encephalic diseases of children, and of none more commonly than of epileptic fits. The second is acidity in the stomach, its distention by wind, or the mere detention in it of crude and undigested aliment. In infants of high natural irritability of frame, these disordered conditions of the stomach frequently lead to paroxysms of convulsion ; and in many cases they recur, and otherwise exhibit all the characters of perfect epilepsy.

At a somewhat more advanced period of life, there is no kind of irritation which so commonly proves the source of epileptic fits, as the presence of *worms* in the intestinal canal ; but almost any disorder of the bowels will, in certain habits and states of body, bring on a tendency to convulsion. The phænomena of cholera morbus will at once suggest themselves as an illustration of this pathological principle. The prognosis, in all the forms of enteric epilepsy, is naturally more favourable than in any other variety of the disease ; because the source of irritation is both more obvious, and more under our control.

The hysteric epilepsy is an equally frequent and much less manageable kind of disorder. It prevails extensively among the most delicate of the sex, at the most interesting period of their lives ; often resisting the most active and judicious treatment, and degenerating into that permanent and almost incurable form of cerebral epilepsy which we are next to notice. Hysteric epilepsy commonly affects females about the commencement of the catamenial epoch, or shortly afterwards, when the flow is scanty and difficult. Occasionally it takes place at a later period of life, in accidental obstructions of the menses. It chiefly prevails among those of sanguine temperament, with full development and vigorous action of the circulating system, and a delicate irritable constitution. There is nothing peculiar in the character of the fits of hysteric epilepsy, except that their recurrence frequently corresponds with the regular catamenial periods.

2. Epilepsy, as I have already hinted, is in some instances de-

pendent upon a *primary* morbid condition of the encephalon, and totally *independent* of disturbed function of the abdominal viscera. Like the preceding variety, cerebral epilepsy is of two kinds ; the one connected with *functional,* the other with *structural* disease of the brain and nervous system.

The obscurity which attaches to the functions of the brain and nerves, makes it impossible to speak with any precision on that difficult point in the pathology of epilepsy at which we are now arrived ; but a variety of arguments might be adduced to show, that there exists primary functional disturbance of the brain, leading to the epileptic paroxysm. The hereditary predisposition to the disease ; the absence of åll appearances after death, excepting such as are common to other forms of chronic disease of the encephalon ; and the recurrence of the fits at irregular periods, and particularly at night are strong confirmations of this doctrine. To these we may add the peculiar character of many of the *exciting* causes of the fit, violent mental emotion, irritation, and the operation of certain poisons, both of the narcotic and morbid kind. Arsenic and the muriate of barytes have been strongly suspected of inducing epilepsy. In children a common effect of the poison of small-pox is an epileptic paroxysm.

It is impossible to overlook the fact, that in a very large proportion of the cases of cerebral or idiopathic epilepsy, and in many of those which are manifestly connected with disturbed function of the bowels and uterus, there is præternatural fulness in some part of the vascular system of the brain. This is an important feature in the pathology of epilepsy ; and if I have reserved all mention of it to this time, it is because I feared that its earlier notice might divert the mind of the student from those other views of the complaint, which though obscure, and therefore less inviting, are yet equally necessary to a thorough understanding of it.

The grounds on which we establish the connection of epilepsy with a state of congestion or over-distension of the cerebral bloodvessels, may be thus briefly enumerated. Epilepsy occurs in persons of full habit of body, and indolent mode of life ; the fit is frequently preceded by head-ache, flushings of the face, and throbbing of the carotid and temporal arteries; it is brought on, in many cases, by great muscular exertion, as in parturition, by stooping, intoxication, heated rooms, and above all by violent fits of coughing, such as occur in severe hooping cough. The hysteric form of the disease is only one of those many consequences of obstructed

menstruation of which the prevailing character is irregular determination of blood. The appearances on dissection, when observed,
are those of sanguine accumulation in the brain; and lastly, we
may bring forward the well-attested good effects which have fol- ·
lowed that depleting system of treatment which I am about to recommend.

While I thus express myself on the subject of epilepsy, as connected with turgescence of vessels, I am not insensible to the fact,
that paroxysms of *convulsion* are occasionally connected with a
state of cerebral circulation, directly the reverse ; as when we see
them following large bleedings at the arm, double amputations, or
excessive purging. Dr. Cullen, indeed, appears to have overstrained his favourite theory of epilepsy from *collapse*, but it must not be
on that account excluded from our reasonings.

The last point which requires consideration previous to entering
on the subject of treatment, is the connection of epilepsy with
chronic disorganizations of some one of the structures within the
cranium.   Those which authors have most usually noticed as producing epilepsy, are spicula of bone detached by some injury from
the internal table of the skull ; ossifications of the falx ; tumours of
various kinds, attached either to the bones, membranes, or parenchymatous substance of the brain ; and lastly, foreign bodies lodged
there. Numerous cases are to be found on record, of epilepsy from
these and similar causes ; but instead of pressing them on the notice
of the student, I would rather wish him to understand how rare they
are in comparison of those which are simply the result of *morbid action*, in many of which we may reasonably hope, by judicious measures and steady perseverance, to produce an alleviation, and even,
in a few, the permanent cure of the disease.

After what I observed in the outset of this chapter, it is unnecessary to state formally the difficulties which the physician has always
to encounter in the management of this obstinate disorder. In many
cases they are such as no skill can overcome. In others, however,
a regular system of treatment, founded on those pathological views
which I have attempted to explain, is productive of decided benefit
whilst a few, which to the pathologist would have appeared hopeless, have yielded to a practice wholly *empirical*.   These considerations should encourage us in our attempts to cure the disease ;
and the following may be viewed as the most important of the
principles on which a rational treatment of epilepsy is to be conducted.

During the fit no remedial measures of any importance are either practicable or necessary. Our efforts are to be reserved for the intervals of the fits, and our aim should be to prevent their recurrence. In effecting this, the following are to be the chief objects of attention :—

1. To remove all sources of irritation.

2. To moderate the afflux of blood upon the brain.

3. To alter that morbid condition of the nervous system, on which convulsion depends ; and to strengthen the body.

To one or other of these principles may be traced the good effects of all the medicines and plans of treatment which have at different times proved efficacious in the cure of epilepsy. They are far from being incompatible with each other. On the contrary, it is often necessary to combine them all in the management of an individual case.

1. Having already described the different kinds of irritation in the body which occasion an epileptic fit, I have only now to state, that in the epilepsies of infants and children, much may be done by free scarification of the gums ; by the administration of an emetic ; by occasional smart doses of purgative medicines ; by the more liberal use of mild aperients and absorbents ; and by strict attention to diet and regimen. Where the concomitant symptoms afford evidence of the presence of worms, anthelmintics are of course to be exhibited, more especially the oil of trupentine in the full dose of six drachms. This medicine exerts, in moderate doses, a power of allaying that irritable state of the nervous system, with which the convulsive paroxysm is so intimately connected. Dr. Prichard adds, that it contributes to produce regular and moderate evacuations. For this purpose it is best administered according to the formula No. 64.

When the irritation is seated in the uterine system, as manifested by the concurrent symptoms (scanty and laborious menstruation, and the peculiar periods at which the fits recur,) our measures must in part be directed to restore the natural determination to the uterus. Recourse may be had to the warm bath, or semicupium, stimulating enemata, relaxing medicines, as the antimonial diaphoretics, and the different kinds of *emmenagogues*. Regular exercise, occasional purgatives, and in some instances an issue or seton in the arm or neck, have also afforded very efficient aid.

2. The second principle in the treatment of epilepsy is the obviating general plethora, and the taking off that peculiar determination

of blood to the vessels of the head, which is one of the most important features in the pathology of the disease.   Such a principle is
equally applicable to the sympathetic as to the primary, or cerebral
varieties of epilepsy.   Where the disease is still recent ; where it
occurs to adults and young persons of robust habit ; and more especially where, in the intervals of the fits, the patient complains of
head ache, giddiness, stupor, or any other mark of permanent fulness in the blood-vessels of the brain, bleeding from the arm is not
to be omitted.   It may even be necessary to repeat it, before the
tendency to accumulation of blood about the head can be thoroughly subdued.

Keeping the same important object in view, the practitioner will
aid the effects of blood-letting by directing a mild and unirritating
diet, early hours of rising and going to bed, regular exercise, abstinence from all fermented liquors, and cold washing of the head
and neck.   Under particular circumstances, he will substitute cupping between the shoulders, blisters to the nape of the neck, and
the steady use of purgative medicines.   For children he will direct
leeches to the temples.   It is hardly necessary to add, that rules can
never be framed for guiding the mere detail of treatment.   This
more particularly applies to a disease which often lasts for years,
and occurs under an infinite variety of aspects.   The judgment of
the practitioner is here alone to be trusted to.

3. Lastly, the physician will attempt to alter that peculiar condition of the brain and nervous system with which the state of convulsion is associated.   Experience has shown, that medicines of
the *narcotic* kind possess a considerable power over it.   Many of
them have accordingly been employed in epilepsy, and with advantage ; more particularly camphor, opium, hyoscyamus, and stramo-
nium.   Further ; there are the strongest grounds for believing, that
the morbid irritability of the brain and nerves, on which spasm
depends, is often connected with general constitutional *weakness*.
Hence it is, that many of the most powerful of the *antispasmodic*
medicines are in fact *tonic*.   Of these I may specify, as having obtained considerable reputation in the treatment of epilepsy, bark,
steel, and valerian.   In the epilepsy of children, after appropriated
purgatives, chalybeates, such as the carbonate of iron, or steel
wine, are decidedly efficacious.

But it must be confessed, that we are too often unable to form any
idea of the precise nature of that morbid state of the nervous system present in convulsive diseases. This feature in the pathology

of epilepsy is important with a view to practice. It shows that some of the medicines which have acquired a character for the cure of the disease, may have deserved it, although the mode of their operation be as little known to us, as the state of brain on which the epileptic paroxysm depends. It is impossible, for instance, to overlook the numerous cases which are on record of the *permanent* cure of epilepsy by the argentum nitratum; and though we were to allow that a large proportion of these are inaccurately reported, still we must acknowledge the *alleviation* afforded by the remedy. Great caution is necessary in the internal administration of the argentum nitratum, from its tendency to blacken the skin, a deformity which does not readily subside. Arsenic, and the oxyd of zinc, have, in the hands of other practitioners, been found not less successful; and upon the whole, we are compelled to believe, that these and similar drugs (properly denominated *nervine*) may really be entitled to that credit which a too scrupulous pathology has often denied them.

CHAP. V.

Controversy regarding the Nature of Maniacal Aberration. Manner in which Mania originates. Progress of the Disease. Varieties in the Maniacal Character. Prognosis. Morbid Appearances. Predisposition to Mania. Exciting Causes, physical and mental. Pathology of Mania. Management of the Insane, moral and medical.

IT is impossible for me to enter on the discussion of this subject without some expression of the reluctance with which I engage in it. Conscious, as I am, that it ill becomes a physician to cherish in the exercise of his duties the refined and delicate feelings of his moral nature, it would yet be affectation in him to overlook the very peculiar character of this branch of his profession,—to reason concerning mental, with the same indifference as on bodily derangements : or, in investigating the nature of mania, to forget the melancholy spectacle of the maniac. But there are other considerations which make me hesitate in entering upon the present inquiry,—the extreme obscurity of the subject, arising from our ignorance of the mode in which the operations of mind and body are connected ;—the remarkable differences observable in the opinions of medical authors concerning mania ;—and the limited extent of my own experience in the disease. On the other hand, it is no small consolation to reflect, that the pathology of mania has little in it which bears upon treatment; and if the student should rise from the perusal of this chapter imperfectly informed of the theory of the disease, he will yet not be the less qualified to appreciate its practical suggestions.

A great deal of metaphysical learning has been displayed in determining the precise nature of maniacal aberration,—in other words, in developing the *theory of diseased ideas*. The object has been to frame from this, some *definition* of mania which may apply to all cases of the disease, and afford to the medical practitioner a certain criterion, by which to determine when a man is actually

deranged, and to distinguish between insanity, and mere singulari-
ty of manner, or waywardness of temper.

The difficulty of effecting this is greater than might at first sight
be apprehended. One class of nosologists define mania to consist
in some error of the judging or reasoning faculty. Mr. Locke
characterizes madness as a disordered state of the association of
ideas. Dr. Cullen, who supports this theory, once said that false
judgments of the relations of things constitute mania. This view
of the subject, however, is in opposition to a principle generally admitted, that madmen reason correctly from erroneous premises;
and moreover it draws no sufficient line of distinction between the
insane, and those who are merely foolish, or capricious.

Dissatisfied with this definition, Dr. Cullen subsequently stated
it as his opinion, that the diseased judgments of the insane were
such as produced *disproportionate emotions*. It is questionable how
far this addition has increased our just notions of the disease. The
emotions of a lunatic are, indeed often vehement and forcibly expressed; but they are probably in due proportion to the impressions from which they take their rise.

Another class of pathologists, therefore, in attempting to establish the nature of madness, exclude all reference to the state of the
reasoning faculty, as well as all notion of a primary derangement
of the emotions or passions, and consider mania as consisting in
diseased perceptions; the mistaking one man for another, a chair
for a throne, a walking-stick for a sceptre. That such false perceptions do occur among maniacs there can be no dispute; but it
may reasonably be doubted whether they are the *essential* circumstances of madness. Many insane persons have the power of perception in a very complete degree; and false or *mistaken* perceptions are among the ordinary occurrences of common life.

Dr. Prichard and others take a somewhat different view of the
subject,—maintaining that the habit which characterizes the lunatic, is that of confounding the results of imagination and memory;
and mistaking the ideas of reverie for the impressions of attentive
and active reflection. This is doubtless a correct and scientific
explanation of a very large proportion of maniacal aberrations;
but whether it includes them all, is a point on which pathologists
continue to differ,

From the diversity of views which have thus been taken of the
precise condition of the mind which constitutes insanity, we may,
I imagine, deduce some very important conclusions: 1st, That all

42

the faculties of the mind are capable of being affected in the maniacal state, though not always equally, or at one and the same
time. 2dly, That it is hardly possible to express in words the nice
distinctions that mark the boundaries of reason and insanity, or to
specify the delicate gradations by which weakness of intellect, depression of spirits, violence of temper and eccentricity of manner,
degenerate into actual disease. 3dly, That in determining the
question of insanity or lunacy, the common sense of mankind must
ultimately be relied on ; and that its decision can receive little or
no assistance from metaphysical speculations.

Passing from these abstruse points, I proceed to give a brief
sketch of the origin and progress of the disease. The manner in
which it makes its approach is considerably diversified. In some
instances the attack is sudden and violent, and perfectly unexpected ; but in others, and probably in a much larger proportion of cases, the advances of the complaint are *gradual*. A certain oddity
of manner has been manifest in the individual, perhaps for years ;
he has exhibited very high or unusually low spirits, been fretful and
irascible on slight occasions, distrustful of his friends, easily intox-
icated, and strongly affected by every emotion or passion of the
mind. The increase of these has prepared the friends of the patient for the complete development of maniacal symptoms.

In the onset of the disease there is generally considerable disorder of the whole system ; much febrile excitement, loss of appetite, a costive state of the bowels, excessive restlessness. There
are present also, very decided evidences of unusual determination
of blood to the head :—flushing of the face, redness of the conjunctiva, contracted pupils, and head-ache. The ideas of the patient are often more incoherent at the commencement of madness
than at a more advanced period. As the general excitement of the
body lessens, they acquire a greater degree of consistency, occurring in trains more evidently connected, though still retaining the
true maniacal character. The patient will now answer questions,
but his replies are vague and unmeaning. Sometimes his delusions
extend to a great variety of subjects. At other times the maniacal
aberration is confined to a single topic, constituting what writers
have called *monomania*.

In this state the maniac remains for a considerable time, the
disease very seldom yielding speedily, or proving immediately fatal. He relapses, perhaps, occasionally into his prior state of complete incoherence, or exhibits the cheering prospect of a *lucid in-*

terval. By degrees his ideas become more settled, until either the morbid impressions altogether disappear, or they remain so indelibly fixed, that he sinks into the condition of a confirmed and incurable lunatic. In its further progress the disease becomes frequently complicated with epilepsy or palsy. After the lapse of some years, the patient dies, and for the most part in a comatose state. When the excitement is violent, and the paroxysms of great length, the patient is sometimes carried off early in the disease, unexpectedly.*

There is a proportion of the insane who can only be restored to a *certain degree* of sanity. While kept quiet and unexposed to any source of irritation, they enjoy a considerable share of rationality and tranquillity. Retaining, however, a morbid susceptibility of all the causes which produce the disease, they are incapable of again mixing with the world without the risk of the total abolition of reason.

From the earliest periods attention was directed, both by the profession and by mankind generally, to the varieties in the maniacal character ; and much importance has always been attached to them. Maniacal aberration exhibits itself under the three great forms of the furious, the gloomy, and the idiotic ; which latter may be either adventitious or congenite. These distinctions correspond with the mania, melancholia, amentia, and fatuitas of nosologists. Although a *popular* subdivision of the complaint, it is certainly superior to that which the old pathological writers chiefly dwelt upon. By them the *extent* of maniacal aberration was assumed as the distinctive character of the species ; and the term *melancholia* was made to bear a reference, not to the concomitant dejection and despondency, but to the *limitation* of the diseased condition of mind to a few objects or trains of ideas, such as religion or love. This, however, appears to be a matter of trifling importance, whether in relation to pathology, prognosis, or practice, and is now in a great measure disregarded. The nymphomania and satyriasis of nosologists are modifications of insanity, constituting the *erotic* monomania of some modern authors.

A detail of the most striking peculiarities in each of these principal forms of insanity would afford ample scope for the display of eloquence, and might prove interesting to the man of feeling, and

* For a fuller detail of the history of Mania, the reader is referred to Dr. Prichard's excellent work on the " Diseases of the nervous System," p. 113.

perhaps useful to the cultivator of intellectual philosophy. To the student of physic, however, it would be of little value, and this consideration deters me from attempting even a faint sketch of it. To him the most interesting subject which the investigation of mania presents is that of *prognosis*, which within the last few years has been prosecuted with uncommon zeal, and has led to results which neither the physician nor the philanthropist can contemplate without much gratification.

It has been satisfactorily proved, in the first place, that mania does admit of cure ; and, provided the disease be brought under treatment at an early period, in a very large proportion of cases. It has been shown, secondly, that a mild and human system of management is that under which the greatest number of cures has been effected ; and that the ultimate good of the lunatic can never be brought forward to cloak the carelessness or ill temper of the attendants. But it is sufficient to examine the reports of any of the great receptacles for lunatics in this country, to be sensible that mania, though curable, is not so in the same degree with many other chronic diseases.

In estimating the probability of *permanent* recovery, many minute circumstances must be taken into consideration ; but we are never to lose sight of the strong tendency which this disease shows to *relapse*, and to rivet itself in the constitution by frequent recurrence. The particular prognosis, or those minute shades of distinction which give us more or less hopes in individual cases, may be comprised under the following heads.—Insane persons recover in proportion to their youth. The chance of recovery diminishes with the length of time that the disorder has continued. Patients who are in a furious state, recover in a larger proportion than those who are depressed or fatuous. Mania connected with palsy or epilepsy is quite hopeless. Mania from physical causes is more likely to be permanently cured than when it arises from mental or moral causes. Puerperal mania is that species of the disease from which *perfect* recovery has taken place in the largest proportion of cases. Insanity is more or less susceptible of cure according as it arises from causes purely *accidental*, or is connected with a greater or less strength of family predisposition.

Much discussion has arisen respecting the morbid appearances observable in those who die maniacal. It has been contended by some, that the brain exhibits certain distinctive characters in all, or almost all cases of mania ; and a peculiar *hardness* of the substance of the brain has usually been regarded as the *common* phæ-nomenon. By others, this is not only denied, but it is actually maintained, on the authority of numerous and accurate dissections, that no alteration whatever from the healthy structure is discerni-ble in the heads of the insane. The truth will be found to lie be-tween these extremes. Morbid appearances are indeed observed, but they are in no wise different from such as present themselves in many other forms of encephalic disease, or even in common fe-vers,—serous effusion, for instance, thickening of the membranes, turgescence of vessels. The notion of the maniacal state being intimately connected with preternatural hardness of the brain, is now abandoned.

In entering on the consideration of the *causes* of mania, my at-tention must first be directed to the important influence of heredi-tary predisposition. It is the most strongly marked and melancho-ly proof which we have of the reality of such a predisposing cause of disease. Struck by its extent and force, some pathologists have even questioned the possibility of mania existing without it, and have alleged, that no combination of circumstances, however pow-erful, can, *per se*, bring on the maniacal state. The phænomena of febrile delirium, however, are strongly in favour of the pre-sumption, that mania is sometimes *acquired*. The instances which appear most unequivocally to prove such a principle in pathology occur in the case of puerperal insanity; and doubtless to this cir-cumstance is mainly to be attributed the greater proportion of re-coveries which distinguish this class of maniacal patients. The predisposition is of course the stronger, as it occurs on the side of one, or of both parents.

The only other circumstance which can be considered to give a predisposition to insanity, is the advanced period of life. As a dis-ease of youth, mania is hardly known. Seldom is it observed be-fore the twentieth year, and it increases in frequency until the fif-tieth year of life. The greater number of maniacal patients have their first attack between the ages of thirty and forty. The fe-male sex has been considered by some as more especially prone to mania, but the disproportion is not very great, and if puerperal insanity is kept out of view, hardly discernible.

The circumstances that more immediately induce the maniacal paroxysm are often obscure, the most accurate inquiries exposing nothing that could have contributed to the event; but at other times it is observed to follow certain physical conditions of the

body, and affections of the mind, which it may be useful to investigate.

Injuries of the head have sometimes brought on mania. A constant habit of intoxication is that which chiefly operates as the
cause of insanity among the lower classes in this country. Such
a result cannot surprise us when we reflect what intoxication is,
how nearly it resembles mania, and how seriously the frequent indulgence of it must injure the vessels of the brain.

I have already alluded·to the numerous instances which occur
of insanity succeeding parturition. Women of *sanguine temperament* are chiefly observed to suffer in this manner, but it is not *peculiar* to such habits; and, altogether, there is considerable difficulty in accounting satisfactorily for puerperal insanity. Maniacal
affections are connected also in other modes with the uterine functions. Irregularity of menstruation, which in many young women
induces symptoms of hysteria, becomes in others the prelude to a
maniacal attack.

Authors are in the habit of illustrating this portion of the pathology of mania by reference to the cases which are recorded of its
origin from *metastasis*, as from repelled eruptions, or the healing
up of old ulcers. I am inclined to think, however, that more importance has been attached to this, than a strict investigation of
the subject warrants. I pass on, therefore, to notice the emotions
of mind, the uncontrolled indulgence of which has brought on insanity; and among these the most common are superstitious dread,
religious fanatacism, intense grief, especially when arising from
domestic calamity, closely allied to which is the despondency of a
hopeless passion. Poets are fond of representing these as the
sources of mental derangement, and there is much less of fiction
here than in other exercises of their genius. Lastly, mania has
often been traced (particularly in commercial countries) to the
constant anxiety of mind connected with an extensive trade and
hazardous speculations. With a view to practice, it is very important to bear in mind, that in maniacal cases most obviously arising
from these and similar violent emotions and passions, there will often be found considerable disorder of the natural functions. Wheth-
ther this is to be regarded in the light of cause or effect may be a
matter of dispute; but it is generally acknowledged that such cases admit of relief by remedies acting through the medium of the
stomach.

Of the actual state of the brain in mania we have no certain knowledge. It is reasonable to presume that in some cases there is *congestion*, or perhaps a peculiar kind or modification of *inflammation*, going on there. Many of the occasional causes of the disease, some of its preceding and concomitant symptoms, its connection with other diseases, the mode by which it proves fatal, and occasionally the appearances found on dissection, correspond perfectly with that notion. We are led to the same opinion by considering the recorded good effects in mania of such measures as are commonly resorted to in encephalic inflammation, compared with the inefficacy of all others.

There are a variety of facts, however, connected with the history of mania, quite inexplicable on such a principle : as, for instance an hereditary predisposition to the disease, and its recurrence at irregular periods from slight and inadequate causes. From these it is to be inferred, that mania is often produced by a morbid condition of the brain, unappreciable by the anatomist, and altogether different from those visible, tangible organic affections, which are the consequences of disturbed circulation within the cranium. Judging from the well-known fact, that mania seldom appears in early life, often not until a good old age ; that it becomes more obstinate as the patient grows older ; and that a modification of mental derangement (imbecility) often comes on in extreme old age, we must infer that the changes which the structure of the brain undergoes in the progress of life tend to increase that peculiar condition of it with which maniacal abberration is connected.*

The treatment of mania is usually discussed under the two heads of moral and medical, and both have been much improved of late years ; the former being more thoroughly investigated, and raised in importance ; the other simplified and regulated by more accurate principles. I begin with the consideration of the *moral management* of the insane ; it being now unreservedly admitted, that on it depends mainly the successful issue of the case. Under this head are included, in public institutions, the classification of patients ; in all situations, the conduct and tone of the medical practitioner and of the attendants towards the patient ; the employment of restraint and coercive measures ; the question of estrangement from friends, and of solitary confinement ; the establishment of a system of regularity in all the actions of the lunatic ; the occupa-

* See Appendix ; Note V.

tion of his mind, religious instruction, amusements ; manual employments, exercise ; the regulation of diet and regimen ; and the
change of scene and association.

A few cursory observations on the principal topics here suggested will be sufficient to point out the spirit and scope of that system
of moral management which is now generally adopted in this country. Firmness on the part of the attendants sufficient to ensure obe-
dience, is found not incompatible with those conciliatory manners
which so commonly win the good will of the patient, and rouse him
from the sullen humours in which he is prone to indulge. The employment of severe bodily restraint is hardly ever resorted to in the
best regulated modern mad-houses. It creates a degree of irritation of mind which impedes advancement, and is at variance with
that soothing and encouraging tone and manner so necessary to
ultimate success. In many cases nothing contributes so essentially to the cure as withdrawing the mind as much as possible from
former scenes and settled associations ; and to effect this, the total
exclusion of friends, and a complete change of scene and habits,
are often found to be measures of indispensable necessity. Amusements of various kinds, that engage attention and promote exercise
in the open air, without rousing the passions or producing fatigue,
should in every way be encouraged. The diet should be simple,
and at the same time nourishing, such as may support the system,
without *healing* it. Regular hours of meals, exercise, and sleep,
should be strictly enforced.

The medical treatment of insanity was at one time conducted in
the most indiscriminate manner, having no reference to the peculiar habits of the patient, the immediate exciting causes of the disease, or the character of the concomitant symptoms. Such an opprobrium is no longer chargeable against those who have the professional care of lunatics. It is now well understood, that though
medicines are of comparatively little service in the relief of mania,
yet when necessary, their administration is to be suited to the complexion of each case, and regulated by the ordinary principles of
pathology. The following suggestions may assist the student in
determining the plan of medical treatment best adapted to the particular state and stage of mania, in which his assistance may be
required.

1. The medical treatment of insanity can alone be entered upon,
with a reasonable prospect of advantage, at an early period of the
disease.

2. It cannot legitimately be employed with any other object than that of relieving the constitutional disturbances with which maniacal aberration is occasionally complicated. When these have ceased, our hopes of success must rest in time, the efforts of nature, and moral management.

3. When insanity first developes itself in a young and plethoric person, it is not uncommonly accompanied with the ordinary marks of phrenitic inflammation ; and here blood letting is often resorted to with very beneficial effects. I am well aware, that among those whose attention is exclusively directed to maniacal disorders, a general belief prevails, that excessive blood-letting rivets the disease, and that the great object of the practitioner should be to support the patient's strength. Acknowledging the correctness of this principle, there are still considerations of great weight to which at times it must necessarily yield. The nature of the exciting cause, for instance, cannot be overlooked in determining the plan of treatment. Where mania is traceable to excessive intoxication, blood-letting, even to a considerable extent, is often required, and for the most part is borne well. The temperament and general habits of the patient are equally to be consulted. Whatever may be thought of general blood-letting, the benefits of *local* blood-letting (whether leeches or cupping) are now fully appreciated in all our best establishments for the insane.

4. One of the earliest means of relief in mania which history has recorded, is the free administration of purgative medicines. There are few who can be ignorant of the presumed virtues of hellebore in this disease ; and though the medicine has sunk in common estimation, the principle upon which it was resorted to is still acknowledged as correct. A disordered state of the alimentary canal is a frequent concomitant of maniacal aberration. So strongly is this marked in certain cases, that pathologists have described a peculiar variety of the disease under the title of *enteric mania*. It is characterized by obstinate constipation, the evacuations when procured exhibiting a most unhealthy aspect, a viscid secretion into the mouth, a failing or depraved appetite, coldness of the skin, scanty and high-coloured urine, and a rapid irritable pulse, with restless nights. In this state of disease the use of purgative medicines is to be long and patiently continued.*

* Consult Dr. Edward Percival's " Report on the Morbid Conditions of the abdominal Viscera in some Varieties of Maniacal Disease, with the Methods of Treatment."—Dublin Hospital Reports, vol. i.

5. The high degree of nervous irritation present in mania has induced physicians, in all ages, to expect relief from narcotic medicines, and most of them have been fully and fairly tried. Those
which have obtained the highest repute are opium, hyoscyamus,
and camphor ; but upon the whole, little reliance can be placed
upon them.

6. It would be improper to pass over without notice the warm
bath, which in the hands of some modern practitioners has been
productive of very marked good effects, and which the concurrent
testimony of several intelligent men has stamped as a remedy of
general and undoubted efficacy in the treatment of insanity.* It
has been found particularly serviceable in cases of uterine or puerperal mania.

The cold bath, or bath of surprise, is mentioned in terms of at
least equal commendation by others ; but its administration requires
to be regulated with a degree of nicety which few can pretend to,
who have not enjoyed extensive opportunities of observation.

Recent enquiries† have satisfactorily shown, that mania, so far
from being as was once apprehended, an increasing malady in this
country, is in reality less frequent than formerly ; and it is not unreasonable to suppose, that this may have in some measure been
the result of those improvements in the medical treatment and moral discipline of the insane, which it is for the honour of the present age to have introduced.

* See " Evidence taken before a Committee of the House of Commons
on Mad-houses," 1815.

† See Burrows's Inquiry relative to Insanity," London, 1820, page 106.

CHAP. VI.

CHOREA.

Literary Notices concerning Chorea. Symptoms and Progress of the Disease. Prognosis. Predisposition. Pathology. Method of Cure. Comparative Efficacy of the purgative and tonic Systems of Treatment. Influence of Arsenic.

CHOREA, commonly known by the name of St. Vitus's dance, received but little notice from the early systematic and practical writers in medicine. This neglect, however, it shared with many other diseases of early life, croup, hooping cough, hydrocephalus, marasmus. It is highly creditable to the pathologists of recent times, that they have extended an equal share of their attention to every form of human suffering, and laboured assiduously in that field which their predecessors had unjustly deserted. From such censure the illustrious Sydenham is, for the honour of this country, exempt. His description of chorea is accurate and spirited, and has served as a model for every succeeding author. No improvement upon it appears to have been made for a long series of years, nor did it again become an object of specific investigation until 1805, when Dr. Hamilton of Edinburgh turned his attention to the complaint, in the course of his enquiries into the utility and administration of purgative medicines. The account of chorea to be found in the useful work of that author* is by far the most precise and complete which has appeared, and leaves me no other task than that of brief analysis.

Chorea usually makes its first attack between the eighth and the fourteenth year of life. Dr. Hamilton mentions having seen the complaint originate between the ages of sixteen and eighteen ; and

---

* Observations on the Utility and Administration of purgative Medicines in several Diseases. By James Hamilton, M. D. Sixth Edition. Edinburgh, 1818. Chap. x, page 134. Chorea.

I once saw it, in a very perfect form, in a young woman nineteen years of age. Its approaches are commonly slow. An awkward dragging of the leg, twitches of the muscles of the face, and un-steadiness of the fingers, precede the more general convulsive mo-tions which characterize the confirmed state of the disease.

The contortions and gesticulations of the patient render him a singular but painful object of observation. All the muscles of vol-untary motion are at different times and in different instances af-fected. Those of the face, neck, and extremities, more particu-larly suffer. The hands and arms are in constant motion. He can grasp no object, even with the strongest exertions of his will; he walks unsteadily; but with all this, there is no symptom of pain or uneasiness. The expression of countenance, though grotesque, is, in the early stage of the disease, that of good humour and content-ment.

The convulsive agitations vary in violence, and are subject to occasional exacerbations. During sleep (unless in very bad ca-ses) they cease altogether. As the complaint advances, articula-tion becomes impeded, and is very often completely suspended. Deglutition also is occasionally performed with difficulty. The eye loses its lustre and intelligence. The face is thin and pale, and ex-pressive of a languor and vacancy, which in severe and protracted cases approaches nearly to fatuity. The mind, indeed, partakes in some instances of the bodily disorder, and the mental faculties retrograde to those of infancy.

With these evidences of disturbance of the cerebral functions, are usually united very unequivocal marks of a deranged condition of the stomach and bowels. A variable and often ravenous appe-tite, a swelling and hardness, or sometimes flabbiness of the abdo-men, with constipation, accompany in a large proportion of cases the onset of the disease. In its advanced periods we may observe impaired digestion, a very offensive state of the alvine evacuations, and flaccidity and wasting of the muscles throughout the body.

Chorea has always been found a tedious disease. The most ex-perienced practitioners admit, that under the best regulated sys-tem of treatment it often continues for several months; and many instances are recorded of its terminating only after a lapse of some years. Occasionally we meet with adults affected with convulsive twitchings of the face and arm originating in early life, and of a nature closely allied to if not identical with, chorea. They often exist, however, with acuteness of intellect, and a perfect state of all the functions, and are viewed rather as peculiarities of habit than as actual disease.

Chorea is not attended with danger. In the few cases which have been recorded of fatal termination, its character had merged in that of epilepsy and it had probably become complicated with organic læsion of some structure within the cranium. It is a very important, but well ascertained feature of the disease, that it admits of a natural cure. I have seen a variety of cases of genuine chorea, which were never subjected to any kind of medical treatment, which gradually yielded in the course of three or four months. The same principle is more generally known as applicable to hooping-cough; and it is interesting in this manner to trace the pathological relations of two diseases, which have little apparent connection with each other.

Experience has fully proved that much may be done by medicines to shorten the duration of this disorder; and the slightest reflection will convince us how requisite it is that they should be had recourse to early. While the disease lasts, an effectual check is put to the improvement of the youthful mind; and though the danger to life from it be but small, yet its continuance for any length of time is attended with the risk of permanent fatuity. The fact of its capability of a natural cure should only be so far impressed upon the physician, as to make him distrustful of some of those medicines which have been brought forward too confidently for the certain removal of the disease.

It not unfrequently happens that chorea, after being to all appearance cured, returns, and perhaps with considerable violence. Still, surrounded as we are in this part of the work with diseases that almost preclude hope, it is consolatory to find one, which, in almost all instances, can be effectually and permanently checked.

The causes of chorea are but little known, and that little is comprised under the head of *predisposition*. It attacks boys and girls indiscriminately, and those chiefly who are of a weak constitution, or whose natural health and vigour have been impaired by confinement, by employments unsuited to their years, or by the use of scanty or improper nourishment.

The pathology of chorea closely assimilates itself to that of the other forms of convulsive affection. It appears to depend mainly upon the peculiar *irritability* or *mobility* of frame which distinguishes the infantile periods of life, and the constitution of the adult female; and which is opposed to the *vigour* of manhood, and the *torpor* of advanced life. That this is a principle of considerable importance in the pathology of chorea, there can, I presume, be no question. I have seen it strikingly illustrated in those cases which originate in young women soon after the appearance of the catamenia, and which bear so strong an affinity to hysterical affections. Chorea, indeed, may without much refinement be characterized as the hysteria of an earlier age. Such an irritable state of body is very frequently associated with real *debility*, and therefore it is that we so commonly find chorea occurring in weakened and relaxed habits, and have so much reason to attribute it, as already stated, to scanty and improper diet. This debility or loss of tone in the general system constituted the leading principle in the pathology of chorea, according to the system of Cullen, and indeed all the professed systems of physic during the last century ; and it naturally led to the exclusive employment of stimulant and tonic medicines in its cure.

In practice, however, it is highly necessary for the student to be aware, that the *irritable habit* of body is compatible with a state of muscular strength, and even of plethora ; and that the convulsive motions, which are among its more obvious marks, originate in some source of *local* irritation. Dr. Hamilton was the first who formally applied this acknowledged principle to illustrate the pathology and direct the treatment of chorea. It was the chief design of his inquiry into the phænomena of this disease to show, that the debility and spasmodic motions, previously so much insisted on, were not its *leading* characters ; but that they depended on an ulterior derangement of the stomach and bowels. Such a view of the nature of chorea has been gaining ground in this country since the publication of Dr. Hamilton's work ; and though it would be contrary to all pathological analogy to expect, and to all observation to maintain that it includes the whole theory of the disease, still it may fairly be assumed as a doctrine of very extensive application.

The general principles of treatment in chorea naturally flow from the considerations which I have now pressed upon the notice of the student. Medicines have been administered with three distinct objects, *viz.*—1. To remove the constipated state of the bowels, and regulate their functions. 2· To strengthen the general system. 3. To break in upon that disposition to habitual recurrence which spasmodic actions, once excited are so apt to leave. On each of these indications of cure, and the best means of fulfilling them, I shall, in conclusion offer a few practical suggestions.

1. The extensive experience of Dr. Hamilton in the administration of purgative medicines in chorea, qualifies him to become a most useful guide in this branch of medical practice. He informs us, that the quantity of fæculent matter collected in the bowels is, in many instances, enormous, and bears no proportion to the fulness and prominence of the abdomen. He imagines it to have a reference to the *duration* of the disease, and its natural consequence, the want of insensibility in the intestines. In the early stage of the complaint, while the bowels still retain their tone, and before the accumulation of fæces is great, gentle purgatives, repeated as occasion may require, will effect a cure, or rather prevent the full development of the symptoms. In the confirmed stage, cathartics of a more powerful kind are demanded; and to ensure success, they must be persevered in steadily, and with a confidence which can be derived only from a conviction of the true nature and causes of the disease.

Here, as in all other cases of extreme debility, the recovery is slow and gradual. A regular appetite for food, a more intelligent eye, and a returning playful temper, are the preludes to that cessation of inordinate movements in the muscles, which we are not to expect as the *sudden* reward of our exertions. The bowels must even continue an object of attention for a considerable time after a salutary change in their state has taken place. The occasional stimulus of a purgative will be necessary to support their regular action, and to provide a security against renewed accumulation, and consequent relapse.

In this disease, and indeed wherever a disturbed state of the natural functions constitutes a *primary* feature in patholgy, it is indispensable that the practitioner should personally inspect the alvine evacuations. The attendants in a sick room are ignorant of the different principles upon which purgatives are administered, and incapable of forming an opinion as to the kind or degree of effect which is contemplated in each particular case. By personal inspection alone can the physician adequately judge of the effect of one dose, or speak with confidence of the necessity and extent of others. From the experience of Dr. Hamilton it would appear, that it is comparatively of little importance what purgative is administered, provided we assure ourselves that the desired effect has been fully procured.

Chorea is occasionally complicated with worms in the intestines. This is not to be considered as a *common*, far less as a necessary concomitant of the disease. It suggests the propriety of exhibitiñg, in suspected cases, the oil of turpentine, in the dose of four or six drachms ; and the effect may be kept up by the terebinthinate emul. sion (No. 64).

2. It is not contended, however, by Dr. Hamilton, nor would it be consistent with common experience to maintain, that benefit may not also be derived from tonic medicines and a strengthening regi. men.   They restore energy to the torpid bowels, aid the operation of purgative medicines, and confirm recovery. Much may be done by light and nourishing food, and regular exercise in the open air. The cold bath has proved a most powerful auxiliary in many cases, and in languid states of the system has often acted like a charm.

Of the tonic *medicines* which have acquired a character in the cure of chorea, deserve especial notice the preparations of steel (R No. 65). I have witnessed the best and most indisputable ef. fects from a scruple of the ferrum ammoniatum, given three times a day.   The oxyd of zinc, in doses of three grains three or four times a day, once enjoyed a high reputation, and it is reasonable to suppose that this was not obtained without some unequivocal ca. ses of success from its use.   The cordial draught, No. 71, con. taining bark and aromatic confection, is well adapted for the ends in view.   The cardamine pratensis, in doses of a drachm every six hours, comes recommended to us on the authority of Sir George Baker. A moderate allowance of wine has proved, in numerous cases, highly beneficial.   It may be remarked with regard to this, as to all other nervous diseases, that the remedy precisely suited to each case can only be determined by actual trial.   One remedy will sometimes succeed where all others have failed, without the reason being discoverable.

3. Like many other kinds of convulsive disease (asthma for in. stance, or hooping cough,) chorea is often kept up in the system by a principle of *habit ;* and in obstinate cases, which resist the plans of treatment now proposed, it becomes an object of impor. tance to interrupt that chain of actions in the body which have been so long associated with convulsive movements of the limbs.   With this intention physicians have frequently prescribed the several kinds of antispasmodic medicines ; more particularly musk, the volatile alkali, opium, assafœtida, ether, and camphor.   But of all the drugs exhibited with this view, arsenic appears to have been the most generally and decidedly successful.   Several cases illus. trating this fact may be found recorded in the Medico-Chirurgical

Transactions.* The medium dose for a child of ten years of age is five drops of the arsenical solution three times a day.

Differences of opinion may exist as to the mode in which arsenic operates. If I might indulge a conjecture, I should be inclined to attribute the influence which it undoubtedly possesses in certain cases of chorea, to the same principle for which we have recourse to it in the treatment of agues. That principle I have already attempted to explain. It is indeed obscure, but there are strong grounds for believing it to have a real foundation in nature.

* Vols. iv, x, and xi.

CHAP. VII.

—————

To mark the very curious analogy subsisting between these diseases, I have placed them in the same chapter; fully aware, however, that there are so many and such important *distinctions* between them, as renders it necessary to give to each a separate consideration.

TETANUS.

In the introduction to the first part of the work, an attempt was made to impress upon the student the impossibility of fixing with any certainty the boundaries of physic and surgery. Among acute diseases, the principle admits of a simple illustration in the phænomena of erysipelas. It is equally well exemplified among chronic diseases, in the history of that singular affection to which my attention is next to be directed.

The nosological character of tetanus is derived from the presence of *tonic* or rigid spasm in the voluntary muscles of the body, more or less general. It is in this manner distinguished from the common form of nervous affection, to which the term *convulsion* is popularly applied, and in which contraction and relaxation alternate in rapid succession. Tetanus, moreover, is characterized by the powers of sensation and thought remaining unimpaired ; and in this respect also, it is strongly contrasted with epilepsy.

Nosologists have been at pains to describe different *species* of tetanus. When the affection is confined to the muscles of the jaw and throat, it has been called trismus, or *locked jaw.* When the great extensor muscles of the back are principally implicated, by which the body is bent backwards in the form of an arch resting on the occiput and heels, the disease has received the name of *opisthotonos.* The term tetanus has been restricted to those cases in which the flexors and extensors being equally affected, the whole body is permanently rigid but straight. These distinctive appellations are so far useful as they express briefly the different *grades* of tetanic disorder; but the student will bear in mind that they are not to be received as indicating any difference in the *kind* of affection. To these acknowledged varieties in the character of tetanus, nosologists have added two others;—the emprosthotonos and the pleurosthotonos, the forward and the lateral tetanic curvature. The former is very rare, the latter is rather the offspring of fancy, than the result of accurate observation.

Other distinctions among tetanic cases have been noticed by authors, infinitely more important than those which have reference to the *seat* of spasm. The one is into the *acute* and *chronic,* according to the duration, and consequently the *intensity* of the disease. The other is into the *idiopathic* and *traumatic* tetanus; a division founded on that remarkable diversity in the *origin* of the complaint, which has been acknowledged from the earliest times. It must, indeed, ever be regarded as a very singular fact in pathology, than an affection of so peculiar a character as this, should have its source in causes apparently so dissimilar;—that the puncture of a nerve, the laceration of a tendon, or an extensive burn, should bring on the same *kind* of nervous affection as that which is the occasional consequence of *cold.*

In the further remarks which I have to offer on the subject of tetanus, I shall principally have an eye to the *idiopathic* form of the disease, as being that to which the attention of the physician is principally called. The *phænomena* of the disease, however, from whatever cause arising, admit of very little variation. The exclusive view which is here contemplated will be principally apparent when the *treatment* of the affection comes under discussion.

The approaches of the disorder are commonly gradual, and it slowly advances to its worst stage. One of the first symptoms of incipient tetanus is a sensation of stiffness about the neck, which increasing by degrees renders all motion of the head painful and difficult. The patient now experiences an uneasiness about the root of the tongue, which soon passes into difficult deglutition.

The aversion to swallowing in this disease is often so great, that the patient refuses all nourishment, and the administration of remedies is rendered equally hopeless. The temporal and masseter muscles are at the same time affected, and the lower jaw being thereby firmly closed, the state of trismus becomes fully developed. In slight cases, the affection does not advance further ; but this can rarely be anticipated. The tetanic disposition once formed, proceeds, with but few exceptions, to exhibit its deeper and more formidable shades of character.

One of the most constant and remarkable symptoms of confirmed tetanus, is a severe pain, referred to the bottom of the sternum, and darting from this point backward to the spine, evidently in the direction of the diaphragm. This *constrictive* pain is the precursor of more violent spasms of all the muscles of the neck and trunk. As these increase in force, the body is raised in the form of a bow ; and thus it remains until the disease has reached its acme, when the flexors act so powerfully as to counterbalance the extensors, and to retain the body in a straight and immoveable position.

In this extreme period of the disorder, every muscle of voluntary motion becomes affected. The eyes are fixed in their sockets ; the forehead is drawn into furrows ; the whole countenance undergoes the most extraordinary change. The muscles both of the upper and lower extremities partake of the general spasm and stiffness. Those of the abdomen are strongly contracted, and the belly feels hard and tense as a board. At length a violent convulsion puts and end to the life and sufferings of the patient. These sufferings are usually greater than it is possible for words to express. Their continuance, even during the ordinary period of the disease, would hardly be compatible with life, but for the occasional *remissions*, which, in common with the spasm, they undergo.* The muscular relaxation, however, is trifling, and the intervals of ease but momentary. The recurrence of aggravated spasm frequently happens without any assignable cause. Sometimes it is determined by the efforts of the patient to swallow, speak, or change his posture.

When the spasms are general and violent, the pulse is contrac.

---

* Sir Gilbert Blane has recorded one very uncommon case of tetanus, in which the spasms were accompanied with a tingling sensation, rather agreeable than distressing. The case terminated fatally, but to the last no pain was experienced.

ted, hurried, and irregular. The respiration, too, is similarly affected; but, during a remission, both usually return to their ordinary state; and feverish symptoms are rarely met with, even in idiopathic tetanus. The same remarkable freedom from disease characterizes the abdominal functions. The appetite not unfrequently
remains good throughout the whole course of the disorder. The
tongue is always moist, and the skin natural in an early period of
the disease. As it advances, however, a cold sweat covers the
surface; and there supervenes obstinate constipation of the bowels,
requiring the most drastic purgatives. The mental faculties are
sometimes preserved entire even to the last. Delirium happily
comes on in other cases.

The duration of these distressing symptoms is various. Dr.
Wells records a case which proved fatal in twenty-four hours. The
usual termination of the disease may be stated to occur on the
third or fourth day; and very rarely it is found protracted beyond
the eighth. I need hardly add how very large is the proportion of
tetanic cases which end unfavourably. It is not improbable that
the immediate cause of death may be the implication of the heart
itself in the general spasm of the body. In a few instances the patient appears to die as if exhausted by the continuance of excruciating pain.

It is a gratifying reflection, that occasionally, even where the
disease has been most fully developed, the event is favourable. In
such cases the decline of the symptoms is gradual, and the patient
long continues in a state of extreme weakness, suffering at the
same time very acute pain in those muscles which had been chiefly
affected during the height of the disorder.

I have already remarked, that a chronic variety of tetanus is occasionally witnessed; and I may now add, that it is of a much milder character than the acute species. It has been known to continue for five weeks, though it seldom exceeds three. Tetanus of
the idiopathic kind has certainly been cured in a larger proportion
of cases than that which follows external injury.

In neither form of the complaint has dissection thrown any light
upon its nature or proximate cause. In many cases no morbid appearances of any kind are discoverable. Sometimes slight effusions
are found within the cranium, and occasionally, but not uniformly,
an appearance of redness is to be met with about the œsophagus
and cardiac portion of the stomach. Traces of disease in the theca
vertebralis have also been recorded, but they are not sufficiently

uniform to authorize our attaching any degree of pathological importance to them.   The body, after death has been observed to be
very prone to putrefaction.

The only known sources of idiopathic tetanus, are cold, and disordered states of the primæ viæ. To generate this form of disease,
however, it would appear that a certain *predisposition* is also requisite, and it is doubtless the same with that which operates as an *accessory cause* of the traumatic tetanus.   The predisposition to tetanic affections is given, in the first place, by warm climates and
warm seasons.   Within the tropics, therefore, it prevails to an extent unheard of in colder latitudes.   Secondly, tetanus is chiefly
observed to prevail when the atmosphere is much loaded with moisture, and particularly where this has suddenly succeeded to a long
course of dry and sultry weather.   Even in this country exposure
to the cold and damp air of the night has occasionally been followed by an attack of tetanus.

In hot climates the ravages of the disease extend to all classes
of persons.   Infants, a few days after their birth, are frequeutly the
subjects of it.   The male sex more commonly suffer than the female; and of the former the robust and vigorous more than the
weak and irritable.   Tetanus from cold occurs for the most part
within three or four days after exposure to the exciting cause. Tetanus from an injury generally comes on about the eighth day.   It
is remarked by Sir James M'Grigor (who gives the results of his
extensive experience in this disease in the Medico-Chirurgical
Transactions,*) that if it does not occur for twenty-two days from
the date of the wound, the patient is safe from its attack.

Among the questions of greatest interest which the investigation
of tetanus presents, are those which relate to the *kind* of wound
which is most commonly succeeded by tetanic symptoms, and to
the *local* means of prevention and relief.   But these are points
which belong exclusively to surgery.   I therefore omit them, and
hasten to the enumeration of the several plans of *constitutional*
treatment which have been proposed for this most painful and fatal disorder.   Their variety must naturally create much perplexity
to the student; and this will be still further increased, when he dis-
covers them to be of the most opposite characters, and that, while
each has occasionally succeeded, it has still more frequently failed.

Reflecting upon the obscurity which involves the proximate cause

* Vol. vi, p. 449.

of tetanic affections, we need not wonder that the practice in them should still be almost empirical. Ignorant of the very elements of their pathology, it cannot be expected that theory should assist us ; and though the most extended trials have been made, experiment has hitherto completely failed in unfolding the secret of their cure. We have no reason, however, to consider tetanus as beyond the reach of medical art. It is our duty, therefore, to persevere in our efforts ; and till a brighter epoch arrives, to employ diligently those means of relief which have hitherto been attended with the great-est degree of *comparative* success.

1. Opium is the remedy on which we are to place our chief, if not our only reliance. To give it a fair chance of success, we must begin its use from the earliest appearance of tetanic symptoms. It must be given in very large doses ; and these doses must be repeat-ed at such short intervals as to keep the system constantly under the influence of the remedy. It is astonishing to observe how the body, when labouring under a tetanic disease, will resist the ope-ration of this and other remedies, which in its healthy state would have been more than sufficient to overpower and destroy it. It is advisable to begin with fifty drops of laudanum, and to repeat this at intervals of two or three hours, or even oftener, if the urgency of the symptoms requires it, until some effect has been produced on the spasms. In the early stage of the disease, we are to bear in mind the approaching closure of the jaw and difficulty of deglu-tition ; and our remedies are to be pushed before such serious ob-stacles to their administration arise. Where they have occurred, and are found insuperable, opiate enemata and frictions may be tried ; but we must not anticipate much benefit from such feeble means.

2. Purgatives claim the next place. Sir James M'Grigor informs us, that the operation of calomel on the bowels was always useful, and singularly so in the mild form of tetanus, distinguished by the spasms coming on *slowly*, and continuing of the *same* violence. A rigid perseverance in the exhibition of purgatives (wherever prac-ticable) is therefore to be advised.

3. Of the remedies which have been employed for the cure of tetanus, none have acquired a higher degree of credit than the cold bath. Dr. Wright has detailed* several cases, both of idiopathic and traumatic tetanus, occurring in hot climates, in which it was

* See Medical Observations and Enquiries, vol. vi.

attended with complete success. Later experience, however, has shown, that in tetanus,from wounds, it is of little or no avail.

The other plans of constitutional treatment which have been devised for the relief of tetanus, may be discussed in a few words. The warm bath is now generally abandoned, after the most satisfactory proof of its inefficacy. Bleeding is equally to be condemned. The employment of wine, bark, and aromatic cordials, comes recommended to us on the strong authority of successful experience. Camphor, musk, and other antispasmodics deserve a trial. Tobacco enemata have acquired some reputation. Mercury has been proved, by adequate observation to be totally inert.

HYDROPHOBIA.

This disease is considered by all pathologists as the consequence of a morbid poison, introduced into the system by the bite of a rabid animal. The general features of the disorder correspond perfectly with such a notion ; but it is not to be overlooked, that a strong analogy exists between hydrophobia and tetanus, and that the former might, with no inconsiderable claim to pathological accuracy, be viewed as a kind of tetanic affection, supervening upon wounds of a particular character. The points of analogy between these diseases will appear as I proceed to describe the symptoms and course of hydrophobia ; but I wish first to call the attention of the student to an important *distinction* that exists between them. Idiopathic tetanus we have seen to be both a frequent and a very fatal disease. Idiopathic or spontaneous hydrophobia has *never* been known to occur in the human subject,—never at least under such circumstances as to remove all suspicion of preceding local injury.

Hydrophobia has certainly existed from a very early period of the world. The first allusion to it is to be found in the writings of Aristotle ; but it is to Cælius Aurelianus that we are indebted for the original description of the symptoms and progress of the disease. From this time, unceasing attention has been paid to every phænomenon which it presents, and nothing is wanting, which observation can supply to perfect our knowledge of it. Like tetanus, however, its cure has hitherto equally evaded the suggestions of pathology, and the blind attempts of empiricism. The investigation of the disease, therefore, must be conducted with a view to elucidate its peculiarities and pathological affinities, without any prospect of practical advantage.

From the most distant times inquiries have been directed to ascertain what animals are capable of originating, receiving, and propagating hydrophobia, and what is the precise mode of its communication from animals to man. The opinions of authors on these subjects have been mixed up with many idle tales, but the following may be taken as a summary of the best established results to which their researches have led. The disease almost always commenees among animals of the canine race. It is questionable how far it ever originates even in those of the cat kind. To them, however, it is readily *propagated*, and they possess, equally with dogs, the power of transmitting it to man, and to every species of quadruped. It is a matter of doubt, whether birds are susceptible of the disease. Herbivorous animals appear incapable of communicating it, and this is even still better ascertained with regard to man. Innumerable attempts have been made to propagate the disease by inoculating animals with the saliva of persons labouring under hydrophobia, but they have always failed.

Of the causes of this peculiar distemper in dogs nothing certain is known. That it originates *spontaneously* in them is now the general opinion ; but it is equally well ascertained that among them it chiefly spreads by inoculation. In respect to the mode of its communication from animals to man, the facts in proof of the reality of a peculiar infectious principle are too numerous to admit of dispute. It is universally allowed, that the poison cannot operate on the sound skin. In many instances, indeed, the wound has been so slight as to escape notice ; but it may be stated as an invariable law, that for the hydrophobic virus to take effect, it must be applied to an abraded, wounded, or ulcerated surface.

A question has arisen, whether the infectious principle resides in the salivary secretion, or in the mucus of the trachea and bronchia. Some have conjectured, that it is more or less diffused through all the solids and fluids of the rabid animal. This latter suggestion may at once be set aside ; but the former opens a curious subject of inquiry. The appearances of inflammation so common about the pharynx, render it by no means improbable that the mucous secretion of that part may undergo a change, by which it is enabled to propagate the disease.

There is some difficulty in ascertaining how it happens, that of a number of persons bitten by a rabid animal, a certain proportion

45

only are subsequently attacked by hydrophobia. The influence of prophylactic measures may be altogether excluded, and differences of constitutional disposition can hardly be trusted to. The circum-stance is probably referable to the ineffectual application of the poison in the cases that escape. This conjecture is rendered the more probable by the acknowledged fact of bites upon the face and hands being always more dangerous than where the tooth had pre-viously passed through cloth or leather.

Hydrophobia, as it affects dogs and other animals, exhibits a very different train of symptoms from that which is observed when man is the subject of the disease. For the former, I beg to refer to a very ingenious paper by Mr. Meynell;* the latter, I shall now proceed to describe, partly from my own observation, and partly from the very admirable memoir on hydrophobia, published by Dr. John Hunter.†

The interval between the bite and the development of hydropho-bic symptoms (in other words, the *latent period* of the virus,) is sub-ject to considerable variation. Among the *genuine* cases which I have seen recorded, the shortest period was twenty-one days, and the longest nine months. Six weeks may be stated as the average; after which time the chances of escape are greatly increased. It is a curious circumstance, that during all this time there is no lo-cal irritation observable in the bitten part nor any derangement of general health, or perceptible change in the constitution, provided the person bitten be not under the influence of fear.

For two or three days previous to the coming on of the more unequivocal symptoms of the disease, the patient often complains of chilliness, some degree of head-ache, languor and lassitude, low spirits, and restlessness. Frequently also a sense of coldness and numbness is experienced in the bitten part, occasionally amounting to actual pain. This, in some instances, extends up the limb, and it has been observed to follow the course of the nerves rather than that of the absorbents. The freedom of the lymphatic glands from disease indeed, has often been noticed, and adduced as an argu-ment that the disorder does not depend on the absorption of any virus.

The second or *confirmed* stage of hydrophobia commences with

---

* Duncan's Medical Commentaries, vol. xix, p. 90.

† Transactions of a Society for the Improvement of Medical and Chirur-gical Knowledge, vol, i, art. 17.

that symptom which gives name to the disease—the horror of li-quids. The distressing sense of suffocation, and the violent spas-modic agitation of the whole body, brought on by the sight of liquids, or the attempt to drink, is unquestionably the most remark-able symptom of the disorder. By degrees the disposition to spasm increases so much upon the patient, that not merely the sight of water, but the least exertion of speaking or moving, the slightest noise, or the entrance of a stranger into the room, brings it on. Extreme irritabillity and sensibility of the whole frame are appa-rent indeed in every action of the patient, and constitute the un-varying feature of the complaint.

It has been erroneously imagined from the very general use of the term *canine madness*, that delirium was one of its usual symp-toms. In a large proportion of hydrophobic cases the mind has continued perfectly clear up to the last moment. In others, where delirium did occur, it was not until a late period of the disease. But though the patient is sensible, he is in the highest degree timid and *nervous*. As the disease advances, the mind is more and more filled with dreadful fears and apprehensions. Excessive anxiety is apparent in the countenance. Almost immediately after the dis-order distinctly manifests itself, the respiration is hurried and *gasp-ing*, and the patient commonly complains of an oppression about the præcordia. The pulse is seldom much affected till towards the latter periods of its course, when it becomes small, irregular, fee-ble, and rapid. Blood has frequently been drawn from the arm; but it has never, I believe, been observed to exhibit any inflamma-tory crust.

The secretions about the mouth are always very much affected. The saliva is usually viscid, and increased in quantity. The pa-tient complains of a parched mouth and thirst, on which account he continually calls out for drink, which yet no persuasions can in-duce him to look at, much less to swallow. A frothy saliva is frequently ejected, to the great terror of bystanders; but it arises merely from the patient's inability to swallow.

Hydrophobia is not characterized by any great degree of dehili-ty : instances have occurred of persons running a considerable dis-tance, and making great muscular exertion, within a few hours of their death. The degree of bodily weakness which has been ob-served in particular cases, is perhaps as much attributable to the remedies employed, as to the natural effects of the disorder. Its duration varies from two to five days, reckoning from the invasion of the *pathognomonic* symptom. The average does not appear to exceed forty hours. The *immediate* cause of death has never been very accurately ascertained, either in the case of tetanus or hydrophobia. Some patients die in a convulsion fit ; the greater number sink under the excessive exhaustion of nervous power.

The prognosis in hydrophobia may be discussed in a very few words. There is not, to the best of my judgment, a single unequivocal case on record, of recovery from this disease. A variety of supposed cures may indeed be found. The second volume of the Transactions of the London College of Physicians contains two ; but the slightest reflection will convince the reader, that neither in origin, symptoms, or progress, did they substantiate their claim to the character of hydrophobia. It must be viewed, therefore, as the only known disease which has hitherto uniformly resisted the efforts both of nature and of art.

This melancholy fact cannot be imputed to any neglect on the part of the cultivators of morbid anatomy ; on the contrary, the appearances on dissection, in those who die of hydrophobia, have been recorded with a degree of minuteness, which, favourably as it speaks for their zeal, is a proof at the same time how little aid their labours are calculated to afford to the mere *practitioner* in physic. The usual, appearances are turgescence of vessels (by some called marks of inflammation) about the pharynx. In some cases, a similar state of parts has been observed about the cardiac orifice of the stomach. Sir Astley Cooper, from a minute examination of several dogs who died rabid, has found reason to believe, that it consists in an effusion of blood into the cellular membrane connecting the mucous and muscular coats of that organ. No morbid appearance has ever been traced in the brain; and though the spinal marrow has been carefully examined, no important læsion has been detected there. These facts, however, are not decisive against the theory which attributes hydrophobia to a disordered condition of the brain and spinal column ; because, from the rapid course of the disease, time is not given for those alterations of structure which are so commonly the results of disordered functions.

A detailed exposition of the different means which have been resorted to for the relief of hydrophobia would be attended with little benefit to the student. It could only impress upon him that which I have already attempted to urge, the uniform fatality of the disease, and the inefficacy of medical art. It will be sufficient to say, that an ample trial has been given to blood-letting, opium, mercu-ry, ammonia, arsenic, musk, and many other antispasmodics ; be-sides a variety of drugs which had nothing to recommend them but the caprice of the practitioner. The latest trials have been made with blood-letting ; and though it acquired a doubtful fame in India, the experience of this country has decidedly proved it to be unwor-thy of general adoption.

Where all plans of treatment have alike failed, it is obviously impossible to offer any useful suggestions for the guidance of the student. *Prevention*, and not cure must be his object. It is unne-cessary with this view to inculcate formally the simple dictate of common sense—a speedy excision of the bitten part. If this is ef-fectually done, the safety of the patient may be considered as en-sured. Instances, unfortunately, are not unfrequent of hydropho-bia supervening after such an operation ; but it is fairly presumable that in such cases some minute wound had escaped the eye of the surgeon. Caustic may come in *aid* of the knife ; but considering that the life of the patient is at stake, it should never be allowed to supersede it.

On the preventive *remedies*, especially sea-bathing, and the Ormskirk and Tanjore specifics, I have of course nothing favoura-ble to report. The whole subject is painful, and I gladly leave it, in the hope that science or chance may one day furnish us with a means of combating, even partially, this formidable malady.*

* Interesting and instructive cases of hydrophobia may be found in the following works. Medico Chirurgical Transactions, vol. i, page 132 ; and vol. xiii, pages 254, 265, and 293. Transactions of the London College, vol. ii. page 46 ; and vol. iv, page 348. Medical Records and Researches, pa-ges 117 and 139. Medical Communications, vol. i, page 215 ; and vol. ii, page 290. Medical Observations and Enquiries, vols. i. and iii. Duncan's Medical Commentaries, vols. iii, xii, and xvii. Memoirs of the Medical Society of London, vols. i, iii, and v. Dr. Pinckard has seen and recorded four cases, which he has collected into one small volume. Three of these and several of the preceding reports, are accompanied by accurate dis-sections.

CHAP. VIII.

Literary History of this Affection. Its nosological Divisions. Neuralgia facialis, or Tic Douloureux. Its Seat and Symptoms. Prognosis. Diagnosis. Pathology. Treatment. By Narcotics. By surgical Operation. Of the Ischias Nervosum.

NOTHING can be collected from the works of any of the ancient authors in physic, regarding that chronic painful affection of the nerves to which the appropriate term of neuralgia is now applied. The first intelligible description of such a complaint, under the title of *tic douloureux,* appeared in the year 1756, forming part of a Treatise on the Diseases of the Urethra, by M. Andre, surgeon of Versailles. In 1766 appeared Dr. Fothergill's full and admirable paper on the subject,* which though partially anticipated by the brief notice of the French author, is well entitled, from its various merits, to be considered as the *original* account of the disease. Since that period a variety of memoirs on neuralgia, and notices of neuralgic cases, have been given to the world in the different periodical journals. Among these an ingenious essay by Dr. Haighton deserves particular mention.†

Nosologists have subdivided neuralgia into different species, cor. responding with the nerves which are the seat of pain. The first, and infinitely the most common form of the disorder, is the neural. gia facialis,—the tic douloureux of the French authors. The se. cond, in point of frequency, is the neuralgia pollicis. Cases are recorded also, in which the same painful affection existed in the nerves of the foot and mamma. They arise without any assigna.

---

* First published in the fifth volume of the Medical Observations and In. quiries. The disease was named by Dr. Fothergill dolor crucians faciei. By Sauvages it was called trismus dolorificus.

† Medical Records and Researches, p. 19. 1798.

ble cause, and are, in the strict sense of the term, *idiopathic* affections. There are, however, others of a very similar character,
which can be traced to injury of a particular nerve. These may
with propriety be classed under the title of symptomatic neuralgia.
For the present I confine my attention to the symptoms, pathology, and treatment of that singular disease to which public attention is now so strongly directed—the *neuralgia facialis*.

This affection has its seat in one or more of those branches of
the fifth and seventh pair of nerves which ramify upon the face.
The nerve most frequently affected is the portio dura of the seventh: next to this comes the second branch of the fifth, then
the first of the fifth, and the least frequent of all is the maxillary neuralgia, in which the third of the fifth is primarily implicated. The pain is of a peculiar kind, shooting in a direction which
corresponds perfectly with the course and communications of the
affected nerve. It will almost always be found to *originate* in-a
single nerve, from the point at which it issues from its bony canal. From this as from a common centre it spreads, until in the
progress of the disease it comes to affect every nerve of the face.

In neuralgia the pain is, in the first instance at least, confined
to one side of the face; it occurs always in paroxysms, which
lengthen and recur more frequently in proportion to the duration of
the complaint. It is often excited to an extreme degree of violence by the least exertion of the body, by speaking, the slightest
touch, or even a breath of wind. When the affection is fully formed,
the pain of it appears to exceed any other variety of human suffering. It occurs with equal severity by day and by night. It is attended with convulsive twitchings of the muscles of the face, which
afford a striking feature of the disease, and often impress upon the
observer a sense of the acuteness of that pain which the patient experiences.

The natural tendency of the disorder is to rivet itself in the habit,
and to terminate only with the life of the patient. It has been
known to last upwards of twenty years, and though it renders life
a miserable burthen, yet has commonly but little influence in sap-
ping its foundations.

The causes of the disease are involved in the deepest obscurity.
Of its immediate exciting causes nothing whatever is known; and
of those which predispose to it, but little. It attacks both sexes,
and apparently in an equal ratio. The robust and delicate are
equally its victims. It rarely originates under thirty years of age.

There is reason to suspect that it is rather on the increase in this country ; but to what circumstance this can be attributed it is in vain to conjecture.

Neuralgia has been in a few cases mistaken for rheumatism of the face, tooth-ache, intermittent head-ache, or abscess of the maxillary sinus. The diagnosis is not difficult, when to the accurate examination of symptoms we add an inquiry into the origin and subsequent progress of the disorder. It would be for the honour of medicine if we could with equal facility unfold its pathology. Dr. Parry has thrown out the hint, that the proximate cause is a chronic inflammation and thickening of the neurilema or vascular membranous envelope of the nerves. Sir Henry Halford has given an interesting series of cases,* tending to show that the disease is often connected with some præternatural growth of bone about the head and face, or with a diseased condition of a bone, or bony canal. Other pathologists have conjectured that neuralgia consists mainly in some obscure affection of the brain. From having known the disease in one instance to terminate fatally by coma, and in another to be followed by amaurosis, I am inclined to look upon this as the correct view of the case, and as fully borne out by the results of experience. The affection has resisted the most vigorous efforts of art with a degree of obstinacy, which can be paralleled only by the want of success which so generally attends us in epilepsy, tetanus, and palsy.

The means hitherto devised for the relief of this disease consist in the employment of narcotics and nervines, local irritants, and the division of the affected nerve. Of the class of narcotics, the principal now in use are opium, conium, and belladonna. Opium constitutes, in fact, the only *effectual* means of relief which we have it in our power to afford. Cicuta was originally recommended by Dr. Fothergill, but his high encomiums have unfortunately not been supported by the results of later experience. Belladonna, in the hands of some practitioners, has been productive of occasional advantage. If a trial of this remedy should be advised, the greatest caution is necessary in the administration of it, so peculiar and so rapid are its effects upon the nervous system.

In the genuine neuralgia the carbonate of iron, in full doses (a drachm or two drachms, repeated every six hours,) has in many cases proved decidedly efficacious ; and when we reflect how much

---

* See London Medical Gazette, vol. i, page 605.

of the pathology of the disease rests upon *irritability* and *debility* of the frame generally, we may account satisfactorily for the result.

Among the nervines which have acquired a character for the relief of neuralgia, may be mentioned bark, arsenic and iron.

The local irritants which have chiefly been employed in the cure of neuralgia are leeches and blisters, embrocations with the cerussa acetata, issues, and electricity. In the case of a y oung woman who came under my care some years ago, having many of the symp.toms of neuralgia, decided benefit was obtained by the application of leeches, a blister, and the free employment of active purgative medicines. The affection under which she laboured is not uncom- mon ; and I particularly allude to it here, having reason to believe that it is sometimes mistaken for *genuine* idiopathic neuralgia. From this, however, it differs in the circumstance of its occurring at an earlier period of life. I have observed it only in young wo. men ; and I believe it to depend chiefly, if not entirely upon a disor- dered and torpid condition of the liver and bowels.

The idea of dividing the affected nerve first occurred to the French surgeons in 1766 ; but was not generally adopted until the result of Dr. Haighton's experiment, in 1788, became known. In that case the operation proved completely successful ; but sub- sequent experience has greatly diminished the hopes that were en- tertained of the probable benefits of such a measure. It has even appeared in some late instances to add to the sufferings of the pa- tient. The excision of a portion of the nerve has been practised in a few cases, but without any corresponding advantage.

For the present, therefore, we can do little more than palliate the symptoms. The discoverer of a medicine worthy of general confidence will have a strong claim upon the gratitude of mankind.

I have too little experience in the other varieties of idiopathic neuralgia to enter upon their consideration with any prospect of utility to the student ; and authors are almost silent on this neglec- ted portion of pathology. One of the most strongly marked among them is that called *ischias nervosum*, a chronic ailment, marked by severe pain in all the branches of the great sciatic nerve, and not always easily distinguished from the rheumatic sciatica formerly treated of. In the nervous affection of the hip joint the efficacy of medical treatment is even less obvious than in the rheumatic.

Little is known regarding the causes of such a complaint. It some-times yields to the mere influence of time. It is happily very rare.

A paper by Mr. John Pearson, in the eighth volume of the Medi-co-Chirurgical Transactions,* gives a detailed account of a painful affection of the extremity of the left thumb, of a decidedly neural-gic character. After resisting a variety of plans of treatment, it ultimately yielded under the use of a liniment, which produced a high degree of irritation in the skin of the arm.

To this paper are annexed some useful reflections on the nature and management of those cases of symptomatic or local neuralgia, which are the consequences of injury to a nerve ; but on a subject which is strictly within the province of the surgeon, the general de-sign of this work relieves me from the necessity of offering any observations.†

* Page 252.

† The reader who may wish for some further information on the subject, may consult with advantage Mr. Swan's " Dissertation on the Treatment of morbid local Affections of Nerves." London, 1820, cap. iv, and v.

CLASS II.

CHRONIC DISEASES OF THE THORAX.

CHAP. I.

BRONCHOCELE.

Nature of the Affection. Symptoms and Progress of the Disease. Speculations concerning its Cause. Treatment. By Medicine. Influence of Iodine. By surgical Operation.

BRONCHOCELE, or the goitres, is a chronic indolent enlargement of the thyroid gland, occasioning swelling of the fore part of the neck, often to such an extent as to produce great deformity. The tumour, however, is quite free from pain, and does not appear to give rise to any degree of constitutional disturbance. There is no malignity in the disease, nor any disposition in the tumour, except from accidental circumstances, to take on inflammatory action.

The precise nature of the swelling which constitutes bronchocele has been a frequent object of investigation. The section of a thyroid gland affected by this disease exhibits a congeries of cells containing a transparent viscid fluid.* The size of these cells differs in different cases ; although externally the tumour shows the same character. It varies even in different parts of the same gland. Some of these cells are sufficiently large to contain a pea ; the generality are smaller. Reasoning from the change of structure thus observed, Dr. Baillie throws out a conjecture, that bronchocele may depend upon an increased and vitiated secretion from the gland, which gradually distends its cells, and forms the swelling which characterizes the disease.

Doubts have been entertained, whether there are not different species of this disorder. Distinctions have been drawn between the

---

* Vide Baillie's Morbid Anatomy, fifth edition, page 91.

sanguineous and the sarcomatous, the common and the scrofulous bronchocele; but these are probably of no real importance. If any essential differences do exist in the morbid changes of structure which the gland undergoes, the appearances presented on dissection are not sufficiently uniform to warrant us in characterizing them with precision.

There are, it is true, some slighter variations in the affection, which have always been acknowledged. The tumour varies, for instance, in point of consistence. It is hard and unyielding, or soft and spongy. In some cases, the whole body of the gland is involved in the disease, while in others the swelling is partial, affecting one lobe of the gland only, or portions of it, so as to occasion tumours that project irregularly over the anterior part of the neck.

In all cases of bronchocele there are grounds for believing that an unusual determination of blood to the gland takes place. There is very often a sensible throbbing of the tumour during life. After death, too, the blood-vessels connected with the gland, both arteries and veins, are found enlarged, and this enlargement is made particularly apparent by injecting them.

The size which the tumour acquires after a lapse of years is often enormous, and its mere weight produces no inconsiderable inconvenience. The adjacent cellular membrane and lymphatic glands in process of time participate in the disease, and the whole neck becomes enlarged. That this should exist without prejudice to the life or general health of the patient, is more surprising than that it should occasionally give rise to alarming symptoms, and be the immediate cause of death. The tumour itself becomes in some instances painful, the veins of the neck enlarge, there is hoarseness and head-ache, and that long train of evils is felt which inevitably results from obstructed respiration.

The causes of bronchocele are involved in great obscurity, and have given rise to much discussion. It has been the object of authors to discover some one cause to which every case of bronchocele may be traced; but such an expectation is neither reasonable nor warranted by pathological analogies. Like swelling of the liver or spleen, bronchocele may have many causes, differing essentially from each other. For all practical purposes it is sufficient to inquire under what circumstances bronchocele shows itself. We may thence deduce some conjectures as to the actual causes of the complaint. The influence of age, of habit, and of climate must be separately examined.

1. Bronchocele is rarely, if ever, observed in children before the ninth year. It commonly makes its first appearance about the period of puberty ; and this leads us to conjecture that it may, to a certain degree, be connected with the change in the whole system observable at that period. The alteration of the voice is a decisive proof that at least the parts in the neighbourhood of the thyroid gland then undergo some peculiar and unexplained change. As life advances bronchocele becomes more and more common ; and in districts where it prevails extensively, few persons reach to an advanced age without experiencing it in a greater or less degree.

2. Bronchocele chiefly occurs in persons of relaxed constitutions, and in such as have fair and delicate skins. It is more frequent in women than men. It often accompanies scrofula, and is by many considered an evidence of the scrofulous habit. Bronchocele has long been known to prevail in particular families, and deserves to be ranked as an hereditary complaint. Where the family predisposition is very strong, the first attack of the disease occurs at a proportionably early period of life.

3. Bronchocele, though not absolutely unknown in any part of the world, yet occurs in some with such extraordinary frequency as to have been considered the great *endemic* of particular districts. In valleys enclosed by lofty mountains, in which the reflected as well as the direct rays of the sun occasion very dense fogs to be raised, this disorder more especially abounds. Hence its frequency in all the valleys of Switzerland ; and, generally speaking, in mountainous rather than in level countries. That its prevalence in these situations is not attributable to the use of snow-water, nor to a poor, unwholesome diet, is now the concurrent testimony of all observers. It prevails in every part of the world, in the hottest as well as the coldest regions, and in every class of persons. It is common in Sumatra, and many other climates, where snow is never seen ; while in Greenland and Lapland, where the inhabitants use snow-water almost exclusively, bronchocele is hardly known. In America it chiefly prevails where the lands are covered with wood. In proportion as the country is cultivated, and the lands cleared, it is found to decline. Goitres have been observed in places particularly open to the influence of southerly winds, in the neighbourhood of rivers and lakes, and generally, wherever much moisture prevails. It chiefly appears among those who are exposed unguardedly to the influence of the weather. All these circum-

stances point out an important connection between bronchocele and some peculiarity in climate. What this is, it would be impossible accurately to specify ; but apparently it is *humidity*. There may, perhaps, be exhalations from damp soils which give rise to bronchocele ; but our ignorance of the nature and uses of the thyroid gland, joined to the obscurity which always attaches to reasonings on the origin of a disease, preclude any degree of certainty in these speculations.

The extensive prevalence of this unsightly disorder proves how little is known concerning the principles of its treatment ; or rather how completely it is beyond the control of medical art. Every plan which ingenuity could suggest, or caprice devise, has been tried, and tried in vain. It is still abundant in all countries ; and, as Dr. Somerville has observed, the families of medical men are not exempt from it. All practitioners however, agree, that to entertain any sanguine hope of a cure, the disorder must be in an incipient state. When the morbid structure of the gland has been thoroughly established, our chance of removing it, even by surgical operation is extremely precarious. The cure of bronchocele has been attempted in two ways, by constitutional and local measures ; and the following are the most approved methods admitted in modern practice.

1. The internal administration of burnt sponge has found many warm supporters, and the instances of success from this remedy are so numerous, as might at first incline the student to believe that the object of his research is found.* No doubt can exist that this medicine has cured many cases ; but it would be much easier to show those in which it totally fails of imparting even the smallest relief. It is said to be most effectual when given in the form of electuary and lozenge, and allowed to dissolve slowly in the mouth. Its use should be continued at least four or five weeks before any opinion is given as to the probability of ultimate benefit from it. The mode of its operation is not at all known. By some, the virtues of the remedy are made to reside in the alkali, or in the charcoal which it contains ; and later theorists would persuade us that iodine is its active principle. These speculations have led to the introduction of different preparations containing iodine, in the treatment of this disease ; but how far they may be administered with

* Consult the papers on the use of burnt sponge in bronchocele, in vols. iv, v, and xi, of the London Medical and Physical Journal, by Mr. Ring.

safety to the patient, and with what real prospect of success, experiments are still wanting accurately to determine. The powers of iodine are certainly very considerable. Its internal use is frequently succeeded by general emaciation. Externally applied, it is much less active, but an ointment, containing the hydriodate of potash, has proved efficacious in the removal of some indolent tumours, and merits a trial in the case of goitre.

2. Some benefit has been derived in bronchocele from the use of deobstruent medicines, more particularly the liquor potassæ, and the carbonate of soda, in conjunction with small doses of calomel, and such gentle aperients as regulate the functions of the bowels without weakening the system. Rhubarb and the neutral salts, in small doses, are recommended for this purpose. Dr. Gibson, of Baltimore, speaking of the value of the extr. conii, states, that when well prepared and diligently taken, it seldom fails to afford relief under favourable circumstances—that is, where the patient is not above twenty years of age, where the tumour is spongy, where the disease has not existed long, and where it occurs sporadically.

3. The application of leeches to the throat has been found useful, but to produce any decided effect upon the complaint they must be frequently repeated.

4. Frictions with mercurial ointment and camphor, or with the soap liniment, may be tried with some prospect of advantage, as calculated to excite the action of the absorbents. With the same view repeated blisters, in the manner recommended by Mr. Benjamin Bell, may possibly be serviceable. Simple but steady pressure upon the gland appears to contribute, in no inconsiderable degree, to the dispersion of the tumour.* The constant use of a neckcloth has sometimes checked the progress of the disease when early resorted to; and to the want of such support I have heard Italian physicians ascribe the greater frequency of the complaint in females.

5. It is a well-established fact that a simple change of residence from the valley where the goiterous person first received the disease, to a different district, or even to a higher spot on the side of the mountain, has in many instances diminished the size of the tumour, and occasionally removed it entirely.

6. When the tumour becomes so large as to produce great deformity, or to endanger suffocation; or when, at an earlier period

* See London Medical Repository, vol. viii, p. 288.

of its growth, the methods now proposed are ineffectual, the aid of surgery has been called in, and relief attempted by an operation. Three surgical plans of treatment have been devised. The first is extirpation of the thyroid gland; an extremely formidable and hazardous operation, of which I know but one successful case on record. The second is tying the superior thyroideal arteries. A case in which this proved for a time successful, is to be found in the Medico-Chirurgical Transactions.* The operation was performed by Mr. Coates in the Salisbury Infirmary, on a young woman seventeen years of age. The artery of the left side only was tried, and in a short time the size of the tumour was reduced one half. The third plan of surgical treatment is the insertion of a seton into the body of the gland. Severel cases of partial, and one or two of complete relief from this remedy, have been lately brought under the notice of the profession ;† but it is doubtful whether the measure be entitled to any large share of praise. In some cases the seton occasioned a high degree of irritation about the throat, rendering its immediate removal indispensable.

Upon the whole, we are led to conclude, that though the means of relief in the hands of the physician are far from possessing any general or very decided efficacy, they are nevertheless preferable to those severe and more doubtful measures which surgery has hitherto afforded.

* Volume x, p. 312.
† Medico-Chirurgical Transactions, vol. x, p. 16.

CHAP. II.

DYSPNŒA AND ASTHMA.

Nosological Difficulties connected with Disordered Respiration. Of Dyspnœa as a Symptom of Disease. Its several Causes. Dyspnœa Permanent and Spasmodic. Asthma. How characterized. Phœnomena of the Asthmatic Paroxysm. Progress of the Disease. Predisposition. Exciting Causes. Pathology. Treatment—during the Paroxysm—in the Interval. Influence of Nauseants. Acids. Narcotics. Antispasmodics. Laxatives. Tonics. Diet and Regimen.

MUCH labour has been bestowed by nosologists in classifying the different kinds of disease which derive their chief character from disordered respiration ; but to so little purpose, that the language of medical men, in regard to them, is even at present hardly more accurate than that of the world in general. The difficulties lie in the very nature of the subject ; which is so extensive, so complicated, and so obscure, as not to admit of that precise elucidation which is indispensable in artificial arrangements. The function of respiration is of such importance in the animal œconomy, and the organs subservient to it (membranes, blood-vessels, nerves, muscles, glands) are so numerous and so variously connected, that it is hardly possible for disease to exist without implicating it more or less. Accordingly *difficult breathing* will be found to be one of the most frequent *symptoms* met with in practice ; and those who have ever experienced a fit of illness will acknowledge it as one which presses upon the patient more heavily than perhaps any other.

The *pathological* considerations connected with dyspnœa *as a symptom of disease* are of the highest importance ; and they demand, from the practical physician, the fullest investigation which the state of the science permits. In the course of the present chapter I shall be led to touch upon most of those interesting topics of general inquiry which this branch of the study of physic in-

47

volves; but a complete discussion of them would far exceed the
limits to which I have here confined myself.

The first questions of the student will naturally be, what are the
immediate causes of difficult respiration, and which of them are
the most frequently met with ? A reply to these inquiries will lead
to a knowledge of the most important *practical* divisions which
have been made among the cases of disordered respiration.

1. Difficulty of breathing, in the first place, is a symptom of
general fever. The increased velocity with which the blood, during fever passes through the great vessels of the lungs, disturbs
their functions, and the natural consequence is dyspnœa. 2. It
occurs as a symptom of the early stage of inflammation in the *mucous* membrane of the lung and air-passages, and is therefore a
leading feature in laryngitis, croup, severe catarrh, and the several modifications of bronchitis. It is attributable here to the *loaded* or congestive state of vessels in the affected membrane. 3. Difficult respiration is a symptom of inflammation in the serous membrane of the thorax ; probably, because by the free expansion of
the lungs the pleura is placed upon the stretch. 4. It is equally
the result of deposition in the parenchymatous substance of the
lungs, and is hence the most important of the early symptoms of
tubercular phthisis.

After this enumeration of only a few of the sources of difficult
breathing, it cannot surprise us that it should be so common a
symptom of acute diseases. We may now observe .the same effect resulting from causes of a more chronic kind.

5. Præternatural secretion from the glands of the bronchia, or
from their secreting mucous surface, is sometimes habitual, and
sometimes the result of accidental inflammation. In either case
it creates dyspnœa, which is felt most oppressively in the morning,
and is only relieved by the labour of long coughing. 6. Permanent dyspnœa is the natural consequence of malformation of the
thoracic parietes. 7. It is a common attendant on hydrothorax,
organic diseases of the heart, aneurism of the aorta, and other
mechanical impediments to the free expansion of the lungs. 8. In
certain cases dyspnœa is believed by many pathologists to arise
from a much less obvious cause, *viz.* some irregular spasmodic action of the muscles concerned in the function of respiration. This
we shall hereafter see to have given occasion to much controversy.
A strong argument, however, in favour of the reality of such a
cause of dyspnœa may be found in the circumstance of its being

traced, 9thly, to the existence of disease within the head. A peculiar modification of difficult breathing is, as I have already stated, a distinguishing feature of apoplexy. It is presumable, that in
this case dyspnœa is owing to impaired function of the *par vagum*
Lastly, dyspnœa has its origin, in a large proportion of cases, from
disturbance in the functions of the abdominal viscera. Sometimes,
as in the case of flatulency of the stomach, a constipated and distended state of the colon, or a swelled liver, this may be imputed
to the mechanical obstruction offered to the descent of the *diaphragm.* In other instances, as in that of worms, the difficulty of
breathing is referable only to the principle of nervous sympathy,—
an explanation which is not to be discarded because less intelligible than some which have preceded it.

This brief and very imperfect sketch of the various causes of
dyspnœa will probably be received as sufficient evidence of the
obscurity in which the subject is enveloped. It results from it :
1, That difficult breathing is equally to be met with in acute and
chronic diseases ; 2. That it arises, partly from causes existing
within, and partly from such as are exterior to the thorax ; 3.
That it admits of a division into the two great classes of *permanent* and *spasmodic.* Upon this latter distinction much stress has
always been laid by nosologists. They have generally agreed in
restricting the term *dyspnœa* to the cases of permanent difficulty
of breathing, while to the spasmodic or recurrent varieties of disordered respiration, they apply the generic term *asthma.* In this
sense, which may fairly be considered as the correct one, dyspnœa
can only be viewed as a symptom, and as such cannot properly be
treated of in this place. The case is different however with regard
to *spasmodic asthma.* This affection of the breathing has long been
regarded as *idiopathic,* and to the title it has unquestionable claims.

ASTHMA.

Asthma was well described by the Greek and Roman authors,
and has always been a favourite topic of speculation among medical writers. The latest and by far the most complete account of
the disease which has ever appeared is that of Dr. Bree,* to which

---

* Practical Inquiry into Disordered Respiration, by Robert Bree, M. D.
fifth edition. London, 1815.

I am chiefly indebted for the following outline of its symptoms, causes, and method of cure.

Symp. of approach of paroxysm

There is often some degree of warning given of the approach of an asthmatic paroxysm, not by thoracic symptoms, but by those of indigestion, heartburn, flatus, itching of the skin, pain over the eyes and sleepiness. The attack most commonly occurs at night and the patient is perhaps waked out of his sleep by it.* To those who experience or witness a paroxysm of asthma for the first time, it appears one of the most formidable diseases to which man is liable. The patient is oppressed by a tightness across the breast, which so impedes respiration, as to threaten the immediate extinction of life. He starts up into an erect posture, and flies to the window for air. For a considerable time his breathing is performed by gasps, slowly and with a wheezing noise; speaking is difficult and even painful to him; there is often present also a propensity to coughing.

In this state of urgent distress the patient continues till the approach of morning, when a remission commonly takes place. However suddenly the fit began, it always goes off slowly. By degrees the breathing becomes less laborious, and coughing and speaking are performed with greater ease. In the generality of cases a copious expectoration of mucus at length takes place, and with it the paroxysm ceases, and the patient falls asleep. During the fit the pulse usually continues of the natural standard, the surface of the body is pale, the muscles appear shrunk, and there is a considerable flow of limpid urine. In a few cases expectoration is very scanty. This, which in itself is an unimportant circumstance, was by the humoral pathologist advanced to a distinguished rank among the symptoms of the disease, and made the groundwork of its division into the two species of *dry* and *humid* asthma.

During the next day, the asthmatic experiences some remaining sense of stricture across the breast, and any exertion of the body increases his uneasiness. At night the urgent difficulty of breathing returns, and in this manner he is harassed for three or four successive days; after which, the symptoms gradually yielding, he enjoys his usual rest without further disturbance. This terminates the paroxysm of asthma.

When it has once taken place, the disease is apt to recur period-

---

* The student will not fail to observe in this circumstance, an analogy between spasmodic asthma and epilepsy.

ically, and when the asthmatic disposition is very strong, to be brought on at all times by some of the circumstances which I shall presently enumerate. I have previously to observe, that a degree of difficulty of breathing, particularly on ascending a hill or flight of steps, is never wanting during the intervals, and respiration is always attended more or less with *wheezing ;* that is, with a morbid accumulation of mucus in the bronchial tubes. Persons subject to asthma acquire a peculiar expression of countenance easily recognised when once observed.

Little is known on the subject of predisposition to asthma. It has some title to rank as an hereditary complaint ; it is not confined to any particular age or sex. The period of youth and manhood is the most prone to it. It is sometimes connected with a deformed state of the chest. The asthmatic disposition commonly exists along with other marks of an *irritable* habit of body. This general principle pervades the whole pathology of asthma. It will be obvious in the strong tendency to dyspepsia which all asthmatics have ; in the slightness of the cause which often induces a fit ; in the great facility, lastly, with which the asthmatic convulsion, when once excited, runs into excess, and rivets itself in the constitution, recurring at last by the mere force of habit.

In ordinary cases, the exciting causes of the paroxysm are sufficiently perceptible, and they exhibit the most singular varieties. Dr. Bree considers them as qualified by their importance to become the basis of a practical division of asthmatic cases ; and he refuses to acknowledge any differences of the *phænomena* of the asthmatic paroxysm calculated to attain this object. From this we may learn to estimate the claims upon our attention which the *exciting causes* of asthma possess.

1. In the predisposed, an asthmatic paroxysm is frequently the result of particular states of the atmosphere, varying however in different cases. One man finds his breathing easy in the most crowded and smoky parts of London, and has a fit the moment he returns into the pure dry air of the country. Some asthmatics can go with impunity into a hot and crowded room, which others would shun as the sure prelude to a paroxysm. Some have their fits in summer, and others dread the approach of cold weather. An asthmatic is a perfect barometer. In a close room he knows when the weather changes, and confidently pronounces the wind in the east.

2. Various sorts of irritating matters conveyed to the lungs by the air, and occasioning, under common circumstances, a fit of sneez-

ing, will, in those predisposed to asthma, bring on a paroxysm. Dust, perfumes, tobacco smoke, metallic fumes, and the vapours of sulphur, have had this effect in many cases.

3. Asthma is often occasioned by whatever quickens the motion of the blood generally, or determines it particularly to the lungs ; such as severe exercise, loud speaking, exposure to cold, and sup. pressed evacuations.

4. A very frequent and important cause of the asthmatic parox- ysm is a loaded, weakened, or otherwise disordered state of the stomach and bowels. This cannot surprise us when we reflect how generally dyspeptic persons, having no asthmatic diathesis, com- plain of difficult breathing, especially in the horizontal posture. The principle is of extensive application in the treatment of asth- matic affections.

5. Asthma is occasionally induced by causes which cannot ope- rate but through the medium of the nervous system.   Of this kind are vehement emotions and passions of the mind, the anxieties of business, or the exertion of deep thought.

6. I have already had occasion to allude to the great law of convulsive motion, viz. that, whatever be its origin, the certain consequence of its repeated attacks will be that increased mobility of the whole frame which occasions a renewal of diseased actions by the mere force of habit.   This principle is particularly applica- ble to asthma, which fixes itself in the constitution with an invet- eracy equalled only by that of epilepsy. Yet with all this, asthma cannot be considered as a disease of danger.   No instance is per- haps on record of a fatal event occurring during the paroxysm ; and though it assuredly in some cases lays the foundation for other diseases (hydrothorax, and perhaps aneurism of the aorta,) yet this is not frequent.   Many confirmed asthmatics have accordingly at- tained a good old age. The gradual inroads however, which, when uncontrolled, it makes upon the constitution, embitter all the enjoy- ments of life, and should be sufficient to induce the patient to sub. mit to any privations that may be necessary towards his cure.

Pathologists in all ages have exerted their ingenuity in determi. ning, if possible, the precise seat of the asthmatic convulsion, and its true nature or proximate cause.   Much controversy has arisen on both these questions, and they are still involved in considerable obscurity.   The bronchial tubes have usually been considered as the primary seat of asthma ; but a difficulty has been experienced in reconciling the notion of spasmodic contraction with their pecul.

iar anatomical structure, nor does this appear to have been hitherto overcome. In the exquisite form of the asthmatic paroxysm, every muscle that can assist in respiration is affected., The great question however, upon which pathologists have divided, is whether the spasmodic action existing in some one of the structures about the chest be the *cause* or the *consequence* of that superabundant mucus in the bronchial tubes, which all admit to constitute so material a part in the phenomena of the asthmatic paroxysm. Dr. Cullen (with other Hoffmannians) contends, that it is the *cause*—that the spasm is the primary feature of the disease, and the effusion of mucus the natural relief of such diseased action. Dr. Bree, on the other hand, joins with the old humoral pathologists in maintaining that the convulsive efforts of the asthmatic are only *secondary* phæ-nomena being set up with the view of throwing off an excessive se-cretion from the mucous membrane of the bronchia.

Dr. Bree has undoubtedly argued the question with great ability, but the general laws applicable to secretion and convulsive action do not appear to bear him out in his conclusions ; besides which, the occasional occurrence of asthma with little or no secretion from the lungs, the very frequent circumstance of excessive accu-mulation there without any spasmodic action excited to disengage it, the phænomena of hooping cough, and the analogy of both asthma and hooping cough to epilepsy, tend still further to the belief, that the first link in the chain of phænomena is convulsive action.

It must be confessed that the question before us is one of a pure-ly speculative nature. Though I have ventured therefore to differ from Dr. Bree in his pathological opinions, I am not the less satis-fied as to the merits of his practical suggestions. Of these I now proceed to lay before the reader a short abstract. The treatment of asthma naturally divides itself, like that of agues, into the two great heads of palliative and radical ; or into that which is to be pursued during the fit, and in the interval. The relative impor-tance of these was long misunderstood. Dr. Cullen distinctly says, that asthma is seldom cured, though it admits of alleviation. Dr. Bree, on the other hand has shown that the paroxysm of asthma is susceptible of but little relief, and that the main object of medical treatment is to prevent the recurrence of fits, and thus to effect a *permanent* cure of the disease.

1. During the paroxysm the indications of cure are to lessen the distension of the blood-vessels of the lungs, and to promote expec-toration. It might be supposed that the first object would at once

be gained by the abstraction of blood, and the relief so commonly afforded by bleeding in most forms of thoracic disease gives countenance to such an expectation. But experience has shown that this evacuation scarcely ever shortens the paroxysm ; while on the other hand it delays expectoration, aggravates the subsequent dyspnœa, and increases that debility which is tbe great obstacle to a speedy and ultimate cure. In place of blood-letting we are to relax the spasm, and unload the vessels by the combined influence of nauseant expectorants, acids, and narcotics.

Where the stomach is much loaded (as when the paroxysm occurs soon after a full meal,) we may begin by directing a gentle emetic (R No 3.) Under common circumstances it will however be sufficient to keep up a nauseant effect by the draught No. 89. If there be suspicion of acidity in the stomach, the draught No. 90. may be substituted. Sir John Floyer's specific in the asthmatic paroxysm was the vinegar of squill, and it is certainly a valuable medicine. The patient should be directed to take at intervals clear coffee, which as an article of diet is peculiarly well adapted to the stomach of an asthmatic. On the second or third day, when the tendency to secretion has increased, some anodyne may be added to the expectorant, and the effect of the whole is much aided by the gentle stimulus of an acid. The formulæ, Nos. 93 and 94, are constructed upon these principles. In the management of this disease the student will bear in mind, that laxity of fibre, and morbid sensibility and irritability, are the predominant features of the asthmatic habit, and he will learn to avoid all violent medicines.

The same considerations might naturally induce him to expect advantage from the administration of *antispasmodics*, more especially ether and laudanum. Though serviceable in a few cases, this combination for the most part fails, in imparting even temporary relief. Dr. Bree has convinced himself that such medicines are useful *only* when the disease has existed long, when the fit recurs from habit and sympathy, and when our object is merely to vary impressions. In this state, opium alone is often useful, but its powers are much increased by combination with ether. The tact of experience can alone teach when the disease has assumed that *habitual* form, in which antispasmodics are indicated.

As the fit of asthma so frequently arises from disordered states of the stomach and bowels, the employment of laxatives during the paroxysm affords an obvious means of relief. In a few cases, the action of a smart purgative carries off the fit ; but, in general, purging, where advisable, should be attempted by rhubarb, castor oil, and the absorbent earths. Dr. Bree has observed the excellent effects which result from the use of chalk and rhubarb. The cold bath has been recommended as a powerful means of directly checking the asthmatic fit. Where the constitution is vigorous, it may occasionally be advisable to employ it, but not otherwise.

2. In the intervals of the paroxysms, attention is principally to be paid to the careful avoiding of the several exciting causes of the disease. Attempts are to be made also to give tone to the capillary vessels of the lungs, and to promote the strength of the stomach and general system. To enter upon such a plan with any prospect of success, co-operation on the part of the patient is indispensable. His health is in a great measure in his own hands. Abstinence from what is hurtful rests alone with him, and this can never be compensated by the prescriptions of his physician. To *aid* the efforts of the asthmatic, preparations of iron, bitters, and the mineral acids, may be advised. A tea-spoonful of the carbonate of iron may be given three times a day, or the pills (R No. 67,) as recommended by Dr. Bree, or the chalybeate electuary, No. 66.

Cold bathing, daily regular exercise, and, where possible, frequent changes of air, of scene, and of amusement, are of real importance. Above all things, attention is to be paid to the regulation of diet. Light and simple food is to be preferred, and always taken in moderation. With this precaution many confirmed asthmatics pass through life in comparative comfort. When the disease is inveterate, the only chance of permanent cure rests in a complete change in all the habits of life, and in Dr. Bree's work* there is recorded a splendid example of what may be effected by such a measure steadily pursued.

*Inquiry into disordered Respiration, page 347.

48

CHAP. III.

HOOPING-COUGH.

On Cough as a Symptom of Thoracic Disease. Early notices concerning Hooping Cough. Manner of its Invasion. Progress of the Disease. Prognosis. Modes by which it proves fatal. Propagation by specific Contagion. Nature of the Affection. Principles of Treatment. Remarks on the Administration of different Remedies. Influence of Change of Air.

Cough and difficult breathing are the leading symptoms of thoracic disease, whether acute or chronic ; but they occur in such very different forms, they are so infinitely diversified in their combinations with each other, and with other local and general symptoms of disease of the chest, in their periods of occurrence and duration, and in the degree of their violence, that no inconsiderable difficulty is experienced in forming a true estimate of their bearing in particular cases. This position I attempted to illustrate in the last chapter, when treating of dyspnœa. It again meets us in our inquiries concerning the nature and varieties of *chronic cough.*

The pathology of cough is much simpler than that of difficult breathing. It always depends upon some morbid condition of the mucous expansion of the lungs and air-passages. This may be either a præternatural *dryness* of the membrane, by which it is rendered unusually susceptible to the stimulus of dust, of vapours, or of a cold moist air ;—or, secondly, inflammation and its consequences ; or, what approaches very near to it, the state of vascular congestion ;—or, lastly, it may be some poison circulating in the system, and possessing, from circumstances unknown, a peculiar disposition to affect the bronchial membrane. Cough as arising from the first of these sources, is a mere symptom of *general fever.* As it occurs in consequence of inflammation, or of any disturbed state of circulation allied to inflammation, it has been already discussed under the title of *subacute* and *chronic* bronchitis. It now remains, that I consider chronic cough as it arises *idiopath- ically* from unknown, or at least, very obscure causes. This sin- gular variety of disease, prevailing chiefly among infants and chil- dren, is well known to the world under the title of *hooping-cough*, and from nosologists it has received the name of pertussis.

Hooping-cough is not described by any of the Greek, Roman, or Arabian authors. It is impossible to suppose that a disease so strongly marked as this, could have escaped the attention of the ancient physicians, had it then existed. We must presume there- fore, that it was not known in Europe before the thirteenth, or per- haps even the fourteenth century. It was first accurately descri- bed by Dr. Willis* in 1664. The most complete treatise on the disease which has since appeared is that of Dr. Watt of Glasgow,† in which the student will find a copious account of the opinions of the best authors.

Hooping-cough begins with the common symptoms of catarrh, from which indeed it cannot be distinguished by any known crite- rion for the first week. It has been observed, that the usual ca- tarrhal symptoms are here accompanied with a more than ordina- ry disposition to sleep, and those which denote general fever are seldom very strongly marked. About the end of the second, or beginning of the third week, the symptoms undergo a remarkable change : the fever declines, and appetite returns ; but the cough continues in paroxysms of extraordinary violence. The child struggles for breath, and appears in danger of suffocation until re- lieved by the long and full inspiration known under the name of the *back draught*, or hoop. The fit of coughing continues for several minutes, and is commonly terminated by expectoration of mucus, sometimes by vomiting, and occasionally by bleeding at the nose, or an epileptic paroxysm. In very bad cases, even this relief is denied to the little patient, whose efforts end only with his complete exhaustion. It is distressing to witness the attempts made to ex- pectorate. The child appears conscious of the benefit thus afford- ed to him, and continues coughing until expectoration is effected.

The fits vary much in frequency. In mild cases they do not oc- cur more than three or four times a day. In severe ones, they harass the patient every half hour. It is very rare to find them re-

* Pathologia Cerebri et Nervosi Generis, cap. 12.
† Treatise on the Nature, History, and Treatment of Chincough, 1813.

curring at regular intervals. They are often brought on by exertions of body, or emotions of mind. It is common, therefore, to find the child averse from moving or speaking. He is often aware of the approach of the fit, and lays hold of any thing near him for support. He finds relief by stooping forward, and by support given to the head and back.

When once the disease has assumed its regular form, the appetite is good; and this is strikingly displayed in the craving for food, which comes on when the fit terminates by vomiting. The tongue is *clean and moist.* There is no difficulty of breathing in the intervals of the fit. Permanent dyspnœa betokens something more than mere hooping-cough, either an inflammatory condition of the bronchial membrane, or a gorged state of the substance of the lungs. The bowels are seldom affected. It is very common to find children with hooping cough complaining of a *tensive* pain of the forehead, and in severe cases this is obviously an *urgent* symptom, and one which demands attention in reference to practice.

The further progress and duration of hooping-cough are subject to great variety. In its mildest form it generally lasts two or three months; and when severe, is often protracted to six or seven. Even after it has wholly ceased, or nearly so, an accidental exposure to cold has occasioned its return. Under the most favourable circumstances the decline of the disease is very gradual, and almost imperceptible. It happens however, but too frequently, that the latter stages of the disease are attended with a formidable train of evils. In some cases a convulsion fit occurs in one of the paroxysms, and carries off the patient when the practitioner is least prepared for it; or genuine hydrocephalus gradually supervenes, and the child dies in a state of coma. This might oftener be anticipated, when we reflect with what force the blood is driven upon the brain, and how much its return is retarded, during a severe fit of coughing. In other cases, from exposure to cold, pneumonic symptoms supervene, and the child either dies with his lungs gorged with blood, or the foundation is laid for a species of infantile phthisis. The last of the modes by which hooping-cough proves fatal, is that by *marasmus and infantile fever.* The child after a continuance of the disease for a certain time, from causes not well understood, loses his appetite, emaciates rapidly, becomes hectic, and dies, *apparently* from pure exhaustion.*

* The deaths by hooping-cough recorded in the London bills of mor-

The danger is not proportioned to the age of the patient. A child of two or three *months* old will struggle through the complaint as well as another of two or three years. When it attacks weakly or scrofulous children, or those labouring under some other disease, it is apt to prove severe, tedious, and therefore dangerous. When hooping-cough begins late in the spring, it is commonly milder than when its approach is towards the beginning of winter. It is always most destructive in cold climates, and in cold and damp seasons.

The appearances on dissection correspond with the views which have been given of the modes by which this disease proves fatal. Dr. Watt has described several cases in which were found the clearest proofs of acute bronchial inflammation, conjoined with more or less *congestion* in the substance of the lungs. In some which have been recorded, serous effusion within the ventricles of the brain has been the predominant morbid appearance ; while to myself and to many others it has occurred to witness numerous in-stances, in which, on examination, nothing preternatural has been observed in either of the three great cavities of the body.

Hooping-cough, though sometimes met with in adults, is for the most part the disease of early life. It is often epidemic. Few children escape it ; but it rarely, if ever, is known to occur more than once in the course of life. From these and other facts which might be adduced, a reasonable presumption exists, that it has its origin in a *specific contagion*, which, like those of the influenza and measles, has a direct determination to the membrane of the bron-chia, though it is not, like them, essentially linked to fever. The contagion of hooping-cough appears to be communicated with great facility. When once it gets entrance into a family, it generally attacks every child.

Different opinions have been entertained regarding the precise nature of hooping-cough. It was originally considered as a spas-modic disease, allied in its more obvious features to asthma and chorea, but acknowledging also many of the laws of convulsive diseases generally. This simple and very satisfactory explanation has latterly been called in question ; and the notion has prevailed, that hooping-cough is an affection of an inflammatory kind, closely allied to the ordinary varieties of bronchitis. In favour of this

tality are always very numerous, averaging not less than five hundred annually.

opinion it has been argued; 1. That common winter cough frequently shows a strong disposition to spasmodic exacerbation ; 2.
That all the more important sequelæ of hooping-cough are of a
decidedly inflammatory character ; and, 3. That inflammatory affection of another mucous membrane (catarrh, and cynanche maligna) are induced by the operation of a specific contagion. These
facts point out a strong *tendency* in the disease to inflammation,
which the practitioner will do well to keep in view ; but an impartial observer will duly appreciate those more numerous considerations which associate it with the class of spasmodic diseases. This
latter view of the character of hooping-cough is supported by the
infinite number of presumed specifics for the cure of the complaint.
That all of them have been at times serviceable it would be in vain
to deny, and such facts are reconcilable only with the notion of the
disease being essentially of a spasmodic nature.

The leading principles to be kept in view in the treatment of
hooping-cough are the following. It is a disease arising from a
specific contagion, over which we have no direct control. Like
small-pox or measles it has a tendency to run a certain course and
to wear itself out. The violence of the paroxysms may sometimes
be moderated by remedies which diminish irritability generally,
and which prove useful in other spasmodic disorders. On the other
hand it is to be remembered, that hooping-cough occurs at a period
of life peculiarly favourable to the lighting up of fever, and to the
engendering local determinations of blood. On this account a
watchful eye must always be kept on the accompanying constitutional symptoms, and antiphlogistic measures adopted in proportion
to their violence.

As to the alleged specifics in hooping-cough, I need not do more
than simply enumerate them. Their very number is a satisfactory proof that no single remedy is of much service. They are, cantharides, cochineal, paregoric elixir, assafœtida, castor, bark, cup-
moss, musk natural and artificial, nitre, arsenic, and prussic acid.
Without detaining the reader by a detail of the relative merits of
these drugs, I shall at once proceed to offer a few remarks on those
means of more acknowledged power which have been sanctioned
by long and general use ; such as emetics, narcotics, expectorants,
stimulant embrocations, laxatives, mercurial alteratives, local and
general depletion, and change of air.

1. Emetics were probably first employed from its being observed
that vomiting is one of the common terminations of the paroxysm,

and that children who vomit, commonly pass through the disease easily. There is a great difference, however, between natural vomiting and that which is the result of an irritating medicine, such as tartar emetic. It will be found in practice, that *frequent* emetics, from their tendency to weaken the stomach, are inadmissible ; but the *occasional* exhibition of a few grains of ipecacuanha may safely be directed.

2. When the disease has subsisted for any length of time, the mild narcotics are decidedly useful. Dr. Butter* recommends very strongly the extr. conii, which may be given according to the form (R No. 51.) Other practitioners have found advantage from hyoscyamus, and the lactuca virosa, (R No. 56.) Opium for the most part confines the bowels, and makes the child feverish.

3. Expectorant medicines, of several kinds, have been tried, and occasionally have proved singularly beneficial. Dr. Richard Pearson† has spoken in high terms of the combined influence of an expectorant (the vinum ipecacuanhæ,) with an anodyne and absorbent. He recommends the formula R No. 91.

4. Stimulant embrocations enjoy a high reputation for the relief of hooping-cough. The formulæ Nos. 110 and 111 may be tried with some prospect of advantage. They should be applied not only to the chest, but along the course of the spine ; and the milder kinds may be repeated frequently during the day.

5. An open state of the bowels is almost essential to the favourable progress of the disease. An occasional dose of rhubarb, in conjunction with the carbonate of potash, or soda, is of decided advantage. Dr. R. Pearson has observed, that the slimy fluid brought up by vomiting has often a sour smell.

6. In the latter stages of hooping-cough, where it becomes combined with symptoms of marasmus, I have derived great benefit from small alterative doses of calomel (a grain twice a day with a little sugar,) and to this may be united very advantageously a few grains of scammony (R No. 10.)

7. In all severe cases, when the cough is accompanied with permanent dyspnœa, much heat of skin, and other febrile symptoms, general or local blood-letting ought never to be omitted. It is frequently necessary to repeat the evacuation of blood two or three times before the symptoms begin to yield. When the child com-

* Treatise on the Kin-Cough.
† Medico-Chirurgical Transactions, vol. i, p. 23.

plains of much head-ache, it will be right to apply a few leeches to the head. It has been observed, that the severity of the *hoop* has been in this way diminished; and the acknowledged influence of certain states of the brain upon the respiratory organs may be adduced in explanation of the fact.

8. When the disease proves very tedious and obstinate, resisting all the common modes of relief, and exhausting the patient by its continuance, we may fairly presume, that it has rooted itself in the system by the force of habit; and to break in upon this, change of air has long been found eminently beneficial. It is often the only thing that gives the patient a chance for life. But it must be remembered in what circumstances it is applicable, and should never be advised where symptoms of bronchial inflammation are present, which a free exposure to cold air would in all probability aggravate.

* See Appendix; Note W.

CHAP. IV.

Sketch of the Objects of Investigation in this and the succeeding Chapter. Functional Disturbances of the Heart. Syncope. Its Causes—and Mode of Treatment. Palpitation. Its several Causes. Angina Pectoris. Literary Notices concerning this Affection. Its Symptoms and Progress. Morbid Appearances. Pathology. Treatment. Structural Diseases of the Heart and great Vessels. Enlarged Heart. Diseased Valves. Aneurism of the Thoracic Aorta. Cengenital Malformations. Symptoms occasioned by them. Morbus Cæruleus.

THERE is no class of diseases which submits to the trammels of nosological arrangement less easily than the chronic affections of the heart. Their characters are so ill defined, so difficult is it to distinguish the idiopathic affections of this organ from those cases in which its functions are sympathetically disturbed, so *impossible* to anticipate with certainty by the symptoms the presence of structural disease there ; in fine, so intimately are the functional disorders of the heart connected with those of the brain, than an attempt to arrange systematically this class of diseases may be considered as almost hopeless. My object in bringing them together is merely to offer a few suggestions upon each, calculated to assist the student in determining the pathological character of particular symptoms, and to impress upon his attention those general views regarding chronic affections of the heart, to which modern pathologists have principally attached importance.

I shall first treat of such as are commonly functional, and comparatively speaking, of little danger, *viz.* syncope and palpitation ; and afterwards advert to those in which disorganization of the heart or great vessels is *manifest.* The link uniting the two will be found in that singular affection known by the popular but unscientific name of angina pectoris. The obscure subject of asphyxia naturally connects itself with our inquiries concerning the morbid con-

49

ditions of the heart; but its bearings are of so very general a kind, that it will be better to refer the consideration of it to a separate chapter.

SYNCOPE.

Syncope or fainting consists, as is well known, in the temporary suspension of the functions of the heart and consequently of every other function of the body. Though commonly considered as an affection of the heart, it is in strict pathology a disease of the brain and nervous system. A dimness comes before the eyes; a deadly paleness overspreads the cheeks; the patient falls down; the pulse fails; respiration is at a stand; sensation and all mental phænomena cease. In some cases indeed, the patient, though incapable of speaking, retains enough of perception and sensation to be conscious of his own disorder, and of what is passing around him. The disease brings with it its own cure. The horizontal position to which it reduces the body quickly renews the supply of blood to the heart, and the fit of syncope is over. In a few cases, recovery is accompanied with a confusion of ideas, vertigo, and head-ache. Much more frequently it is described as being attended with very *painful* feelings. Fainting, viewed in the light of a *disease*, must always from its very nature terminate favourably. I shall have occasion indeed, in the next chapter to speak of death by *syncope*, that is, of a sudden and *permanent* check given to the heart's action; but to such a state, the term fainting, in its common acception, is obviously inapplicable.

Nosologists have attempted to distinguish different degrees of swooning, to which they have applied the terms leipothymia, leipopsychia, echysis, syncope, and apopsychia; but there are certainly no real grounds in nature for any such distinctions. Syncope may be considered, in a pathological point of view, as arising from two different sources,—imperfect supply of blood to the heart, and defect of nervous power: and in one or both of these ways it will be easy to understand the operation of the several predisposing and exciting causes of fainting, which systematic writers have enumerated.

A predisposition to fainting is given by original delicacy of organization. Hence it is so much more frequent among woman than men. Weakness of constitution, the result of long illness, or of

scanty nourishment, may be viewed in the same light. In conval-
escents from typhoid fevers, the exertion of getting out of bed is
often followed by a fit of syncope.

The most common exciting causes of a fainting fit in persons
otherwise in good health are, violent and long-continued exertion,
long continuence in the erect position, violent and protracted pain,
excessive evacuatious, whether of blood or by purging, external
heat, the sudden operation of a depressing passion, and in very delicate habits of body certain objects of dread and antipathy.

The treatment applicable to the state of syncope is very obvious
and simple, and, excepting in the case of syncope from flooding,
rarely, if ever, demands the exercise of professional skill. The
horizontal posture, a free current of cold air, sprinkling a little
cold water over the face, and hartshorn held to the nostrils, will
be sufficient to re-excite the circulation in common cases. In those
severe ones which are the consequence of excessive evacuations
of blood, the most powerful stimulants (ether and brandy) are often required, and an unremitted perseverance in them can alone
ensure the safety of the patient.

There are few sensations better known, and which create at the
same time more uneasiness, than that to which the term PALPITA-
TION is popularly applied ; it is not therefore surprising that pathologists should have directed so large a share of their attention towards it. By some it has been advanced to the rank of an *idiopathic* affection, and considered in the light of a *convulsion.* By others,
and certainly with more justice, it is viewed merely as a symptom,
arising from various causes, sometimes quite unimportant, but sometimes indicating, in conjunction with other symptoms, disease in
different parts. A few observations on the nature and sources of
palpitation may be of some assistance to the student with a view
to the diagnosis of disease, and the administration of remedies.

When the action of the heart becomes, from any cause, perceptible to the individual, he is said to have *palpitation.* Such irregular action may be either sharp and strong, when it is called *throbbing* of the heart ; or it may be soft and feeble, when it is called a
fluttering. The sensations of the patient are obviously to be aseri-
bed to the rebound of the heart against the inside of the chest.
With a view to practice, a distinction is to be drawn between *per-
m anent* and *occasional* palpitation. The former is always, or nearly
always, the result of organic disease existing within the chest, more
especially of water accumulated in the cavities of the pleura or pe-

ricardium, ossified valves, pericarditis acute and chronic, and its
consequences. The latter also may sometimes indicate structural
derangement, but is far more commonly the evidence merely of
sympathetic disturbance in the action of the heart. To this variety
of palpitation I confine my attention for the present.

1. Every one must be sensible of the influence of strong emotions and passions of the mind over the actions of the heart ; and
palpitation from such causes is very frequent. Dr. Cullen entertained the idea that this arose from the too rapid influx of nervous
power into the muscular fibres of the heart, but the notion is too
hypothetical to require discussion. Palpitation is frequently observed in persons of *irritable* habit, and is often connected with amenorrhœa, chlorosis, and hysteria, of which latter disease the *animus
various et mutabilis* constitutes so striking a feature. 2. Palpitation
is owing, secondly, to *a plethoric* state of the body, the heart labouring in its functions from over-distension of its cavities ; and
sometimes to preternatural increase in the velocity of the blood,
without augmented bulk, as where it is brought on by violent exercise. 3. It arises thirdly, from sympathy of the heart with a deranged condition of the abdominal viscera, and consequently is a
frequent symptom of dyspepsia, constipation, and diseased liver.
It is hardly consistent with sound pathology to attempt any more
precise explanation of this phænomenon, than what the term nervous sympathy suggests. 4. The last proximate cause of palpitation to which I shall allude, is weakness of the heart's action. It
seems to be a law of the human economy, that debility in the ex.
ercise of any function often produces temporary efforts at more vigorous exertion, and commonly in a convulsive manner. Hence it
is that syncope and palpitation are so often associated together.

It is hardly necessary to lay down any precise rules for the guidance of the student in the treatment of palpitation. An affection
arising from such various and even opposite causes, must be met
(where any treatment is required) by measures adapted to the particular circumstances of each case. I shall only advert to the
benefit experienced from taking away a small quantity of blood
from the arm, which, either as a means of temporary relief or of
permanent cure, generally deserves a trial. Where the stomach
is in fault, the decoction of aloes (R No. 32) is eminently serviceable. In that most common variety of palpitation which occurs to
delicate females from the age of fifteen to five-and-twenty, rest of

of body, quiet of mind, and a very temperate diet, are the chief means of relief in our power. Under this plan of management the complaint will generally subside in the course of a year or two.

***

ANGINA PECTORIS.

To a disease exhibiting many uniform and characteristic symptoms, and usually considered as depending on some chronic derangement in the heart, either functional or structural, Dr. Heberden, in 1768, gave the name of ANGINA PECTORIS.* Dr. Parry, of Bath, has treated of it fully, under the title of syncope anginosa.† In Dr. Cullen's nosology it has received no place, although it might readily have found one next to asthma, to which, in many of its characters, it bears a strong analogy. Modern writers have added but little to the observations of the distinguished author who first described this disease.

Angina pectoris consists of repeated paroxysms of violent pain or uneasiness about the chest, occurring principally when the patient is walking up hill, or soon after eating. The feeling of pain is so acute as to make him instantly stand still, and even to give the apprehension of immediate death ; it is referred to the sternum a little inclined to the left side ; from this point it shoots across the breast to the left arm, and appears to terminate at the elbow. In some cases it shoots to the right breast, and passes down the right arm in a similar manner. At first the paroxysms do not last more than a few minutes, and occur only at long intervals. Gradually they lengthen, and recur too with increased frequency ; being brought on, not only when the patient is walking, but when sitting or lying down, and by the slightest bodily exertions, or even anxiety of mind. The duration of the paroxysms has been, in some very severe cases, protracted to half an hour or more, the face and extremities becoming pale and bathed in a cold sweat, and the patient, for a while perhaps, deprived of the power of sense and voluntary motion.

The character of the pulse during the fit is apparently subject

***

* Transactions of the London College of Physicians, vol. ii, page 59. " Some Account of a Disorder of the Breast." By Dr. Heberden.

† Inquiry into the Symptoms and Causes of the Syncope Anginosa. 1799.

to considerable variety. Dr. Heberden found it sometimes, though far from uniformily, affected. Dr. Fothergill reports, that in his cases it was commonly intermitting or irregular. There is always some difficulty of breathing, or at least a distressing sense of *suffocation*, present at the same time ; and in the advanced periods of the disease the stomach becomes unusually irritable. Angina pectoris has been known to last for many years ; yet the prognosis is very unfavourable. In the larger proportion of cases it proves fatal *suddenly*, giving rise to the suspicion that apoplexy has taken place, or that the heart itself has given way, but which upon dissection nothing will appear to corroborate. The diagnosis has often been looked upon as a matter of considerable difficulty, but I think without sufficient reason. Angina pectoris derives it character from symptoms present during life, and not from any appearances found after death; and if the former are observed, the disease is at once entitled to such a denomination.

It has indeed been attempted by some pathologists to attach the peculiar symptoms of angina pectoris exclusively to an ossified state of the coronary vessels of the heart ; but this is taking too confined a view of the subject. More enlarged experience will show, that this state of disease is connected with several kinds of structural derangement within the thorax, though certainly this is the most frequent of them all ; but to prove that the restricted notions of the disease entertained by Dr. Parry and others are not correct, it is sufficient to state, that in many cases (and very remarkably in that described by Mr. H. Watson*) a most extensive ossification of the coronary arteries existed without giving rise to a single symptom of thoracic disease. Dr. Latham, in an interesting communication to the London College of Physicians,† has described two cases of enlarged liver, in which all the genuine symptoms of angina pectoris were observed. Both patients died suddenly.

But further, this disease has proved fatal where the most accurate anatomists have failed in detecting any morbid alteration of structure ; and it has been observed, during life, in combination with certain other symptoms denoting general constitutional disturbance,—such as are sometimes designated by the title of *flying gout*. Upon the whole, therefore, we must conclude, that angina

* Medical Communications, vol. i, p. 234.

† College Transactions, vol. i, p. 278. " Observations on the Angina Pectoris notha."

pectoris is, in strict pathology, a chronic functional derangement of the thoracic organs, frequently associated with, but not directly depending upon, disorganization of the heart.

The objects of medical treatment in this affection are limited to affording some degree of relief while the paroxysm is actually present, and to the avoiding as far as possible all those circumstances which occasion its renewal. With a view to immediate relief we have recourse to a small blood-letting, carminative draughts, and opiates. The more important object of preventing the gradual inroads of the disease upon the constitution, is to be attempted by strict attention to diet and regimen, the regular use of aromatic laxatives, and the insertion of an issue or seton. All practitioners agree in the benefit which is derived from using the lightest and most digestible food, with perfect abstinence from fermented and spirituous liquors. Even in the latter periods of a protracted paroxysm, when the prostration of strength appears extreme, we should hesitate in giving wine and cordials. The heart is here oppressed, not weakened.

Any thing that hurries the circulation is sufficient to bring on a paroxysm. The patient should therefore be cautioned to keep his mind quiet, and to refrain from all severe exercise. Flatus in the stomach and a torpid state of the bowels are so commonly found accompanying this disease, and either inducing or aggravating paroxysms of it, that the practitioner will do well to obviate, by the use of aromatics, bitters, and laxatives, any irregularity in the action of the chylopoietic viscera, which he may observe. Where sleep is interrupted, he may with propriety exhibit some narcotic —the extract of hyoscyamus for instance, or opium. Dr. Heberden says, that he has known opiates given at night, in many instances, prevent the accession of a paroxysm.

The symptoms occasioned by the several kinds of *structural* disease of the heart and great vessels, have been closely investigated by modern pathologists. Inquiries, however, have rather tended to show that they are obscure, than to establish their uniformity; and as the whole subject is one of curiosity more than of practical interest, I shall be very brief in my notices concerning it.

1. The simplest, and one of the most frequent structural derangements of the heart is dilatation, either general or partial, of

its cavities. This sometimes takes place without any increase in the muscular parietes of that organ. At other times the heart is enlarged by an addition of solid substance, cellular and muscular ; , its cavities remaining little, if at all, more capacious than usual. The symptoms vary according to the *nature* of the enlargement which the heart undergoes. Simple dilatation of its cavities (sometimes called aneurism of the heart) is attended with a sense of oppression about the chest, a full, slow, soft, occasionally even an *imperceptible* pulse. Persons have lived in this state for many years. The disease goes on, in almost all cases, to produce dropsy, and most remarkably dropsy of the pericardium, and consequently urgent dyspnœa. In somé instances chronic inflammation (with adhesion) of the pericardium supervenes a short time before death, when the character of the symptoms very essentially changes. Nothing is known regarding the causes of simple dilatation of the heart. It has been observed in young persons, without any disease of the valves, or other mechanical impediment to the transmission of blood. A disposition to it may be be traced in particular families.

2. Where the heart is enlarged by increase of its muscular parietes, the symptoms are nearly the same with those formerly described as attending chronic inflammation of the pericardium. To this affection the name of hypertrophy of the heart has been given. It is characterized by a *constant* sense of struggling in the thorax, with inexpressible anxiety referred to the heart. The pulse is quick, hard, and *jarring* ; and when the hand is applied to the chest, the stroke of the heart seems restrained, and is succeeded by a kind of *thrilling*. Such cases are truly deplorable, and much more formidable than those of simple dilatation. The bodily strength becomes rapidly exhausted, the faculties of the mind are overpowered, and the patient is debarred from every source of enjoyment. Dropsy commonly supervenes in this as in the former case.* The solid enlargement of the heart is believed to be always dependent upon some mechanical impediment to the free transmission of the blood, and is therefore often found united to a diseased state of the

* Consult Mr. Allan Burn's " Observations on some of the most frequent and important Diseases of the Heart." Edinburgh, 1809. To this work I am indebted for the attempt now made to establish the diagnosis between *active* and *passive* enlargement of the heart ; but it cannot be relied upon in all cases.

valves. This suggests the pathological principle (warranted certainly in many cases,) that in proportion to the resistance offered to the passage of the blood, the circulating powers have their strength augmented.

3. Much importance has always been attached by pathologists to the changes of structure which the valves of the heart and large arteries frequently undergo, and to the symptoms thereby occasioned. That in many cases diseased valves are the direct cause of various marks of obstructed circulation there can be no doubt ; but it is not to be forgotten, that they are often found where no symptoms had led to the suspicion of them. It is, I believe, quite impossible to ascertain with any degree of precision during life the existence of diseased valves, as separate from every other variety of disorganization of the heart. Still more hopeless is any attempt to determine what valve or set of valves are affected. The general symptoms of obstructed circulation by which we are led to form a plausible conjecture as to the existence of ossified valves, are, according to Dr. Baillie,* frequent palpitations, a difficulty of breathing, a weak and often irregular pulse, and in some cases a disposition to fainting. To these symptoms other authors have added, and I believe justly, hæmorrhage from the lungs, and dropsy.

4. Aneurism of the thoracic aorta is a frequent and most distressing state of disease. It can never be distinguished with any degree of certainty until it has attained to such a size that a tumour begins to be formed externally, accompanied with a strong pulsation. Dr. Baillie cautions us against supposing, that strong pulsation in the chest indicates necessarily *disorganization* of the heart or great vessels. Aneurism of the aorta is generally attended with more or less pain in the tumour, shooting to the arm of the same side ; and in proportion to the advances of the disease the breathing becomes disturbed. It sometimes proves fatal *suddenly* by the bursting of the sac, but in many cases the patient is destroyed more gradually by interruption to the respiration.

The unpleasant symptoms occasioned by aneurism of the aorta admit of very essential relief, and perhaps even the growth of the tumour is sometimes checked, by medicine. Repeated leeches to the chest have proved serviceable in many cases, and the application of cold to the tumour has been occasionally productive of advantage. Digitalis unquestionably possesses a very considerable

* Morbid Anatomy, p. 49.

50

power in moderating the urgent symptoms ; and if to the occasional employment of this drug be added a strict attention to diet and re-gimen, the patient may often pass the remainder of his days with tolerable ease.

5. Congenital malformations of the heart and large blood-ves-sels are of various kinds, and they have been ably described by Dr. Farre,* to whose work I beg to refer for the anatomical peculiari-ties of the several cases. They all agree in one result,—the inter-mixture of venous with arterial blood throughout the body. It is certainly a curious fact, that life should be compatible with such a state of the circulating system ; yet it is so, and persons have been known to live for many years with it, and even ultimately to die of a disease unconnected with such deviation from ordinary struc-ture.† The great source of mischief and danger, as Dr. Farre has pointed out, is not the mere mingling of black and red blood, but the *difficulty* with which the circulation is generally carried on by a malformed heart. This is connected, in many cases, with the comparatively small size of the pulmonary artery ; the consequence of which is, that the *full* proportion of blood is not circulated through the lungs.

The principal symptom of malformed heart is a permanent blue colour of the skin ; from which circumstance the term *blue disease, or cyanosis,* has commonly been applied to these cases. The oth-er symptoms to which it gives rise are general weakness of the whole frame, permanent or spasmodic dyspnœa, palpitation, an ir-regular, weak, or intermittent pulse, and in some cases coldness of the skin, and emaciation. Persons who have malformed hearts are liable to hæmorrhages, dropsical effusions, attacks of syncope or of epilepsy, and occasionally to the unequivocal symptoms of op-pressed brain.‡

* Pathological Researches by J. R. Farre, M. D. Essay i, on Malfor-mations of the human Heart. London, 1814.

† See Medico-Chirurgical Transactions, vol. xi, p. 296.

‡ See Appendix; Note X.

CHAP. V.

Extent and obscurity of the Doctrines connected with Asphyxia. Their Application to the Phenomena of Disease. Animal and Organic Life. Of the several Modes of Death. Sudden Death, beginning at the Lungs —at the Brain—at the Heart. Exemplified in the Cases of Drowning, Hanging, the Narcotic Poisons, Irrespirable Gases, Cold. Death by a more general Effect upon the System, instanced in the Case of Arsenic and Lightning. Of the immediate Causes of Death in Acute and Chronic Diseases.—Treatment of Cases of Suspended Animation. Effects and Application of Artificial Respiration.

THE term asphyxia (literally signifying want of pulse) has commouly been appropriated to those cases in which animation is for a time suspended, from some violent cause impeding respiration, such as strangulation, drowning, or exposure to mephitic gases; but in the present instance I propose to employ it in a much more extended sense. My intention is to include under this head all those investigations which are connected with sudden death, from whatever cause arising, and without reference to the possibility of subsequent reanimation. Asphyxia, in this acceptation opens a most extensive field of curious investigation, which on many accounts deserves the attention of the physician. Setting aside the importance of the *pathological* doctrines which it directly embraces, or to which it more distantly refers, it is interesting as being one of the most frequent subjects on which judicial examinations of medical men are required. It is no less important as connecting itself very intimately with the more familiar objects of medical inquiry. Asphyxia cannot be considered as a disease, but it is a state nearly allied to it, in which the sources of life and health are suddenly and violently invaded; the different kinds of sudden death being merely the simplest cases and the best illustrations of those termi·

nations of disease, which it is the object of the art of medicine to avert.*

It is hardly necessary to enumerate the many difficulties with which the subject of asphyxia is surrounded. From the remarks already offered, it must be seen to involve a number of the most abstruse questions both in physiology and pathology. To such inherent difficulties is doubtless to be attributed the neglect which asphyxia has experienced from the systematic writers of former times. Bichat, in his Essay on Life and Death, first placed the inquiry upon a scientific basis ; but much still remains to be done with regard to it, and that, without overstepping those boundaries which physical science ought always to prescribe to itself, in investigating the phænomena of life. Conscious of the difficulties, but aware of the importance of the subject, my endeavour will be to lay before the student such an *elementary* view of the leading principles which it embraces, as may enable him to appreciate more fully its bearings, and to prosecute the inquiry hereafter with a more definite understanding of its objects. The principal points to which my attention will be directed, are the causes of death from hanging, drowning, mephitic gases, lightning, and poisons ; the causes of sudden death which are independent of external agency ; the causes of death in acute and chronic diseases generally ; and the means of restoring suspended animation.

The foundation of almost all reasonings concerning asphyxia is laid in the mutual relations and connections of the three great organs of the body, the heart, the lungs, and the brain ; and the consequent division of the phænomena of the living system, into those of *organic* and *animal* life.* It will be sufficient for me here to remind the student, that the heart and arteries are the bases of all the operations of vitality, and the grand source therefore of *organic* life. Fœtuses have been born without a brain, but never without an arterial system. Next to circulation, the most important function in the body is respiration, because by it the *arterialization* of the blood is effected. The third in the series is the brain and nervous system, the origin of *animal* life, and necessary to respiration, inasmuch as that function is carried on by means of *sensations,*

---

* For much assistance in the composition of this chapter, I beg to express my obligations to Dr. Allison, Professor of the Theory of Physic in the University of Edinburgh.

† This great principle in physiology was partially known to some of the older authors, but was first fully developed by Bichat.

which in all cases depend upon a peculiar condition of the brain and nerves. Respiration, therefore, is the link uniting the phænomena of organic and animal life.

All sudden deaths are of one or other of the following kinds : 1. Death beginning at the lungs; 2. Death beginning at the brain ; 3. Death beginning at the heart ; 4. The simultaneous destruction of animal and organic life. The two first may be considered as modifications of each other ; and as they are the most usual modes by which death is effected, whether suddenly or in the progress of disease, they well merit a priority of discussion.

1. An accurate observation of nature will show, that in many kinds of death (well exemplified in that by suffocation) two distinct stages are perceptible. In the first, sensations, thought, and voluntary motions are destroyed. In the second, circulation and the organic functions cease. In common language, the term *life* is annexed to the presence of mental phænomena, and death to their absence. In a strictly physical sense, however, the body is said to be alive, so long as actions are going on in it, differing from any which chemical and mechanical principles can explain. In considering therefore the order in which the functions cease, we do not stop when we come to the cessation of all indications of mind, but we pursue the changes as long as any movements take place in the body inexplicable by such laws. In other words, the body is not pathologically considered as dead, until *organic* as well as *animal* life has ceased.

Many theories have been proposed to explain the mode by which *suffocation* proves fatal, and some of them obtained credit from their apparent simplicity. We are indebted to Bichat, however, for proving that the changes in *pure asphyxia* are more complicated than had generally been supposed. He distinctly ascertained that the heart continues to act *after* respiration has ceased ; that the left ventricle propels venous blood to all parts of the body ; that when a very few waves of unarterialized blood have circulated through the brain, insensibility takes place, and animal life ceases ; and, lastly, that the penetration of venous blood gradually destroys the action of the heart itself, and of every other contractile part through which it circulates. Death by pure asphyxia, therefore, is attributable to venous blood acting as a poison, first, upon the nervous, and secondly, upon the muscular textures of the body. Here animal life (with which suffering is connected) ceases before organic life, and doubtless this is a benevolent provision of nature.

That this is a correct description of the order in which the functions cease in asphyxia, will be rendered apparent by the following
considerations. In animals which have been made the subject of experiment, the heart has been seen contracting after the diaphragm
has ceased to move. Dark-coloured blood is found in the left side
of the heart and in the great arteries. The large veins on the *right*
side of the heart are always the most full of blood. The skin and
different other organs assume speedily a livid colour.

The principle in pathology now adverted to, admits of a further
illustration from what happens in a few cases of drowning, and
more frequently after exposure to carbonic acid gas. The action
of the heart is renewed, but insensibility continues, and the patient,
after remaining in a perfectly apoplectic state for some hours, dies.
In some instances, these comatose symptoms have subsided, and life
has been preserved. It is fairly presumable, that in cases of this
kind the quantity of venous blood which had circulated through the
brain, had been sufficient to injure seriously, though not totally to
destroy, the functions of the brain.

The sort of death that I have now described as beginning at the
lungs, takes place not only in hanging and drowning, but by cutting the spinal cord in the upper part of the neck, whereby the
muscles of respiration are paralysed, and by confining an animal
in vacuo, or in a simple irrespirable gas, such as nitrogen.

2. Death beginning at the brain is closely allied to that which
has been just explained. In this instance, the functions of the
brain cease first, sensibility, thought, and voluntary motion. Respiration, which is an action dependent upon sensibility, fails next.
The blood not being arterialized, the functions of the heart cease
as in the former case. The only difference between death beginning at the brain, and that by suffocation is, that the circulation of
black blood through the arteries is in the present instance the effect, and in the other the cause of the cessation of animal life.
This at least is one mode by which death takes place from causes
operating immediately on the brain. I shall hereafter have occasion to point out that it is not, as Bichat imagined, the only one.
It remains to state, that the first link in the chain of phænomena,
the cessation of animal life, is not always *instant* and *complete*,
Respiration, performed, it is true, slowly and with difficulty, sometimes continues after voluntary motion, and all other marks of sensibility, have ceased. This constitutes, as the student will at once
anticipate, the state of coma or apoplexy.

Instances of *sudden* death, beginning at the brain, occur in the cases of severe injuries to the head, epileptic fits ushering in the attack of small-pox, poisoning by opium, woorara, and the greater number of the narcotic poisons.

3. Sudden death beginning at the heart opens a field of inquiry not less interesting than that which has already engaged our attention. Here the order in which the functions terminate is reversed. The pulsations of the heart are first stopped ; and as the brain ceases to be excited by the stimulus of blood, sensation and voluntary motion and the mental phænomena gradually fail, and with them respiration and the contractile power of moving parts. In this case breathing is the latest act of life, and therefore here only can an animal, in strict pathological language, be said to *expire*.

There is an important principle in pathology involved in this consideration ; *viz.* that the mere cutting off the supply of arterial blood is not so detrimental to the brain, nor so speedily and certainly fatal, as the penetration of its substance by venous blood. This is the reason why persons recover so easily from fainting, even though sensation and thought be there as completely at a stand as in the case of a drowned man.

On opening the bodies of animals who are killed by some poison acting directly on the heart, *scarlet* blood is found in the left side of that organ, and the heart and large arteries appear turgid. The skin does not become livid as in death by suffocation. Very often, indeed, no perceptible change in the body takes place for many days. In most of these cases the blood is found *uncoagulated*, a phenomenon not yet satisfactorily explained.

Sudden death beginning at the heart occurs from the action of certain *poisons*, as the upas antiar, and tobacco ; in particular diseases affecting the heart, as angina pectoris ; apparently in some cases from a *paralytic* state of the heart, and lastly, from extreme cold. It is well known that animals exposed·to a certain degree of cold, perish. There is some doubt, however, as to the precise mode by which it destroys life. Some imagine that it operates by *coma* ; and others that it enfeebles, and ultimately checks altogether, the contractile power of the heart. In either case it merits great attention from the practitioner, being frequently associated as the cause of death with simple suffocation.

4. It might be imagined, that excessive hæmorrhage proves fatal by its suddenly checking the heart's action. But it has been shown that the heart continues to contract after all supply of blood to it

is cut off, and hæmorrhage therefore is the cause of death by a very obvious but more general effect upon the *whole* system. It is not indeed to be supposed that all cases of sudden death can be classed under one or other of the heads to which I have now adverted. Such a contracted view of the subject of asphyxia might tend rather to embarrass than to assist the inquiries of the student. He must be aware, that there are, fourthly, cases of sudden death in which all the powers of vitality are at once destroyed, or at least in which the functions of animal and organic life are so equally impaired, that it is impossible to ascertain the order of their cessation. Such cases are far from being rare. The most familiar instance which can be given is that of poisoning by *arsenic*, taken in large quantities. The same principle is exemplified where death takes place from lightning, and exposure to the vapours of sulphur; and lastly, it is occasionally in certain violent impressions made on the brain and spinal marrow, where death both of the heart and brain ensues instantaneously, without the intervention of the respiration.

Such are the modes by which the different kinds of sudden death are brought about; and the deviations from these, in the case of death from acute and chronic diseases, are not so great as might at first be imagined. If attention be paid to the series of symptoms, that mark the close of life, different sets of phænomena will present themselves. In one instance *dyspnœa* will be observed, followed by delirium and coma. As this becomes gradually more and more intense, respiration proportionably labours, and at length stops altogether; the extremities grow cold, and the heart ceases to beat. This is plainly death beginning at the lungs. It takes place in almost all diseases affecting the lungs primarily (most obviously in hydrothorax, vomica, and acute pneumonia,) and in many of those which affect the lungs secondarily, such as fever, smallpox, and measles.

In another instance *coma* occurs first, and the pulse often continues firm and unaltered in its character, and the extremities are warm, up to the period when respiration ceases, and when, in the common acceptation of the term, life is at a close. This mode of death (by coma) is witnessed in common cases of apoplexy, in hydrocephalus, phrenitis, and fevers complicated with local determination to the head.

The attentive observer will lastly have occasion to notice many cases where the first symptoms of approaching death are *feeble.*

ness of the pulse and *cold extremities*, respiration being still free, and the functions of the brain unimpaired. In such cases, it is not uncommon to find the mind perfectly clear, even up to the last breath which the patient draws. Here, in the language of the common people the patient is said *to die very hard.* It is unnecessary to say, that this is death beginning at the heart, in which no admixture of unarterialized blood overpowers the operations of the nervous system. Such a mode of death is often observed in those who labour under peritonæal inflammation affecting a *large surface* of the membrane, in the case of extensive and violent injuries inflicted upon any part of the body, in severe burns, in ileus, in organic affections of the stomach and other viscera, and I believe also in tetanus and hydrophobia. In all these instances, the heart appears to be affected *sympathetically.* This is one of the modes too, by which confluent small-pox proves fatal. We are, lastly, indebted to Mr. Chevalier,* for pointing out to us another occasion in which this mode of death takes place. It is where a woman dies soon after child-birth, especially of twins, without any great degree of hæmorrhage. Here the heart and whole system languish under the efforts of parturition. The blood is detained in the capillaries, and the heart ceases to contract from *exhaustion.*

The only case of disease which occurs to me as illustrating the contemporaneous destruction of the brain and heart is that of gangrene, which, like lightning, or arsenic, appears to overpower equally every part of the animal œconomy.

The last topic to which I proposed to advert was the treatment of genuine asphyxia. Animation is here considered to be only *suspended*, and from very early times a notion has prevailed that in such cases the powers of medicine might be signally displayed in the resuscitation of life. It must be obvious, however, to the student, that much caution is here required. While the doctrines connected with asphyxia are involved in such obscurity, it is impossible to suppose that our practice can or ought to be, regulated by the conjectures of persons, who, whatever be their claims to humanity, have none to physiological knowledge. In cases of such imminent danger as those of asphyxia, a measure not founded upon thorough acquaintance with the subject may very probably add materially to the danger of the patient, check those ill-understood efforts of nature, from which alone real benefit could have been de-

* Medico-Chirurgical Transactions, vol. i, p. 157.

51

rived, and thus tend only to *extinguish* the glimmering flame of life. When we find blood-letting, cold affusion, the warm bath, tobacco glysters, galvanism, and artificial respiration, recommended without discrimination in the treatment of asphyxia, it is obvious that no just understanding can exist of the nature of those changes which are taking place in the body, nor of the operation of each remedy. In the few remarks which I have now to offer on the management of persons in the state of asphyxia, I shall be careful not to exceed those limits which the present state of physiological science prescribes.

The first question that naturally occurs is, for how long a time may breathing be impeded, and the body remain susceptible of re-animation? Instances are recorded of the recovery of persons after being half an hour under water; but in a scientific investigation no credit can be given to such statements. It is confidently said, that even the most experienced divers of Ceylon cannot remain under water an entire minute; and it is therefore a reasonable supposition, that if respiration has ceased during three, or at furthest four minutes, life is irrecoverably lost.* It is probable that something depends on the *temperature* of the water. An animal immersed in a freezing mixture, but with the respiratory organs free, speedily dies. This suggests the important practical inference, that during the state of asphyxia the body is to be kept in a warm atmosphere: and here we may observe how closely the dictates of science correspond with those of common humanity.

The application of artificial respiration in cases of pure asphyxia, holds out, in every point of view, a reasonable prospect of success; and that it has been effectual in restoring suspended animation, numerous observations concur to assure us. Bichat maintained, but apparently on theoretical grounds only, that this operation can never restore circulation that has once ceased; in other words, that it is effectual only in those instances where the heart still pulsates, though carrying on a circulation of venous blood. According to the statement of persons worthy of credit, however, the action of this organ has been renewed by artificial respiration, after all marks of it had *wholly* ceased; and here it is probable that the left side of the heart, which could no longer be excited to contrac-tion by venous blood, was stimulated by blood which had been ren-

* Dr. Davy informs me, that he has not been able to recover dogs that have been under water *two* minutes, even by means of artificial respiration and galvanism employed immediately.

dered arterial. Mr. Brodie has shown, that this process will support circulation for many hours in small animals, even after the
complete destruction of animal life by cutting off the head. We
should thus be encouraged to persevere in its employment so long
as any marks of pulsation in the heart remain, under the hope that
the brain may gradually be restored from that state of *oppression*
into which it was thrown by the influx of venous blood. Artificial
respiration, therefore, appears well adapted to those cases of apoplexy succeeding asphyxia, to which I formerly referred. Reasoning from these principles, Mr. Brodie has conjectured, that artificial respiration might be successfully applied in the case of animation suspended by opium, woorara, and such other narcotic poisons
as operate first upon the brain, and through it upon the respiration.
Some experiments recorded in the Phil. Trans. for 1812, give
countenance to this expectation.

From the preceding remarks it will be obvious that artificial respiration is wholly inapplicable to those numerous instances of sudden death which *begin at the heart.* Scarlet blood is here already
present in its left cavities, and means of relief for such cases, if any
exist, must be sought for elsewhere. In the same manner, it will
not be difficult to convince the student how great is the danger
which attends an indiscriminate employment of tobacco glysters,
and cold affusion. These have a direct power in checking the
heart's action, and must, in a great majority of cases of asphyxia,
be positively injurious. Galvanism holds out a better prospect of
advantage ; but the experiments hitherto made with the view of determining the kind and degree of influence which it possesses, are
not sufficiently accurate to induce me to hazard any decided opinion of its value.

The opening of a vein has been frequently resorted to, both in
the asphyxia of drowned persons, and in that which arises from the
inhalation of carbonic acid gas. In the former case, if a flow of
blood can be obtained, the operation may possibly be useful, by
relieving the oppressed state of the heart and great vessels. In
the latter case, great caution is required, as we may gather from
the experience of Dr. Babington, recorded in the Medico-Chirurgical Transactions.[*] The remarks of this author on the state of
asphyxia, and the remedies proposed for its relief, are well deserving the attention of the student.

[*] Vol. i, p, 83, "Case of Exposure to the Vapour of burning Charcoal."
1806.

CLASS III.

CHRONIC DISEASES OF THE CHYLOPOÏETIC VISCERA.

CHAP. I.

DYSPEPSIA.

Frequency of dyspeptic Complaints. Symptoms of dyspepsia. Physiological considerations connected with Digestion. Dyspepsia, primary and secondary. Exciting Causes of primary Dyspepsia. Sympathies of the Stomach. Varieties of secondary Dyspepsia. Prognosis. Principles of Treatment. Diet, Regimen, and Medicine. Other morbid Affections of the Stomach. Spasm. A state of continued Vomiting. Decay of Nature. Scirrhous Pylorus. Erosions of the Stomach.

INDIGESTION is certainly the most frequent of all diseases. It is met with in every country, in every class of society, in every season of the year. Devoid of the danger which attends other diseases, it is nevertheless equally distressing to the patient, poisoning all the sources of his enjoyment, and leading, in many instances, to the miseries of confirmed hypochondriasis. Long as it has been made the subject of inquiry by medical authors, it remains involved in much obscurity. The pathology of the disease is little understood ; the method of its treatment is still imperfectly known ; and the most remarkable diversities of opinion are entertained regarding the extent to which it influences the production of other disorders. On these various accounts, indigestion may justly lay claim to a full and accurate investigation.

By dyspepsia, in its most precise sense, physicians understand that state of the stomach, in which its functions are disturbed, without the presence of any other disease. In practise, however, it will be found impossible to restrict the meaning of the term within such narrow limits. The stomach being one of the great centres of the system, its functions are more or less disturbed in every disorder to which the human body is subject ; and thus to confine the acceptation of dyspepsia, would be to presuppose our knowledge of the diagnostic features of many very obscure forms of disease. It will be sufficient, therefore, to limit the term dyspepsia to those cases in which the functions of the stomach are impaired, without the presence of well-marked general fever, of local inflammation in the organ itself, or of any very obvious *cognizable* disease in a distant part. So far from indulging a too strict adherence to nosological accuracy, it will be advisable to acknowledge a distinction between *primary* and *secondary* dyspepsia. In the latter case the dyspeptic symptoms, though in reality secondary, yet often occupy the first place in the mind of the patient, those of the distant organ being either very obscure, or but little troublesome, or manifesting themselves only in the *progress* of the disorder.

The symptoms of dyspepsia are extremely diversified. They may be divided into such as are referable to the stomach itself, or to its sympathies with other parts of the body, especially the colon, kidneys, heart and lungs, brain, and nervous system. Among the first may be enumerated, nausea, pain in the epigastrium or hypochondria, called *gastrodynia*, heart-burn or cardialgia, a sense of fulness, distension, or weight in the stomach, a feeling as if a ball were lodged in the œsophagus, acid or fœtid eructations, pyrosis, or the vomiting of a clear liquor, sometimes of an acid quality and often in vast quantity, a sensation of *sinking* or fluttering at the pit of the stomach, and lastly loss of appetite. To the second head of dyspeptic symptoms may be referred, among many others, costiveness, or an irregular state of the bowels, with a morbid appearance of the evacuations, pain of the back and turbid urine, a disagreeable taste in the mouth, especially on first waking, tooth-ache —palpitation, pulsation in the epigastrium, irregularity of the pulse, a short dry cough, and occasional difficulty of breathing,—giddiness, and head-ache, sometimes referred to the fore, but more commouly to the back part of the head,—languor, lassitude, and great depression of spirits, with fear of death, or of impending evil, in one word, hypochondriasis. These last evidences of affection of the nervous system indicate a very aggravated state of the disease, and the probability of a protracted recovery.

The tongue is generally referred to as affording evidence of the state of the stomach ; but it will often be found that the tongue is perfectly clean when the stomach is most incontestably disordered.

It would seem, indeed, as if the morbid appearances of the tongue (its fur, dryness, præternatural redness and smoothness, and its chapped aspect) and referable to the state of the constitution rather than to any particular derangement in the stomach. When, however, we observe the tongue *furred and moist* (its true character in common dyspepsia,) that is to say, when the secretions of the mouth are depraved, we may reasonably presume that there exists a similarly disordered state of the *secretions* of the stomach.

In adults, dyspepsia occasionally produces a state of ephemeral feverishness. In infants this is very commonly observed, and it often increases to a state of high and formidable excitement. Very anomalous pains, too, sometimes arise from simple dyspepsia, but these it is obviously impossible to specify.

In order to form a just idea of the connection of these various symptoms with a disordered state of the functions of the stomach, —to illustrate the modes in which the several exciting causes of the disease, hereafter to be mentioned, operate,—still more with the view of explaining how dyspepsia becomes so frequently a concomitant or cause of local disease in a distant part, we must advert to a few facts connected with the physiology of the stomach.

There appear to be three important stages in the process of digestion. The first of these is an intimate mixture of the food with certain *fluids* of the body, particularly the saliva, and secretions of the stomach. It is probable that these have a higher office than merely lubricating the coats of the first passages, and moistening the morsel of food; but physiologists are not agreed as to their exact operation. The notion of a *chemical* solution of the food in the gastric juice is still entertained by some; but it is at variance with the results of chemical analysis. It is not unreasonable to believe, that the animal fluids act to a certain degree as *ferments*, approximating the food taken in to their own nature, by means peculiar to the operations of life, but analogous, as we may presume, to some acknowledged chemical phænomena.

The second important step in the function of digestion is the detention of the food for a certain length of time in the cavity of the stomach, in which stage of the process the food is brought by degrees into contact with its coats, and exposed to the influence of its *nerves*. Here that peculiar vital action is exerted upon the food which renders digestion so totally different from a chemical operation, and which actually suspends ordinary chemical agency. In this stage of digestion too it appears that the food is reduced to its proper consistence as to *fluidity*, the absorbents of the stomach rap-idly removing any superabundant fluid, and thirst being excited when the gastric secretions are insufficient for the due moistening of the mass.

The third step in the progress of digestion is the propulsion of the chyme into the duodenum, where it becomes mixed with the bile and pancreatic juice. The length of time during which the aliment remains in the stomach has never been very accurately de-termined. It probably varies in different individuals, according to the *energy* of the stomach, and in the same individual at different times, according to the nature of the food, and its greater or less facility of digestion. From three to four hours is perhaps the ave-rage. At the end of this period, the pyloric orifice, which had previously been closed, gradually dilates, so as to allow the mass of food to pass in the duodenum, the stomach remaining perfectly empty until the next meal. In the duodenum the chyme, mixing with the bile and pancreatic juice, certainly remains a considera-ble time, and changes in it there take place which are necessary to the full completion of digestion. The important influence of this organ has procured for it the appropriate name of *ventriculus succenturiatus*.

From this brief statement of the steps in the progress of diges-tion, we shall be prepared to give an explanation of the several modes in which dyspepsia may be brought about.

1. It may depend in the first place, upon a morbid state of the *glands* subservient to digestion. The saliva may be deficient,—the gastric juice may be either deficient, or secreted in too large quantity, or vitiated in quality, whereby the coats of the stomach become enveloped with a thick tenacious mucus.* Lastly, the bile may get into the stomach, and there interfere with the *first* steps in the digestive process.

2. Dyspepsia may arise from a morbid condition of the *nerves* of the stomach,—or from general torpor, or defect of the *whole* ner-vous system.

3. Dyspepsia may in some cases be owing to such morbid states of the *muscular* coat of the stomach as cause the food to be detain-ed too long there, or which hurry it too soon into the bowels.

---

* This appears to take place in some cases of dyspepsia connected with pregnancy, but certainly not in all. Occasionally such a state of the stom-ach would seem to depend upon a low degree of inflammatory action.

4. Dyspeptic symptoms, lastly, may originate, independant of all disease in the stomach, from the functions of the duodenum being imperfectly performed. Morbid accumulation in the duodenum is justly reckoned the immediate cause of that pain high up in the back which sometimes accompanies, but it is often observed independent of the more common dyspeptic symptoms.

All practitioners must acknowledge the necessity of distinctions among the numerous cases of dyspepsia ; but great difficulties have been experienced in establishing any which may have a practical application. Dr. Pemberton* attempted to found a division of dyspeptic cases upon the *pathological considerations* which I have just adverted to ; but though we may acknowledge, in theory, an independent affection of the *glands*, the *nerves*, and the *muscles* of the stomach, yet, in practice, it will be found impossible to trace their diagnostic symptoms, or to ground upon such views any important differences of treatment.

The older nosologists almost uniformly agreed in looking upon *symptoms* as the best ground-works of distinction among dyspeptic cases, the most prominent being pain, vomiting, flatulence, and loss of appetite. The views now taken of the theory of indigestion may assist in explaining these symptoms. Gastrodynia, or acute pain in the stomach, is sometimes owing to inflammation of its mucous coat, but more commonly to the excessive acrimony of the gastric secretions. Pyrosis, or the water brash, indicates the *irritable* state of the stomach. Flatulence is the opposite condition, marking loss of tone, the lodgment of food, and consequent fermentation. Lastly, anorexia, or loss of appetite, indicates the total failure in the supply of nervous influence. Such distinctions as these, however, are ill calculated as indications for the permanent cure of the complaint. All they can do is occasionally to guide the practitioner in the employment of measures of temporary relief. With a view to practice, I have always felt the absolute necessity of paying attention to the *causes* of the affection ; and there can surely be no better basis of distinction, than such as is fitted to facilitate treatment. The causes of dyspepsia therefore are next to be investigated.

There are undoubtedly persons who possess, and perhaps, even inherit *constitutional weakness* of the stomach ; but such a predisposition to indigestion is happily not common, and being altogether

* Practical Treatise on various Diseases of the abdominal Viscera. 1814, p. 99.

beyond the reach of art, may without impropriety be discarded from our present consideration. It remains, then, only that the *exciting* causes of the primary form of dyspepsia be enumerated, and the following will, I believe, be found the most important.

Tabular View of the Varieties of primary Dyspepsia.

1. Dyspepsia from occasional overloading of the stomach.
2. ————— from habitual overfeeding.
3. ————— from habitual indulgence in spirituous liquors.
4. ————— from want of air and exercise.
5. ————— from excessive or long-continued evacuations.
6. ————— from cold.
7. ————— from anxiety of mind.

1. The first and most simple cause of dyspepsia is the occasional *overloading* of the stomach ; or the taking in of some indigestible substance, which, even in small quantity, offends the nerves of the stomach such as tainted meat ; or, lastly, an accidental debauch of wine. This form of dyspepsia is commonly attended with a sense of oppression at the stomach, *nausea*, and that peculiar species of headache called the *megrim*. It is carefully to be distinguished from every other, because it demands a particular mode of treatment.

2. The second cause of dyspepsia is habitual full living, particularly the too *frequent* indulgence in animal food. This is one of the most common sources of dyspepsia in the upper classes of society, and is easily distinguished from all others by its occurring along with *gout*.

3. The third is the abuse of spirituous liquors. This is the prolific source of dyspepsia in the lower ranks of life, in comparison with which all the other causes of the disease are of little importance. Dyspepsia from this cause is often a very *severe*, and always an obstinate complaint. It is attended in most cases with a very acute pain in the region of the stomach (*gastrodynia*,) and tenderness of the epigastrium. It may be distinguished also by the trembling hand which never fails to accompany it. This and the preceding form of dyspepsia may so far be considered as connected, as the remedy for the disease is in both cases obvious ; and as any plan of treatment, which does not make the removal of the exciting cause an indispensable condition, will be either ineffectual, or serve only in the end to aggravate the evil.

4. The fourth cause of indigestion is the want of air and exercise. Torpor and inactivity of the body naturally extend their in-

52

fluence to internal organs, and the stomach is the first to suffer. Hence it is that dyspepsia is the frequent concomitant of a sedentary profession, and that it prevails not only among the luxurious and dissolute, but amongst the most industrious and sober classes of the community. Distension of the stomach by wind, particularly after meals, eructations, and a torpid state of the bowels, usually prevail, and constitute the *urgent* symptoms in this form of the complaint. To a certain extent it admits of relief by remedies, but the least irregularity of diet is often sufficient to renew the unpleasant symptoms.

5. Another cause of primary dyspepsia may be found in excessive evacuations, such as flooding, and large bleedings at the arm; or in more moderate evacuations, if long continued, as for instance, leucorrhœa, or protracted suckling. The practice of keeping strong children at the breast for a year and a half or two years is very common in the lower orders in this country, and leads, particularly in weak habits, to some of the most distressing forms of dyspepsia which are ever witnessed. The peculiar characters of this variety of dyspepsia are a sense of *sinking* at the pit of the stomach, giddiness, dimness of sight, a feeling of different objects dancing before the eyes, and a *small*, often *imperceptible* pulse. It admits of very essential relief from medicine.

6. In the next place, dyspepsia may be traced in very many cases to the influence of cold and moisture. The general effect of cold, when long continued, is to depress the nervous power, and this is often manifested in the temporary loss of the functions of the stomach. Hence it happens that dyspeptic ailments are so frequently met with when the cold weather first sets in. This kind of dyspepsia may usually be distinguished by the thirst, the restlessness, the white tongue, and other marks of general though slight febrile disturbance which attend it. Its usual duration, when left to itself, is about three weeks or a month; and though several of the concomitant symptoms admit of essential relief by medicine, yet its course (in those weakly habits in which it commonly occurs) can seldom be much shortened. The symptom that most attracts the notice of the patient, and for which he specially solicits the aid of the physician, is loss of appetite (*anorexia*.)

7. The last source of primary dyspepsia which requires notice, is mental emotion, particularly the depressing passions, fear, grief, but above all *anxiety*. This, though very common, can only so far become a practical consideration, as it may lead to the propriety of

recommending, in some cases, change of air, of scene, and of habits, as essential to recovery. That such a cause is operating may
generally be inferred from the circumstance of the dyspeptic symptoms continuing for a great length of time uninfluenced by medical
treatment.

The various *sympathies* of the stomach have frequently been described, and every one is sensible of the intimate connection of
dyspepsia with local disease in other parts. In many of these instances the affection of the stomach has been viewed as the primary complaint, upon the principle that such states of local disease are
best combated by remedies which *apparently* act on the stomach.
It has been well observed, however that when a disordered state of
the digestive organs, and local disease in a remote part, are concomitant, they may be but effects of some distant and unknown irritation, perhaps proceeding from the nervous system. The medicine therefore which *appears* to act beneficially on the local disease, through the medium of the digestive organs, may in fact
operate by correcting that more *general* derangement of the health,
of which, disorder of the chylopoietic viscera is but one of the effects.

Tabular View of the Varieties of secondary Dyspepsia.

1. Dyspepsia symptomatic of habitual constipation.
2. ———— of chronic disease of the liver.
3. ———— of chronic disease of the spleen.
4. ———— of functional disturbance of the uterus.
5. ———— of obscure disease of the kidney.
6. ———— of chronic affections of the bronchia.
7. ———— of chronic cutaneous diseases.

1. Dyspepsia is in many instances accompanied by a costive
state of the bowels, to which, when present, the patient himself is
generally disposed to refer all his symptoms. The student, however, will remember, that the functions of the stomach and great
intestines are very different, and that disturbances in them are by
no means necessarily associated. Costiveness frequently exists
without indigestion, and dyspepsia without constipated bowels. The
contrary indeed sometimes happens ; but whenever habitual costiveness is the *direct cause* of dyspeptic symptoms, the circumstance
will generally be made manifest by the hardness or fulness of the
abdomen, and by those inquiries into the present and *previous* state
of the alvine evacuations which the practitioner will in no instance

fail to make. 2. In some cases dyspepsia will be found dependent upon chronic diseases of the liver; but assuredly not to the extent which is frequently imagined. When a defective or vitiated state of the bile, that is to say, *functional* disturbance of the liver, exists; still more, when structural disease of that organ is present, accurate investigation will commonly lead to the detection of some of those symptoms formerly enumerated as *characteristic* of hepatic affections. 3. There can be little doubt, that dyspepsia, is in certain instances, symptomatic of an affection of the spleen. It would be contrary to all analogy to suppose that this organ is not subject to some primary forms of disease; but very little appears to be known concerning them. Dr. Bree has described an affection of this kind,* which he imagines to consist in a *congestive* state of the vessels of the spleen. It is probable, that an acquaintance with the physiology of the spleen might enable us to separate and refer to their true source some other cases now classed under the general head of dyspepsia. The peculiar symptoms of *splenic* dyspepsia, as far as I have been able to trace them, are fulness and sense of weight in the region of the spleen (without corresponding flatulence,) a sallow countenance, loaded tongue, and occasional hæmorrhages. It chiefly occurs in young women, particularly in female servants who have over-exerted themselves, and is very obstinate and difficult of cure. 4. Dyspepsia is a frequent concomitant of disturbance in the uterine functions. It is a leading symptom in chlorosis and hysteria, and is well known as one of the earliest evidences of pregnancy. This form of the disease is easily distinguished from all others by the *habit of body* in which it occurs. Vomiting of the food half an hour after it has been taken (marking the great degree of irritability prevailing in the stomach) will generally be found characteristic of *uterine* dyspepsia. 5. Indigestion is a well-marked symptom in diseases affecting the kidney, the *local* evidences of which are often very obscure. Hence it is that the original complaint is sometimes overlooked; but the error is fortunately of no material importance. 6. The functions of the stomach are frequently impaired in chronic affections of the bronchia, and this complication of a disease is very formidable particularly in old people. 7. A remarkable connection has long been observed between dyspepsia and several varieties of chronic cutaneous dis-

* Medico-Chirurgical Transactions, vol. ii, p, 84, " On painful Affections of the Side from tumid Spleen;" also vol. iii, p. 155.

ease ; but this is chiefly deserving of notice as it bears upon the pathology of the latter affections.

Such are the most important distinctions which I have been enabled to trace among the several kinds of dyspeptic complaints. Their variety may, perhaps, at first, occasion some embarrassment to the student ; but experience has assured me, that an imperfect investigation of the subject would be productive even of greater difficulties. Before entering on the treatment of dyspepsia, a few observations may be useful with reference to prognosis.

In all forms of dyspepsia the prognosis is, favourable ; even though of very long continuance it does not appear to induce any serious or permanent mischief. In particular habits it gives rise to, or aggravates, calculous disorders ; but there seem to me no just grounds for the notion entertained by a late author,* that it lays the foundation of *organic* diseases in distant parts, particularly in the lungs. The view which has been taken of its exciting causes will show that some cases admit only of temporary relief, but by far the larger proportion of dyspeptic patients may, by moderate attention to diet, medicines, and the regimen of mind and body, be permanently and effectually cured.

It is unnecessary to say, that there is no one drug which will fulfil the great object of treatment, that of giving *tone* to the weakened stomach of a dyspeptic patient. This can be obtained only by measures calculated to avert the *cause* which may have excited the disease. The tone of the stomach never fails without some *assignable* reason, which strict inquiry will detect, and the knowledge of which will point out the proper means of relief. Nor is it often that these will fail of success, provided the patient have sufficient firmness to submit to them, and afterwards remain sensible that his health is in his own hands. The assistance of the physician, however, is very often required where the patient either *cannot* or *will not* submit to the measures which prudence dictates. In such circumstances we must endeavour to aid the digestive process by *medicines ;* but I would wish to impress upon the student the impropriety of trusting to them in dyspeptic cases. He should remember, that almost any drug will injure digestion in a healthy state, and learn from hence to be sparing of medicine when the stomach is weakened by disease.

* Dr. Wilson Philip, in his " Treatise on indigestion and its Consequences." London, 1821.

In every form of dyspepsia attention to diet is *indispensable*, and the patient must have regard, not to its quality only, but to its quan. ty. In a weakened state of the stomach it must have little given it to do. The body is strengthened, not in proportion to the quantity of food taken in, but to that which is *thoroughly* digested. Diffe. rences in the habits of life will of course lead to important diffe. rences in the *kind* and quantity of diet which should be permitted to a dyspeptic patient; but the following may be regarded as rules of very general application. It should consist in a due mixture of animal and vegetable food, but the former should be eaten only *once* a day. It should be thoroughly masticated. Great varieties of food at any one time should be prohibited, as leading to an in. dulgence of the appetite beyond the wants of the system. Arti. cles of difficult digestion should be carefully avoided; such as all kinds of smoked, hard, dried, salted, and long-kept meat; all those dishes where too much nutritious matter is collected in a small space; eggs, for instance, potted meats, strong soups, and prepara. tions of suet, fat, and butter; lastly, all raw vegetables whatever, with the exception of ripe fruits. Regularity in the hours of meals should be rigorously enjoined, and the patient directed to abstain from food at *all other times*.

Of the necessity of regular exercise to the due performance of the functions of the stomach, every one must be fully sensible. Walking is of all exercises the best. It is that which nature intends for us, and can never be compensated by what are called the *pas. sive exercises* of the luxurious. Pure air is eminently conducive to healthy digestion.

The objects to be kept in view in the treatment of primary dys. pepsia are, first, to free the stomach from offending materials, se. condly to improve the tone or energy of the stomach, and thirdly to relieve painful and distressing sensations. The medicines cal. culated to fulfil these several intentions are emetics, purgatives and laxatives, bitters and stimulants, absorbents, mercurial al. teratives, and narcotics. I proceed to point out to what cases each of these classes of medicines applies, and upon what principles they may be supposed to act. Much of what is important in regard to treatment resolves itself into the avoiding of *exciting causes*; but it is necessary also to keep in view the duration of the disease, or the difference between *occasional* and *habitual* dyspepsia. Lastly at. tention is to be paid to the degree of *strength* in the patient's gene. ral habit.

1. In the *acute*, or occasional dyspepsia, the object is to free the stomach at once from offending matters, and afterwards to permit it gradually to recover its tone. Where full vomiting has not taken place by the efforts of nature, the emetic draught No. 1, may be given, followed the next morning by the purging draught, No. 21. This is one of the cases of dyspepsia to which emetics are applicable. Their frequent use is undoubtedly to be condemned, as weakening the tone of the stomach and ultimately increasing the disease ; but it is right to know that long continued atony of the stomach leads to the collection of thick and vitiated mucus there, which sometimes renders necessary the aid of a gentle emetic.

2. Occasional brisk purgatives, such as the draught now recommended, or that containing rhubarb (R No. 18,) or the powder No. 12, and pills No. 7, will be found highly advantageous in dyspeptic cases which are not of long standing and which occur in persons of robust habit. Half an ounce of Epsom salts in two ounces of warm water, or the draught No. 20, is often sufficient to carry off a mild attack of the complaint. Where any considerable degree of feverishness exists (provided the stomach be not *irritable*,) much advantage will be derived from the strong cathartic pills, R No. 6. Calomel, as a purgative, is well adapted to *sudden* attacks of dyspepsia in persons not habitually liable to it. In weakened habits it frequently irritates the stomach and aggravates the symptoms.

3. Laxatives in small doses, just sufficient to keep up a gentle peristaltic motion through the whole alimentary canal, are highly serviceable in *common* or habitual dyspepsia. Rhubarb in conjunction with an aromatic (as in R No. 35,) given a short time before a meal, is useful to persons of weak stomach and sedentary occupation, by preventing a lodgment of food in the stomach and deodenum after the first processes of digestion are over. With the same view the tonic aperient draughts (R Nos. 33 and 34,) or the pills (Nos. 28 and 36,) may be administered.

4. Bitters, astringents, stomachics, aromatics, and other stimulating medicines, known under the general denomination of *tonics*, have been extensively employed in cases of dyspepsia ; but they too frequently disappoint the expectations of the physician. It must be recollected, that even the lightest bitters (camomile, orange-peel, or gentian) are stimulant and *heating*, and therefore wholly inapplicable to those numerous cases of dyspepsia which are connected with a *feverish* and *irritable* habit of body. The following plain maxims for the employment of such medicines may perhaps

be of some use. Bitters are adapted to those forms of dyspepsia
in which the tone of the stomach has been weakened by previous
disease, or by long and severe evacuations. When pyrosis is the
urgent symptom, astringents are often serviceable such as the pulvis kino compositus in doses of ten grains three times a day. In
that kind of dyspepsia which arises from the habitual use of spirituous liquors, bitters are sometimes borne, but the gentler stimulus
of an acid is often preferable. In that species of dyspepsia which
occurs to women who have suckled an infant too long, recourse
must be had to the more powerful of the class of tonics. The mistura ferri composita, in doses of ten drachms three times a day, is
very efficacious in such cases, a gentle emetic powder being first
premised, to clear the stomach of tenacious mucus. Bark and the
aromatic confection may be substituted, as in R No. 71. The volatile alkali is useful under the same circumstances, and may be administered in the form No. 79. When pain is occasioned by taking any thing *warm* into the stomach, the aromatic confection (R
No. 61) is singularly beneficial. Where languor and the feeling
of sinking at the stomach are very urgent, we may direct a tea-
spoonful of the cordial drops (R No. 80) to be given occasionally ;
or, without the formality of a prescription, some ginger may be
taken at the time of a meal. The power of any stimulant in promoting digestion *to a certain extent*, is well known, and may legitimately be turned to advantage in the treatment of dyspepsia.

In that variety of dyspepsia which occurs about the beginning of
winter, and which is probably owing to the influence of a reduced
temperature upon the body, a mixed plan is requisite. The treatment should commence by an emetic, followed by two or three
doses of purgative medicine ; after which some aromatic and bitter aperient, as an infusion of cascarilla and rhubarb (R No. 34)
should be taken, and persevered in for two or three weeks. The
compound decoction of aloes (R No. 32) and the formula No. 78,
carrying with it a drachm of the sulphate of magnesia, are also
well adapted to this state of disease.

5. Absorbents, as lime-water, magnesia, and the carbonate of soda, may be combined with other medicines (as in R Nos. 33 and
75) where heartburn and acid eructations are particularly distressing ; but it must be remembered, that their good effects are always
transitory, and often precarious, and that they can never be relied
on for the *permanent* removal of the disorder.

6. Mercurial preparations are frequently resorted to in *simple*

dyspepsia; not as purgatives, but in small doses, for their specific, or, as it is said, *alterative* effect upon the secretions of the body. Three grains of the blue pill, given at bed time certainly prove serviceable in some obstinate cases, especially where the stools are clay-coloured ; but it is difficult to define otherwise under what circumstances such a plan of treatment is *essentially* required.

7. There are, lastly, certain medicines employed for the cure of dyspepsia, whose agency is apparently upon the nervous system. Of these I may first specify the oxyd of bismuth given in the quan. tity of five grains three times a day, with ten of the compound pow- der of tragacanth ; the sulphate of zinc in small doses, and the hy- drocyanic acid. They deserve a trial in severe and obstinate cases. Opium, or the extract of hyoscyamus, are requisite when the sto- mach is very irritable, or when severe pain is complained of. I have never observed however that opium possesses that decided power of checking inordinate secretion of the gastric juice which Dr. Pemberton attributed to it. Blisters applied to the pit of the stomach are often useful where there is much pain with disposition to vomiting.

Such are the most important of the means by which we attempt the relief and cure of *primary* dyspepsia. They are equally appli- cable to all the secondary varieties of the same affection ; but are then, of course, to be adopted in union with other measures which the nature of the original disease suggests.

As a sequel to this account of dyspepsia, I shall notice certain affections of the stomach, closely allied to it, but which appear to have something peculiar in their pathology.

1. Spasm of the stomach is a disease of very rare occurrence, but of formidable character. Its attack is sudden and attended with acute pain. It generally arises from some error in diet, and is, for the most part, connected with that ill-defined state of con- stitution, called the *gouty diathesis*. The remedies on which we are to place reliance, *in the first instance*, are ether, laudanum, wine, brandy, and aromatics, taken internally ; and fomentations or stim- ulating epithems to the epigastrium.

2. Dr. Pemberton was, I believe, the first to describe a disease of the stomach, characterized by *incessant vomiting*, unattended by

53

pain, or any symptoms of diseased structure in the organ itself.[*] It has frequently *proved fatal*, and the cause of the disease has remained, in many instances, undiscovered after dissection. I believe it to be, in all cases, symptomatic of some obscure affection in a distant organ. In a case that fell under my own observation, it appeared to depend upon a morbid condition of the ovarum. In another, described in the Medical Communications,[†] it was connected with a diseased state of the kidney. D. Baillie has described[‡] a similar affection of the stomach, in which this organ throws up a fluid like cocoa, in large quantity, a quart perhaps at a time, and perhaps for many days together. This fluid is a diseased secretion from the inner coat of the stomach, and the disease is sometimes (though not invariably) connected with a diseased state of the liver. In some instances it proved fatal. According to Dr. Baillie's experience, it is but little influenced either by diet or medicine. The tincture of kino or catechu with laudanum afforded some relief, with the aid of an occasional mild aperient.

3. In some cases the stomach loses, almost entirely and very rapidly, the power of digestion. The only complaint of the patient is want of appetite (*anorexia.*) He becomes pale and emaciated, and appears as if affected by some fatal visceral disease. Dr. Baillie informs us, that some of these cases have been completely restored to health by a course of the Bath waters, but in most instances the disease proceeds to a fatal termination, cough and delirium coming on as it advances. It is one of the most striking evidences of that general state of constitutional weakness which is known to the world under the name of the *decay of nature.*

4. The most dangerous, however, of all the diseases of the stomach, is that of organic læsion of its coats. Ulcers of the stomach (sometimes partaking of a cancerous nature,) stricture of the cardiac orifice, and scirrhus of the pylorus, are the common appearances on dissection. The symptoms will, of course, vary with the situation of the organic disease. In the case of scirrhous thickening and consequent *stricture* of the pylorus, the symptoms are pain, often very acute, shooting to the back, and aggravated by taking food; vomiting, generally occurring from one to three hours after a meal, the matter rejected being for the most part dark-co.

* Diseases of the abdominal Viscera, page 132.
† Vol. i, page 127.
‡ Lectures and Observations on Medicine, London, 1825.—(Unpublished.) Page 192.

loured; and, lastly, emaciation. These distressing cases are some-times very rapid in their progress, at other times tedious, equally resisting however every plan of treatment that can be devised.

Dr. Pemberton has remarked, that it is not very uncommon to find extensive mischief in the structure of the stomach, without the constitution being sensibly affected by it ; that is, provided the disease was so situate as not to interrupt the passage of the food.

Nothing appears to be known regarding the *causes* of organic disease of the stomach, further than that it is connected with an ad-vanced period of life.

5. Erosions or perforations of the stomach, without thickening of its coats, or any surrounding inflammation, have been occasion-ally found upon dissection; and they were attributed by John Hun-ter, to solution of the stomach in its own juices *after death.* More recent observations, however, have tended to show, that such an occurrence sometimes takes place *during life;* more especially in infants. The circumstances, however, which favour it are not well understood, and the whole subject is certainly still involved in con-siderable obscurity.*

* The student is referred for further information on this curious point in pathology, to a paper by Dr. Gairdner, in vol. i, Transactions of the Medi-co-Chirurgical Society of Edinburgh, page 311.

CHAP. II.

MANY very intricate questions, both in physiology and general pathology, are intimately connected with the consideration of jaundice. How far the further advances which science is destined to make will throw light upon these, and consequently upon the nature and treatment of the several varieties of jaundice, it would be in vain to conjecture. It is sufficient for my purpose, if the student, in entering upon the investigation of this disease, is thoroughly convinced of the difficulties which assail him at the very threshold of inquiry, and is content, therefore, with those qualified and imperfect opinions concerning it, which are alone consistent with the present state of our knowledge. As this notion may perhaps appear to some overstrained, and hardly compatible with the ideas commonly entertained on the subject, it may be right to begin by pointing out briefly the different physiological difficulties which will meet us in the several steps of our progress.

Jaundice obviously arises from some obstruction to the passage of the bile into the intestines; but to understand *correctly* in what manner this takes place, and to appreciate fully the symptoms which accompany it, we ought to be tolerably well informed of the mode in which the bile, in a state of health, passes through its ducts; of the use of the gall-bladder; of the use of the bile; and of the extent to which the nerves influence the secretion of the bile. None of these points have been determined with that degree of accuracy which is desirable ; but, obscure as they are, there is at least equal difficulty attaching to most of the *pathological* discussions into which we shall soon be led.

In all systems of nosology, different *species* of jaundice have been described ; but in many cases it would appear as if the ingenuity of authors had rather been displayed in enumerating the several ways in which obstruction *might* take place, than their experience adduced in determining which of them are the most frequent and important in practice. An useful distinction may, in the first place, be drawn between those cases of jaundice which arise from *mechanical* impediments to the natural course of the bile, that bile being secreted of a healthy quality, and such as are connected with impaired *function* of the biliary ducts, the secretion of bile being more or less faulty. To the first class belong, 1. The passage of gall-stones. 2 Enlargements of neighbouring organs. 3. Accumulation in the duodenum. To the second class belong, 1. Spasm of the ducts. 2. Inflammation of their coats. 3. Preternatural viscidity of the bile, with *atony* of the ducts. Each of these will require separate investigation.

1. Some physicians have attempted to simplify the pathology of jaundice by ascribing all cases of it to the passage of gall-stones. Dr. Heberden, whose account of the *symptoms* of the disease is so generally accurate,* seems to have acknowledged no other cause for it ; and Dr. Cullen's views were warped by a similar persuasion. That it is an *occasional* source of jaundice must undoubtedly be acknowledged ; and therefore it becomes an object of importance to inquire into the *nature*, *origin*, and *consequences* of gall-stones. It should however be well understood at the outset that the connection between jaundice and gall-stones is more *accidental* than *essential*.

Chemists have long been diligently occupied in the analysis of biliary calculi ; but this portion of animal chemistry has not hitherto attained such perfection as enables us to state with any degree of certainty their constituent parts. They appear to contain all, or most of the ingredients of bile, and not to differ in any *essential* characters from each other. They vary of course very much in number, size, and figure. Several of their properties, and their peculiar crystallized structure, are sufficient to prove that something more than mere *inspissation* of bile is requisite for their

---

* Commentarii de Morborum Historia et Curatione. Lond. 1802.

formation. What that is, however, pathologists have not hitherto succeeded in detecting. It is an important and apparently well-ascertained fact, that biliary concretions are always formed in the gall-bladder. The circumstances which determine their formation there are not well known; but a life of indolence seems particularly to predispose to them. They are much more frequent in women than men, and chiefly are met with in those who have passed the middle and active period of life.

Impacted in the gall-bladder, biliary calculi are productive of no inconvenience. They are often found upon dissection where no symptoms during life had given occasion for the least suspicion of their existence. When, from some cause unknown to us, they pass into the ducts, especially if their size be large they create intense pain in most cases, and jaundice, for a time at least in all. The pain is usually felt about the pit of the stomach, and is often described as more excruciating than that which attends acute inflammation, even in the most sensible parts of the body. The pain recurs at intervals. When the pulse is felt during one of these severe attacks, it is perhaps found to be accelerated in a very trifling degree; but generally, it is not more frequent than in health, and sometimes it is even slower.* There are at present also at the same time, nausea, and vomiting, and extreme languor.

The further progress of the disorder is subject to considerable variety. In some cases the gall-stone passes through with rapidity; in others it appears to meet with great difficulty in its passage. I have seen a gall stone, weighing six drachms, passed by stool after a long continuance of the symptoms now enumerated. It has been made a matter of question, whether the gall-stone is propelled forward by the contraction of the coats of the ducts, or by the pressure of accumulated bile. Some have indeed imagined, that the gall-ducts could never dilate sufficiently to allow a stone of large size to pass through them, and that it is more reasonable to suppose it ulcerates its way directly into the colon, or duodenum. Such a notion is certainly borne out by the fact, that in some cases this process has been *distinctly* ascertained to take place; the gall-stone working its course to the parietes of the abdomen, and being there extracted.† This, however, is one of the *many* doubtful points in the pathology of jaundice.

* Baillie's Morbid Anatomy, p. 268.
† An instance of this kind once fell under my own observation. On ex-

2. Enlargements of the neighbouring parts such as schirrhus of the pancreas, and scrofulous enlargements of the mesenteric glands, have occasionally been found after death so situated as to press on the biliary ducts, and to obstruct the passage of the bile. In some cases during life the same thing may reasonably be *presumed* to have taken place, from observing jaundice in connection with scro. fulous disease of the inguinal or cervical glands.

3. There is reason to believe, thirdly, that impediments to the course of the bile, occasioning jaundice, have in many cases existed in the duodenum, and we can readily understand how mucus or sor. des accumulated there may so press on or clog the mouth of the common duct as to produce such an effect. The opinion is rendered probable by the rapidity with which the disease sometimes yields to a single dose of purgative medicine. It is not unlikely that in. fantile jaundice, the *yellow gum* of the lying.in room, has its origin in such a cause.

4. Spasm of the gall.ducts is another cause of obstruction strong. ly insisted on by some and as strongly denied by others. The ar. guments in favour of such an opinion are, that jaundice has been observed to attend hysteria, and other spasmodic affections; that occasionally its attack is transitory, and frequently, where the dis. ease proves fatal, dissection fails to show any concretions, or me. chanical impediment to the passage of bile. The only one of these arguments that can be relied on is the first; but the combination of hysteria and jaundice is so very rare, that it should rather be viewed as an accidental circumstance, than as tending to establish a great pathological principle.

5. A much more probable occasion of obstruction to the descent of the bile is inflammatory action in the coats of the ducts, either originating in them, or spreading to them from the liver, or from the mucous surface of the intestinal canal. The grounds on which such a proximate cause of jaundice has been built appear to me well established, and they are important, as bearing immediately on practice. It has been observed, that jaundice often arises from exposure to cold, more especially from taking large draughts of cold water while the body is overheated; that it begins, under such circumstances, with rigors, and is attended with many symptoms of general fever; that it is frequently complicated with *tenderness*

tracting the gall-stone, the ulcer healed up, the jaundice went off, and the patient, who had suffered excessively for several months, got rapidly well.

of the epigastrium, or of the right side ; and that after death, inflammation of the liver, or of the mucous coat of the intestines (and
their consequences,) have been sometimes distinctly traced.*

6. Præternatural viscidity of the bile has frequently been adduced as the cause of jaundice, and the opinion has been supported
by the tenacious and pitchy stools which are often passed after the
obstruction has been removed. It is highly probable that some of
the milder cases of jaundice, beginning without pain, and attended
with general sluggishness in the action of the stomach, bowels, and
heart, and torpor of the whole nervous system, have really such a
state of the biliary secretion for their proximate cause. Hardly any
thing is known regarding the causes of this morbid condition of the
bile. It has been stated to arise from indolent habits, as well as
the too free use of ardent spirits. I have frequently observed it
in opening the bodies of those who die during the autumnal months,
and it appears to be concerned in the peculiar character of the fevers of that season.

Jaundice is often met with as one of the symptoms of *diseased
liver*, and upon dissection no *mechanical* source of obstruction in
the ducts can be detected. These are the cases to which nosologists have given the name of *icterus hepaticus*. No very defined
views have ever been taken concerning its nature. The most reasonable explanation of the phænomenon is, that the ducts participate in the general disturbance of function throughout the hepatic
system, and that they are in a state of *atony*, or inaction.

To complete that brief outline of the general pathology of jaundice which it is my object here to give, I must advert, lastly, to
the curious but well-ascertained connection existing between it and
certain states of disease in the brain and nervous system. From
the earliest periods of medicine, we find such an opinion avowed,
and it may be illustrated in a variety of ways. Jaundice has been
observed in many cases to arise most incontestably from mental
emotion, more especially from intense domestic grief. It is frequently complicated with decided proofs of disease of the encephalon, and in severe cases it has been observed to prove fatal by
the supervention of *apoplexy*, Inflammation, and abscess of the
liver, and jaundice, have often succeeded to injuries of the head.
The fevers of hot climates, in which the brain and nervous system

* See a paper on "Jaundice," by Dr. Marsh, in the Dublin Hospital
Reports, 1822, vol. iii, pp. 298 and 302.

are so deeply involved, are frequently complicated with yellowness of the skin. These phænomena probably admit of no more precise explanation than that of *mutual sympathy* existing between the brain and all parts of the animal economy. With reference to prognosis they are of much importance to the observing physician.*

The views which have now been taken of the pathology of jaun. dice, lead to the distinction of it into the two great classes of idio. pathic and symptomatic. Idiopathic or genuine jaundice is that which *commences* with yellowness of the skin, and is attended with constitutional symptoms obviously referable to the morbid course which the bile takes. Symptomatic jaundice, on the other hand, is that in which yellowness of the skin occurs *subsequent* to, and is in its progress complicated with, *unequivocal* evidence of local disease, either in the liver or in some distant part. In describing the *symp. toms* and progress of jaundice, I of course confine my attention to the *idiopathic* form of the disease.

The only symptoms necessarily present in every case of jaun. dice, are discoloration of 'the skin and urine, and a corresponding absence of the natural colour of the stools. These vary, however, greatly in intensity. Sometimes the yellow tinge is so slight as to be perceptible only in the conjunctiva. At other times the whole skin becomes deeply imbued with it. Popular opinion long ago di. vided jaundice into three kinds, the yellow, the green, and the black, according to the intensity in the colour of the skin ; and with it Dr. Baillie's experience (recorded in the College Transac. tions†) in some measure coincides. He considers the *green jaun. dice* as a less frequent, but much more severe form of disease than the common or yellow jaundice. It is in most cases connected with an enlarged, hard, or tuberculated state of the liver. The progress of the disorder is slow, but its fatal issue is almost cer. tain.‡ In a few instances persons have lived for many years (en. joying even tolerable health) with the green tinge of bile in the skin. After a time, however, the body becomes emaciated, drop.

* If we could place any reliance on that theory, which makes *secretion* a mere *separation* from the blood, and which considers bile as existing at all times in that fluid, it might be said, that in these cases there exists some oppressed state of the brain, which suspends the functions of the liver, and causes an *accumulation* of bile in the blood-vessels.

† Volume v, p. 143.

‡ Of all the cases of green jaundice which fell under Dr. Baillie's notice, he remembered only two that recovered.

sy perhaps supervenes, the powers of the constitution give way, and
at length sink altogether.

In all the varieties of jaundice the stools are pale, and the urine
loaded with bile, so as to tinge linen which is immersed in it of a
yellow colour, more or less deep according to the severity of the
case.   Other secretions, however, are supposed to be similarly impregnated ; the saliva, and the perspirable matter.   This however
is doubtful.*   The milk of a jaundiced nurse, at least, is never discoloured.   The yellow dye pervades the internal parts of the body,
but it does not appear to attach itself equally to all structures.   The
substance of the brain has never, as far as I know, been found to
assume the yellow hue.   In like manner it will be observed, even
in very severe cases, that the upper surface of the tongue is not
perceptibly affected, although its lower surface may be deeply tinged.

But independent of symptoms obviously referable to the presence
of bile in the circulation, there are others of a different character,
very frequently met with in jaundice ; such as languor and lassitude, lowness of spirits, an itching of the skin (often exceedingly
obstinate and troublesome,) a sluggish pulse, and great debility.
Jaundice too is commonly attended with the usual marks of indigestion ; loss of appetite, flatulence, and acid eructations.   It is
generally stated, and as generally believed, that costiveness is a
necessary consequence of a want of bile in the alimentary canal ;
and it has hence been argued, that the great use of the bile is to
stimulate the intestines.   But the fact is not so.   Very often the
bowels act as under common circumstances, and sometimes diarrhœa prevails.   In one case which I attended, the mucous secretions from the bowels were so dark and depraved, as to give to the
motions the appearance of being tinged by *bile*.

It is certainly a singular circumstance, that in some cases, where,
judging from the colour of the skin and of the evacuations, the disease must have gone to a great extent, the general system has yet
not at all sympathized.   I have seen young persons continue busily

* Much ingenuity has been displayed in ascertaining by *experiment* as
well as by reasoning, how the bile gets into the circulation ; whether by the
medium of the thoracic duct, or by the hepatic veins ; by *absorption*, that
is to say, or *regurgitation*.   The determination of this point is of no importance to the pathologist, and the theory of jaundice is already sufficiently obscure.   It obviously merges in the more general questions connected
with the physiology of absorption.

engaged in an active employment—their appetite, sleep, pulse, and tongue, remaining healthy, where yet the jaundiced colour of the skin was intensely deep. This appears to prove, that the mere presence of bile in parts not destined to receive it is of no serious detriment to the system, and that many of the constitutional symptoms attending jaundice are attributable to some *ulterior* cause. It concurs too with many other phænomena of this disease, in leading to the belief, that the bile while circulating in the blood-vessels is still capable of exerting a degree of influence over the digestive process. In no other way can we satisfactorily account for the nutrition of the body so often going on but little disturbed, even in obstinate cases.

The remarks already made will preclude the necessity of detailing minutely the usual progress, and of laying down the *prognosis* in this disease. Almost every thing depends, as Dr. Heberden remarked, on the circumstance of the liver being in a healthy or morbid state. If jaundice arises from *simple* obstruction of the biliary ducts, and if the bile continue to be secreted of a *healthy* quality, it is a disease of little or no danger. Hence it happens that the jaundice of infants and *young persons* so generally ends favourably, while that which occurs in advanced life is very often the precursor of worse evils, dropsy and apoplexy, and in fact becomes one of the strongest evidences of a broken-down constitution. No definite period can be assigned for the continuance of the disease. It frequently recurs in those who have once suffered an attack of it.

The works of medical authors are not wanting in remedies for the jaundice; but some of them are very inert, and others of such opposite characters, that it is difficult to suppose they can be productive of any real benefit. If the views which have been here taken of the pathology of jaundice be correct, it is easy to perceive that the treatment must vary essentially in the different varieties of the affection. All that I now propose, is to offer a few reflections on the general principles which have usually guided physicians in their attempts to afford relief in this obscure disease.

I need hardly remark, in the first place, that where the nature of a disease is little known, *symptoms* must be the guide to practice. Where jaundice occurs, therefore, without giving rise to any local pain or constitutional disturbance, we should *abstain* from medicine, and allow nature to work the cure. Where pain is urgent, it must, if possible, be relieved; and when it is reasonable to pre-

sume that such depends on the passage of a gall-stone, opium must
be resorted to. Two or three grains of opium in the solid form,
or forty drops of the liquor opii sedativus, may be given in the first
instance, and repeated according to the urgency of the symptoms.
A warm bath is sometimes, of great use ; and under very aggravated circumstances, blood must be taken from the arm. A brisk
purgative is often of essential service in the jaundice of young
persons ; but a continued exhibition of aperient medicines, under
the impression of thus affording a substitute for the *natural* stimulus of the bile has been productive of serious inconvenience. An
emetic, in like manner, has sometimes proved useful, apparently by
emulging the biliary system, but in most instances it is of little or
no avail.

A generous diet, cheerful company, change of scene, and moderate exercise in the open air, especially riding on horse-back, by
promoting the general health, will go far towards effecting a cure
in obstinate chronic cases, and are frequently perferable to the
best-regulated course of medicine. The dyspeptic symptoms under
which the jaundiced patient so often labours, sometimes admit of
relief by the moderate and judicious use of bitters and aromatics.

The great desideratum, however, has been to discover a medicine which has the power of dissolving the biliary calculus, or at
least of altering that morbid condition of the bile which leads to the
formation of the gall-stone. Specifics for the jaundice were at one
time in great vogue, but of late they have been deservedly neglected. The remedies which are now chiefly trusted to for *resolving
the obstruction* are alkalis, soap, the nitric acid, taraxacum, the natural mineral waters, especially that of Cheltenham, its artificial
substitute, and lastly, mercury.

Of the influence of mercury in certain states of diseased liver
with which jaundice is often associated, I have already expressed
my opinion, and in such a combination of disease this remedy
may unquestionably be employed with advantage ; but in simple
jaundice from obstructed ducts, it is difficult to understand on what
principle it can legitimately be resorted to.

Lastly, the practitioner will bear in mind, with a view to practice, that jaundice sometimes presents itself under the aspect of an
inflammatory affection ; and he will see the propriety of treating
such cases by local blood-letting, fomentations to the side, and saline aperients.

HEPATALGIA.

There is a chronic complaint, characterized by severe pain in the side, which may be alluded to in this place. It is peculiar to females from the fifteenth up to the thirtieth year of life. It is extremely tedious and difficult of cure, recurring often with unconquerable obstinacy for a series of years, until some change in the constitution has brought with it a natural cure. From its leading symptom, it received from Sauvages the appropriate name of *hepatalgia* ; but as the seat of pain is often on the left side of the body, that of laterodynia is perhaps more applicable. Of its intimate nature little or nothing is known with certainty. That it is not of an inflammatory character may be inferred from its duration, from the absence of constitutional excitement, and from the small benefit which blood-letting affords. Some pathologists consider the affection as of a rheumatic kind. I have sometimes been inclined to view it as depending in some degree upon a distended state of the gall-bladder. To this opinion I am led, first by the circumstance of its occurring frequently in young women of sedentary occupations or of inactive habits ; secondly, from its being sometimes accompanied with a waxy or sallow expression of countenance analogous to that which occurs in jaundice ; and thirdly, from the benefit afforded by such medicines as excite the torpid action of the liver and its ducts.

I am well aware, however, that it is also a frequent complaint with young women who have over-exerted themselves, and that the left side is perhaps as often the seat of pain as the right. It will therefore be more consonant with sound pathology to consider this affection as depending upon a congested state of the vessels of the liver, spleen and neighbouring parts. It is sometimes accompanied with hæmatemesis, and other marks of irregular distribution of blood.

This complaint, though very distressing, is not dangerous. When the pain is very urgent, relief is obtained by the application of leeches to the side, of cupping glasses, and of blisters ; occasionally it is necessary to take ten ounces of blood from the arm. Active aperients, such as the powder No. 12, or the pills, Nos. 4 and 15, should be given, so as to produce a free action on the bowels, which is afterwards to be kept up by the daily use of some bitter aperient, such as the draught Nos. 29 or 32, or the mixture R No. 23. Electricity would probably be useful in some of these cases. Certainly much benefit is derived from regular exercise, either on foot or horseback ; and change of climate has proved in many instances efficacious, not merely in the relief, but even in the permanent cure of the complaint.

Diagnosis of the several kinds of Disease attended with purging. Patho-logical Considerations connected with it. Causes of Diarrhœa. Ingesta. State of the Atmosphere. Diarrhœa independent of external Agents. Prognosis. Treatment. Of Cholera, as it occurs in temperate Climates —as it occurs epidemically in hot Countries. Pathology of epidemic Cholera. Treatment.

WE are now to enter on the consideration of that important class of disorders which are known to the world under the familiar de-nomination of *bowel complaints.* The distress which they occasion is far greater than what attaches to diseases of more real danger; and from a general belief prevailing that their treatment is very simple—at least, that the influence of medicine upon them is great, the patient is dissatisfied unless he experiences speedy and effect-ual relief. To meet this (not ill-founded) expectation, the practi-tioner must be aware of the several kinds and causes of bowel complaints, and have rendered himself familiar with those minute shades of difference in symptoms, on which the successful admin-istration of remedies so essentially depends. By nosologists they are distinguished by the names of diarrhœa, cholera, colica, and ileus.

Opposed as these diseases *apparently* are to each other in the prominent symptom of the state of the alvine evacuation, the stu-dent must yet be apprised of their intimate pathological affinity, and of the necessity of considering them, not only in their relation to each other, but as connected with dyspepsia, and with every va-riety of abdominal inflammation. I am fully sensible, indeed, that such enlarged views of disease are scarcely reconcilable with the simplicity required in *elementary* instruction ; but it will be neces-sary to keep them in mind from the moment the student enters on the practice of his profession, and gradually to allow the artificial

distinctions of diarrhœa, dysentery, colic, and enteritis, to merge
in the wilder notion of *disturbed function of the intestinal canal.*

The characters of enteritis and of dysentery have been already
discussed. It will be remembered, that the former is attended generally with a costive, but sometimes (especially where the mucous coat of the intestines is primarily affected) with a relaxed
state of the bowels ; while the latter is uniformly characterized by
purging, the stools being slimy or bloody, without any admixture
of natural fæces. Purging is a symptom of disease greatly diversified in its degree, causes, concomitant symptoms, and the appearance of the matter evacuated. When it occurs without fever, and when the evacuations consist of a watery secretion from
the bowels more or less mixed with their natural contents, it constitutes an idiopathic complaint, and is termed diarrhœa. When
the upper viscera of the abdomen (the stomach and liver especially) are implicated, and when to purging is added vomiting, with
a copious, or perhaps vitiated, secretion of bile, the affection is of
a more formidable kind, and, according to the degree of its violence, is called either *bilious diarrhœa,* or cholera. To the highest grade of this disorder, when it becomes complicated with spasms
and excessive exhaustion of the whole system, the term *spasmodic
cholera* is applied.

Diarrhœa, even in the limited sense in which it is now taken, is
yet a disease presenting itself under very different aspects. To
decide, therefore, in any particular case, upon its nature, and to
direct its treatment with success, it is necessary to investigate accurately its rise and progress, its probable cause, its preceding
and concomitant symptoms ; but, above all, it is requisite to have
clear notions of the pathology of purging.

The increased irritability in the intestinal canal which leads to
purging is commonly (though not necessarily) associated with increased secretion from the vessels which open on its internal surface. Such a state of disordered function in the bowels may be
the result of causes acting on them *directly,* or *indirectly* through
the medium of the general system. To the first of these heads we
refer,—stimulating matters taken into the stomach either as food
or medicine. To the second,—particular states of the atmosphere,
diseases of other parts of the body, and mental emotion.

1. Diarrhœa is, in the first place, a frequent consequence of aliment, taken either in too great quantity, or improper in point of
quality. Being imperfectly digested, it is sent in a crude and pro-

ably *acrid* state to the intestinal canal, the delicate mucous membrane of which it irritates, and thereby occasions a purging. Diarrhœa arising from this cause is usually accompanied with the common symptoms of *dyspepsia*, and not unfrequently with severe *vomiting*. The appearance of the matter evacuated is often sufficient to characterize this form of the disease, without reference to its immediate exciting cause. It is attended with griping pains of the bowels, but the pains are perfectly relieved by the evacuation. It commences suddenly in almost all cases, though it barrasses the patient for a time, it carries with it its own cure. This is the *diarrhœa crapulosa* of nosologists. It is unnecessary to add, that the same kind of diarrhœa is frequently induced by design, and that there exists in nature a variety of substances, both vegetable and mineral, which have the property of producing, even in very small quantity, purging. Should the bowels be peculiarly irritable, or, under common circumstances, when taken in excess, these drugs produce that species of diarrhœa which has been termed hypercatharsis.

2. A most important feature in the pathology of diarrhœa is its connection with particular states of the atmosphere; but the same general principle is applicable to almost every other disease attended with purging. We have already had occasion to notice it when illustrating the dependence of dysentery upon a moist and heated atmosphere. We shall presently see it constituting all that is known of the causes of cholera; and we may now perceive it influencing the phenomena of diarrhœa. This disease chiefly prevails in the autumnal months, and after any very remarkable changes in atmospheric temperature; as for instance, on the breaking up of a long frost.* Such a condition of the atmosphere is sufficient of itself to produce diarrhœa; but it most commonly acts as a predisposing or *accessory* cause, augmenting the irritability of the intestines, and rendering them susceptible of stimuli, which under other circumstances, would have occasioned no inconvenience. We presume that it operates like an accidental exposure to cold, by altering the distribution of the fluids, and determining them in increased quantity upon the mucous membrane of the intestines.

3. I have stated, that there are other causes of diarrhœa which act through the medium of the general system. Sometimes they

---

* This was strikingly exemplified in the general prevalence of diarrhœa in London, in February 1823, after one of the longest and severest frosts which have occurred in this country for many years.

operate singly ; but more commonly, as just hinted, in combination
with certain conditions of the atmosphere. Of these the most important are, mental emotion, especially the anxiety of mind arising
from the embarrassments of business, excessive fatigue, late hours,
and irregular habits. Lastly, diarrhœa occurs *symptomatic* of certain diseases in other parts of the body with which the intestines
sympathize. This is strikingly displayed in the diarrhœa which
attend the process of dentition, ulcerated lungs, suppressed cutaneous eruptions, and chronic diseases of the liver.

Diarrhœa connected in this or any of the preceding ways with
general disturbance in the *whole* system, is often a severe and very
troublesome complaint, frequently recurring after it appears to be
effectually suppressed, and giving rise, by its long continuance, to
loss of appetite, languor, lassitude, great debility, and emaciation.
The *weakness* induced by a severe purging that lasts only twenty-
four hours, is often extreme ; and, while it shows us the necessity
of giving opiates and astringents in this disease, should teach us
also the value as well as the *danger* of purgatives in *others.* Diarrhœa is not, however, a disease of danger except in the case of
children and of old persons. The exhaustion produced by it in
children has often occasioned a fit of convulsion which proves fatal.
Dr. Baillie has described* a particular species of *chronic* diarrhœa
occasionally met with in elderly persons, and in those who have
lived in warm climates, and suffered from diseases of the liver. It
consists in a copious evacuation of a matter resembling a mixture
of lime and water (sometimes of the consistence of pudding,) and
very frothy on the surface. It occasions great debility, is very
liable to recurrence when the mind is harrassed, is little under
the control of medicine and ultimately wears out the constitution.
Persons have lingered under it, however, for several years. The
peculiar nature of this variety of diarrhœa does not appear to be
accurately known.

The treatment of diarrhœa must be regulated by a consideration
of its cause, of the age, constitution, and previous state of health
of the patient, the concomitant symptoms, the manner of invasion,
its duration, and effects upon the general habit. Much importance
has always been attached, by nosologists, to peculiar appearances
in the evacuations. These will afford some instruction to the practitioner in reference to the severity of the disease, and the progress

* Transactions of the London College of Physicians, vol. v, p. 166.

made towards a cure, but they are incapable of any immediate practical application.

1. Diarrhœa in young persons of robust habit may very often be permitted safely and with propriety to wear itself out. It should be remembered, however, that where the disease is sufficiently ac‑tive to effect its own cure, it will do so *speedily*. The continuance of the complaint for more than twenty-four hours must have some latent cause, which it is necessary to detect, and to obviate by me‑dicines.

2. Diarrhœa, from whatever cause it may arise, leaves the bow‑els morbidly *irritable ;* and this it is proper to check by an anodyne given either with a demulcent, as in R No. 48, or with a gentle tonic and absorbent, as in R No. 47. In severe cases it is ne‑cessary to repeat a draught of this kind after every loose motion.

3. The diarrhœa of children being often connected with imper‑fect digestion and the formation of *acid* in the stomach, it is right in such cases to begin by exhibiting a gentle emetic of ipecacuan‑ha, and subsequently, small doses of chalk mixture, with syrup of poppies ; or of the hydr. cum creta with Dover's powder. This plan of treatment is applicable also in many instances to the diar‑rhœa of adults.

4. Where the disease continues long, with griping pains and much *tenesmus,* it is presumable that there are acrid fæces pent up in some portion of the canal, which the natural action of the bowels is unable to dislodge ; and here a purgative medicine is in‑dispensable. Half an ounce of the tincture of rhubarb is a popular and useful remedy. Twenty grains of powdered rhubarb in an ounce of peppermint water, or the powder of calomel and rhubarb (R No. 12,) may be given in like manner, so as to ensure a free discharge from the bowels. I have seen the same treatment requi‑red, where the disease, in the first instance, was too speedily check‑ed. Under other circumstances, purgatives are either unnecessa‑ry or absolutely hurtful.

5. When diarrhœa can be distinctly traced to arise from cold, when it occurs in variable states of the weather, or when it is com‑plicated with restlessness, a white tongue, or other marks of gene‑ral fever, it will be right to commence the treatment by the com‑bination of some diaphoretic (antimony or ipecacuanha) with calo‑mel as in the formulæ Nos. 6 and 13, followed by the demulcent mixture R No. 58. If, in addition to the diarrhœa, there be any con‑siderable fulness of the pulse with tenderness of the abdomen, the

student will bear in mind the possibility of its being connected with an inflammatory condition of the mucous membrane of the bowels ; and he will obviate this, as circumstances may require, either by bleeding at the arm, leeches, and fomentations, or the milder discipline of confinement to bed, and the pediluvium. It is unnecessary to add, that here, as in every other form of diarrhœa, the diet should be light and easy of digestion, and may consist of grit gruel, rice gruel, panada, sago, or chicken broth.

6. Lastly, when diarrhœa resists the medicines now recommended, especially when it occurs to elderly persons in that chronic form lately described, more powerful astringents become necessary. I have derived great advantage from a mixture (No. 100) containing the compound powder of kino. The conf. opiata (R No. 53) is adapted to these cases as well as to those of hypercatharsis. The sulphate of copper, in doses of three grains twice a day, made into a pill with extract of hyoscyamus, may be tried. Starch injections, containing laudanum (R No. 107) are sometimes required once or even twice during the day.

———

The leading features of CHOLERA, and its pathological relation to diarrhœa, have been already pointed out. From the earliest times, it has been acknowledged as one of the most dangerous diseases to which the human body is subject ; but the extreme malignity of which it is susceptible was never thoroughly known until within these few years, when it has been seen to spread with an uncontrollable violence, unequalled, except in the records of the most dreadful plagues.* Cholera must be distinguished, as it occurs in this country *sporadically*, and in hot climates *epidemically*.

1. Cholera, as *here* observed, makes its attack in almost all cases suddenly and unexpectedly. It commences with nausea, unremitted and violent vomiting, severe griping pains of the bowels, and generally purging ; the matter ejected consisting partly, if not principally, of *bile*. In its progress, it is attended with great thirst, a coated tongue, a small, frequent, and feeble pulse, a cold skin, and a hurri-

* Cholera prevailed epidemically in the island of Ceylon during the first six months of the year 1819. Out of 160 soldiers attacked by it (including Europeans, Caffres, Malays, and Indians) 88 died.—Vide Marshall's Medical Topography of Ceylon, 1821, page 200.

ed irregular respiration. The prostration of strength which accompanies it, and the rapidity with which it advances, give to this disease a peculiar character, and render it one of very urgent danger. In many cases, when unchecked, it proceeds so rapidly, that in a few hours the patient is brought into a state of considerable risk. Cramps of the legs, extending to the thighs, abdominal muscles, and diaphragm, combine with the incessant vomiting and purging to exhaust the patient's strength; and if relief be not speedily obtained, coldness of the extremities and of the whole skin, extreme restlessness, clammy sweats, and hiccup follow, and are the immediate precursors of the fatal event. In general there is no pain of the abdomen on pressure, and little or no delirium; the patient dying from exhaustion of nervous power. Cholera is not usually attended by febrile symptoms, unless indeed we acknowledge that to be a febrile state which the ancients call *lipyria* where the inward parts burn and the skin feels cold. In this country cholera has proved fatal in twenty-four hours, and it seldom lasts longer than three or four days. It occurs principally in the months of July and August, and appears to be altogether dependent upon some peculiar influence of a heated atmosphere on the system, more particularly on the functions of the chylopoietic viscera. The violence of the disease is almost always proportioned to the heat of the preceding summer.

2. It was a general belief among the older pathologists, that cholera depended primarily upon an *increased* and vitiated secretion of bile, irritating the stomach and bowels. The more enlarged views of the complaints, which have been taken since cholera has prevailed so extensively in India, enable us to correct this notion, and to show that the proximate cause of the disease is still unknown, though, whatever it be, it operates *equally* on the stomach, liver, and upper intestines. The peculiarities of that highly malignant form of cholera which has lately been observed in India, may be thus briefly enumerated.

The disease began for the most part suddenly, sometimes after two or three days of previous illness. When it ran its full course, it was divisible into two stages. The first was that of oppression or collapse, characterized by a pulse hardly to be felt, cold and clammy extremities, universal cramps, excessive weakness, an expression of deep anxiety, unquenchable thirst, restlessness, and the purging of thin, watery, or starchy stools. If the patient survived this stage, lasting from twenty-four to forty-eight hours, a *reaction*

came on, amounting to fever, which was in itself a source of imminent danger. During this time, the bowels threw off a load of vitiated bile, the stools being dark and pitchy; and if due attention
was now paid to keeping up the strength by light nourishment, the
system recovered by degrees from the shock it had experienced.
Where the onset of the disease had been so violent as to occasion
death during the first stage, the appearances presented on dissection were those of *congestion* in the branches of the vena portæ,
viz. the liver enlarged and gorged with blood, the gall-bladder full
of dark green or black bile, and the inner surface of the stomach
studded with tissues of enlarged vessels.

The cholera of India, when in its greatest violence, has been
known to prove fatal in a few hours, and sometimes without even
the appearance of spasm; the pulse sinking at once, and all the
secretions being entirely suspended. Every phænomenon connected with the disease denotes a highly deranged state of the whole
nervous and vascular system of the body, the blood being thrown by
the contraction of the vessels of the surface upon the deeper and
larger organs. Of the remote causes of this extraordinary disease,
further than its general dependence on the heat of the climate, nothing is decisively known. Some circumstances led to the belief
that it was propagated by a specific contagion, but others might be
mentioned irreconcilable with such a supposition. The notion of
its dependence upon a *malaria* or exhalation from the soil has lately
been revived.

The treatment of cholera as it occurs in this country, under an
aspect so much less formidable than that which it assumes in India,
is to be conducted on the following principles. The patient's strength
is to be supported by drinking freely (but in small quantities at a
time) of broth, or beef tea, which will serve also to dilute the depraved secretions which are poured into the intestinal canal. At
the same time the morbid irritability of the bowels, and of the
whole nervous system, is to be allayed by opium given in doses
proportioned to the violence of the disease. Fifty drops of laudanum may be given in the first instance, and repeated to the extent
of ten or fifteen drops every quarter of an hour, either in camphor
mixture or cinnamon water, until the violence of the vomiting
abates. It is obvious, that as the medicine is thrown off the stomach, it should be speedily and steadily renewed. Where the pulse
is feeble, and the general debility is great, warm negus must be
administered freely. Where the surface is cold, a warm bath has

been employed with very beneficial effects. Hot bottles to the feet, and wrapping the patient in hot blankets, is a very excellent substitute. The necessity of instant attention and unceasing superintendence in all cases of cholera must be apparent. Without such care the powers of life may quickly sink beyond the reach of medical aid.

As the disease subsides, the tone of the stomach is to be supported by an allowance of wine. The decoction of bark, or an infusion of the aromatic bitters, cusparia, calumba, and cascarilla, should be taken twice or three times in the day.

A similar system is to be pursued in that aggravated form of the disease which prevails in hot climates. A draught, with sixty drops of laudanum in an ounce of peppermint-water, is to be administered at the very onset of the complaint, and repeated as circumstances require. The tone of the heart and arteries is to be supported by external warmth, stimulating frictions, and the liberal use of brandy, ether, ammonia, camphor, and other diffusible stimuli. We are informed that a warm bath appeared in many severe cases to augment the distresses of the patient. When the stomach is quieted, a full dose of calomel appears to be useful by *emulging* the biliary system.

An ample trial has been given to blood-letting, but in many cases no blood could be obtained, and in others where it did flow, the evacuation served only still further to depress the powers of the system. Occasionally a happier result was experienced. The gorged vessels of the liver acquired a freer play, and the system rallied; but still, in the commencement of a disease possessing such pathological characters as the Indian cholera, general blood-letting is not indicated.

General Character of these Diseases. Division of Colic into four Species. Common or Accidental Colic. Other effects of Simple Constipation. Bilious Colic. Symptoms and Progress of this Disease. Its pathological Relations. Mode of its Treatment. Colica Pictonum. Its Symptoms and Method of Cure. Of Ileus. Its Causes and usual Termination.

THERE is but little in the history of these affections which is novel or interesting, either to the practitioner or the pathologist. A few observations, therefore, on their general character, causes, and methods of treatment, will include all that seems essential to be known regarding them.

Colic and ileus are to be considered as *gradations* of the same state of disease ; *viz.* of a spasmodic constriction of some portion of the intestinal canal. They are equally characterized by griping pains and distension of the lower bowels, a sense of twisting or wringing round the navel, and spasmodic contractions of the abdominal muscles, with *costiveness.* When these symptoms continue obstinate, and when there is added to them *vomiting,* particularly of matter having the appearance or odour of fæces, the disease is in its highest degree, and is called *ileus,* or the iliac passion.

Nosologists have been at great pains to describe different *varieties* of colic, but they have extended them beyond all reasonable bounds. It will be found in practice, that colic admits of a four-fold division, according to the nature of the remote cause. The first is the *accidental* colic, arising from some acrid ingesta, which irritate the bowels without producing diarrhœa. The second is the *bilious* colic, a form of disease closely allied to bilious diarrhœa and cholera, occurring along with them, principally in the autumnal months, and apparently differing from them only in some unessential features. The third is the colic *pictonum,* the well-known painter's colic, arising from the poison of lead. The fourth is *ile-us*, from disorganization of the abdominal viscera, or some mechan-ical impediment to the due exercise of their functions.

1. Common or accidental colic is frequently occasioned by im-proper articles of diet, or acescent wines. It is usually attended with some symptoms of indigestion, and is hence called the *flatu-lent colic*. The pain of which the patient complains is often very acute, but seldom permanent, and is in almost all cases *relieved* to a certain degree by pressure. These circumstances, joined to the natural state of the pulse, and the absence of all febrile heat of skin, will seldom fail to constitute an obvious diagnosis between colic and *enteritis*, the only disease with which it is likely to be con-founded. The student, however, will bear in mind, that the cau-ses of colic prove also in some cases those of abdominal inflam-mation, and he will be prepared to find the one merging occasion-ally in the other. He will not hesitate, therefore, to take away blood, if the severity of the attack, or the habit of the patient, lead to the probability of inflammatory action.

Under common circumstances, the treatment of this variety of colic is sufficiently simple. In many cases, the spasm is relieved by a carminative draught (R No. 81), or a small portion of bran-dy. A table spoonful of the tincture of rhubarb is a familiar and useful remedy. Where these fail of the desired effect, the aperient draught, No. 19, containing rhubarb and the aromatic confection, may with propriety be given or stronger purgatives if necessary, and their operation promoted by a purging enema. This species of colic is frequently observed in women of an *hysterical* habit, and the term *hysteric* colic has often, but unnecessarily, been applied to it.

Simple constipation frequently exists without giving rise to the ordinary symptoms of colic. It is not uncommon to observe *tho-racic* symptoms emanating from such a source, such as tightness across the chest, difficulty of breathing, and a hard, dry cough. These effects of constipation are, perhaps, referable to distension of the great arch of the colon, and consequent impediment to the free motions of the diaphragm. Active purging by the pills No. 7, and the mixture No. 14, will in all such cases effect a speedy cure. In like manner a constipated state of the body gives rise to head-ache, giddiness, and other sympathetic affections of the brain. The purgative powder No. 9 is admirably adapted to these cases.

2. The second species of colic is that to which the term *bilious*

is popularly, and, I believe, justly appropriated.   It is one of the
common autumnal epidemics of this country, and will generally be
found to prevail after a long continuance of a hot and moist state of
the air.   It occurs at the same time with diarrhœa, cholera, and
jaundice, and may fairly be imputed to an increased and vitiated
secretion of bile.   It would appear as if the bile under such circumstances wants that cathartic quality with which it commonly
possesses, and acquires some præternatural acrimony, which, irritating the intestinal canal, throws it into spasmodic contractions.
Acrid bile pent up in the intestines, becomes literally a *poison* to
the system, and is the occasion of many very anamolous symptoms.

Bilious colic is ushered in with head-ache, loathing of food, a
bitter taste in the mouth, and very often bilious vomiting ; but the
urgent symptoms are distention and griping pains of the bowels,
urgent pain of the loins, and obstinate costiveness, or at most *tenesmus*, the motions being very scanty and partly slimy.   The continuance of such an irritation for a short time usually leads to fever ; and bilious colic is therefore frequently complicated with the
more general affection, *bilious fever.*   In this particular variety of
fever, there is often considerable head-ache, for the most part referred to the occiput.   The tongue is loaded, the fur upon it being
often yellow, and in streaks.   There is besides, much thirst, a short
dry cough, restlessness, and exceeding languor and lassitude, the
the pulse being seldom much accelerated, or the heat of skin very
apparent.   In irritable habits, hysterical symptoms frequently show
themselves.

In this state of disease, if a discharge of fæculent bilious matter
can be obtained, the symptoms generally yield ; but it is often exceedingly difficult to procure evacuations of this character, on account of the irritability of the stomach.   Where bilious stools are
not brought away, it is common to find chocolate-coloured motions
passed, often in vast quantity, reducing the patient to a state of
great weakness.   If by the fortunate combination of medicines, or
by the efforts of nature, the irritating cause is removed, the tongue
becomes clean, appetite returns, and the patient recovers strength.

Such is a brief sketch of the bilious colic, as it prevailed in London in 1821.   It closely resembled that described under the same
name by Sydenham, as occurring in London in 1670-71.   The observations formerly made on the causes of bilious diarrhœa apply
equally to this case.

In the treatment of bilious colic, the object is to free the bowels from the load which oppresses them; but the practitioner must also keep in view that *irritable* state of the whole tract of the alimentary canal, which is so prominent a feature in the disease. Opium at once suggests itself as a ready means of allaying this morbid irritability of the bowels; but experience will show, that though it affords relief in the first instance, its exhibition is in most cases succeeded by increased feverishness, and an aggravation of head-ache and uneasiness of the bowels.

Unless full vomiting has already taken place, it will be advisable to begin by giving ten or fifteen grains of ipecacuanha, which may be followed by a pill containing calomel and rhubarb, a dose of castor oil, or the common senna draught. If there be much irritability of stomach, it is better to commence with a saline medicine, in a state of effervescence, containing a few drops of laudanum. This will enable the practitioner to administer his aperient subsequently with more advantage. When the operation of the purgative upon the bowels is manifest by the appearance and odour of the evacuations, a full dose of laudanum may be given with the best effects. For several days afterwards it becomes necessary to exhibit, occasionally, some gentle aperient, which may prevent *accumulation* and reaction. During the convalescence, which is sometimes very tedious, advantage will be derived from a light tonic, such as equal parts of camphor mixture and decoction of bark.

COLICA PICTONUM.

3. There is a species of colic which has been proved by ample evidence to arise from the gradual absorption of lead into the system. Little mention is made of such a disease in the writings of the ancient authors, though many of them were sensible of the generally deleterious effects of lead upon the body. Paulus Ægineta is the first who distinctly describes the disease, without however being aware of its true cause. For many years afterwards it was attributed to *acidity.* It was first called colica pictonum by Francis Citois, in 1617. The discovery of its real source was made by some German physicians in 1696, who in attempting to investigate the origin of an epidemic colic then prevailing, ascertained that vintners had been in the habit of making their wines palatable by throwing into the casks *litharge.* The first author who drew the attention of the profession to the subject in this country was Sir George Baker, who in the most elaborate manner* traced the disease to lead in a variety of situations where it had not previous-ly been suspected.

This complaint has little to distinguish it from the more common varieties of colic. There is the same violent and almost constant pain about the navel, with a retraction of the integuments of the abdomen towards the spine, pain in the small of the back, tenesmus and sometimes, though not constantly vomiting. The patient ex-periences a degree of relief by keeping the trunk bent upon the knees. The constitution suffers but little, even in aggravated cases of this affection. The pulse and tongue are unaffected, and no de-bility is produced by it. Instances of a fatal termination to colica pictonum however are by no means uncommon, and this has oc-curred even after the bowels have been opened by medicine. On dissection nothing has been observed calculated to throw light on the immediate cause of death.

Colica pictonum, when once established, is very liable to relap-ses. In the course of time it assumes a chronic character, and is accompanied with a remarkable palsy and wasting of the muscles of the fore-arm and hand. The joint of the wrist becomes loose and flaccid, and a tumour is often perceivable in the back of the hand. In the worst cases, a more formidable affection of the ner-vous system is met with, evinced by the occurrence of delirium, convulsive fits of an epileptic character, and even confirmed coma. If these complaints concur with such habits of life as expose the patient to the influence of lead, the true nature of the disease is placed beyond the possibility of doubt.

The only peculiarity that I am aware of in the treatment of sa-turnine colic, is the greater necessity of employing *opium* along with the purgative. In the more common varieties of colic, it is often advantageous, though not absolutely necessary, to *allay* the pain in the first instance ; but here the spasm is so fixed (appa-rently in the circular bands of the colon,) as generally to defeat the operation of a purgative, unless it be aided by the relaxation which an opiate produces. If the stomach be in a state to allow the administration of a purgative in a *liquid* form, it should always

* Transactions of the London College of Physicians, vols. i, and ii, 1767. A series of six papers.

be preferred. The draught No. 26, containing castor oil and opium, may be repeated every six hours, until the bowels are freely
moved, or the common senna draught may be given with a proportion of laudanum. Where the stomach is irritable, attempts should
be made to procure stools by pills of colocynth, calomel, and opium, as in R No. 5 ; but the practitioner will be careful not to persevere too long in the use of calomel, as the system is very susceptible of the influence of mercury in this, and, I may add, in all other states of spasmodic disease. Fomentations to the abdomen, the
warm bath, and emollient injections containing laudanum, will contribute materially to a speedy and successful result. In some cases,
blood must be taken from the arm before the spasmodic constriction of the bowels will relax, but in general bleeding is not required, and in a few instances it seems to have even proved hurtful.
When the bowels are once freely moved, the pain, which had previously perhaps been excruciating, quickly subsides. A return of
the disease, so much to be dreaded, is to be guarded against by the
constant use of some aperient medicine. The draughts R No. 29
and pill R No. 15 are well adapted for this purpose.

ILEUS.

4. One of the most distressing states of disease which the physician has ever occasion to witness, is that of ILEUS ; but happily it
is very rare. The complaint usually begins with the ordinary symptoms of colic, and is perhaps, in the first instance, relieved by the
means now recommended. Continuing to recur however, the time
at length arrives, when purgative medicine ceases to have its effect. Day after day passes without relief to the bowels, which remain painful and *distended*. Vomiting succeeds, and stercoraceous
matter is sometimes rejected. The distress of the patient under
these circumstances can be equalled only by that of his friends and
medical attendants, and his release from suffering is all that can be
desired. Life is often protracted, however, in this state of disease
to a painful extent, and the mind in many cases continues clear up
to the last moment.*

---

* Dr. Baillie has described (Transactions of a Society for the Improvement of Med. and Chi. Knowledge, vol. ii, p. 174) the case of a man who

Dissection will generally unfold, in a satisfactory manner, the source of mischief; but there is considerable variety in the circumstances which will occasion this total derangement in the functions of the bowels. In some very rare cases, the canal is rendered impervious by mechanical obstructions, such as intestinal calculi and polypi. ·More commonly a scirrhous tumour will be found, affecting, probably, every portion of the structure of the intestines, and occasioning ulceration of a cancerous character, and *stricture* of the gut. In a third set of cases *intussusceptio* will be obseved. Such an appearance indeed is often met with, particularly in children, where no symptoms of obstruction appeared during life ; but at other times, so large a portion of the gut passes within another that it cannot be disentangled. It is certainly a curious circumstance, that this state of disease has, in one or two cases, been removed by the efforts of nature, adhesions being formed, the intussuscepted portion of intestine sloughing off, and being afterwards passed by stool. A distinction has been made between *progressive* and *retrograde* intussusception, but for obvious reasons it can never be applied in practice. It is worthy of notice, that occasionally, after death by ileus, the intestines have been found, not contracted, but inordinately *distended*. It has hence been conjectured, and with great appearance of reason, that their muscular fibres may, by the overdistension either of fæces or of flatus, become paralysed, as often happens to those of the bladder of urine from a similar cause. The last source of ileus meriting particular mention is chronic inflammation and general thickening of the peritonæal coat of the intestines. This I have seen in two cases to produce all the symptoms of ileus, without any constriction of the intestinal canal in a particular part.

Recoveries from ileus are very rare. It arises, as we have seen, in most instances, from local causes, obviously unsusceptible of relief; but in those cases where it depends upon more general disturbance in the intestinal functions, the disease, before it assumes a decided character, has probably attained a height which will baffle all the resources of medical art. The remedies which have been chiefly resorted to with the view of overcoming the obstruction, after the failure of purgatives, are, dashing cold water upon the ex-

had no evacuation from the bowels for nearly fifteen weeks before his death.

tremities, injections of tobacco-somke, or of tepid water in large quanitity, and the exhibition of crude quicksilver. It is hardly to be expected, that a disease which in its early stages has resisted a *well-directed* course of medicinds, should yield in its latter periods to such bold but unscientific treatment.*

---

* A case is recorded, in which ileus was relieved by the employment of an exhausting syringe introduced into the rectum. This remedy appears to be deserving of further trial.

CHAP. V.

Notice of the several Varieties of intestinal worms. The Lumbricus. The Tænia. Ascarides. Symptoms occasioned by them. State of the System, and of the intestinal Canal, leading to their formation. Theory of the Generation of Worms. General Principles of Treatment. Varieties of anthelmintic Medicines Mode of their Operation.

THE presence of worms in the intestinal canal carries with it such decided evidence of the existence of disease, that it has from the earliest ages been a constant object of anxiety in the world, and a favourite subject of investigation with medical authors. Hippocrates and Galen have written concerning worms; and in our own times the attention of many distinguished pathologists has been directed to the same inquiry. With all this, it is singular how little is really known concerning them, which may illustrate their origin, or direct us in our methods of treatment. It is true, indeed, that their varieties, and every thing relating to their *natural history*, has been fully and ably detailed; but to the practitioner in physic these are mere objects of *curiosity*, which may claim attention in an hour of leisure, but are wholly useless as applied to practice. That which to him would be desirable —a knowledge of the general pathology of worms, of the state of body in which they originate, of the symptoms which they *immediately* excite, and of the extent to which they influence the production, or modify the symptoms and progress, of other diseases,—is, it must be confessed, still involved in very great obscurity. Yet these are points which I am well persuaded will be found in practice of essential importance, and the investigation of which appears to require only patient attention. I cannot doubt that the subject will one day receive that *full* investigation which it merits.

The intestinal canal in man is infested by five different kinds of worms; *viz.* the ascaris lumbricoides or lumbricu teres, the ascaris vermicularis or common ascaris, the trichuris, and two varieties of tænia. Of these the trichuris and the tænia *lata* are so rare as not to require a detailed notice in an elementary work. Our attention may be confined, therefore, to the three varieties well known under the familiar appellation of the round worm, the tape worm, and the thread worm. In treating of them, I shall briefly allude to such circumstances only in their history as appear susceptible of practical application.

1. The lumbricus teres, or round worm, resembles in its general aspect the common earth worm; but there are many points of difference between them, as well in their external appearance as in their internal structure.* It is from twelve to fifteen inches long, and infests principally the jejunum and ileum. It sometimes ascends to the stomach, and has even been taken out of the mouth. A few instances occur of its being *solitary.* In the generality of cases, however, there are at least two; and occasionally thirty or forty have been found together. They are much more common in the intestines of children than in those of persons full grown, or advanced in life. In fact, they are rarely met with after fifteen years of age.

2. The tænia, or tape worm, is frequent in this country, both among children and adults. The worm is often very long, extending in many cases to twenty or thirty feet. It occupies the upper part of the intestines, and feeds on the chyle. It is commonly imagined to be solitary, and has from this circumstance been called the tænia *solium.* This is not however, strictly the case. The detached joints of this worm have the appearance of gourd-seeds, and it has hence received the name of the vermes *cucurbitinus.* It has been supposed, that each joint possesses a kind of independent life; but this notion if altogether unwarranted.

3. Ascarides, or thread worms, are about half an inch in length, of a yellowish white colour, and remarkable for their very quick motion. Their true domicile is the mucus and thin fæces of the rectum and colon. From this they sometimes wander, and are found in the vagina and about the thighs. Mucus is probably the food by which they are nourished.

The symptoms occasioned by worms are often very indistinct. Their general characters are those of dyspepsia, irregular action of

* The reader will find these fully detailed in Dr. Baillie's Morbid Anatomy, p. 194. For the anatomy of intestinal worms I beg also to refer to Dr. Hooper's paper on the subject, in the Memoirs of the London Medical Society, vol. v.

the bowels, and nervous irritation. A sense of tightness across the epigastrium, with inability to swallow, although the appetite was good, were the characteristic symptoms of tape worm in a very severe case which once fell under my care. I am not aware that it is possible to distinguish between the symptoms occasioned by the round and tape worm. It can only be stated generally, that the former produces symptoms of greater intensity, and being so much more generally found in children than the tænia, may commonly be suspected at an early period of life. In adults, on the other hand, affected by symptoms of worms, the presence of tænia is rendered probable.

Children who are troubled with worms complain of a gnawing uneasy feeling about the stomach, which is removed, or diminished, by eating. The appetite is deranged and variable, often more than ordinarily voracious. The belly is hard and swelled. There is picking of the nose, hiccup, disturbed sleep, and grinding of the teeth. The countenance acquires a peculiar character (smooth and livid), not easily described, but well known to those who have the care of children. Irregularity of the pulse, a slow remitting fever, and emaciation are also observable in some cases. The irritation which worms occasion in the delicate constitutions of children has frequently brought on symptoms marking an affection of the brain and nervous system, such as giddiness, dilated pupil, and epileptic fits.

Nothing perhaps more strikingly characterizes the presence of worms than certain *anomalous* symptoms, not observed in other diseases, or not accompanied by those which under common circumstances would appear along with them. A short dry *sympathetic* cough, or pains in the thorax without corresponding dyspnœa or affection of the pulse, are among the most unequivocal symptoms of worms which I have ever witnessed. In like manner I have seen worms occasion every symptom of peritonæal inflammation, with the exception of buffy blood. The difficulty of making an accurate diagnosis between the symtomatic *nervous* affections brought on by worms, and genuine hydrocephalus, has long been acknowledged. In many cases, I presume it to be quite impossible ; the two diseases existing together, and probably standing in the relation of cause and effect to each other. Worms will not only *produce* other diseases, but they will serve to modify the symptoms of such as may accidentally arise. This I have frequently noticed in the case of hooping cough. It appears, therefore, difficult to assign any limits

to the degree of constitutional disturbance which worms may occasion.

There can be no doubt that worms frequently exist in the intestines of adults (and even sometimes of children) for a very long
time without giving rise to the least uneasiness. In this way only
can we account for the extraordinary length which the tape worm
has frequently attained. In many cases the first notice of the complaint which the patient has, is the passing of some portions of the
worm by stool. I have seen a person from whom they dropped on
any exertion of walking. In other instances, adults having worms
suffer some of the inconveniences usually attendant on dyspepsia
or colic. It is not often that the nervous system sympathises at
an advanced period of life.

Ascarides seldom occasion any thing more than local uneasiness,
—a constant, often intolerable itching about the anus and puden-
da, with a sense of heat in the parts, tenesmus, and slimy stools.
These uneasy sensations almost always come on towards evening,
and prevent sleep for several hours. Although ascarides do not
produce much constitutional disturbance, yet they have been known
to give rise to itching of the nose, restlessness, head-ache, giddiness, and some symptoms of dyspepsia. They are easily got rid
of for the time by some bitter or oily injection.

I have already had occasion to remark, how little is known regarding the state of the general system, and of the intestinal canal
in particular, which leads to the formation of worms or encourages their lodgment. They are commonly met with in persons of
weak, enfeebled, or irritable habits : and therefore prevail much
more extensively in children than in adults, in women than in men.
Yet many persons in the prime of life are subject to worms who
have no obvious marks of general weakness about them. Further,
it cannot be doubted that a weak state of the digestive organs is
that which principally leads to the production of worms ; and this,
as we shall presently see, is an object of the first importance with
a view to treatment. The disposition to form worms, when once
begun, is with difficulty removed. In some habits it appears to be
almost unconquerable, and this I have observed to apply more particularly to the case of tænia.

There is nothing in all pathology more obscure than the *origin*
of intestinal worms. The theory which ascribes them to ovula
which are taken into the body along with the food and drink, and
find a nidus in the mucus and imperfectly assimilated food of a

weakened intestine, might be supported if we found such animals in other situations. But this is not the case : they are incapable of existence for any length of time, except within a living animal body. Another supposition has therefore been started, that they are formed independent of ova, from matter contained in the intestines, having previously no regular organization. This idea, however, is contrary to all analogy in the production of animals, where any, satisfactory opportunity of investigating the subject exists. The origin of intestinal worms, therefore, is still involved in great difficulties, and probably will not soon have any satisfactory light thrown upon it.

The treatment in worm cases has usually been conducted upon very empirical principles. The only object sought has been the expulsion of the worms, and this has in many instances been effected by medicines which have a tendency at the same time to weaken the action of the stomach and intestines, and thus to increase the disposition to form them.

It would be tedious and useless to enumerate all the *anthelmintic* remedies which have been recommended even upon high authority. Some of them are simply drastic cathartics ; such as colocynth, scammony, gamboge, calomel, and jalap. These medicines, in spite of their debilitating effects, are certainly of great importance, and it will be right in all cases to commence the treatment with some mixed purgative powder. That which operates briskly, and which brings away most mucus, will answer the best. The legitimate reason, indeed, for exhibiting active purges, is to free the intestinal canal from that load of mucus in which the worms burrow, which is thrown out perhaps, in some measure, as a defence against them, but which in its turn interferes seriously with the process of digestion, and prevents the due action of tonic remedies.

The second class of anthelmintic medicines includes the oils, fixed and volatile, especially castor oil and oil of turpentine. They have been supposed to operate by blocking up the respiratory pores of the worms ; but this theory can hardly be supported. The oil of turpentine, first recommended by Dr. Fenwick, of Durham, in 1810,* is undoubtedly the most certain of all the means we possess of directly removing worms. The full dose (in which it may *safely* be given even to children) is six drachms, in milk, or mixed with water either by means of mucilage or honey. It generally pro-

* Medico-Chirurgical Transactions, vol. ii, p. 25.

duces an intoxicating effect that quickly passes off. The tænia seldom or never resists it. The student will remember that this is of all worms the most difficult to remove. The round worm, on the other hand, possesses great sensibility, and is very easily got rid of; and hence it is that such a variety of medicines have been found useful in its cure.

The third class of vermifuge medicines includes those which are bitter, acrid, or astringent, and which may be imagined to act either by a direct effect upon the worm, or more probably by virtue of some tonic property. Of this kind are the artemisia santonicum or worm-seed, the male fern root, the spigelia marylandica, and geoffræa inermis.

Lastly, there are certain anthelmintics admitted into common practice, whose operation it would be difficult to explain on any ascertained principle; such as the dolichos pruriens, tin powder,* strong brine, and assafœtida. Some powerful drugs have been recommended with a view of *poisoning* the worm, such as tobacco, arsenic, and hellebore. The remedy, however, is here worse than the disease.

Too much stress has undoubtedly been laid on the administration of these *direct* vermifuges. Practitioners seem to have lost sight of those greater principles which should regulate their treatment, and which are fairly deducible from the views already taken of the *habit* of body in which worms appear. The principal object should be to strengthen the system generally and the digestive organs in particular; and to excite that energy in the constitution which may enable the intestines to expel the worms, and to *resist* their subsequent formation.

The means by which these ends are to be obtained are the same which apply in ordinary cases of dyspepsia. The diet of the patient is carefully to be regulated. Digestion is to be promoted in languid habits, by the use of bitters and stimulants. A regular action of the bowels is to be kept up, and accumulation prevented, by small doses of rhubarb in combination with the extract of chamomile. The general system is to be strengthened by daily exercise in the open air, by the cold bath when the season permits, and partly too by the use of some preparation of steel.

* The practitioner will cautiously refrain from exhibiting the *filings* of tin, which have been known to prove highly irritating aud deleterious. Even the tin powder is a medicine of questionable safety.

CHAP. VI.

In all systems of nosology, *atrophy*, or emaciation, has been considered as a disease comprehending under it a great variety of species. In practice, however, it can never be viewed but as a *symptom*, referable to some ulterior cause, and never of itself leading immediately to treatment. Of all the species of atrophy which have
been described, there is none so common, or so uniform in its accompanying symptoms, as that which occurs in early life. The
general wasting of the body is then attended with fever of a slow
remitting kind, which being an equally prominent feature of the
complaint, has in many cases given a name to it. The student will
accordingly find the disease described in different works, under a
variety of scientific names, according to the views which have been
taken of it :—infantile hectic, infantile remitting fever, worm fever,
atrophia infantilis, tabes mesenterica, mesenteric fever, diseased
mesenteric glands, marasmus. It is certainly a curious circumstance considering the frequency of this complaint and the period
of life at which it prevails, that no *familiar* denomination should
ever have been found for it in the language of the nursery. All
authors have agreed in acknowledging its close connection with a
disordered condition of the abdominal viscera, either structural or
functional : and as it is strictly a *chronic* disease, this is obviously
the right place for entering on its investigation. The title which I
have preferred is that which is now commonly adopted in this country. In its early stages, while fever gives the disease its character, it is natural also that it should give it its name. At a more ad-

vanced period, particularly when *structural* derangement of the abdominal viscera has supervened, it is usual to call it marasmus ; but the denomination is of course of trifling importance, if the true nature and causes of the disease are well understood.

The following may be taken as a general outline of the symptoms of this complaint. It makes its advances very gradually, manifesting itself by irregularity in the bowels, and slight daily accessions of fever, during which the patient is drowsy.* The appetite is variable, the tongue often unaffected, but the pulse is præternaturally quick. In the intervals of the paroxysms the child appears perfectly well. After a time, varying from one to three, or even four weeks, feverish symptoms come on, of a more violent kind, perhaps lasting for several days, during which the cheeks are flushed, the skin is exceedingly hot and dry, and the pulse a hundred and forty in the minute. There is also very often delirium.

Digestion appears now to be perfectly at a stand. The food passes off without undergoing any change but what results from its exposure to heat and moisture. The fæces are altogether devoid of their natural smell and appearance. The appetite is so totally destroyed, that for many days toast and water, or the juice of an orange, constitute the whole nourishment. It is not to be wondered at, that under such circumstances emaciation should take place, and even go on rapidly. The child loses all spirits and strength, and refuses to be moved from the bed. There is a very striking symptom of the complaint too, which all authors have noticed,—an incessant picking of the skin of the lips and face, and fingers, apparently connected with their dry and rough state.

The presence of so much disease, if unchecked, still more if aggravated by improper management, brings in its train consequences of even a more formidable character. In some cases the brain and nervous system particularly suffer, and there come on symptoms so closely resembling those of genuine hydrocephalus, that it would be a waste of time to attempt a diagnosis between them.

At other times the brain is unaffected, and the violence of the disease falls upon the abdominal viscera. There is pain in the bowels, more or less constant, often very acute, and causing the child to keep his legs continually drawn up towards the belly. The

---

* In one case I saw the disease ushered in by an attack of *acute* peritonæal inflammation. The child ultimately recovered.

lips are of a deep red colour, the angles of the mouth beset with small ulcers, or the whole lip divided by fissures. The bowels are variable, though commonly relaxed. The abdomen gradually en-larges, and feels full and tense, while the other parts of the body waste. Emaciation indeed goes on in this state of the disease very rapidly and extensively, and gives a well-marked character to it. The cheeks fall in, and, unless flushed with fever, are of a marbly whiteness. The nose appears lengthened ; the eye glassy and sunk in its socket. The same whiteness is observable over the whole frame, and the superficial veins are therefore more than commonly distinct.

Lastly, it is not uncommon to find the thoracic viscera implica-ted, either with or without the mesenteric obstruction now describ-ed. The child is said to *catch a fresh cold.* Cough comes on, with some shortness of breath and expectoration of puriform mucus, and ultimately the child becomes decidedly *consumptive.*

It is an object of importance to determine under what circum-stances this peculiar combination of symptoms occurs, for by this we shall be led to form a just estimate of the causes and general pathology of the affection. It never occurs to children at the breast, where the mother is healthy, and the milk abundant ; but they often suffer from it, when the milk of the mother is insufficient for the support of the infant. It requires but little acquaintance, how-ever, with infantile remitting fever to know, that it is after weaning that it chiefly prevails, and that its principal cause is improper feeding, and consequent bad digestion. From the moment the child is taken from the breast it becomes exposed to it. It may then be supplied with food unfitted for its age, though otherwise whole-some ; or with food unwholesome at all ages. Its nourishment may be given too thick or too thin,—too frequently or too rarely,—too much or too little in quantity. It is very difficult for an adult (at least without experience) to form an accurate notion of what is fit for the stomach of a *child.* But of this we may be sure, that what-ever is given to the child that is not digested, may justly be con-sidered as sowing the seed of subsequent disease. If not quickly discharged from the body by diarrhœa or vomiting, it injures by slow and often imperceptible degrees the digestive organs, *depraves* the humours, weakens the general habit, developes the scrofulous taint, brings on worms in some cases, and in the end, remitting fe-ver, diseased glands, and a fatal marasmus. A thorough convic-

tion of this should be impressed on all those who are in any manner entrusted with the management of children.

But while I am thus advocating the extensive influence which
derangements of the stomach and bowels have in the production of
infantile hectic and its consequences, I am not insensible that other
causes are also to be taken into consideration. It appears to me,
indeed, that modern pathologists are *too exclusive* in their opinions
concerning the origin of this disease. It cannot, for instance, be
overlooked, that it is in the period of dentition that this disorder, in
many instances, first manifests itself. The disturbance which difficult dentition produces in the infant constitution is often extreme ;
leading to general feverishness, hydrocephalus, convulsions, peripneumony. Its influence upon the abdominal viscera is equally
apparent in the disposition which it gives to diarrhœa. That it may
serve as an *accessory* cause to genuine remittent fever, cannot, I
should suppose, be doubted. In like manner, it is very common
to find the most unequivocal symptoms of *marasmus* supervening
on hooping-cough. In some cases I have seen these connected
with *worms*, and disappearing when they were expelled ; but it cannot thereby be argued that they were owing to the worms. It is
more consonant with sound pathology to consider them both as
effects, depending on general derangement of the digestive organs,
and of the whole system, and therefore removed by the same treatment.

Whether the constitutional irritation brought on by hooping-
cough and painful dentition be of itself sufficient to induce remittent fever, without the intermediate state of disturbed digestion, is
well worthy of consideration. It probably is so, considering how
much in the pathology of this disease depends on the higher degree of irritability in the infant than in the adult frame. The
notion of an *idiopathic* hectic was entertained by John Hunter ;
and, though difficult to reconcile with commonly received opinions,
is probably correct. In determining the causes of infantile fever
we are not to neglect the strongly predisposing influence of a scrofulous or naturally delicate habit ; and indeed much more depends
upon this than is generally imagined. How else can we explain
the fact, that among so many thousand children who are improperly fed, a small number only are attacked by infantile fever?
Such a weakened habit is in some instances the consequence of a
poor diet, bad air, and scanty clothing; but the disease prevails
also among children in the first ranks of society. Its first ap-

58

proaches are attributable, in many instances, to the cold of winter;
and this consideration may serve, among other arguments, to show,
that the sources of infantile and of the more common varieties of
continued fever are more nearly allied than modern pathologists for
the most part admit.

Infantile hectic proves in many cases very obstinate, and in no
small proportion fatal. The chance of recovery varies with many
circumstances which hardly admit of precise detail ; such as the
natural strength of constitution, the time which the disease has
lasted, and the attentions of those about the patient. In its early stages, it is not difficult of cure ; but when, commencing gradually, it has at length come to disorder the whole system, it requires constant and *close* attention to ensure the safety of the child.
It frequently subsides for a time, and then recurs with even increased violence, not merely from irregularities in diet, but at a moment
perhaps when the greatest attention is paid to diet and regimen.
Under the best management, indeed, infantile remittent fever occasionally proves fatal, and that without any structural derangement.
In such cases the constitution appears to sink under the exhaustion consequent upon long-continued excitement. On dissection,
the bowels have sometimes been found greatly distended with air,
sometimes more than commonly empty.   :

When the disease is more rapid in its progress, it is not uncommon to find, on examination after death, extensive ulceration of the
mucous membrane of the bowels, with or without disease of the
mesenteric glands. Sometimes the only morbid appearance has
been enlargement and ulceration of the mesenteric glands, of a
scrofulous character. This circumstance has induced some pathologists to describe an affection having its *primary* seat in those
glands; and Dr. Pemberton* has been at pains to *distinguish* such
a disease from infantile remitting fever, though I think unnecessarily. In many cases the lungs are found studded with tubercles,
more or less advanced to suppuration.

That there exists a primary chronic inflammation of the *peritonæum*, attended with hectic fever and emaciation, I am well persuaded ; and the peculiarities of this form of marasmus will be
found desribed in the Medico-Chirurgical Transactions.† It appears to occur only in scrofulous habits, and to have for its diag-

---

* Treatise on the Diseases of the abdominal Viscera, p. 194.
† Vol. xi, p. 258.

nostic symptoms excessive tenderness of the abdomen, paroxysms of
acute lancinating pain, and after a certain time, the evacuation by
stool of very large quantities of a thick white matter, wholly dif.
ferent both from the usual appearance of fæces, and from the slimy
stools tinged with bile which accompany the common form of infantile hectic. On dissection the viscera of the abdomen are found
united together into one undistinguishable mass. The mucous
membrane of the bowels appears ulcerated through, in various
places, and communicating freely with the thickened and ulcerated
peritonæum. The matter observed within the abdomen corres.
ponds perfectly with that passed during life by stool. The disease
appears to be uniformly fatal.

The principles of treatment in infantile remitting fever are now,
and have long been well ascertained. To establish a good digestion, to allay that morbid irritability which prevails in the whole
system, and to resolve mesenteric obstruction, are our primary objects ; in accomplishing which we have recourse to aperients, tonics, narcotics, and deobstruents, either separately or combined,
according to the state of the patient and stage of the disease. It
is easier, however to lay down indications of cure than to carry our
views into practice. The fretfulness of the child, the irritability of .
the stomach, the perverseness of attendants, unite with the natural
obstinacy of the disease in opposing the most serious obstacles to
our success. In the treatment of all diseases attention to detail is
useful, but here it is *indispensable*.

Calomel is often resorted to as a *panacea* in this complaint, and
under judicious regulation it is of infinite service, both as aperient
and alterative ; but if given in too large doses, or too frequently,
or when the stomach and whole system are labouring under high
irritation, it will only aggravate the evil. It must always be employed with great caution, and its effects *carefully* watched. Where
the disease is recent, and the strength not much impaired,it may be
given advantageously in full doses twice in the week, along with
scammony, under the old form of the *pulvis basilicus* (R No. 10.)
When very high febrile excitement prevails, it will be advisable to
substitute the blue pill with ipecacuanha (R No. 17). A moderate action on the bowels may be kept up in the interval by small
doses of rhubarb, given at night, in combination with the sulphate
of potash (five grains of each ;) but the student will remember that
active and *frequent* purging is far from being desirable. It tends

to weaken the stomach and bowels, and therefore impedes the great object, a return to healthy digestion.

Where much irritability prevails, advantage will be derived from some of the mild narcotics. Three grains of the extr. conii may be given according to the formula R No. 51. When the parox-ysms of fever are less severe, it will be right to commence the use of a light tonic, such as the infusion of calumba or cascarilla (R No. 78), in which some gentle aperient may, if necessary, be dis-solved. Where we have reason to believe that the mesenteric glands are becoming affected, half a grain of calomel should be giv-en every night.

It is unnecessary to say, that the most scrupulous attention must be paid to the regulation of diet. It should consist chiefly of farina-ceous food, but a small quntity of plain-dressed animal food may be allowed when the age of the patient permits it.* Wine is hardly ever required. When the strength of the system has been a little recruited, gentle exercise in the open air will contribute materially to the recovery. Change of air is very advisable where it can conveniently be obtained.

This very imperfect sketch of the treatment to be pursued in in-fantile fever and marasmus, is intended only to impress upon the mind of the student, how many objects must engage his thoughts, and how essentially necessary in the management of all the dis-eases of infantile life, is a strict attention to minutiæ.†

* It may be right to mention, that genuine infantile hectic has been ob-served to *commence* as late as the ninth or tenth year of life.

† See Appendix; Note Y.

CHAP. VII.

ABDOMINAL HÆMORRHAGE.

Varieties of abdominal Hæmorrhage. Hæmatemesis. Passage of Blood by Stool. Their Causes and Mode of Treatment. Hæmorrhois, or Piles, a functional and structural Disease. Causes of Piles. Symptoms occasioned by them. Treatment.

In the present chapter I propose to direct the attention of the student to hæmorrhage as it occurs from the stomach and intestines. The former has been well denominated hæmatemesis. The term hæmorrhoids, or piles, is appropriated to that form of the disease where hæmorrhage takes place from vessels on the verge of the rectum. To the flow of blood from the intestinal canal generally, no appropriate designation has ever been given. The terms *melæna*, and *hepatirrhæa* have occasionally been applied to it; but I would venture to suggest that of *entirrhæa*, as, upon the whole, more advisable. In all cases the blood escapes from the minute vessels ramifying on the mucous surface of the bowels. The peculiar disposition of mucous membranes to the effusion of blood has been already exemplified in the case of epistaxis and hæmoptysis. The principle is equally well illustrated in the phænomena of abdominal hæmorrhage; and it will be a chief object with me to point out under what circumstances of disease, either in the system generally, or in the abdomen in particular, the mucous expansion of the alimentary canal becomes so disturbed in its function that hæmorrhage takes place from it. An affection of this kind is sometimes primary and idiopathic, arising from accidental causes, such as severe horse-exercise, or a blow on the stomach; but it is chiefly a consequence of different kinds of functional disease in *other* organs, of which the following are most important.

1. Vomiting and purging of blood occur, in the first place, symptomatic of general febrile disease, of a highly *malignant* or typhoid character. Under such circumstances they are usually

associated with petechiæ, and a *dissolved* and putrid state of the blood ; and constitute but a part of the symptoms which mark that very peculiar and most formidable state of the nervous and vascular system.   I have seen them usher in the attack of small-pox, as well as of idiopathic *petechial* fever.   It is unnecessary to say, that such symptoms indicate the greatest danger, and are seldom, if ever, subdued.

2. Hæmorrhage from the stomach and bowels occurs, in the second place, as a consequence of inflammatory action in the mucous expansion of the alimentary canal, and is met with therefore as a symptom of abdominal inflammation, of dysentery, and of hectic fever.   As such, it has already been noticed.   On dissection of those who die under such circumstances, the mucous coat of the intestinal covering is found highly vascular, and almost always ulcerated in particular parts.

3. Hæmatemesis, with which entirrhœa frequently concurs, has long been known to be a complaint of young women, chiefly the unmarried, between the ages of fifteen and five-and-twenty, more especially such as are of a full plethoric habit.   The matter rejected is seldom pure blood.   It rarely coagulates, and should rather be characterized as a morbid secretion of the stomach *tinged* with blood.   This hæmorrhage is seldom attended with danger, and in many instances, even though profuse, is unaccompanied by any signs of debility.   It has been observed to last for a great length of time uninfluenced by medical treatment, and to yield spontaneously. In a large proportion of cases it is unquestionably connected with, and *probably* dependent upon, a deranged state of the uterine functions, more particularly amenorrhœa.   In some instances the vomiting even seems to be *vicarious* to the menstrual discharge.

4. Hæmorrhage from the stomach occurs, in the third place, along with costiveness, colic, and other marks of simple functional derangement of the *bowels*.   In this and the following varieties, the discharge is often of pure blood, and is succeeded by faintness, a feeble pulse, and other alarming symptoms.   The complaint has not unfrequently been mistaken for hæmoptysis ; from which, however, it may always be distinguished by accurate inquiries.   It occurs to young females, sometimes with, sometimes without irregular menstruation ; and to elderly persons of both sexes.   It is commouly preceded by languor and oppression about the præcordia, cough and dyspnœa, head-ache, vertigo, and disturbed sleep, a dulness of the eye, and feeble pulse.   Constipated bowels, how-

ever, appear to be the *leading* feature of the complaint. The fæces, when brought away, are unnatural in colour, consistence, and
smell.

5. Hæmorrhage from the stomach and bowels sometimes proceeds from disease (chiefly organic) of the liver, and is here referable to the difficulty experienced in the transmission of blood
through the vena portæ. These cases of hæmatemesis are generally attended with dropsy, and a swelled state of the veins of the
abdominal parietes. The discharge of blood is often one of the immediate forerunners of death ; and I have noticed, that in cases of
this nature nothing is observed on dissection which can lead to a
knowledge of the *immediate* seat of the hæmorrhage. The mucous membrane has been observed softened, as if chemically acted
upon.

6. Hæmatemesis and entirrhœa, lastly are to be traced in a few
instances very distinctly to disease of the spleen. This organ may
then be felt more or less enlarged ; and the discharge of blood
from the stomach is complicated with epistaxis, petechiæ, and other marks of irregular action of the vascular systam generally.
The intimate connection subsisting between the spleen and stomach by means of the *vasa brevia*, will sufficiently explain the manner in which the intestinal hæmorrhage occurs. In this and the
preceding varieties of abdominal hæmorrhage the matter discharged has often the appearance and consistence of *pitch* ; the term
melœna, or *morbus niger*, was given to it. Such a disease is frequently to be traced to the excessive use of spirituous liquors, and
is then, for the most part, preceded for several days by very acute
pain about the præcordia.

The treatment of these different varieties of abdominal hæmorrhage will depend on the nature of the exciting cause, and the habit of the patient. In young woman it is often useful to take away
blood by the arm, and to repeat this evacuation occasionally, according to the urgency of the symptoms. Purging is adapted to all
the forms in which the affection occurs independent of fever ; and
provided the strength of the patient be not much impaired, full
purging may be safely restored to. Where the liver is diseased,
and the constitution seriously weakened, the bowels should be simply unloaded by castor oil, or gentle doses of Epsom salts. In a few
cases it may be necessary to employ astringents. The mineral
acids, alum, and the combination of kino and opium, are those
upon which our chief reliance may be placed. The oil of turpen-

tine, in moderate doses, has sometimes been found of service in checking the disposition to hæmorrhagy, but it cannot generally be relied upon.

HÆMORRHOIS OR PILES.

The hæmorrhoidal flux occupied an important place in all the old systems of physic. It was believed to be a salutary provision of nature, a special effort of the vis naturæ medicatrix, for the advantage of the constitution. The sudden suppression of it, therefore, was highly dreaded. These notions have passed away; and piles are now considered as a painful and disagreeable complaint, arising in most cases from local causes, the cure of which should never be delayed.

It is a curious circumstance, that pathologists are not yet agreed regarding the true nature of hæmorrhoidal tumours. According to some, they are varicose expansions of the veins of the rectum. The more general, and doubtless the more correct opinion is, that these tumours are formed by blood extravasated under the mucous coat of the rectum, and that the cyst of the tumour consists of this membrane rendered tense by pressure. Hæmorrhoids have been divided into the external and the internal, the blind and the bleeding; but these distinctions are of little use in practice, and of no importance whatever in pathology. The only division of the disease which has any practical bearing, is into the functional and structural; or, in other words, the *accidental* and *permanent piles*. Whatever notion may be entertained regarding the *essential* nature of hæmorrhoidal tumours, all authors agree, that in cases of long standing their contents coagulate and become solid, their coats increase in thickness, and they resemble pendulous excrescent tumours in other situations in the body.

Hæmorrhoids vary very much in size and form. Some are hardly larger than a pea, while others exceed a hen's egg in size. The symptoms which they occasion may be divided into such as occur in accidental piles (which are obviously referable to the same condition of the body which produces the tumours,) and such as attend permanent piles (as plainly referable to their bulk and mechanical inconvenience.) Accidental piles are frequently attended with a sense of heat and pain at the extremity of the rectum and in the loins, head-ache and giddiness, flatulence, and not uncommonly marks of general feverishness, such as dryness of the mouth and fauces, scanty and high-coloured urine, with a frequent desire to void the urine and fæces. The evacuation by the bowels is pain-ful, and very often occasions the tumours to bleed. In many cases they inflame, sometimes without any obvious cause, but more us-ually from becoming strangulated by the sphincter ani. The pain which they then create is often extremely acute.

The permanent *organized* piles produce in many instances a de-gree of inconvenience which interferes most seriously with the ac-tive duties and comforts of life. Even when altogether *internal*, they impede by their bulk the passage of the fæces, give rise to se-vere pain whenever the bowels are emptied, and gradually bring on that train of evils which necessarily follows long-continued consti-pation. The extent of hæmorrhage from them is also such as to oc-casion in many cases considerable uneasiness. This state of the disease arises, it may be presumed, from a continuance of the same causes which lead to the accidental, or acute hæmorrhoids. With these alone the physician is concerned. When the internal mem-brane of the rectum has become permanently thickened, the dis-ease can be relieved only by surgical operation. In this place, therefore, my attention will be directed exclusively to the conside-ration of the causes and method of treatment of the primary or *ac-cidental* hæmorrhoids.

I. Piles are frequently a symptom of general febrile excitement. They arise from over-indulgence in food of a too stimulating qual-ity, and the free use of heating wines, such as Champaign. They occur, therefore, along with common febrile symptoms, and for the most part yield spontaneously on a recurrence to a mild and unir-ritating course of diet.

2. Piles arise, in the second place, from any circumstance that impedes the regular action of the great intestines, so as to cause *straining*. They may concur, therefore, either with costiveness or diarrhœa. A confined habit of body is that which of all others is most disposed to hæmorrhoids. Hence it is that they are so fre-quently met with in persons of *sedentary* occupation. But the con-tinued use of aloes and other purgative medicines has been often followed by piles. It is fairly to be presumed, therefore, that straining at stool from any cause forces out blood into the cellular membrane at the extremity of the rectum, constituting an hæmor-rhoidal tumour.

59

3. Piles appear to be connected in some cases with the local irritation occasioned by horse exercise, and the long continuance in a
particular posture. It is a common complaint, therefore, with caval-
ry soldiers, and mail-coach travellers. I traced it in one instance,
to the too frequent use of a bougie. Lastly, hæmorrhoids have been
owing to causes impeding the free return of blood by the great abdominal veins. Hence they occur symptomatic of pregnancy, and
a diseased state of the liver.

The treatment of hæmorrhoids may be discussed under the two
heads of curative and palliative. When the disease arises from a
heated state of the system, it will be proper to give ten grains of
antimonial powder with two of calomel, for three successive nights
on going to bed, with a gentle dose of some neutral salt (R No.
20) the following morning. The diet should consist entirely of
vegetables and puddings. When it depends upon a naturally costive
habit of body, the regular use of some mild aperient, which operates gently and without sraining, is indicated. Sulphur has long
been recommended for this purpose, and may be given in combination with the electuary of senna, as in R No. 25. Regular
walking exercise is often indispensable to that due action of the
great intestines which is the surest preservative against piles.

The local or palliative treatment consists in the employment of
leeches and cold lotions, when much inflammation is present, with
confinement to the horizontal posture ; the careful return of the
tumour within the sphincter ani, whenever it has been prolapsed ;
and the application of an astringent ointment (R No. 108), where
the membrane of the rectum is much relaxed, with profuse bleeding. It is difficult to define in what cases, and on what principles,
such stimulating substances as the conf. piperis nigri, or Ward's
paste (an electuary composed of black pepper, fennel seeds, and
elecampane root), prove useful ; but experience has fully demonstrated their power. Under the same circumstances, small doses of
balsam of copaiba (R No. 63) have been employed with advantage. Injections of cold water have frequently proved serviceable.

When piles and hæmorrhage from the rectum become complicated with a thickened, or otherwise diseased state of the coats of
the mucous membrane, the efforts of the *physician* must be confined
to keeping the bowels in a natural state, and to the avoiding of all
such causes as may aggravate the sufferings of the patient. The
daily passage of the fæces may be assisted by injections of warm

water. Where the gut is in a state of ulceration, and blood passes with each stool, nothing can be done but to palliate the symptoms by narcotics, and to enforce the most rigid attention to a mild, un-irritating diet.

I beg to refer to surgical works, more especially to Mr. Aber-nethy's observations on hæmorrhoidal complaints,* for the most efficient mode of operating upon hæmorrhoidal tumours.

* Abernethy's Surgical Works, vol. ii, p. 231.

CLASS IV.

CHRONIC DISEASES OF THE URINARY AND UTERINE SYSTEMS.

CHAP. I.

LITHIASIS.

Objects of Investigation in this Chapter. Depositions from the Urine, primary and secondary. Lithic Diathesis. Circumstances tending to induce or increase it. Depositions of Oxalic Acid and of the Cystic Oxyd. Phosphatic Diathesis. Principles of treatment in calculous Affections generally—where the Lithic Diathesis prevails—where the Phosphatic Diathesis prevails. Application of these pathological views to the determination of Questions connected with the operation of Lithotomy.

The frequency of calculous disorders, and the distress which in their confirmed stages they create, have long made them an object of attention to surgeons; but it is only of late years that the *general pathology* of these affections (with which the physician is chiefly concerned) has been prosecuted with any degree of scientific precision. Scheele, in 1776, paved the way to a correct understanding of the subject by the discovery of uric acid; but it was reserved for Dr. Wollaston, in 1797, to complete the groundworks of this branch of medical inquiry by his masterly analysis of urinary calculi, published in the Philosophical Transactions of that year. The investigation has been followed up in this country with equal diligence and success; and the writing of Dr. Marcet,* Mr. Brande,†

------

* An Essay on the chemical History and medical Treatment of calculous Disorders. By Dr. Marcet. Second Edition. 1819.

† Observations on the medico-chemical Treatment of calculous Disorders. By W. T. Brande. (Quarterly Journal of Science and Arts, vol, viii; and in Phil. Trans. for 1810.)

and Dr. Prout,* have put us in possession of a number of important particulars, bearing on the formation and pathology of depositions from the urine, which seem well calculated for discussion in an elementary work. It will be my endeavour in the present chapter, to lay before the student a brief outline of the opinions of these authors, on the general questions connected with lithiasis.

Depositions from the urine are of three kinds ; 1. Pulverulent or amorphous sediments ; 2. Crystalline sediments, usually denominated sand and gravel ; 3. Solid concretions, or calculi formed by the aggregation of these sediments. The same pathological doctrines are applicable to each of these forms of urinary deposition, which obviously can never be understood without a knowledge of the constituent parts of the urine, and of the changes which that fluid undergoes in the body, from agents which either act upon it chemically, or by laws peculiar to vitality. It is this which gives to the consideration of lithiasis an interest so much greater than could have been expected to belong to it. The inquiry, in fact, will be found to have a bearing upon *general disease*, as much as upon the deranged operations of the urinary organs, and to connect itself intimately with some of the most intricate points in physiology and pathology. It affords a remarkable instance of the application of chemistry to the theory and practice of physic ; and though it would be highly unphilosophical to maintain that the history and treatment of calculous disorders depend entirely on chemical principles, yet it cannot be forgotten, that before this branch of science was cultivated, our notions of lithiasis were vague and incorrect, and that now, the best pathologist, unacquainted with animal chemistry, is continually exposed to the risk of error.

The most general principle which can be taken as the foundation of our reasonings concerning lithiasis is the division of calculous deposites into *primary* and *secondary*, or those which take place when the disease *first* developes itself, and after it has subsisted for a considerable length of time. The primary consist of the lithic acid (either simple, or in combination with ammonia,) and of oxalic acid in union with lime ; the secondary, of the phosphoric acid combined in various proportions with lime, magnesia, and ammonia.

* An Inquiry into the Nature and Treatment of Gravel, Calculus, &c. By Dr. Prout. London. 1825. Second Edition.

In the outline here given of calculous affections I have chiefly followed the views and arrangements of this last author.

The former derive their chief character from the acid which they contain, the latter from the earthy matters. The first are principally formed in the kidney, the second in the bladder. Hence the distinction into the primary and secondary deposites is nearly equivalent to *acid* and *earthy, renal* and *vesical*; but in the present state of our knowledge all these views of the subject require to be taken with certain limitations, nor do I propose them except as the basis of *elementary* instruction.

1. Under the general denomination of a *lithic* diathesis, we may arrange with Dr. Prout, all those states of the system in which lithic acid is either contained in the urine in more than its natural quantity, or in which the urine acquires a peculiar disposition to *deposit* it, even though its quantity is not morbidly increased. Such a disposition is given to the urine by a very slight excess of *free* acid,—either the phosphoric, sulphuric, or carbonic. These conditions of the urine may exist independently of each other; but in most instances they are present at the same time, constituting the *perfect* lithic diathesis. *Sediments* from the urine, having a lithic character, are usually of a brickdust or pink colour though this is liable to some variation. They consist of the lithate of ammonia. The *crystallized* deposites, commonly called *red gravel*, are lithic acid nearly pure; and many calculi of a large size are composed of the same material.

Several circumstances tend to produce an excess of lithic acid in the urine, and these it will be proper to enumerate.

1st. The presence of fever and of inflammatory action in some part of the system, is always indicated by *lateritious* or pink sediments of the urine, and the deeper the colour the more severe in general are the symptoms. The latter are especially observed to occur in rheumatic, gouty, and hepatic affections. The pathological connection of gout and gravel has long been noticed, and their mutual dependence on predominant acidity in the system was a favourite speculation with many old authors. This theory has certainly received some degree of support from the inquiries of modern pathologists. That excess of lithic acid, however, which is the consequence of *fever*, can hardly be viewed as a source of the chronic calculous deposites which it is my object now to investigate. I pass on therefore, to notice those states of the body independent of fever, which lead to such a result.

2d. Of these the most commonly witnessed are simple errors in diet, which may be, either the mere excess of wholesome food; or the partaking of food decidedly unwholesome or peculiarly difficult of digestion; or such as uniformly disagrees with a particular sto. mach; or lastly, the indulgence in food at unusual hours. This principle in pathology points out the intimate connection that sub. sits between gravellish and *dyspeptic* complaints, to which almost every thing that is important in the treatment of the disease has a reference. It may perhaps be asked in what *manner* these derange. ments of the digestive organs come to increase the formation of lithic acid by the kidney. The question is one of very considera. ble difficulty. It is not exactly known whether the kidney partakes of the diseased action or not. Dr. Prout is disposed to consider that it does not; and that the mere circumstance of imperfectly assimi. lated matter being brought in the course of circulation to the kid. ney, is sufficient to cause the formation of a more than ordinary quantity of lithic acid.

3d. Irregularity in exercise, great fatigue, depressing passions of the mind, inordinate mental exertions, all tend in like manner to produce turbid urine from excess of lithic acid. From these re. marks it will appear that the tendency to lithic deposition may of. ten be *acquired* (like gout) by indolent habits and excess in eating and drinking. But there is still another view of the subject which requires to be taken, before it can be appreciated in its several bearings.

4th. The disposition in the urine to superabundant lithic acid is sometimes *natural*, and not unfrequently *inherited*. Under such circumstances it is usual to see it deposited in the shape of *crys. talline grains*, and there is every reason to believe that these are in most instances formed in the kidney. Such a morbid state of the urine often continues for a great length of time, without occasion. ing any symptoms of peculiar severity; but sooner or later the constant deposition of crystals of lithic acid in large quantity ends in the formation of a calculus. It is a singular circumstance, that in certain countries and districts of countries, the disposition to lithic deposites from the urine is particularly strong, and calculus therefore is considered as *endemic* in such situations. A remarka. ble instance of the kind occurs in an extensive tract of this country, of which Norwich may be taken as the centre, in which more cal. culous cases occur than in the whole of Ireland or Scotland. The water, temperature, and peculiar habits of the district, have each

in their turn, been accused as the exciting cause, but the circumstance is still unexplained.* It probably depends upon the diet.

2. Very little is known regarding that state of body in which
depositions of oxalic acid take place. It appears, that in this diathesis there is little or no sand voided, and the urine is generally
clear. The calculi which contain it are probably formed in the
first instance in the kidney, though afterwards increasing to a considerable size in the bladder. Dr. Prout has shown,† from the examination of *alternating* calculi, that the deposition of oxalic acid
is both preceded and followed by that of lithic acid ; from which
it may be inferred that they are of the same general nature. Oxalic acid is formed in the kidney instead of the lithic, where, combining with the lime naturally existing in the urine, it lays the
foundation of those rough, hard, and very troublesome concretions,
to which the term *mulberry* calculi is usually appropriated. It is
a curious circumstance, that in the district of which Bristol may
be considered as the centre, this species of urinary calculus is
more frequent than any other ; at any rate, that it much exceeds
its usual relative proportions, as observed in other parts of the
kingdom.†

3. The *secondary* deposites from the urine are commonly *amorphous*, but occasionally also they appear *crystalized*. The former
consist chiefly of the phosphate of lime, but with this is generally
to be found some portion of the triple phosphate of magnesia and
ammonia. The latter consist *invariably* of the triple phosphate.

It has long been observed that a deposition of the earthy phosphates is attended with a very peculiar set of constitutional symptoms, differing both in *kind* and *degree* from those which accompany the lithic diathesis. They may be characterised as indicating
great derangement of chylopoietic viscera, with general irritability
and debility of the system. Among the most prominent of these
symptoms may be noticed nausea, flatulence, costiveness alternating with diarrhœa, the stools having an extremely unhealthy appearance (black, clay-coloured, or yeasty ;) a sense of uneasiness
and weakness in the back and loins, a sallow haggard countenance,

---

* See Dr. Prout's Inquiry, page 139 ; and Dr. Marcet's Essay, page 28.
† Prout's Inquiry, pages 106 and 159.
‡ I omit the consideration of that deposite which Dr. Wollaston denomi-
ated cystic oxyd, on account of its great rarity, and the scantiness of our
information concerning it.

languor and 'a depression of spirits, coldness of the extremities. The urine in this state of disease is pale, and more copious than natural. After standing for a short time it becomes opaque, and deposites a copious precipitate of the mixed phosphates in the state of an impalpable powder. It is extremely prone to decomposition, becomes speedily alkaline by the evolution of ammonia, and emits a very nauseous smell. The following appear to be the most im- portant of the pathological principles connected with *phosphatic* de- positions.

1. They are very seldom, if ever, formed in the kidney; nor do they often take place in the bladder without a previous deposite of lithic acid. It has been satisfactorily proved, that very few phospha- tic, or white calculi, are to be met with, which have not a lithic or oxalic nucleus. Hence it is, that to this species of urinary deposite we apply the term *secondary*. It is not contended, however, by any means, that a *natural* or primary disposition to depositing the phos- phates is not *occasionally* observed.

2. The deposition of the phosphates is connected with debility of the whole frame, the result of long-continued dyspepsia, diar- rhœa, excessive fatigue, or protracted mental anxiety. It is fre- quently present at an advanced period of life, and is one of the strongest proofs of the *breaking-up* of the constitution. Whatever may have been the previous nature of the calculus, the phospha- tic diathesis always prevails when the patient's general health gives way.

3. Phosphatic depositions are sometimes the result of a long course of alkaline medicines. Mr. Brande has detailed some ex- periments,* which he considers highly important as showing the danger of administering alkaline remedies where there is a ten- dency to the production of the phosphates. Dr. Prout also acknow- ledges their mischievious effects, in common with all medicines which act as diuretics.

4. A disposition to throw down the phosphates is given, not only by these *general* causes, but by many which act *locally* on the uri- nary organs, more particulary injuries of the back, and irritations about the bladder, kidney, or urethra, when operating without in- termission, and for a considerable length of time. That injuries of the back produce *alkaline* urine, is a very old observation, but it was not known until lately that this was merely a symptom of that

* Philosophical Transactions, 1810, p. 143. et seq.

60

phosphatic *diathesis* which such a cause induces. Hence too it is, that the presence of a small uric calculus in the bladder comes at length to produce a decided deposition of the phosphates.

5. It is very seldom observed that phosphatic calculi are encrusted by layers of *lithic* acid ; and it is argued, therefore, that the phosphatic diathesis is rarely succeeded by any other. Upon this subject, however, the great authorities are not in strict accordance. Mr. Brande asserts, that such a sequence may sometimes be observed, more particularly after a free use of acid medicines given incautiously while the phosphates are in excess. Dr. Prout, on the other hand, maintains confidently, that a decided deposition of the mixed phosphates (particularly in advanced life) is never followed by other depositions, and that the few exceptions to this law which have been observed are more apparent than real.

6. The question has frequently been discussed, how far depositions from the urine are ever of a *mixed* character. Pathologists are not agreed on this point. Mr. Brande informs us (on the authority of chemical analysis,) that cases of mixed sabulous deposite are by no means unfrequent ; while Dr. Prout, from an attentive examination of what have been called *compound* calculi, believes that such mixtures are very rare. He states,* that he has never seen an instance of the pure lithic acid intimately *mixed* with the phosphates, nor does he believe that such a compound ever existed in nature.

I have now to add a few words respecting the period of life at which calculous complaints occur, and the prognosis which may be formed under the different circumstances in which they prevail. Every one must have observed how liable the urine is at an early age to every species of deposite. This particularly happens in children of delicate constitution and weak stomach. In most cases the deposite is white and consists of the phosphates, but in the very beginning of the complaint it is often lithic. The irritability of habit, however, at this age is so great, that the character of the sand frequently changes with rapidity. From tables which have been drawn up, it appears that nearly *one half* of the whole number of stone cases occurring in this country take place prior to the age of puberty. Of the remainder, a large proportion have their origin in early life ; but the constitution being then sound, the general health good, and the calculus small, no symptoms are produced.

* Inquiry, p. 113.

The next period of life most prone to calculus occurs about the age of forty, when gout begins to make its inroads on the constitution. A calculus previously existing in the bladder will rapidly increase at this period, or a nucleus will now be formed for that of advanced life.

The phosphatic diathesis occurs most frequently in childhood and old age. Where its exciting causes, however, are strong, it may occur *as an original disease*, even in the prime of life. When the deposition of the phosphates is merely occasional, it is hardly an object of attention ; but if it invariably follows meals, still more if it occurs as *white sand*, subsiding *immediately* to the bottom of the vessel into which the urine is voided, it becomes a serious disorder. When *thoroughly* established in the system it is very difficultly got rid of ; and to this circumstance we may trace the large size which white calculi have sometimes attained, rendering their removal from the body, in neglected cases, hazardous, or even impossible.*

The infinitely greater frequency of calculous diseases in the male than the female sex, as well before as after puberty, has been clearly established. It may be ascribed in part to the shortness of the female urethra; but some other circumstances probably concur, which have hitherto eluded the researches of pathologists.

The generally received opinion, that an accurate acquaintance with the chemistry of urinary deposites would lead to clear and definite views of treatment, is founded upon very imperfect observations. The chemical treatment of lithiasis indeed, though much talked of, is, comparitively speaking, of but little service. The practitioner who aims at general success, must be guided by pathological considerations of a higher character. He must look to the state of the whole system, and to that of the chylopoietic viscera in particular. He must bear in mind, that while the urine is in its natural state, no deposition from it will take place ; or if such has already occurred, that the calculus will not increase in size. His object, therefore, must be to keep the urine, as well as other secretions, in a healthy condition, and this is to be done, not simply by an acid, or an alkali, but by strict attention to all that can improve health, or ward off disease. The deranged operation of the urinary organs must certainly be broken in upon, in the first in-

* In the Philosophical Transactions for 1809 (p. 303,) is an account, by Sir James Earle, of a phosphetic calculus, sixteen inches in length, and weighing *forty-four ounces*. Lithotomy was performed, but the stone could not be brought away, and the patient died ten days afterwards.

stance, by *medicine* ; but the effect is to be kept up by *diet* and *re-gimen*.

1. Where the lithic diathesis prevails, laxatives and alteratives are to be employed, so as to promote a due action of the digestive organs ; and after them, or occasionally along with them, may be exhibited with advantage some form of alkaline medicine. Five grains of Plummer's pill, or the pill R No. 15, or in robust habits, the more powerful combination in R No. 7, may be given at night, fol-lowed the next morning by a Seidlitz powder, or the alkaline ape-rient No. 74. This plan may be pursued every night, or every other night, according to the urgency of the symptoms. Once or twice during the day a tea-spoonful of magnesia may be taken in a glass of soda water, or the liquor potassæ in the dose of twenty drops. This last medicine is best given in barley-water, and liquo-rice assists in covering its nauseous flavour. All alkaline medi-cines, whether in a pure or carbonated state, are apt, when long persisted in, to disagree with the stomach. They should there-fore be frequently varied.

Much has been written concerning the mode in which alkalis op-erate in the relief of calculous disorders. The notion of a *solvent* power, so long and so confidently maintained, is now laid aside by the best pathologists, and their use (which none can dispute) is as-cribed to their action on the digestive organs ; where, either by obviating the formation of acid, or by neutralizing it when formed, they prevent its secretion in the kidney. Dr. Prout considers al-kaline remedies as *palliatives* only, allaying irritation, and in the case of magnesia, promoting a laxative operation.* He further gives it as his opinion, that *general* remedies (especially purgatives, judiciously administered, and never carried to excess) are those upon which reliance is chiefly to be placed.

The remarkable exemption from calculous complaints enjoyed in hot climates, has been frequently mentioned as a hint in prae-tice. It has been attributed to the uniform moist state of the skin, and certainly points out the propriety of attention to exercise and warm clothing, and perhaps the occasional use of a warm bath.

2. The treatment of those calculous cases where a *phosphatic* diathesis prevails, must vary with the duration of the disease, and the consequent degree to which the general health has suffered. They will often be found to yield to the same remedies as have

---

* Medico-Chirurgical Transactions, vol. viii, p. 549.

been already recommended ; proving that the two great forms of urinary deposition are much more intimately connected than is commonly imagined. In children, and adults, where the general health is little impaired, the occasional use of rhubarb and calomel in moderate doses will prove highly serviceable. In the majority of cases benefit will be derived from *tonic* medicines ; and the peculiar advantages of *acids* are equally suggested by chemical and pathological considerations. The mineral acids (sulphuric and muriatic) have been most usually employed ; and where they agree with the stomach, often give a decided check to the symptoms in a few days. Uva ursi, bark, and other astringent vegetables, may be had recourse to with the best effects in protracted cases, where the tone of the stomach is weakened, and the constitution much reduced. Saline purgatives, active diuertics, and alkaline remedies, must be carefully avoided, both with reference to the general and urinary system. Above all, during the presence of a phosphatic diathesis, the *mind* is to be set at rest. Absence from care, change of scene, the sports of the country, and regular hours, have an influence upon the disease quite astonishing, and often prove effectual where medicines have failed.

In every variety of calculous deposition strict attention is of course to be paid to diet : but we can hardly concur with those modern pathologists who have attempted to regulate this also by chemical principles. The excrement of animals feeding solely upon animal matter, contains uric acid in considerable quantity. It has been argued therefore, that vegetable food should be preferred where the lithic, and animal food where the phosphatic disposition exists. The fact is curious, but the practical inference incorrect. That diet is in every instance to be preferred which agrees best with the stomach.

In the treatment of calculous cases, it is necessary to look to the degree of *irritation* prevailing in the system generally, in the kidney particularly. Opium, hyoscyamus, and other sedatives, are often *indispensable*, and in *most* cases will be found useful auxiliaries. Where there is much pain in the loins, a galbanum or opium plaister may be recommended. If manifest injury has happened to the back, an issue or seton should be had recourse to.

It is hardly necessary to remark, that these observations on the treatment of lithiasis are intended to apply to those cases which are strictly *constitutional*, where no actual calculus has formed, and where no disorganization of the urinary organs has taken place.

The treatment of such only is in the hands of the physician ; but it will be obvious that the same general principles must apply in every variety and stage of the disease.   This may be illustrated by showing how the doctrines now delivered become subservient to the determination of questions connected even with the operation of lithotomy.   It is to be recommended, for instance, without delay, whenever a calculus, no matter of what species, is ascertained to exists in the bladder *before puberty ;* and in after-life, when the phosphatic diathesis is *fully* formed.   It is worthy of remark, that children upon whom lithotomy has been performed are not more liable than others to calculous complaints, at an advanced period of life.   On the other hand, the operation may be safely postponed when the calculus is small, and the lithic disposition steadily pres-ent,—provided the patient be in the prime of life, his *general* health sound, and he himself willing to conform to regular living.   Under all other circumstances, the retention of a calculus in the bladder is to be dreaded, not only on account of present suffering, but the probability of its future increase.

DISEASES OF THE KIDNEY.

Nephralgia. Symptoms and Mode of Treatment. Nephritis. Abscess of the Kidney. Hæmaturia. Ischuria Renalis. Its Causes. Prognosis. Method of Treatment.

NEPHRALGIA.

THE presence of a calculus in the kidney is not necessarily followed by distressing symptoms. Instances are recorded where a calculus of considerable size, nay even a large collection of calculi, have been found, after death, distending the kidney, without any one symptom having occurred which could lead to an idea of disease in the urinary organs. In most cases, however, when a calculus becomes *impacted* in the kidney, suppuration and gradual wasting of that organ takes place. This is generally accompanied by an *obtuse* pain, or sense of weight in the lumber region, aggravated ' by exercise, especially by riding on horseback. There is also retraction of the testicles, and a sense of numbness extending down the inside of the thigh on the affected side. The urine is commonly a deep red colour, depositing either sand or sediment. It is voided frequently, and in small quantity at a time. A person may exist for a great number of years with this affection, without materially suffering in his *general* health ; but in most instances it brings on bloody urine, and ultimately proves fatal.

The *retention* of a calculus in the kidney is, after all, a rare occurrence. Far more commonly, while yet of moderate size, it quits the pelvis of the kidney, and descends into the bladder. There can be no doubt but this has *sometimes* taken place without pain or uneasiness, even where the stone was of considerable size. In the majority of cases, however, the descent of the calculus along the

ureter is accompanied by well marked symptoms, constituting ne.
phralgia, or in common language, *a fit of the gravel*. There is a
sudden attack of very acute pain in the region of the kidney, with
violent sickness and vomiting. The pain extends to the groin, and
is generally attended by *numbness* of the thigh, and retraction or
pain of the testicle. The urine is discharged in small quantity,
high coloured, and often mixed with blood, or with mucus tinged
with blood. Dr. Pemberton has noticed, as occasionally accompa.
nying this state of disease, a sympathetic pain on the skin of the
abdomen midway between the os ilium and navel, increased by
pressure, and in some cases so acute as to arrest the whole attention of the patient.

The distressing symptoms now enumerated are of very variable
duration. They usually terminate as suddenly as they began,
marking the moment at which the calculus escapes from the ureter
into the bladder. There it remains for a longer or shorter time,
when it either enters the urethra, and is ultimately discharged from
the body, or begins to occasion some of the symptoms of *stone in
the bladder*. In a few unfortunate cases the calculus becomes permanently retained in the contracted portion of the ureter, producing that train of symptoms which usually attends disease of the
urinary system, and terminating in disorganization of the kidney,
and eventually the death of the patient.

A fit of the gravel has been mistaken for lumbago. It is to be
distinguished by the nausea which attends it, by the changes observable in the secretion of the kidney, the affection of the testicle, and the pain cotinuing unaltered by any variations in the posture of the body. Attention to the same symptoms will serve to
distinguish nephralgia from a fit of the colic, with which also it is
liable to be confounded.

In the treatment of nephralgia the principles laid down in the last
chapter for the relief of the lithic diathesis may be applied ; recol-
lecting, that here high irritation and feverish action are superadded
to great excess in the formation of uric acid. An active purgative
is often of essential service. When the pain is very acute, blood
may be taken from the loins by cupping, or even from the arm.
The patient should be placed in a warm bath, and a full dose of
opium given every second or third hour, according to the urgency
of the symptoms. Starch glysters, with laudanum, contribute materially to the patient's relief, but opium should not be employed
until the lower bowels have been freely emptied by the extr. colo-

cynth. comp. aided by a brisk purgative enema, which, of itself, will generally afford considerable ease. Stimulating diuretics are to be carefully avoided.

NEPHRITIS.

Nephritis, or inflammation of the kidney, may have its seat either in the substance of that organ, or in its capsule and surrounding cellular membrane. The former occurs only as a consequence of calculi retained in the kidney, and wherever met with has, I believe, always a *chronic* character. The latter has been observed in a few instances, as an *acute* idiopathic affection, arising from exposure to cold, or severe horse exercise.* The symptoms in no respect differ from those of nephralgia, except that the pulse is here frequent and hard, and the tongue loaded, with other marks of inflammatory fever. The treatment of inflamed kidney must be conducted upon the usual principles. General and local blood-letting, mild purgatives, frequent emollient glysters, demulcent drinks, and the warm bath, are our principal resources. Blisters should of course be avoided. Opiates may be administered where we have reason to suspect the presence of calculus.

Inflammation of the kidney duly treated may subside without any serious consequences; but in most instances, in spite of every care, it terminates in *abscess*, a lamentable and not uncommon state of disease. Dr. Baillie observes,† that no considerable gland of the body is so liable to form abscesses as the kidney. In some cases which he has seen, they appeared to be of a common kind, but the greater number partook of the nature of scrofula. He considers it probable, that calculi in the kidney are the immediate cause of the inflammation, which, however, receives it character from the constitution of the patient. The existence of abscess of the kidney may be known by the voiding of pus with the urine, subsequent to, or accompanied by, the usual symptoms of diseased kidney. We further learn from the same experience, that renal abscess is sometimes complicated, with enlargement of the kidney. Patients may

* See particularly a case by Dr. Turner in the College Transactions, vol iv, p. 226.

† Morbid Anatomy. page 288.

continue to live with this complaint for a very long time. The formation of matter will sometimes be suspended for several months, but very trifling circumstances will renew the symptoms. Permanent recovery from renal abscess is rarely witnessed. Medicine produces little or no effect upon it. A seton in the loins with the uva ursi have occasionally proved serviceable. Great quiet of body and uniform temperate living are useful in mitigating symptoms and retarding the progress of the disease.

A predisposition to ulcerated kidney, and generally to disease of the urinary system, is given by the decline of life. A very large proportion of old people suffer under some morbid affection of these organs. In one it takes the form of calculus, in another of diseased prostate, in a third, of irritable bladder, in a fourth, of chronic inflammation and abscess of the kidney.

The researches of pathologists, and particularly of Dr. Cheston,* have proved the dependence, in many cases, of abscess of the kidney upon the presence of a stone in the bladder. Dr. Cheston adds, that the sympathy is mutual, and that abscess in the kidney leads, in its turn, to diseased and irritable bladder.

The complete destruction of one kidney is not necessarily fatal. Where the constitution is sound, the other kidney has sometimes enlarged so as to do the office of both, and life has been preserved, and even rendered comfortable, under such circumstances. Occasionally a true *scirrhous* enlargement of the kidney takes place; and though instances are not wanting of such a disease remaining unsuspected during life,† yet in most cases, it is attended with the voiding of bloody urine, a constant pain in the loins aggravated by the slightest motion, and a lingering death.

HÆMATURIA, or hæmorrhage from the urethra, sometimes occurs along with hæmatemesis, and other marks of a general hæmorrhagic tendency. But in the majority of cases it is symptomatic of local disease in some part of the urinary system. I have seen it occur with fever, pain about the region of the bladder, constant desire of micturition, and other unequivocal evidences of inflammation of the bladder. It is seldom, however, of sufficient violence to

* Cheston's " Pathological Inquiries," chap. ii.
† See Medical Observations and Inquiries, vol. vi, page 236.

prove hurtful by the mere quantity of blood lost. The prognosis, therefore, and treatment of this hæmorrhage, merge in those of the primary affection, and hardly merit a more specific notice.

ISCHURIA RENALIS.

If the importance of any disease could be estimated by the survey of a system of nosology, ISCHURIA would stand foremost among the disorders of the human race. Subdivisions of this disease have been made with tedious minuteness, but they are altogether useless in practice. The only species with which the physician is concerned, is the ischuria renalis ; a few observations on the history of which, will conclude what I have to offer on the chronic diseases of the urinary system.

Ischuria renalis is a very rare form of disease, in which the functions of the kidneys are suspended, and the urine is retained in the blood. The accompanying symptoms are, a dull pain, or sense of weight in the iliac regions, with great anxiety ; nausea, vomiting, hiccup, cramps, general irritability and restlessness, or sometimes delirium, lethargy, and coma. It is occasionally attended with a constant desire to void the urine, though the catheter proves that none is in the bladder. The tase of the urine has been discerned in the mouth, and in many instances a remarkably strong urinous smell has been perceptible in the perspiration.

The causes of this affection are various. It seldom occurs except in advanced life. It has been traced to cold in habits of body liable to gravellish complaints. A more common cause of the disease may be found in local irritations in one kidney, operating by sympathy on the other; such as calculi, hydatids, and schirrhus. Lastly, it would appear from the progress of the disease, that it has originated, in a variety of cases, from some affection of the brain and nervous system. It is an important pathological fact, that this paralytic state of the kidney is almost always succeeded about the second or third day by marks of oppression on the brain.* Dr. Heberden indeed relates a case where the retention existed seven days, and the patient recovered ; but it has been well remarked by

* See a paper by Sir Henry Halford on "The Necessity of Cautious Prognosis ;" College Transactions, vol. vi, p. 398.

Sir H. Halford, that a very small measure of urine is sufficient for the exigencies of the constitution, and that it is the *total* cessation of the secretion which is so uniformly fatal.

The treatment of ischuria renalis, consists in the employment of the warm bath, of the stimulating diuretics, and terebinthinate injections. Opium has been advised, on the principle of some spasmodic stricture existing in the vessels of the kidney. Cupping from the back of the neck, and a brisk purgative, appear more consonant to the suggestions of general pathology,

CHAP. II.

THE high importance of the uterine functions of the animal œconomy cannot be doubted; and from the earliest ages ingenuity has been taxed to explain them, and to ascertain the extent of their influence both in health and disease. The menstrual flux, the most obvious of the uterine phænomena, has afforded a wide field for pathological discussion; and being a constant object of attention to females, has thus acquired a consequence which fixes it upon the notice of the medical practitioner. Its overflow or suppression are continually adduced as the causes of disease; and in different ways it has become interwoven with the opinions entertained of almost every complaint to which the female sex is exposed. Before entering on the consideration of the diseases of the uterine system, a few remarks, calculated to place this subject in its proper light, may not be without their use.

The functions of the uterus are veiled in almost impenetrable obscurity, and it is hardly possible for us to reason at all concerning them without falling into error. Much caution at any rate, is necessary, that the natural bias on our minds in regard to the menstrual flux does not induce us to impute to it an influence in disease greater than it really possesses; and thus to withdraw our attention from considerations more general, better ascertained, and therefore more practical. So strongly has the necessity of this caution impressed itself on some late pathologists,* that they have been

---

* See Hamilton on Purgative Medicines, pages 93, 110, and 126.

tempted to exclude entirely, from their speculations on the origin
of disease, the influence of the uterine system. This view of the
subject, however, cannot be supported. Every one must admit,
that there are certain combinations of symptoms (independent of
the menstrual discharge,) which occur *only* to women, and not to
them except at particular periods of their lives. The strictest pathology would authorize us in attributing such phænomena to what
constitutes the peculiar feature of that sex and age,—the uterine
system. Upon the whole, therefore, I am inclined to think that
the influence of the uterine functions in the production of disease
is unquestionable ; though fully satisfied, as I shall hereafter point
out, that the consideration is of pathological rather than of *practical* importance.

Amenorrhœa is of two kinds ; the first where the menses do not
begin to flow at the period of life when they usually appear in other women ; the second, where, having occurred and continued for
some time, they are interrupted. Nosologists distinguish these two
states of the disease by the terms amenorrhœa emansionis, and sup-
pressionis. In common language they are called *retention* and *suppression* of the menses. In neither a pathological nor practical
point of view do these species of the disease differ essentially from
each other. Their accompanying symptoms are nearly alike. They
arise, as far as we can form a judgment, in a great measure from
the same causes, and their treatment is to be conducted on the
same principles.

There is considerable diversity in the period at which the menstrual flux first appears, depending partly on the climate, and partly on the habit of the individual. In this country, and in healthy
constitutions, it commonly shows itself about the age of fourteen ;
but the delay of some months, or of one or two years, is not to be
viewed as a source of uneasiness. Retention of the menses for
even a longer period than this, is not always to be considered as a
disease. It is compatible with a state of robust health. Notwithstanding this, the anxiety of mothers frequently prompts them, under such circumstances, to solicit the advice of a physician. It is
scarcely necessary to say, that these cases are on no account to be
interfered with. A practitioner could hardly flatter himself that he
understood better than nature the management of the female constitution.

Circumstances, however, are widely different when, about the

age of seventeen, a young woman who has never menstruated begins to droop in her general health. The symptoms which accompany this state of the uterine functions are very various, but they
may be characterized generally as the indications of a weak and
irritable habit. Those of dyspepsia and hysteria predominate, and
the system sinks into that state which nosologists have very aptly
designated by the term *chlororis*. The phænomena, which present
themselves in this condition of body, will soon be described. In
the mean time I may notice all that appears to be known regarding
the causes of *retained* menses. In almost every case which requires
medical assistance, this symptom will be found associated with
some unequivocal marks of scrofula. It is frequently followed by,
or connected with, *consumption*, and it must therefore be viewed in
a great measure as depending on the *scrofulous* habit of body.

Suppressed or obstructed menstruation may be either acute or
chronic. The acute or accidental obstruction arises from cold, or
perhaps some strong mental emotion, is attended with slight feverish symptoms, and is for the most part relieved in a short time by
a gentle diaphoretic. Chronic obstruction of the menses, on the
other hand, is a complaint of a more serious kind, and is accompanied by two very different trains of symptoms.

In one variety there are marks of plethora, or of irregular distributions of blood. Sometimes the head is affected, and constant
excruciating head-ache, with giddiness on stooping, and paroxysms
of epilepsy or mania, are the urgent symptoms. At other times
the stomach principally suffers ; and there occur loss of appetite,
flatulence, fits of dyspnœa, and a very disturbed state of the alvine
evacuations, but without corresponding emaciation. In a third set
of cases, the arterial system is that on which the violence of the
disease falls, and the leading symptoms are hæmorrhagies from the
stomach, nose, or lungs, with a frequent and often full pulse, a
flushed face, and a constantly loaded state of the tongue. In very
many instances, symptoms are present referable to each of these
classes. Perhaps the most common combination of symptoms giving evidence of an obstructed condition of the uterine system, is
pain of the left side (about the region of the spleen,) head-ache,
and occasional epistaxis. The pathologist will remark, with surprise, to what an extent the symptoms may go in this state of disease, without any cause for immediate alarm ; and how long they
will continue without serious injury accruing to the constitution.
He will frequently have occasion too to notice, that the same ano-

malous train of symptoms occurs, not merely with complete obstruction, but with *irregular* states of the menstrual secretion.

In the other variety of chronic obstruction of the menses, we
may observe all the most unquestionable evidences of a *weakened*
state of body. It is to this very remarkable combination of symptoms, seldom if ever, witnessed, except in young women, and in
them, for the most part, under these circumstances of the uterine
function, that nosologists have given the name of CHLOROSIS. It
has received this appellation from the appearance of the skin,
which loses its natural mixture of red and white, and acquires a
pale, sallow, or sodden aspect, generally attributed to a diseased
secretion of the sebaceous glands, and sometimes, though I believe
very unjustly, to diseased liver.

The eyes are *pearly*, and appear sunk in their orbits. A dark
circle is particularly apparent beneath them ; the lips lose their
colour ; there is a degree of anasarcous puffiness over the whole
body. The eyelids are swelled in the morning, and the patient
complains of a weight in the loins from œdematous accumulation
there. There is great langour and listlessness, and aversion to all
kinds of motion or exertion. Pains of the side, loins, and legs,
are complained of. The least exercise occasions fatigue and accelerated respiration, frequently amounting to dyspnœa. This is
particularly apparent on going up stairs. A sense of suffocation
or tightness across the chest too is frequently noticed ; and these
symptoms render it probable that some accumulation of serum has
taken place in the air-cells of the lungs.

The heart is liable, from very slight causes, to palpitation and
syncope. The pulse is quick and small, or sometimes natural in
point of frequency, but *very feeble*. Occasionally there may be observed that throbbing of the temporal arteries which is very common in cases of great general weakness from profuse bleeding. The
appetite is bad, often entirely lost, and sometimes strangely depraved. Dyspeptic symptoms are particularly distressing.

The mind sympathizes with 'this morbid condition of the body.
The patient gradually falls into that irritable state when slight and
trivial causes produce great uneasiness ; when the opening of a
door, or the entrance of a stranger, hurries the pulse and aggravates the symptoms. In common language, she is *nervous* and hysterical.

This state of things may last for a great length of time,—a
twelvemonth or more ; sometimes aggravated, but never entirely

subsiding. By degrees, if no relief is obtained by the efforts of art or nature, the symptoms occasionally assume a more serious character. Anasarca supervenes, or a genuine hectic is at length developed; and the patient after a most painful and protracted illness, dies consumptive. More frequently, the disease, in the course of two or three years, wears itself out. The whole train of symptoms denotes a weakened state of the general system and great laxity of fibre. Very little is known regarding the causes of chlorotic amenorrhœa. It seldom originates after the age of twenty-three It may sometimes be traced to circumstances which obviously debilitate the body, such as want of air and exercise, sedentary employments, bad food, and bad air; but it often takes place where these causes cannot operate, as in the upper ranks of life. It is a frequent complaint among the domestic servants in this town soon after their arrival from the country, and it may reasonably be attributed to the sudden change from the active employment and pure air of a farm-yard, to the close confinement and heated atmosphere of a London kitchen.

The treatment of amenorrhœa is to be guided altogether by a consideration of the character of the attendant symptoms without reference to the state of the uterine functions. To the practitioner, therefore, it is a matter of indifference, whether the obstructed menstruation is the *primary* cause of all the symptoms, or only one in the general series. Such an opinion, indeed, is in direct opposition to a long-established theory in medicine. It was at one time a prevailing belief, that certain drugs possessed a peculiar property of exciting the uterine vessels to action, and the treatment of amenorrhœa was thus reduced to a fixed principle. Juster notions of pathology have banished the tribe of emmenagogue medicines. It is now acknowledged that the uterine functions can be restored only by measures possessed of *general* efficacy; and that when the system returns to a healthy condition, menstruation, which is a healthy action, will in most cases naturally follow. To bring the system into this desirable state, we must, in some instances, have recourse to lowering, in others to *tonic* remedies. Symptoms must be closely watched and treated as they rise. Unbiassed by theory, the student must learn, that in this disease, more perhaps than in any other, he may require to take blood one day while he supports the system the next.

When obstructed or irregular menstruation is attended with

62

marks of strength of the general system, and local determination of blood, great benefit is derived from a small bleeding at the arm. It is in fact, in many cases, the only means in our power of relieving the urgent symptoms. A hip-bath is useful with the view of diffusing the circulation generally, and of taking off any spasmodic constriction or chronic inflammatory action which may exist in the vessels of the uterus. Low diet, saline purgatives, but above all regular exercise in the open air, will contribute to a favourable result. I have noticed in several cases, that nothing tended so effectually to assist the constitution in throwing off this disease, as change of climate.

Many cases, however, of obstructed, and *almost all* of *retained* menstruation, are attended with those marks of languid circulation and of debility or atony, which we generalized under the title of chlorosis. This state of body demands a very different system of management. If, as generally happens, there are evidences of accompanying disorder in the stomach and primæ viæ, a gentle emetic or a mild purgative may with propriety be premised. But the great object of treatment is to give tone to the system. Systematic writers add, that we are further to attempt to excite the uterine vessels to action.

The first indication is fulfilled by directing moderate exercise, a nourishing diet, change of air, cold bathing during the summer season, and the use of some bitter medicine that may improve digestion, or of a more powerful *tonic*, that may strengthen the constitution generally. A weak infusion of calumba and cascarilla (R No. 78) may be given in the first instance, and the more powerful bitters afterwards, as the tone of the stomach improves. Attention must be paid to secure regularity in the alvine evacuation, and the bitter purgatives combined with myrrh have long enjoyed a high reputation in the treatment of this disease. Five or ten grains of the pil. aloes c. myrrha may be directed every night, or a dose of the tonic aperient pills (R No. 36) containing myrrh and rhubarb.

Steel possesses the most unquestionable power over this form of constitutional weakness. In no other state of disease, indeed, is its direct tonic virtue so unequivocally demonstrated. Six drachms of the mistura ferri compositi, with an equal quantity of cinnamon-water, may be given twice a day, and the dose gradually increased. The pilulæ ferri cum myrrha, in the dose of ten grains twice a day, may be substituted if this should disagree with the stomach.

The *form* of the medicine may be frequently varied; and as all tonics lose their effect by long continuance, their employment should be occasionally suspended. Where great languor and low-ness of spirits prevail, camphor and the volatile alkali, as in R No. 82, are serviceable.

Of the influence of *direct* emmenagogues I have already ex-pressed my total distrust. In cases, therefore, where we have suc-ceeded by these means in strengthening the system, and the men-ses still remain obstructed, time, and those inexplicable changes which take place in the constitution in the progress of life, can, I believe, be alone relied on. But their operation is commonly too slow for the anxieties of parents, and a variety of *stimulating* drugs have been resorted to with the view of *forcing* the uterine vessels to action. Of these the most in repute are the tincture of helle-bore, the powder and oil of savine, the tincture of cantharides, galbanum, the secale cornutum and the oil of turpentine. That they have occasionally succeeded it would be in vain to deny; but in many cases they disorder the stomach and bowels, and are much better avoided. Electricity has been recommended with the same intention, and has proved useful in a few cases. The cheerful amusements of society, however, have an influence over the ac-tions of the uterus, much greater than what belongs to any means of a more directly *remedial* character.

DYSMENORRHŒA, or painful menstruation, is a state of disease, which, though not associated pathologically with amenorrhœa, may be mentioned here, as my notice of it will be short. It is a com-mon, and, though not dangerous, very distressing state; in which medical assistance is frequently solicited. The pain in the loins is often in the highest degree acute, lasting two, or perhaps even three days. Small portions of coagulable lymph are sometimes discharged along with the menses, which are usually scanty. It sometimes happens that dysmenorrhœa is attended with several of those symptoms of general constitutional disturbance described as accompanying chronic obstruction of the menses in plethoric ha-bits. Under such circumstances, the occasional use of aperients, with regular exercise, will contribute to the relief of the patient. The disease too admits of some relief from a small blood-letting,

the hip-hath, sitting over the steam of hot water, and other relaxing measures. The volatile tincture of guaiacum has been found
useful. Narcotics are generally resorted to ; as Dover's powder,
in the dose of ten grains, given alone, or (as in R No. 50) in combination with the extract of conium. They are certainly of some
use; but in very many cases the disease recurs with unconquerable obstinacy, and baffles for a time every effort of medical skill.

On the cessation of the menses, which usually happens between
the forty-fifth and fiftieth year of life, complaints often make their
appearance, the system being then left extremely susceptible of
morbid impressions. To such a disorder, whatever be its nature
or character, the term *turn of life* is commonly applied. For the
most part, the symptoms are such as indicate plethora and irregular determinations of blood, giddiness, for instance, head-ache or
sleepiness, dyspnœa, with fulness of pulse, or pains in the belly.
Sometimes dyspeptic symptoms predominate. At other times le-
prous affections occupy the skin. Diseases of the liver, schirrus
of the uterus and mammæ, and chronic ailments of every description, are liable to originate, or at any rate to develop themselves,
at this particular period.

The treatment must vary according to the character of the symptoms and the habit of the individual. In almost all cases.some
blood may be taken from the arm with manifest advantage. An
issue is often serviceable. Attention must be paid to diet and regimen, with the view of avoiding the more direct causes of disease.
Lastly, the system must gradually be strengthened by bark, bitters,
and chalybeates; taking care to regulate the bowels by apropriate
aperients.

MENORRHAGIA.

Division of Menorrhagia into Species according to the State of the Uterus —and of the general System. Phœnamena of the common or active Form of Menorrhagia. Of passive Menorrhagia. Their Causes and Consequences. Treatment. Pathology and Treatment of Leucorrhœa.

THE pathology of menorrhagia is very complicated ; and before entering on the consideration of that variety of it which strictly falls within the province of the physician, I shall attempt to explain under what different circumstances it occurs, and how necessary in practice is a division if it into species.

1. The term menorrhagia is, in the first place, applied both to profuse menstrution, and to actual hæmorrhagy from the uterus. I take it for granted that the student is informed of the *physiology* of the uterine functions, and is sensible that the menstruous fluid is not pure blood, but a peculiar *secretion* from the vessels of the uterus. Menstruation is considered as *profuse*, either when the quantity is greater than natural, or when the intervals are shorter. This state of the function is sometimes, but by no means, always, an object of medical care. There is great diversity in the *quantity* of the menses in different women, in different climates, and in the same woman under different circumstances ; and this must be borne in mind when estimating the degree in which menorrhagia exists. Here, as in the case of obstructed menstruation, *accompanying* symptoms must be looked to ; and an inordinaate flow of the menses is not to be viewed as a *disease*, unless coupled with pain, fever, weakness, or disturbance of some other function.

2. The dircharge of *blood* from the uterus is to be distinguished as it occurs connected or unconnected with pregnancy. The former opens one of the most extensive and interesting fields of inqui-

ry in the obstetrical department of medicine. It requires, however, a previous survey of the physiology of the impregnated uterus, and is therefore unfitted for investigation in this work.

3. Cases of hæmorrhagy from the unimpregnated uterus admit of an important practical distinction, into such as are purely functional, and such as are connected with organic disease of the uterus, more especially cancerous or malignant ulceration about its cervix. Nothing can be imagined more distressing than this latter state of disease. One of the first evidences of it is a gush of blood from the uterus, which recurs at intervals. In its progress it is attended by severe pains of the loins and thighs, failure of the appetite, extreme weakness, and emaciation. The flooding at length is almost constant and the patient after the lapse of some months dies bloodless and exhausted ; but with a mind painfully sensible to the miseries of her own situation. Such a case can be relieved only (and that partially) by the internal administration of narcotics, beginning with cicuta and ending with opium, and by the use of astringent and anodyne injections.

4. Hæmorrhage from the uterus, strictly functional, occurs in two different states of the general system. It is sometimes attended with marks (more or less distinct according to the period of the disease) of increased action throughout the body, and is undoubtedly *dependent upon* such a state of constitution. This is the *usual* form in which menorrhagia, occurs in the practice of the physician. It may be distinguished by the name of *active* or common menorrhagia, and it is to this variety of the disease that my attention will principally be directed. On the other hand, it is *occasionally* observed in connection with general weakness. There is here however, an obvious source of fallacy, to which I shall presently advert.

5. Lastly, menorrhagia requires to be considered in some degree as a *local* disease, and it will be found to concur with very opposite states of the uterine vessels. It is sometimes the result of local increased action, independent of any general febrile disturbance. On this principle we explain its being a sequel of frequent miscarriages, and a common complaint among prostitutes. At other times, it is as obviously connected with a morbid degree of relaxation in the uterine vessels. The parts are relaxed to the touch. Instead of the firm feel of health, the uterus gives to the finger the sensation of œdema or flabbiness.

After this enumeration of the several circumstances, both con‑
stitutional and local, under which menorrhagia appears, I recur to
that form of the complaint in which I have stated that the advice of
the physician is most usually sought. The *active* hæmorrhagy from
the uterus is attended with fever. It is ushered in by rigors, head‑
ache, severe *bearing‑down* pains of the loins, foll‑wed by a hot skin,
thirst, restlessness, and a frequent hard or full pulse. The dis‑
charge of blood varies in quantity, but is often very profuse. The
same habit of body continuing leads to many symptoms of *debility*
—œdematous feet, cold extremities, paleness of the skin, a weak
pulse, lassitude on taking exercise, dyspepsia, palpitations, and a
sensation of sinking at the pit of the stomach. In this sate of *ap‑
parent* or febrile debility, the patient may perhaps *first* come under
the notice of the practitioner ; and he will then often find it diffi‑
cult to divest himself of the feeling that these symptoms indicate
the true nature of the disease, and the necessity of *tonic* medicines.
Such cases however, are very different from those of *passive* or
atonic hæmorrhagy, and they may commonly be distinguished by
tracing the symptoms to their origin, and by some still *lurking*
proofs of the existence of feverish action. The tongue perhaps is
white, and the urine high‑coloured and scanty, or there is thirst,
and disturbed sleep, These are the symptoms which in such cases
should be the guide to our practice.

The genuine *passive* hæmorrhagy from the uterus is a much
rarer species of the disease. It occurs principally to women in the
lower ranks of life, and arises from a scanty and impoverished diet,
laborious exercise, bad air, and long watching. I have noticed in
dispensary practice, that washerwomen and night nurses who live
much upon tea, and undergo great bodily fatigue, are those who
chiefly labour under it. Whatever debilitates the body generally,
will under certain unfavourable circumstances of the uterine sys‑
tem, bring on atonic menorrhagia.

Common or active menorrhagia, on the other hand, has for its
exciting causes whatever will increase plethora, and determine the
blood with more than ordinary force into the vessels of the uterus.
In the upper ranks of life it is brought on by too full living, heated
rooms, late hours, and the want of sufficient exercise ;—in the low‑
er ranks, by the abuse of spiritous liquors ;—and in both by expo‑
sure to cold. Akin to these causes of menorrhagia are those which
operate locally,—excess in venery, costiveness, and consequent

straining at stool, severe exercise, and even long-continued dancing.

Other circumstances, however, must be taken into consideration in developing the causes of uterine hæmorrhage. It is a very rare complaint with young unmarried women, and it cannot be doubted that frequent child-bearing gives a predisposition to it. It seldom originates even with married women before thirty years of age ; but from that time to the period when the menstrual discharge ceases, the tendency to it greatly increases. Many women, indeed, who had never suffered from the disease before, experience it to a greater or less degree at the time of the cessation of the menses. It is well ascertained also, that there exists in some women a *natural* inherent weakness of the uterus, and consequent proneness to menorrhagia.

Functional hæmorrhage from the uterus is not a dangerous disease. When very obstinate, it saps the foundations of the constitution, and induces more alarming complaints ; but a fatal event from the mere loss of blood is hardly upon record.

Menorrhagia, when it occurs as an active hæmorrhagy, attended with fever and bearing-down pains, must be combated by *depleting* measures adapted to the violence of the disease. Blood-letting is often necessary. If there is much pain in the loins, we should direct cupping in that part to the extent of ten or twelve ounces. Saline aperients should be given so as to ensure an open state of the bowels. A light spare diet is to be enjoined, and confinement to a bed or sofa. The bed-clothes are to be as light as is consistent with comfort. Napkins dipped in ice-cold water are to be applied to the lower parts of the abdomen. Cold injections holding in solution alum, or the sulphate of zinc, may be thrown up three or four times a day ; or in slighter cases the parts may be frequently moistened with a sponge dipped in some astringent lotion, such as the liquor aluminis compositus.

If the stage of active excitement requiring these vigorous measures should have passed by before assistance is required, the praetitioner will be careful to regulate his treatment on the same principles, while he proportions his means to the strength of the patient's habit. Saline draughts, containing Epsom salts and antimonial wine, will now be required, and the same attention must still be paid to diet and *regimen*. If all marks of feverish action have subsided, the mineral acids, which are both astringent and tonic, will be found eminently serviceable. They are commonly given in the infusion of roses, as in R No. 99. A proportion of Epsom salts may be added, so as to act gently on the bowels. The de. coction of bark with acid (R Nos. 68 and 69) is a favourite and very efficacious formula in these cases, especially where the con. stitution is much enfeebled. In the event of its failure, we must attempt to check the hæmorrhage by more powerful astringents, as alum (R No. 97,) or the cerussa acetata (R No. 98.) Decoctions of pomegranate or oak-bark, containing alum, should be frequently used in the form of injection. If the discharge be so profuse as to create alarm for the safety of the patient, she should be freely exposed to cold air, and a lump of ice applied within the vagina.

To diminish the general irritation that often prevails in the pas. sive forms of uterine hæmorrhagy, opium may be advantageously given. Five drops of tinct. opii, or a drachm of the tincture of hyoscyamus, may with this view, be added to any of the astringent draughts already recommended.

An increased secretion of mucus from the vagnia constitutes LEUCORRHŒA, or fluor albus; a very frequent, troublesome and obstinate complaint. In several respects its pathology is associa. ted with that of menorrhagia. It frequently accompanies profuse menstruation and is one of the most constant attendants upon the natural decline of the menstrual discharge. It appears also in many cases to depend upon the same causes. Slight symptoms of fever. ish excitement attend it, or sometimes the more obvious marks of *plethora*. Occasionally, but I believe more rarely, it is connected with general weakness, as indicated by palenesss of the skin, a weak pulse, and œdema. Lastly it depends in certain cases on *local* irritations.

The treatment of leucorrhœa must of course vary with the char. acter of the accompanying symptoms, but will be readily under. stood from the remarks already offered on the management of me. norrhagia. Where the system is heated, antimonial diaphoretics, laxatives, and cupping-glasses to the loins, are indicated ; the cold bath, tonics, and astringent injections, when the constitution is de.

63

bilitated. In some cases the checking of the discharge might possibly be prejudicial. In many this fear is groundless, the disease continuing, but without injury to the general health, in spite of every effort.

CHAP. V.

Marks of an hysterical Habit. Phœnomena of the hysterical Paroxysms. Prognosis. Diagnosis. Pathology. Dependence of Hysteria on the State of the nervous System—of the uterine Functions—of the Stomach and Bowels. Treatment. Influence of Antispasmodics.

OFTEN as I have had occasion to animadvert on the inconveniences and difficulties of nosological arrangements, in no instance, per-haps, are they more strikingly displayed than in that before us. Hysteria, indeed, has in all ages proved a fertile theme of nosolo-gical controversy. So various are its symptoms, so widely exten-ded and so obscure its pathological relations, that the very assign-ing to it a situation, presupposes some *theoretical* notions concern-ing its nature, which have been, and may still be disputed. I have here placed it among the diseases of the uterine system, following, in this respect, the opinions, (or perhaps what some might call the *prejudices*) of an early period of medical sicence. The objections, however, which may be urged against this arrangement will be of little moment, if the student derive his notions of the disease from the pathological views which will be taken of it, rather than from the division of the work in which they happen to be discussed.

The symptoms of hysteria may be subdivided into such as mark the hysterical habit, or constitute the hysterical paroxysm. The *hysterical habit* is characterised by great irritability both of body and of mind. There occur sudden fits of laughing and crying, without any cause, or from causes wholly inadequate ; the patient crying where she ought to laugh, and laughing where she might be expected to cry. There is great dejection of spirts, a cause-less dread of evil, a hurried manner, and a variable temper. With this morbid condition of the mind are associated many symptoms of bodily derangement—dyspepsia in all its shapes, the *globus hys-tericus,* or sensation of a ball rolling about in the stomach and gradually ascending to the throat, costive bowels, fits of difficult breathing, palpitations, a peculiar kind of nervous head-ache com- mouly called the *clavus hystericus*, and a copious flow of *limpid* urine.

These symptoms afford, of themselves, sufficient evidence of the hysterical disposition, but in all severe cases the more striking characters of the disease are developed by the occurrence of par- oxysms of *convulsion*. These are often very violent, evincing a force that overcomes all opposition. The trunk of the body is writhed to and fro, and the limbs are variously agitated. The fists are closed so firmly that it is difficult or even impossible to open the fingers. A frequent symptom is that of beating with the closed fist upon the breast violently and repeatedly. There is an involun- tary utterance of shrieks and screams, with fits of laughing and crying, sometimes accompanied with, or succeeded by, an obstinate and distressing hiccup. In this state the patient continues for a longer or a shorter time ; often for twenty-four hours, though of course with occasional *remissions*.

More or less suddenly, and frequently with repeated sighing and sobbing, the patient returns to the exercise of sense and motion, generally without any distinct recollection of the circumstances of the fit. For some time afterwards she appears quite spent, and lies stupid, and careless of what is going on around her.

Formidable as these symptoms appear to the bystanders, they are attended with no real danger, at least for the time. Where the hysterical habit, indeed, is very strong, the fits gradually acquire more and more of an *epileptic* character, until at length (though probably not until after two or three years) the disease merges al- together in epilepsy. It cannot therefore surprise us, that in many cases the diagnosis of epilepsy and hysteria should be a matter of considerable difficulty. I believe it to be often impossible. The symptoms which are chiefly to guide us, are the globus, the variable mind, the flow of limpid urine, and the degree of coma subsequent to the convulsive paroxysm. But it is not only from epilepsy that hysteria is difficultly distinguished. There is hardly a disease in the whole nosology of which it has not imitated the symptoms, and that with surprising accuracy. I have seen hysteria accompanied by constant vomiting ; by a complete ischuria renalis ; by the most obstinate colic ; by all the symptoms of genuine asthma. I have seen it assume, with most deceitful accuracy, the symptoms of ap-

oplexy. Authors have described in like manner an hysterical jaundice, an hysterical mania, an hysterical diabetes. These circumstances require to be borne in mind with reference to *prognosis*.
It is hardly necessary to apprize the student, that the danger in
these cases is to be estimated, not from the violence of the leading
symptoms, but the character of the *habit* in which they occur.

Such are the phænomena of the *hysteric passion*. Its pathology is
complicated and difficult ; for in attempting to investigate its causes
we must direct our attention *equally* to the nervous system generally, to the uterine functions, and to the state of the stomach and
bowels. It is only by taking this enlarged view of the subject that
we can arrive at any adequate explanation of its varied appearances, or reconcile the conflicting opinions of authors of acknowledged merit.

1. Hysteria is scarcely ever observed except in females whose
nervous system is peculiarly irritable. This is by no means a necessary concomitant of a *delicate* frame of body. It frequently exists along with a full *plethoric* habit, and is brought on by a life of
dissipation and inactivity, late hours, and heated rooms. At other
times it is manifestly connected with a want of tone in the general
system. Hysteric symptoms, therefore, occasionally accompany
the convalescence from acute diseases, and co-exist with severe
diarrhœa, and such chronic ailments as produce much constitutional debility. In this *irritable* state of the nervous system (whether
dependent on plethora or weakness) the hysteric paroxysm once
excited, is often renewed by very slight causes, which under other
circumstances would have produced no effect, such as mental emotion, irritation or fatigue. In fact, it becomes by habit riveted in
the body.

2. The connection of hysteria with morbid states of the uterine
system has given a name to the disease, and it is undoubtedly an
important consideration. This may be illustrated in a variety of
ways. Cases of hysteria in males have been recorded, but upon
no very good authority. The complaint is in truth *peculiar* to the
female sex. It commences at the age of puberty, and seldom occurs after the thirtieth year of life. Its attack frequently coincides
with the menstrual period. It chiefly prevails among unmarried,
or barren women. It accompanies chlorosis, amenorrhœa, menorrhagia, and all irregularities of the menstrual function.

3. Hysteria is intimately connected with disordered states of the

stomach and bowels. The nervous system may be irritable, the menstrual discharge may be obstructed, but it often requires a fit of dyspepsia, or a very costive state of the bowels, to develop the hysteric paroxysm. Of late much importance has been attached to this feature in the pathology of hysteria, and by some it has even been supposed to supersede every other. This confined view of the subject, however, is neither consonant to general pathology, nor is it borne out by the results of experience. A practitioner who trusts to purgatives alone will *sometimes* succeed,—but he will occasionally fail, where another of more enlarged views is happily successful. In the treatment of hysteria, all the views which I have now taken of the disease merit an equal share of attention.

The first object is the relief of the patient during the actual paroxysm of convulsion. Little, however, can be done at this time. Where the attack is very severe and long-protracted, the patient young and plethoric, and the pulse full, blood may safely be taken from the arm ; but we must not anticipate much benefit from the measure even under these favourable circumstances. Its good effects are for the most part only slight and temporary. Cold water to the face, volatile alkali to the nose, and æther to the temples, are often equally effectual. Turpentine or assafœtida glysters have sometimes succeeded in cutting short the fit. The power of swallowing being usually lost, or at any rate, the teeth firmly clenched, the attempt to give medicines internally during the fit is commonly fruitless. This must be reserved for the interval of the paroxysms, at which time they may be resorted to with a fair prospect of advantage. The *indications* of cure are to allay the excitability of the nervous system, and to improve digestion. The state of the uterine functions may in some cases also become an object of attention.

In full plethoric habits the irritable state of the whole frame is best combated by purging, low diet, and regular exercise. Purgatives have been found very useful in the practice of Dr. Hamilton,[*] who has noticed, that in this disease the bowels are often so torpid as makes it necessary to give them in full and frequently repeated doses. He observes, that the first purgatives may appear to aggravate the symptoms ; but a perseverance in their use removes a mass of accumulated fæces, and with it the general irritation.

* See Hamilton on Purgative Medicines, page 131.

The hysteric paroxysm being very frequently brought on by sordes in the stomach generating wind and acid, a gentle emetic is indicated, and may often be given with the best effect.

In languid habits *tonics* are called for,—myrrh, steel, and bark ; a course of mineral waters; regular hours, cold bathing, horse exercise and a generous diet. In every state of body in which hysterical symptoms arise, advantage is derived from the use of the fœtid gum-resins, assafœtida, galbanum, and sagapenum ; as also from castor, musk, camphor, valerian, æther, ammonia, and the essential oils of amber and cajaput. The utility of these medicines in the slighter forms of convulsive disease is unquestionable, and has procured for them the generic appellation of *antispasmodics*. The mode of their operation is but little understood. They are all stimulating or heating drugs, possessed of strong sensible qualities. They may be exhibited in various forms of combination. The pilulæ galbania compositæ in the dose of five grains three times a day is an approved and elegant formula. In the Appendix I have inserted specimens of the more common antispasmodic juleps, which may be given at the option of the practitioner (R Nos. 84, 85, and 86.)

Dyspeptic symptoms constitute so essential a part of the hysteric character, that the physician must naturally direct much of his attention to them. Flatulence so generally prevails, that the aromatic distilled waters (R No. 81,) which possess in so eminent a degree *carminative* qualities, will be found very serviceable.

The remarks already offered on the treatment of primary dyspepsia preclude the necessity of my entering more at large on this branch of the medical treatment of hysteria. I have only further to add, that some management of the *mind* is also necessary. A woman can often by a little exertion resist the tendency to the fit, and by well-timed *firmness* on the part of the practitioner, the same desirable object may be sometimes obtained.

CHAP. VI.

Varieties of Ovarial Disease. Phænomena of Dropsical Ovary. Appearances on Dissection. Treatment.

MORBID anatomy has proved that the ovaria are liable to several kinds of disease. They have been found greatly enlarged, and converted into a firm white mass, feeling like cartilage, more or less intersected with membranous septa. At other times, one or both ovaria appear ossified. Still more frequently this organ is converted into a fatty substance, enclosing teeth and hair, the whole being surrounded by a firm membrane. The theory of the production of these latter tumours is very obscure, and has given rise to some curious speculations.* But these subjects can hardly be considered proper for investigation in this work. The symptoms which attend such diseased conditions of the ovarium are quite unknown, and can never therefore become an object of practice. I allude to them only in so far as they suggest the probability of their being *functional* diseases of the ovarium, of which these disorganizations are the results. Pathologists have long entertained the suspicion that such affections exist, and certain diseases of the uterine system (hysteria in particular) have been by some ascribed to this cause. The opinion can never, from the very nature of the subject, be viewed except as a plausible conjecture.

Omitting then these topics as being too imperfectly known to admit of discussion, I proceed to the consideration of the only diseased state of the ovarium which is ever likely to become an object of *practical* interest,—I mean that of dropsy. The symptoms that mark the early stage of dropsical ovary are very obscure, nor can the existence of the disease be ascertained, until it has made

* See Baillie's Morbid Anatomy, page 410

such a progress as to have formed a swelling at the lower part of the belly. This swelling is attended with a sense of *weight* in that part, and according as the right or left ovarium is affected, the tumour and hardness are perceptible in one or other groin. When the disease is somewhat more advanced, fluctuation may generally be felt, sometimes nearly as distinct as in common ascites, but more usually obscure. Probably this depends on the degree of tenacity in the contained fluid.

The great mark of distinction between ovarial dropsy and common ascites, is to be found in the little disturbance which the former occasions in the constitution. The appetite remains good. There is no thirst, and the urine continues to flow as in health. Neither weakness nor hectic are produced, at least in the early stages of the complaint, and the menses are unaffected. So little does the disease influence the general health, that instances are on record of a woman becoming pregnant and bearing a child to the full time, while one ovary was enormously distended by dropsy. When the disease has reached a certain point, it produces many very unpleasant symptoms from its mere bulk,—difficult breathing, amounting often to what is commonly called orthopnœa, dyspepsia, costive bowels, swelled legs, with cramps, and a varicose state of the veins.

The progress of dropsical ovarium is subject to great variety. Instances have been met with where it proceeded rapidly, and proved fatal in one or two years. Much more commonly its advances are very slow, and life can often be preserved under it with tolerable comfort for many years.* Very few cases are recorded of a cure of this disease, either by the efforts of art or nature. It would appear as if the absorbents of the ovarium were hardly capable of being excited to the degree of action necessary for the removal of the fluid. In one instance only have I ever known such absorption to occur, and the relief prove permanent. In most instances the ovarium again fills, and the patient ultimately dies. Death takes place sometimes from *exhaustion*, and sometimes from inflammation supervening on the sac in consequence of tapping.

On dissection, the ovarium is found converted into a capsule, often of enormous size, and of variable thickness, adhering in some cases, but not universally, to the peritonæum lining the abdominal parietes. It is sometimes so large as to occupy almost the whole

* A short time ago, I saw an elderly woman who had laboured under ovarial dropsy for thirty years. She died without having been ever tapped.

64

cavity of the abdomen. In other cases, instead of a single bag, the ovary is converted into a congeries of cysts, either separate or communicating with each other by considerable openings, and containing at times fluids of different kinds. Occasionally tumours of a firm texture are found attached to the inner surface of the capsule,

The fluid of a dropsical ovary is almost always mucilaginous, and of a bluish or sometimes, chocolate colour. Without experience in the disease, it is difficult to give credit to the statements which have been published of the *quantities* of fluid observed in different cases. On the 9th January 1822, I drew off after death, from a single thin membranous cyst, eighty-two pints. I have heard of a hundred and twenty pints having been drawn off at once during life. The rapidity with which the fluid accumulates varies in different cases. In the Medical Communications (vol. ii, p. 123) will be found an interesting case of dropsy of the ovarium, in which nine hundred and sixty-four pints were discharged in the course of one year, at fourteen tappings, making on an average a daily secretion of nearly two pints and a half. The disease lasted five years, during which time the patient was tapped forty one times, and two thousand seven hundred and eighty-six pints of fluid were taken from her. In general it will be found, that when twenty-five or thirty pints are accumulated in the sac, the uneasiness from distension becomes so great that paracentesis is rendered necessary.

Of the causes of dropsical ovary very little is known. It does not appear that impregnation gives any peculiar disposition to it. Among the recorded cases many occurred among unmarried women. It has commenced as early as the twentieth year of life; but it is most frequent after thirty. Some cases may possibly have their origin in chronic *inflammation* of the ovarium. This opinion is supported by the fact, that in several instances the disease has been attributed by the patient to a contusion or fall.

Little need be said on the subject of treatment. Mercury has been tried and found to be useless. The operation of tapping affords the only effectual relief which it is in our power to hold out. A *radical* cure of the disease has been attempetd by making a large opening in the cyst, with the view of inducing inflammation and adhesion, as in the case of hydrocele. Very powerful reasons have been urged against this operation by Dr. W. Hunter,[*] and it appears in every respect unadvisable.

See Medical Observations and Inquries, vol. ii, page 41.

CLASS V.

CHRONIC CONSTITUTIONAL DISEASES.

CHAP. I.

SCROFULA.

General Outline of the Pathology of Scrofula. Marks of Scrofula in the healthy conditions of the Body. Characters of Scrofulous Disease. Structures affected by Scrofula. Causes of scrofula. Hereditary Predisposition. Acquired Scrofulous Diathesis. Causes leading to the development of Scrofulous Disease. Principles of Treatment. Importance of pure air. Sea Bathing. Nourishing Diet. Influence of tonic, alkaline, and other Medicines. Treatment of Scrofulous Inflammation of the Lymphatic Glands.

THE pathology of scrofula is altogether *sui generis*, not assimilating with that of any other known disease. It is moreover a subject of very great difficulty. A full investigation of it presupposes an acquaintance with almost all forms of disease, and of the modifications of which they are susceptible. Its extent is unbounded. To the physician and the surgeon it is equally an object of attention. Whether we regard symptoms, causes, or treatment,—whether we view diseases as external or internal, acute or chronic, a knowledge of the several doctrines connected with scrofula is indispensable to their complete elucidation. It may be considered, in fact as the most important of those great links which bind together the infinitely varied ramifications of medical inquiry.

Interesting as scrofula is to the *general* pathologist, it cannot be denied that it is more especially essential in the inquiries of the surgeon. The principal forms of scrofulous disease being external fall under his cognizance, and from them the chief characters of the affection are necessarily derived. These considerations will point out how little calculated is this investigation for a work so brief in its plan, and so confined in its design, as the present. We may even go further, and say, that a subject of such extent and difficulty is ill suited for elementary works generally, and that the student should at first content himself with a superficial examination of it. Such at least is all that will here be attempted.

Scrofula is usually designated by nosologists as a morbid state of the *lymphatic glandular* system, but our notions of the affection would be very imperfect were we to view it only in this light. On the other hand, some have altogether denied to scrofula the name of a *disease*, and have considered it only as a peculiar habit of body giving a *predisposition* to morbid action. Without waiting to discuss a point which resolves itself into a mere dispute about words, I proceed to state, that independent of the unequivocal characters of scrofulous *disease*, there are marks by which, in the very healthiest conditions of the body, the scrofulous disposition may (not indeed with certainty, but with a reasonable share of probability) be distinguished. Of this kind are, a fair, thin, smooth skin, in which the blood vessels are particularly apparent ; light and soft hair ; large blue eyes and a blooming complexion ; the upper lip, columna nasi, and lower part of the nostril, more tumid than natural ; fulness and turgescence of the veins ; long and slender fingers ; and lastly, a narrow chest, and prominent shoulders. The scrofulous habit is thus characterized by a geneal laxity of muscular fibre, and delicacy of organization throughout the body. The mental faculties are usually developed early. The intellect is acute and lively.

The scrofulous diathesis, however, can never be decisively proved by the concurrence even of all these appearances. There must be superadded to them certain *morbid* phenomena, before its presence in the system can confidently be pronounced ; and these will seldom fail to exhibit themselves, for scrofula is marked by a peculiar disposition to morbid action in the body. Among the earliest, the most frequent, and most characteristic symptoms of the disease, are swellings of the absorbent glands, particularly those of the neck. This too is the mildest form under which scrofula ever appears. Such tumours sometimes continue for a long time, neither advancing nor receding, unattended by pain or any constitutional disturbance. Sometimes they subside spontaneously, but more frequently suppuration of an imperfect kind gradually takes place in them, followed by open ulceration. The ulcers heal slowly, leaving ragged and unsightly scars, and are succeeded by other tumours, which run a similar course. In this manner the disease is often kept up for a series of years, until at length the constitution strengthening either throws it off, or it appears under some of its more severe and dangerous forms.

An opinion has been entertained, that in scrofula a *morbid matter* is generated which has a *specific* influence on the lymphatic system; but there are no sufficient grounds for this notion. What the circumstances, however, are, which in a scrofulous habit render the lymphatic system so peculiarly liable to inflammation we know not. Scrofula affects equally many other structures,* and in all cases the inflammation which is excited has the same general character. It is of a chronic, languid kind. The scrofulous abscess is distinguished by its jagged and uneven sides. The pus which it contains, instead of having a bland, uniform, cream-like appearance, is thin, or *ichorous*, and mixed with curdy flakes. The ulcer by which it is succeeded has a smooth, obtuse, and overlapping margin. The surface of the sore is of a light red colour, and the granulations are flabby and indistinct. For a great length of time, in spite of every care, it remains indolent, neither increasing nor diminishing in size.

There is hardly an organ or tissue of the body which can be considered free from the occasional ravages of scrofula. It appears sometimes in the head, in the form of small tumours, attached to the membranes, or imbedded in the substance of the brain or cerebellum, and laying the foundation of hydrocephalus. In the lungs, scrofula exhibits itself in the form of tubercles, scattered through their substance, modifying the character of inflammation in that organ, and producing genuine consumption. Scrofula, in like manner, attacks in their turn all the viscera of the abdomen, the liver, the peritonæum, the kidney, the ovaria, and above all the mesenteric glands.

Of the external parts of the body liable to scrofulous disease (independent of the lymphatic system) may be particularly specified, the tarsi, the thyroid gland, the mamma, the testicle, and lastly, the bones and other structures connected with joints. These varied forms of scrofulous disease constitute a very large proportion of the objects of a surgeon's attention. Scrofula predisposes to infantile remitting fever, to chorea, and to several other kinds, of *consti-*

---

* The gradual expansion of the opinions of pathologists regarding the nature of scrofula, will be found ably detailed in an article in the Edinburgh Medical and Surgical Journal, xviii, p. 121.

tutional ailment it would be desirable certainly, to ascertain, and strictly according with the design of this work to point out, the unvarying, the *pathognomonic* characters of scrofulous complaints generally, and thus to limit the application of a term which is now perhaps employed too extensively. The task, however, is a very difficult one, and in the present state of the science hardly to be effected. I pass on therefore, to the consideration of the *causes* of scrofula, a branch of the inquiry involving many interesting but doubtful points.

All periods of life are liable to scrofulous disease, but the tendency to it is certainly greatest in childhood, and again when the growth of the body is completed. If a person, most obviously scrofulous, passes his thirtieth year, he may then in a great measure consider himself secure from its ravages. Age has a singular power in modifying the liability which particular structures have to this disease. In early life the lymphatic glands, the tarsi, and the joints, are those which chiefly suffer. After puberty the lungs are principally affected. In advanced life the disease, when, it does, occur, has a tendency to disorganize the abdominal viscera,—the liver, kidney, and prostate gland.

Much discussion has arisen regarding the propriety of calling scrofula an *hereditary* complaint ; but the general observation of mankind has decided this question. It is not contended, that all the children of scrofulous parents are *necessarily* scrofulous, that the scrofulous taint can never be eradicated from a family, or that the disease is not occasionally generated in persons whose parents were free from any suspicion of it. The opinion must be received with limitations. Scrofula is hereditary as far as any disease can be so, as far as any kind of temperament or constitutional peculiarity can descend from parents to their offspring. Children of scrofulous parents undoubtedly often continue through their whole lives entirely free from the disease ; but the spirit of the doctrine is this: —of two families of children, the one born of scrofulous, the other of healthy parents, the probability is strongly in favour of the disease breaking out in the former, rather than in the latter.

That the scrofulous diathesis may be *acquired*, is a point which no one, I presume, would venture to dispute. The very notion of hereditary transmission presupposes some one in whom the morbid phænomena primarily appeared. The same causes which, operating in a minor degree, lead to scrofulous disease in those hereditarily predisposed, will, in a higher degree, *generate* it. It appears indeed to be satisfactorily ascertained, that no purity or strength of original constitution will exempt from the ravages of scrofula those who have been long and repeatedly exposed to its exciting causes. In considering what the circumstances are, which lead to the development of a scrofulous diathesis, we should direct our attention principally to climate, town air, diet, mode of life, and lastly, previous disease.

1. The influence of climate is immense, and may be estimated by the following facts. In the East and West Indies scrofula is hardly known, but when the natives of either are brought into this or any European country, they suffer from it severely.* The prevalence of scrofula is directly proportioned to the coldness, or, more properly, to the *variableness* of the climate. Scrofulous affections are principally met with in all countries during the winter months. They rapidly improve, or disappear altogether, on the approach of summer, and this effect of warm weather upon scrofulous ulcers is important in *diagnosis* as well as in practice. 2. Among the causes of scrofula, the close confined air of a town appears to merit especial mention. The complaint is infinitely more common among the inhabitants of a town, than among those of a corresponding class of society breathing the pure air of the country. It is notorious, that the population of our large manufacturing towns (Manchester for instance,) pent up during the day in cotton-mills, are of all others most afflicted with it. 3. Certain modes of life contribute also in no small degree to the development of scrofula,—confined habitations, want of cleanliness, sedentary occupations, irregular habits, but, above all, deficient or unwholesome diet. They concur in reducing the tone of the system below that healthy standard, which is the surest preservative, not only against the attacks of scrofula, but of every other disorder. The extensive influence of debilitating causes, lastly, is demostrated by the prevalence of scrofulous affections subsequent to small-pox, measles, hooping cough, and other diseases which most unequivocally impair the energies of the constitution. Of late years, attempts have been made to connect the scrofulous diathesis in a peculiar manner with *primary* derangement of the digestive functions, but no sufficient reasons have been adduced in support of this opinion. It appears to me to be founded on very imperfect views of the mu-

* This was strikingly exemplified in 1816, when one of the West Indian regiments was stationed at Gibraltar.

tual influence of the different parts of the animal œconomy upon
each other.

These pathological considerations lead directly to practice. It
is obvious, that the *prevention* of a disease, and in a great degree
also the principles of treatment when it has broken out, must depend
on a knowledge of its causes. The time is past when direct or
specific remedies for the scrofulous diathesis could be proposed,
with any prospect of obtaining the confidence of professional men.
All that is now attempted is to avoid the obvious exciting causes,
and to place the system in that state, in which it may best resist
the operation of such as are more obscure, or altogether beyond
our control.

Climate cannot, except in a few instances, be changed ; but attention to clothing, more especially the use of flannel, will go far
towards obviating many of the injurious effects of that in which
we live. The importance of a pure country air, still more of the
air of the sea-side, has been long and very generally acknowledged.
There have been differences of opinion, however, as to the value
of *sea-bathing* in scrofula ; but it is hardly possible to entertain such
now, after the ample experience of its power, which has been afforded since the establishment of the Margate Sea-Bathing Infirmary. Some caution is of course necessary in its application.
The constitution must have vigour to support the shock of immer-
sion, and the system must be free from fever or latent visceral disease. In some cases, the warm salt bath may be preferable to
the open sea ; but there are few, even of the most aggravated forms
of the disease, which are not benefited by sea bathing under judicious management. There is even strong reason to believe, that
a perseverance in it for two or three years during the summer
months, has materially contributed to assist the constitution in ·
throwing off the disease altogether.

Regular exercise and early hours will of course be enjoyed ;
but attention to diet is of all measures perhaps the most important
with a view to the permanent security of the patient. The value
of a wholesome nutritious diet in scrofula can hardly be overrated,
but the *asthenic* nature of the disease has often led both parents and
practitioners to a hurtful extreme. They have overloaded a delicate stomach with full meals of stimulating food, wine, and fermented liquors ; and thus, in their attempts to strengthen the system, have brought on the very condition of the stomach and bowels, in which the seeds of scrofulous action are most effectually

laid. It should be remembered, that there is no morbid state which is not, in one sense, debilitating, and in which, by parity of reason, the same treatment is not requisite. The diet of a child liable to scrofula, then, should be nourishing, not stimulating, and given only in such quantity, and at such regular intervals, that the stomach may never be *oppressed*.

I would not wish to undervalue the influence of *remedies*; but it requires only a very superficial knowledge of the disease to be convinced, that in comparison with those other means of relief which have been recommended (warm clothing, pure air, cold sea bathing, and nutritious diet), they are of little avail. Those which chiefly deserve confidence, are occasional gentle purgatives containing a small proportion of calomel, followed by the use of bitters and the carbonate of soda, when the functions of the stomach and bowels are impaired; the more powerful tonics, steel, bark, or the mineral acids, when the constitution is much debilitated; and certain mild alteratives, such as the decoction of sarsaparilla, and the liquor potassæ, in states of the system not so well defined. To these a long catalogue of drugs might be added, which have acquired reputation in the hands of different practitioners. Dr. Cullen recommended the coltsfoot, and Dr. Crawford the muriate of baryta. Dr. Storck had equal confidence in hemlock. These remedies however have followed the fate of others which preceded them, and are now almost discarded from common use.

It remains only that I advert briefly to the treatment of that characteristic form of scrofula, to which the term king's evil is specifically appropriated, and in which the lymphatic glands of the neck become enlarged, with or without supervening inflammation. Besides the general measures already recommended, and which of course are equally serviceable in this as in every other variety of scrofula, advantage has been derived, where the tumours are indolent, from stimulating or *discutient* remedies, such as lotions and poultices made of sea-water, mercurial plaisters, and friction. When the tumour has advanced so as to form an abscess, and the skin is so far destroyed as to leave an open sore, the case is purely surgical; and for its management under these circumstances I refer to the writers on surgery, who abound in directions for the treatment of scrofulous ulcers.

CHAP. II.

————

Literary History of this Disease. Symptoms of Rickets. Its supposed Causes. Its Dependence on bad Nursing. Pathology. Treatment.

It is a singular circumstance, that a disease arising, as we have reason to believe, from causes which must have operated in all ages and countries, should not have attracted attention until a very recent period. That it must have existed previously can hardly be doubted; and we are reduced therefore to the alternative of either imputing great negligence to the early observers in not having noticed it, or bad pathology in having confounded it with scrofula. The first account which we have of rickets was drawn up by Glisson, in conjunction with two other English physicians, in 1650, and it is both copious and accurate. Their inquiries tended to prove, that the disease first appeared in the western counties of England about the year 1620, whence it spread over the whole of Europe. A long controversy succeeded on the question of its modern origin. Zeviani and De Haen attempted to trace it in the writings of Hippocrates, but failed.

Rickets is, comparatively speaking, a rare disease. We meet with but few deformed persons in the streets, and there can, I believe, be little doubt that it is now much less frequent than when it first attracted the notice of English physicians. A very short description of it therefore will suffice on the present occasion.

Rickets never appears in children at birth, and very rarely indeed before the ninth month, or after the second year. The advances of the disease are gradual, and at first hardly perceptible. One of the earliest symptoms is an unnatural softness and flaccidity of the flesh. The body emaciates, although the appetite be good, and food perhaps be taken in sufficient quantity. The cheeks are wan and sallow; the abdomen protuberant; the stools unhealthy in their aspect; the urine turbid. Dentition goes on slowly: the teeth which appear are unsound, and speedily become loose and carious. The process of ossification is peculiarly imperfect, and this leads to many of the most characteristic features of the complaint. The fontanelles and sutures are more open than is usual with healthy children of the same age. The head appears large with respect to the body, and the forehead prominent. The ribs flatten at their sides, and the sternum projects into a ridge. The epiphyses of the long bones become spongy, and the joints therefore appear swelled. This is particularly manifest in the wrists, ancles, and knees. If the child had begun to walk, he daily becomes more feeble on his legs; he waddles, and speedily returns to his nurse's arms. As the disease advances the bones are rendered soft, and being unable to resist the weight of the body, or of the muscles inserted into them, are strangely and frightfully distorted. The spine particularly suffers. The dorsal vertebræ are forced out of their places by the weight of the head, and the child becomes hump-backed.

It is frequently remarked, that the evolution of the mental faculties does not correspond with this *stagnation* of the assimilating functions. In many cases, the child learns to talk with surprising rapidity, and enjoys an acuteness of intellect much beyond his age. The same thing is equally observable in *scrofulous* cases. The phænomenon is not, however, of invariable occurrence. In that highest grade of rickets, which occurs in some of the valleys of the Alps and Pyrenees, and to which the term CRETINISM has been applied, the mind becomes completely imbecile and fatuous.

It is seldom that rickets prove fatal. Usually after the lapse of two or three years the constitution acquires sufficient strength to put a check to its further advances, and at length the general health is thoroughly re-established. If the distortion of the limbs had not proceeded very far, it will often be remedied in after-life in proportion as the bones lengthen; and it is surprising to see how much nature will sometimes effect in such cases. But where the distortion has been very great, particularly, as Glisson remarks, if the child passes his fifth year without any decided symptoms of improvement, he will continue a miserable object through life. Dissections of those who have died of rickets do not unfold any peculiar affection of the viscera.

Some very extraordinary opinions have been entertained regarding the origin and pathology of rickets. It was at one time supposed to be allied to syphilis ; and more lately a pathological connection between scrofula and rickets has been insisted on, hardly supported, however, on better authority. From the circumstance of its frequently appearing among the children of the same family, it has been considered as *hereditary*. All the older writers agreed in the belief that the constitution of parents had much to do with the appearance of rickets in their offspring, and the opinion received the high sanction of Dr. Cullen's authority.

There appears little occasion, however, for accusing the *constitution* of parents. Their inattention and neglect are quite sufficient to account for the phænomena. Pathologists are now, I believe, well satisfied that rickets is the disease of bad nursing. The child is kept on a bed instead of being tossed about in the arms. It is confined to a close ill-ventilated small room, instead of ranging at large in an airy one. It is scarcely ever carried into the open air. The child's body is neither washed nor rubbed as it should be. When it has arrived at the eighth or ninth month, it is taken from the breast, and crammed with all manner of unwholesome food. That this system of management, persevered in for several months, should end in great constitutional disturbance, can hardly surprise us ; and that these are the real efficient causes of rickets will be obvious from this,—that the disease appears only among the lower orders of the people, who cannot afford the time to nurse their children properly, or among those of an upper rank who are put out to nurse, where the same interest cannot be taken in the welfare of the child as if it were brought up at home.

Various conjectures have been offered as to the proximate cause of rickets. A depraved state of the blood and humours, with a laxity of structure in the solid parts, was the suggestion of the early writers. Dr. Cullen attributed every thing to debility of the digestive organs. A chemical theory in later times has made the disease depend on a deficient formation of the phosphate of lime. The theory of constitutional diseases is necessarily obscure, and nothing appears to be gained by the display of pathological learning which has been made in the case of rickets. Every function of the system languishes. Digestion, assimilation, nutrition, absorption, are equally impaired ; and as the whole system is in fault, from causes which operate widely, so must the cure be attempted by measures of general application.

Strict attention to regimen is above all things to be insisted on. Daily washing, cool and fresh air, exercise suited to the age of the patient, and either breast-milk or a nutritious unirritating diet, are to be rigorously enforced. If the system be not exceedingly reduced, cold bathing during the summer months, and tepid bathing in the winter, will conduce essentially to recovery. Frictions are of some use. Bandages I believe to be altogether ineffectual.

Tonic medicines, in moderate quantities and not too long continued, may be exhibited with some advantage. Steel wine is a favourite and useful domestic remedy. A powder containing the carbonate of iron and calumba (R No. 65, or the tonic electuary (R No. 66,) may be substituted. Cascarilla and the Peruvian bark, with acid, have been serviceable in many cases. An occasional dose of rhubarb or of scammony, with calomel prevents the accumulation of sordes in the stomach and bowels, promotes digestion, and thus tends materially to invigorate the general system. In slighter cases it will be sufficient to direct, along with the steel wine and daily cold washing, five grains of hydrag. cum creta with three or four of rhubarb, to be given every other night at bed-time.

CHAP. III.

Of Cachexia. Character of the Class Cachexia. Of Scurvy. Its Symptoms and Causes. Speculations on its intimate Nature. Treatment. Influence of Antiscorbutics. Of the Cachexia Africana. Of Beriberi.

THE term cachexia was employed by Dr. Cullen and some other nosologists to express that depraved condition of body which is the result of depressing causes long operating, without fever. Of such a kind are deficient nourishment, food of an improper *quality*, want of exercise suitable to the age and circumstances of the individual, irregular hours and modes of life, habits of intemperance, the venereal poison, a long and ill-conducted course of mercury, and lastly, a bad condition of the air. There are the strongest grounds for believing, that the intimate nature of cachexia is a deterioration in the qualities of the blood, a favourite doctrine with the humoral pathologists, in support of which many very powerful arguments might still be adduced.

Several diseases exist, having for their characteristic feature such a depraved or *cachectic* state of the system. Rickets, of which we have already treated, is the principal form of infantile cachexia. In the present chapter, I shall treat of some affections occurring to adults, in which cachexia is manifestly present; and first of SCURVY.

A variety of cutaneous eruptions, supposed to be dependent on a morbid condition of the blood, are familiarly called *scorbutic*; but in strict nosological language, the term scurvy is appropriated to a disease seldom met with except among seamen. It has been designated as one of the great *sea endemics*, and has proved, even up to a late period, the destruction of many a fleet.* Of a disease

---

* The ravages of this disease are finely pictured in the " Account of Lord Anson's Voyage round the World in 1743."

which I have rarely seen, and can hardly expect to see, I would willingly omit the consideration; but to complete the plan of the work, I shall venture on a very brief sketch of its symptoms, causes, and treatment, abstracted from the essay of most repute on this subject.*

The scurvy comes on gradually, with lassitude, disinclination to motion, and difficulty of breathing on slight exertion. The face assumes a pale or yellowish hue. The gums swell and bleed upon the slightest friction. They appear soft, spungy, and sometimes livid. The breath is offensive. The skin is dry and rough or sometimes smooth and shining. It will generally be found covered with livid spots, which coalesce into large blotches (particularly about the legs and thighs,) and obviously arise from the effusion of blood. The legs swell, and ultimately the whole body becomes œdematous. The patient complains of a pain in all his bones, with tightness and oppression about the chest. Any sore which may happen to be on the body acquires the peculiar character de-nominated *scorbutic*. It discharges a fœtid or bloody sanies. The base of the sore is covered with sloughs. Its edges are livid, and lined with a soft bloody fungus that increases rapidly.

In what has been called the second or aggravated stage of the complaint, the patient loses all use of his limbs; the tendons in the hams are contracted, with swelling and pain of the knees and oth-er joints. General emaciation ensues, with a tendency to syncope on the slightest exertion. Hæmorrhages break forth from the nose, ears, and bladder. Diarrhœa supervenes, and the stools are offen-sive and bloody. The patient either dies dropsical, or exhausted by some sudden effort.

Very ample experience has proved that scurvy arises from de-ficiency of proper nutriment. It occurs to sailors when living on salt provisions, more especially such as have been long kept, and which, therefore, contain very little nourishing matter. All obser-vations tend further to prove, that the disposition to the disease is greatly augmented by neglect of cleanliness, imperfect ventilation, want of proper exercise, and a cold damp atmosphere.

The whole train of symptoms manifestly points out extreme fee-bleness of the powers of life, as the leading principle in the patho-logy of scurvy. Attempts have been made, however, to define more accurately the *seat* of the disease. Dr. Lind is of opinion,

* Treatise on the Scurvy, by Dr. James Lind. 1772.

that scurvy consists mainly in a weakened and relaxed state of the *solids*. Dr. Cullen, on the other hand, imagines that a putrescent state of the *blood* (the result of its complete impregnation with salt) is the true proximate cause of the disease. How far the latter opinion is correct, it is hardly possible to determine, for we have no authentic accounts of the disease appearing, where salt provisions could fairly be considered as the *sole* agents in its pro- duction. Common sense and pathology equally teach us, that in scurvy there is laxity of the solids and putrescency of the fluids, and that in fact every function and structure of the body partici- pate in the general weakness.

Whatever difficulties may be experienced in determining the theory of scurvy, few points in medicine are less susceptible of dispute than its treatment. In fact, scarcely any thing else is re- quisite than a return to wholesome diet, particularly to the use of fresh vegetables. For this hardly any thing will compensate. The great object of navy surgeons is not to cure, so much as to *prevent* the scurvy; and this is now effected by an admirable system of regulations, in which *diet* and *regimen* are equally looked to. To unfold these is out of the scope of a strictly medical inquiry. It is sufficient to say, that they comprise attention to personal clean- liness, clothing, ventilation, exercise, with the means of avoiding cold and damp. To these may further be added the daily use of what are called *antiscorbutics*. Substances of this class have long and justly enjoyed a reputation in the world as *purifiers* or *sweeten- ers* of the blood. Those which the experience of the navy has shown to be most deserving of confidence, are lime-juice, pre- served fruits, sugar, infusion of malt, spruce beer, and vinegar. The power of lime-juice in preventing and checking scurvy has been proved by the most ample experience, insomuch that this remedy well deserves to be called a *specific*.

Where the disease has made its appearance, and the true anti- scorbutics (fresh vegetable and animal food, or, in their stead, lime-juice) cannot be procured, bark, the mineral acids, and medi- cines of the alterative kind may be tried; but the prospect of suc- cess from them is small. Scorbutic ulcers are improved by local applications of an astringent and antiseptic nature; but it is obvi- ous that their cure must equally depend on the employment of the proper *constitutional* means.

CACHEXIA AFRICANA.

This term has been appropriated to a very singular disease of negroes, met with in the West Indies, but more especially in the island of Trinidad. It is there called *mal d'estomac*, from one of its most remarkable features, an oppressive weakness of the stomach. The other phænomena of the disease, pointing out its truly cachectic charac'er, may be thus described.

After various attacks of intermittent or remittent fever, of dysentery, or pneumonia, by which the health of the individual is manifestly impaired, he becomes pale, and squalid, and unable to take exercise. The feet and legs swell, especially towards evening. There is palpitation, and occasional vomiting. As the complaint advances, these symptoms increase in severity. The stomach rejects all kinds of food and medicine. The most moderate exercise, especially in ascents, occasions a sense of urgent suffocation and even syncope. On one remarkable occasion, witnessed and described by Dr. Ferguson, when the Royal West India Rangers after a long residence in Trinidad were marching along the level parade of St. Ann's, Barbadoes, the men dropt and fell out of the ranks by dozens, as if under a murderous fire of musquetry. Their quivering bloodless lips, ghastly looks, and hurried convulsive breathing, presented a striking image of the mortally wounded. By degrees the cellular membrane becomes everywhere distended with serum, and a peculiar white adipose substance may be observed in its cells, through the distended and almost translucid integuments. Its presence gives to the face and whole body that whitish colour, which is the common pathognomonic symptom of the complaint.

On dissection, this white matter is seen deposited in the cells of the cellular membrane. Serum is accumulated in the ventricles of the brain, and in the serous cavities of the thorax and abdomen. But the most peculiar appearance is a diminution, or rather an abolition of the muscular substance of the heart. The heart, often enlarged and overloaded with fat, when taken in the hand, yields to the slightest pressure, and its ventricles, like membranous sacs, are easily pressed together.

* Dissertatio Medica Inauguralis de Sanitate et Vi animi inter Tropieos. Edin. 1819.

Dr. M' Cabe, to whose treatise* I am indebted for this description of the complaint, attributes it to the frequent changes of temperature and the extreme moisture of the air which distinguish the climate of Trinidad. To these sources of the disease must be added frequent intemperance. Dr. Ferguson ascribes it to the gradual action of a malaria on the human constitution. It is very common on the swampy banks of the great rivers of Guiana, and in the marshy districts of Trinidad at some distance from the sea coast. The soldiers of the black regiments stationed in Trinidad are its principal victims.

The proximate cause of this disease is doubtless a cachectic state of the blood. Imperfectly formed, and wanting its natural proportion of red globules, it communicates neither energy nor density to the musculur fibre. The treatment must of course consist in change of climate, and in the exhibition of nourishing food and tonic medicines.

The complaint known in the East Indies under the name of BE-RIBERI is perhaps of the same nature. It has for its principal symptoms an enfeebled paralytic state of the lower limbs. The patient staggers in his walk, in a manner not unlike the gait of a sheep. This is succeeded by an œdematous swelling of the extremities, with oppressed breathing, and the bloated leucophlegmatic countenance of hydrothorax. The danger attending it does not appear to be so great as might have been expected. Beriberi, in the Singhalese tongue, means *very weak*, and it is doubtful whether this term be not also applied to some other complaints which have *weakness* for their characteristic feature.

CHAP. IV.

States of the System in which cutaneous Hæmorrhagy takes place. Malignant Fever. Plethora, with Congestions or iregular Distributions of Blood. Exhaustion. Phænomena of chronic cutaneous Hæmorrhage. Prognosis. Treatmeut.

IN several parts of this work allusion has been made to the occurrence of hæmorrhage from the cutaneous capillaries; and as the pathological doctrines which it involves possess considerable interest, it will be right to bring them before the student in a connected manner. Independent of their more obvious bearings, they will serve to impress upon his mind principles, which, of all others, it appears to me of importance to inculcate; the *constitutional* disturbance present in a greater or less degree in almost every variety of disease, and the dependence of the same phænomenon upon very opposite states of the general system. I shall first point out the several conditions of the body in which cutaneous hæmorrhage has been observed to occur, and then detail the phænomena and treatment of that affection to which the terms *hæmorrahæa petechialis, petechiæ sine febre,* and *purpura hæmorrhagica,* have been commonly applied.

1. Purple spots on the skin, constituting petechiæ and vibices, are in the first place the result of febrile action, generally of a typhoid or malignant character. They occur sometimes at the very onset, sometimes towards the close of the fever. In the former case they often acquire an undue importance in the eyes of the practitioner, who is apt to overlook the febrile state by which they are accompanied. They are in strict nosological language cases of *petechial fever*; but the terms purpura contagiosa, and purpura maligna, have been frequently applied to them. Fevers of this class will commonly be found associated with great disturbance of function in the brain and nervous system, upon which, in all probabili-

ty, the cutaneous hæmorrhage immediately depends. It is hardly
necessary to add, that the occurrence of petechiæ in an early stage
of fever is a symptom of urgent danger. It denotes either uncommon malignity in the contagion, or a peculiarly depressed and languid state of the body in which the contagion operates. On opening the bodies of those who die of the disease, it will generally
be found that the hæmorrhagic tendency displays itself equally in
some of the internal organs. I have noticed effusions of blood in
the heart and mesentery.

2. An eruption of purple spots in every respect resembling those
which occur in fever, is sometimes met with accompanying plethora ; still more decisively in connection with symptoms denoting
congestion of blood in some of the great organs of the body, or irregular distribution of blood throughout the body generally. It has
been observed along with, and probably depending upon, thoracic
disease of an obscure kind, marked by dyspnœa and an oppressed
pulse, and commonly described as a state of congestion about the
heart and lungs. Dr. Batemen* details the particulars of a case
that fell under his own observation, in which the disease appeared
to arise from an enlargement of the thyroid gland. I observed it,
in one instance, succeeding measles.

Again, chronic cutaneous hæmorrhage has frequently been
found associated with *abdominal* disease. It has long been known
that morbid states of the spleen are attended with different forms of
hæmorrhage, and among others with that from the cutaneous capillaries. Cases not unfrequently occur in which purpura is connected with hepatic obstruction (the result of habitual spirit-drink-
ing,) evidenced by the jaundiced hue of the skin and eyes, pain of
the side, and dry cough. Some recent observations have led to the
belief that purpura occasionally depends on a morbid condition of
the villous coat of the intestinal canal. It would be more correct,
perhaps, in this and other cases, to consider both the abdominal
and cutaneous disease as *effects* of an ulterior but obscure cause
influencing the *whole habit of body.*

3. A disposition to petechiæ appears, in the third place, as a consequence of deficient nourishment, and other most unequivocally
debilitating causes. It has been met with in children ill fed and
nursed, and among persons of all ages who live in close situations,
enjoying but little exercise in the open air, whose chief diet is tea,

* Practical Synopsis of cutaneous Diseases, page 111.

and who are exposed to much fatigue, long watching, and great mental anxiety. It is not uncommon in the last stages of infantile marasmus ; and it has been observed in adults exhausted by any severe or protracted illness, especially dropsy.

4. Cutaneous hæmorrhage, lastly, is in some instances altogether *constitutional* ;—that is to say, it depends upon a natural inherent weakness of the circulating system. In such habits of body, attacks of petechiæ are *habitual*, whereas in all the cases hitherto alluded to they are *accidental*. They then occur on very slight occasions, and not unfrequently without any apparent cause. Errors in diet, unusual fatigue, or exposure to cold are sufficient to induce them. In aggravated cases the gentlest pressure on the skin will occasion a purple blotch like that which is left after a severe bruise. In constitutions so disposed, the drawing of a tooth is sometimes followed by alarming hæmorrhage. Instances are even on record of death from such a cause.

The first of these states of disease does not require further investigation. The other three constitute the different species of that complaint which received from Dr. Adair, in 1779, the name of hæmorrhœa petechialis. There is the utmost variety both in the manner in which the hæmorrhage commences and ceases, and its accompanying symptoms. It sometimes occurs suddenly ; but more commonly is preceded for a week or two by great lassitude, faintness, and pain of the limbs. In its progress it is attended with extreme debility and depression of spirits, and a pulse generally feeble. After the disease has continued for some time the patient becomes sallow, and much emaciated, and a degree of œdema appears in the lower extremities, which gradually extends to other parts. The effusion of blood commonly commences in the legs. The spots are at first of a bright red colour, but soon become purple and when about to disappear, change to a brown or yellowish hue. The cuticle covering them is smooth, and not sensibly elevated, except in a few rare cases, which Dr. Willan distinguished by the name of purpura urticans. They vary in size, from the minutest point to that of streaks and large blotches. They are neither itchy nor in any way painful.

Discharge of blood take place at the same time from some of the great mucous surfaces,—from the gums, nostrils, lungs, stomach and bowels, or urethra. These hæmorrhages are often profuse, and not easily restrained. The disease is extremely uncertain in its duration. Where the hæmorrhagic diathesis is constitutional, it may continue to harass the patient, more or less, through life. Where it arises from accidental causes, its severity and termination are in some degree under our own control. When the disease ends fatally, it is often by a copious and sudden discharge of blood from some important, organ—the lungs, the stomach, or the uterus.

In the treatment of hæmorrhœa petechialis, no rule of practice can be laid down which shall be universally applicable. We have improved certainly upon the notions of the older physicians, in admitting that cutaneous hæmorrhage does not necessarily preclude the application of the lancet; but further than this it would be unsafe to go. The idea of treating all, or even the majority of cases of this disease by depleting measures, is hardly less blamable than the blind adherence to astringents and stimulants which characterized the practice of an earlier age. A *constitutional* tendency to ecchymosis is best combated by those tonic means which are of slow operation, but of undoubted efficacy,—I mean pure country air, regular exercise, nourishing food, early hours, and such amusements as withdraw the mind from the cares and fatigues of business or study. The use of the mineral acids, bark, and a moderate allowance of wine, will coincide with the general indication. The same plan of treatment is applicable to such *accidental* cases of purpura as arise in debilitated habits, and are accompanied by a weak pulse, a sallow dirty complexion, and a tendency to syncope or œdema. In many of these, wine and beef tea are required, with stimulating remedies in full doses.

No theoretical views of laxity or debility, however, are to prevent our having recourse to a different system of management, when the disease occurs under opposite circumstances. If petechiæ appear in persons already enjoying pure air, and suffering no privation of diet; if they are accompanied by a sharp pulse, a white and loaded tongue, with occasional chills; and if, at the same time, there are fixed internal pains, cough, dyspnœa, or other symptoms indicating the existence of some local visceral congestion, tonic medicines will be ineffectual, if not actually injurious. Depleting measures proportioned to the urgency of the symptoms must here be promptly resorted to. Blood may be taken from the arm, in the first instance, with safety and advantage. Free purging is well suited to these cases. Calomel and jalap in active doses may be liberally given.

The convalescence will generally prove tedious; for the disease is one which denotes, under all circumstances, very deep and extensive disturbance throughout the whole animal œconomy.

CHAP. V.

DIABETES. .

Division into the insipid and saccharine Varieties. Symptoms of the true Diabetes Mellitus. Prognosis. Appearances on Dissection. Causes. Conjectures concerning the Nature and Seat of Diabetes. Proposed Plans of Treatment. Influence of Drugs on the Secretion of Diabetic Urine.

THIS singular disease has excited a more than common interest among the pathologists of modern times. The original description of it is to be met with in the writings of Aretæus ; but though it has been known from so distant a period, few attempts were made until lately to investigate its nature. That they have not been followed by all the success which might be desired, may be attributed in part to the rarity of the complaint; but much curious information has been collected concerning it, and many ingenious conjectures have been thrown out regarding its remote and proximate causes, which may prove useful to the student. These it is my present object to lay before him in a condensed form. The leading symptoms being an increase in the quantity, and an alteration in the quality of the urine, diabetes has usually been considered as a disease of the kidney ; but this is merely a conjecture, into the merits of which we may hereafter inquire. The phænomena which it presents ought, in the first place, to be studied without reference to any peculiar pathological opinion.

An increased flow of urine accompanies several disorders, especially such as are of a convulsive, or *hysterical* character. These, however, are not included under the head of *diabetes*. Nosologists have confined this term to cases in which the increased flow of urine is *permanent*, and with which are associated constitutional symptoms usually designated by the term *cachexia*. Two *species* of diabetes have been described, the *insipidus*, and *mellitus* ; and it

has long been a question, whether these differ in any *essential* cir.
cumstances from each other. Dr. Prout is inclined to believe
they do, and recommends, that the term diabetes should in future
be restricted to those affections in which the urine is *saccharine.*
I shall principally direct my attention to the phænomena of the
genuine diabetes mellitus, noticing incidentally the peculiarities of
the other variety of the complaint.

Diabetes makes its approaches very insidiously. The first symp.
toms usually complained of are lassitude, weakness, a disposition
to sweating on slight exertions, and head-ache. Sometimes a diseased state of the urine advances to a considerable extent, and
subsists for some time, without being accompanied by any strongly-
marked constitutional disturbance, and occasionally even without
attracting the notice of the patient. The most striking symptom
of the disease is an increase in the *quantity* of the urine. This va.
ries very much in different cases, and is for the most part a good
index of the violence of the disease. The largest quantity which
I have seen recorded as having been passed in twenty-four hours
is thirty-six pints ;* and it is no uncommon thing to find from twenty
to thirty pints discharged daily for weeks, or even months togeth.
er. The average quantity may perhaps be stated at twelve or fifteen
pints; and it is a remarkable fact, that in many instances it exceeds
the whole amount of ingesta, solid and fluid. The secretion of so
much urine is almost necessarily attended with a frequent desire to
pass it. The patient is generally compelled to rise three or four
times in the night for this purpose.

The urine of diabetes is of a pale straw colour. Its smell is
commonly faint and peculiar, sometimes resembling sweet whey
or milk. Its taste is, with few exceptions, decidedly saccharine,
in a greater or less degree.† Even if this should not be percepti.
ble in the first instance, it may often be detected when the urine is
concentrated by evaporation. In many cases the saccharine qual.
ity of the urine is occasionally suspended ; and this happens both
spontaneously, and from the influence of medicine. Of the fact,
that sugar is secreted by the kidney in this disease, no doubt can
be entertained. It is confirmed by the repeated experiments of
chemists in all countries. The quantity of sugar formed is in most
instances directly proportioned to the degree of *diuresis*, and may

---

* See Bardsley's " Medical Reports," page 103.

† This remarkable quality of diabetic urine was first noticed in 1684, by
Dr. Willis.

always be estimated by the specific gravity of the urine. We are indebted to Dr. Henry, of Manchester, for the following table, showing the quantity of solid extract in a pint of urine of different specific gravities.

Specific Gravity of the Urine at 60° compared to Water as 1000.	Quantity of solid Extract in a Wine Pint (in Grains.)	Quantity of solid Extract in a Wine Pint (in Ounces, Drachms, Scruples, and Grains.)			
		oz.	dr.	scr.	grs.
1020	382.4	0	6	1	2
1025	478.4	0	7	2	18
1030	574.4	1	1	1	14
1035	670.4	1	3	0	10
1040	766.4	1	4	2	6
1045	862.4	1	6	1	2
1050	958.4	1	7	2	18

Healthy urine has a specific gravity of 1012, and contains seven parts in a 100 of solid matter.

From this table it appears, that if a patient passes twelve pints of urine in a day, of the specific gravity 1035, he voids in that time above sixteen ounces and a half of solid matter. The quantity, however, is in many cases much greater than this.

Other important symptoms occur in diabetes besides those now specified. The appetite is usually much greater than in health; though digestion is seldom if ever perfect. There is uneasiness therefore in the stomach after meals, with flatulence, acid eructations, and irregular bowels. Thirst is a never-failing source of complaint, and often attracts the notice of the patient before he is sensible of the true nature of his case. The skin is dry, and has a peculiarly rough and parched feel from the total want of perspiration. The gums are often swelled, tender, and red; sometimes ulcerated. The breath has a subacid odour. The tongue is white and foul in the centre, with bright red edges. The mouth is dry and parched, and the taste depraved. The patient will generally be found to complain of some pain or sense of weakness in the loins. Phymosis and excoriations on the penis are frequently noticed. Besides these, there occur in almost all cases symptoms indicating general weakness or exhaustion—such as swelled legs, emaciation, coldness of the feet, dyspnoea on the slightest exertion, a sense of weight at the epigastrium, with tendency to syn-

cope, general languor, lassitude, and depression of spirits. Early
in the disease the pulse is seldom affected; but in its progress hectic fever supervenes, and the pulse becomes frequent, feeble, and
irritable.

The duration of diabetes is very variable. An instance is recorded where it ran its course, and proved fatal, in five weeks.
On the other hand, it has been known to last for several years, and
ultimately to wear out the constitution. The prognosis indeed, under all circumstances, is very unfavourable. A few well-authenti-
cated instances of recovery might be quoted; but they are too rare
to redeem the disease from the character of danger which it has so
long borne. It has proved fatal in three ways; first and most frequently by the supervention of either acute or chronic inflammation
in the chest; secondly, by dropsy and exhaustion; while in a few
cases the patient has been cut off suddenly. The distinction between the insipid and saccharine forms of diabetes to which I formerly adverted, is chiefly of importance with a view to prognosis.
The danger is certainly much greater where the saccharine quality
of the urine is thoroughly established.

Dissections of those who die of diabetes have been diligently
practised; but hitherto they have thrown no light whatever on the
nature of the complaint. The lungs are often found diseased. The
kidneys in a few cases have exhibited their usual healthy appearances; but commonly they are more or less affected. Their texture is more flaccid than natural, or they are turgid with blood,
though seldom enlarged in size. The cellular membrane surrounding the kidneys, that of the abdominal parietes, and of other parts
of the body, is frequently found loaded with a gelatinous substance.
I have seen the same, in a different form of chronic ailment, lining
the inner surface of the bladder; and it appears to be a diseased
secretion, occurring generally in worn-out constitutions.

In investigating the pathology of diabetes several curious questions occur. It may be right to remark, previously, that it is a disease observed in all ranks of society. No employment or profession
can be stated as particularly liable to, or exempt from it. It is met
with in both sexes, and at various ages; but it chiefly prevails
among men, and in the middle or advanced periods of life. It would
appear to be more frequent in cold than hot climates. Dyspeptic
complaints long continued may perhaps favour the disposition to
diabetes; but little or nothing is known regarding its remote or occasional causes. Intemperance, severe evacuations, hard labour,

and exposure to cold, have been accused of bringing it on, but I believe without any very adequate reason.

One of the first objects of pathological inquiry is to determine whether the saccharine condition of the urine is a primary feature in the complaint, and if it ever exists independent of increase in its *quantity*. Dr. Prout* is inclined to the opinion that it does, and that the increased flow of urine is referable to an *irritable* state of the system, which forms part of the disease, and resembles that present in hysteria and other nervous affections. Some of the constitutional symptoms attendant on diabetes are perhaps owing to the vitiated quality of the urine ; but the most distressing are doubtless to be referred to that enormous *drainage* from the system, both of fluid and solid matter, which takes place when the disease is severe. Differences of opinion are entertained regarding the origin of the sugar which exists in diabetic urine. Some imagine it to be formed in the stomach, and others in the kidney. Dr. Wollaston has rendered the latter the more probable opinion, by showing (Phil. Trans. 1811,) that sugar does not exist in the blood of diabetic patients whose urine is at the same time sweet. Many persons indeed have been inclined to consider the stomach as the *primary* seat of diabetes, and they support the opinion by reference to the thirst and inordinate appetite which attend it. Such symptoms, however, are more probably the result of excessive discharge.

A suggestion has been thrown out, that the functions of the lungs are primarily implicated, and that diabetes consists in perfect *animalization* of the blood, whereby sugar is formed instead of the true *animal* principles. The abettors of this opinion rely for its support, partly on the fact that diabetes is frequently succeeded by unequivocal affections of the lungs, and partly on the appearance of the blood drawn, which in some cases does not coagulate, and in many can be preserved a long time without putrefaction. Dr. Cullen looked upon diabetes as a disease of the kidney, and some later pathologists have revived the notion. Morbid anatomy does not favour it ; and I am disposed to think, that in this theory stress is laid on a single symptom to the neglect of others which equally tend to illustrate the real nature of the disease. No view of diabetes hitherto proposed appears so reasonable as that originally

* Inquiry concerning the deranged Operation of the urinary Organs, page 66.

suggested by Galen, who considered it as a disease depending on general constitutional disturbance, and allied pathologically to dropsy.* This indeed is not advancing far in the way of explanation, but it may still be preferable to simpler though less accurate hypotheses.

Where pathology is obscure the principles of treatment are necessarily deficient. To this we may ascribe the very opposite plans which have been devised for the cure of diabetes. The practice in this disorder, in fact, is almost purely empirical ; and, considering its great fatality, little else is requisite than a mere enumeration of the several kinds of treatment which have been proposed and a brief notice of the influence which medicine exerts upon it.

Astringent remedies were early resorted to, more particularly lime water, alum whey, kino, and catechu. On the supposition of diabetes being mainly a disease of debility, bark, chalybeates, and the mineral acids, have been extensively used. In 1776 Dr. Rollo suggested the employment of animal diet, and experience has shown that it possesses an undoubted power of diminishing the *quantity* of urine. It will be found, however, in practice, that this plan of treatment can never be rigidly enforced. Blood-letting has been tried by some practitioners, and has proved serviceable in one or two cases ; but it cannot be recommended for general adoption. Cupping from the loins has been practised with the view of diminishing the morbid excitement of the kidney. Opium is the latest and most esteemed remedy ; but upon this, and upon all other remedies for the cure of diabetes, one remark may suffice. Many drugs exert a *certain* power over the disease, which after a time fails. A blister to the loins will occasionally check, in a remarkable manner, the inordinate secretion of urine. Uva ursi, alum, and opium, will do the same in other cases ; but the relief they afford is temporary ; and when the influence of the drug goes off, we are still as far removed as ever from the cure of the complaint.

Pathological considerations lead to a doubt, whether a remedy for diabetes, in its confirmed stage, can ever reasonably be expected.

* Galen informs us that the complaint was known in his days under the names of *diarrhœa per urinas*, and *hydrops ad matulam*.

CHAP. VI.

FEW topics in medicine have received more attention from systematic writers than dropsical effusion. The frequency of the complaint, the very striking influence exerted upon it by medicine, and the marked character of the symptoms, have contributed to obtain for it, in all ages, this share of attention. The subject being one of great extent and difficulty, it is not surprising that the notions concerning it, entertained by the older writers, should have been imperfect. Even with all the assistance which the labours of modern pathologists have afforded, it still continues obscure and incomplete. Their improvements, however, are undoubted ; and that the student should be able to appreciate their value, and at the same time form for himself correct notions of the nature of dropsy, he must, in the first instance, take a general survey of its *pathology.* Without this, his views of the disease must necessarily be limited and confused ; while, by its help, the details of symptoms, causes, and treatment in each of the principal varieties of dropsy are easily comprehended. The *nosological* division of dropsies are very necessary in practice, and will hereafter be adverted to, but there are certain *pathological* distinctions among them, which are at least equally important. With these I shall commence ; and to explain them shall, in the first place, direct the attention of the reader to the proximate causes of dropsy, and secondly, to that of the *appearances after death.*

The first distinction to be made among dropsies is, into such as are connected with general constitutional disturbance, and such as are strictly *local* (employing, of course, that term in the qualified sense in which it can alone be properly received in medical disquisitions.) Of the latter there are three principal forms,—cbro-. nic hydrocephalus, ovarial dropsy, and hydrocele. The two former have been already treated of. The latter is exclusively surgical. They may without impropriety, therefore, be excluded from our present consideration.

When dropsy exists along with constitutional derangement, it is reasonable to suppose that all the functions of the body participate, and doubtless this is a correct view of the case; but a notion has always prevailed, that the absorbent and sanguiferous systems are those which principally suffer. In former times, *diminished absorption* was viewed by pathologists as the leading feature of the complaint; and in the eyes of practitioners, the great principle of treatment was to stimulate the absorbents. More recently the circulating system has chiefly been looked to, and *increased exhalation* has been held up as the proximate cause of dropsy. We are too imperfectly acquainted with the physiology of the *absorbent* system, to determine what share it has in the production of dropsy; but the dependence of this disease on disturbance of the *sanguiferous* system is obvious, and of the first importance in practice. Dropsy is observed in two very opposite conditions of the vascular apparatus: of which the one is, sluggishness in, or actual interruption to the passage of blood through the *veins*. The other is increased action of the heart, or arterial capillaries, or both. The first of these may be called dropsy of the right side of the heart; the second, dropsy of the left side of the heart; and they require to be separately noticed.

I. Dropsical effusion (œdema, as it is here called) may be traced in many instances most distinctly to mechanical causes interrupting the steady flow of blood though the veins, as where it follows ligatures placed on veins, enlarged absorbent glands pressing on them, or the gravid uterus. But pathologists ascribe to the same proximate cause some more obscure cases of dropsy, such as that which accompanies enlarged and tuberculated liver, and that also which occurs occasionally in the latter stages of consumption. In both of these cases it is supposed that the venous circulation throughout the body generally is impeded.

2. Dropsy attended with increased vascular action is very com-

mon, and either general or local, according as the heart or the arterial branches are affected. The morbid action of vessels which gives rise to it, may be either actual *inflammation* or high *irritation,* or *congestion.* Hydrocele and hydrocephalus may be taken as instances of local dropsies of this kind. Ascites sometimes accompanies chronic inflammation of the peritonæum, and hydrothorax that of the pleura. Various examples might be offered of *general* dropsy, arising from, or intimately connected with, this state of the circulation. The most common are anasarca from exposure to cold, frcm the excessive use of spirituous liquors, from oppressed uterine functions (amenorrhœa,) and from scarlet fever. In all these cases, the disturbance of the heart's action is functional, and admits of a permanent cure. The principle, however, is perhaps most incontestably displayed in the disposition to dropsy, which comes on in the course of structural diseases of the heart (especially enlargement or hypertrophy,) when that organ labours exceedingly in its functions.

To this species of dropsy pathologists have given the name of acute, active, inflammatory, or *plethoric.* * We might call it with some propriety, *arterial,* as it is not necessarily accompanied with plethora or with feverish symptoms, nor does it always run a very rapid course. In this kind of dropsy the pulse is for the most part full and active, but sometimes hard, wiry, and incompressible. There is commonly also cough and head-ache, aggravated by a full inspiration. Dr. Blackall † has attached much importance to the coagulability of the urine in these cases on exposure to heat, a phæ-nomenon very frequently but not universally observed. The exciting cause, where it can be ascertained, and the previous history of symptoms, assist materially in establishing the diagnosis. Arterial dropsy occurs, for the most part, at an early period of life, and may often be traced to cold. Its attack is sudden, and it usually proves fatal by the supervention of apoplectic symptoms.

3. There is still however a third proximate cause of dropsy to be investigated ; one in which the heart and the different organs and functions of the body mutually participate—*viz.* relaxation or atony of the whole system, and especially of the exhalant vessels. This

* This term was introduced about thirty years ago by Dr. Grapengiesser, who appears to have the merit of having accurately described such a form of dropsy.

† See " Observations on the Nature and Cure of Dropsies." By Dr. Blackall, of Exeter. London, 1813.

form of dropsical effusion corresponds with that colliquative sweating, which is the frequent consequence of great or repeated losses of blood. It is very often to be observed, therefore, in the latter stages of chlorosis, diabetes, consumption, and hectic fevers of all kinds. Atonic dropsy occasionally follows flooding, great and sudden abstractions of blood by the lancet, and protracted fevers. It is sometimes brought on in the lower ranks of life by the want of proper nourishment, and in all persons it may be induced by a long-continued state of disordered stomach and imperfect digestion. Dropsy from relaxation was a favourite doctrine with the early schools of medicine. They admitted indeed, of no other species, and were at any rate unaware that the doctrine of atony and debility applies only to a small proportion of the cases of genuine idiopathic dropsy which are met with in common practice. Dropsies of this kind are attended with a weak and languid pulse, night-sweats, cold extremities, and in many cases, a strong disposition to erysipelas, petechiæ, and gangrene. They chiefly occur in elderly persons whose constitutions are worn out. They commence imperceptibly, and are not traceable to any obvious cause.

It cannot be denied however that there is something still imperfect in our analysis of the proximate causes of dropsy. A high degree of arterial action may exist, or the powers of life may be excessively reduced, without dropsy supervening. As under certain circumstances of disease there is a peculiar tendency to hæmorrhage, so in others there is a tendency to dropsy. In what the *hydropic diathesis* consists, it is impossible to define with strict accuracy. The notion that it is essentially *pressure on venous trunks* is ingenious, and apparently borne out by experiment, but certainly is neither applicable to inflammatory dropsy, nor to that which attends hæmorrhage, or chlorosis. Possibly it may depend on some condition of the nerves; or on some want of *consent* between the functions of the capillaries, and those of the great arterial and venous trunks. To pursue these speculations, however, would be useless. It will be more advisable to direct the attention of the student to the *symptoms* of this hydropic disposition, which are few in number, but very distinct. They are,—diminished secretion of urine, thirst, œdema of the feet and ancles, and a peculiar expression of countenance, to which the term *leucophlegmatic* has been applied.

Having now pointed out the divisions of dropsy founded on the consideration of symptoms, I proceed to such as may be referred to the diversity of appearances observed on dissection.

Two sets of morbid appearances present themselves in those who die of dropsical, the one thoracic, the other abdominal; and this furnishes a most useful distinction in practice. In the thorax we meet with enlargements of the heart, diseased valves, adhesions of the heart to the pericardium, ossification of arteries, inflammation of the internal coat of the great arterial trunks, aneurism of the aorta;—or sometimes diseased states of the lungs, such as tubercles, vomicæ, and hepatized induration, independent of any disease about the heart and great vessels. Lastly, we find malformations of the chest generally. When dropsy occurs connected with any of these conditions of thoracic disease, it assumes the form of hydrothorax, hydropericardium, anasarca, or their combinations.

In many cases, the thoracic viscera are found without the smallest trace of disease; instead of which we meet with marks of inflammation (acute or chronic) of the peritonæum,—adhesion, thickening, or tuberculated accretion of that membrane;—or we find enlargement and disorganization of the solid viscera; tuberculated liver, swelled spleen, diseased mesenteric glands; the stomach scirrhous, tumours attached to the omentum, thickened and ulcerated intestines. When dropsy occurs complicated with any of these varieties of abdominal disease it appears in the form of. ascites, or of anasarca and ascites combined. Abdominal dropsy is much more common than thoracic, in the proportion of about three to one.

Sometimes we have occasion to notice thoracic and abdominal appearances present in the same subject, and lastly, instances are not wanting of dropsy connected with mere *functional* disturbance of one or more organs proving fatal, and leaving behind it no trace of morbid structure.

It follows from what has been said, that though a few cases of dropsy are local, partial, temporary, and therefore of no material importance, yet the greater number of them are extremely dangerous. The prognosis in general dropsy indeed should always be most strictly guarded, and for many reasons. It is, as we have seen, connected with states of thoracic and abdominal disorganization, over which we have no control. It indicates great *severity* of disease, and shows that the *whole system* is deeply involved. It is often the strongest mark of a worn-out constitution, and of failure of the *vis vitæ*. In all forms of dropsy there is a remarkable liability to relapse.

68

The duration of the disease varies with many circumstances which it is impossible to enumerate, but which have all an important influence. There is an acute form of dropsy which has proved fatal in a few weeks, and there are instances on record of persons living for a long series of years labouring under a greater or less degree of it. Ascites is perhaps the most generally fatal of all the forms of dropsy, and certainly that over which medicine exerts the least power. It is hardly necessary to say, how much, in the successful issue of a dropsical case, depends upon bringing it early under medical treatment, before the foundations of health are sapped, and the disease advanced to that point, where from being one of function, it becomes complicated with structural derangement.

The remarks now offered have been intended to show, that, the pathology of dropsy assimilates itself very closely with that of other diseases. No sufficient grounds have been advanced for connecting it peculiarly (as the old pathologists did) with the absorbent system, or with a state of morbid tenuity of blood.

In the treatment of dropsy we are to aim, in the first place, at restoring a due state of the circulating system. Secondly, where this cannot be done, or while the measures for effecting it are in operation, we are to promote, the temporary absorption of the effused fluid. Thirdly, where the powers of the system are inadequate either to the one or the other, recourse must be had, when practicable, to surgical aid.

1. The means of relief calculated to attain the first object vary of course with the kind of dropsy present. In the acute, plethoric, or arterial dropsy, we are to lower the tone of the arterial system, and to lessen the impetus of the circulating fluids upon the exhalant capillaries. For this purpose, it is sometimes necessary to have recourse to blood-letting, or to local depletion by cupping, or leeches. At other times the object may equally be gained by brisk purgatives, nitre, cream of tartar, and other relaxing saline medicines, by antimony, or colchicum. The utility of blood-letting in certain forms of dropsy has been established on the clearest evidence; but it is right to add, that so powerful a remedy is not *lightly* to be resorted to. In all cases of disease not accompanied by fever or inflammation, great caution is required in the management of the lancet. In the case of dropsy this is peculiarly necessary; first, on account of the debility, which, if carried too far, blood-letting produces; and secondly, from its being so often associated with that *passive* enlargement of the heart, which does *not* admit of the de-

traction of blood. Bleeding in dropsy should never be pushed therefore to such an extent as to endanger the occurrence of syncope.

In dropsy from relaxation, or glandular obstruction, the indica-tion of cure is to support the tone of the system, and to rouse the action of the absorbents. Among the *tonic* medicines most ser-viceable in dropsy, are the infusions of several bitter and acrid herbs, the aromatic confection, camphor mixture, bark, steel, and wine. Of *deobstruent* medicines, the most powerful are mercury, squill, and ammoniacum.

2. With the second intention (that of promoting the temporary absorption of effused fluid,) recourse is had to medicines which determine to the bowels and kidneys. The cathartics most useful in this view are those called *hydragogue*, in which class are ranked jalap, cream of tartar, elaterium, and gamboge. It is a remarkable fact, that in almost every case of general dropsy, active purging will do something towards the relief of the patient. It appears in a peculiar manner to excite the absorbent system to action. Of the diuretic medicines employed in dropsy, some are weakening, as digitalis, the acetate of potash, nitre, and colchicum. Others are stimulating, such as the spiritus ætheris nitrosi, the oil of tur-pentine, squill, and juniper berries. The former are chiefly ser-viceable in thoracic, the latter is abdominal dropsy.

Great advantages are derived from combining these remedies. Where blood-letting is indicated, digitalis and occasional purging are applicable. The best effects have followed the union of digi-talis or squills with mercury (R No. 105). There is probably no plan of treatment adapted to such a variety of cases as this. Digi-talis may often be given with perfect propriety in combination with aromatics and tonics. Lastly, the powers of diuretic medi-cines are much heightened by mixture.

3. The surgical means of relief in dropsy are tapping and scari-fications. Of their value, I shall have a fitter opportunity to speak in the next chapter, when treating of the three principal varieties of dropsical effusion.

CHAP. VII.

---

*Ascites. Its symptoms. Causes. Peculiarities in its Treatment. Diag-
nosis of Hydrothorax. Symptoms of Hydropericardium. Remedies
peculiarly applicable to Thoracic Dropsy. Phænomena of Anasarca.
Its Causes. Peculiarities in its Treatment.*

HAVING explained in the last chapter the pathology of dropsical
effusion, I proceed to offer a few observations on the chief varieties of general dropsy which meet us in practice. I shall principally direct my attention to the *symptoms* of these diseases, and to
the selection of remedies for their removal.

I. ASCITES, or dropsy of the peritonæal cavity. This form of
dropsy is readily known by the concurrence of the common symptoms marking the hydropic diathesis with swelling and fluctuation
of the belly. Simple as these characters appear, there are occasions in which the diagnosis is difficult. Ascites has been mistaken for dropsical, or otherwise diseased ovarium ; and physicians
have occasionally erred in their attempts to distinguish it from the
tumour of pregnancy. Ascites in a few cases occurs alone, but
more frequently it is associated with a degree of anasarca, and
sometimes also with hydrothorax. The quantity of water collected in the belly is often enormous, amounting in some instances to
upwards of a hundred pints. It is curious to observe how little inconvenience this occasions to the viscera among which it floats.
The functions of the stomach and bowels are performed in most
cases of ascites with tolerable regularity. The disease may occur
in either sex, and at any age ; but like the other forms of dropsy,
it is chiefly to be met with in advanced life.

The causes of ascites may be reduced to the following heads.
It is, in the first place, a sequel of peritonæal inflammation, both
acute and chronic, diffused and circumscribed. This form of ascites
is accompanied with tenderness in some part of the abdomen, more

especially in the right hypochondrium. It arises, in the second place, from diseased conditions of the solid glandular structures of the abdomen—the liver, spleen, and pancreas. In by far the larg. er proportion of cases the liver is the organ affected. On dissec. tion it appears enlarged, schirrhous, tuberculated, or studded with hydatids. It is a commonly received opinion, that the dropsy which attends diseased liver is referable to the difficulty with which the blood is transmitted through the vena portæ, and its consequent stagnation, or congestion in the capillaries. This notion is in some measure confirmed by the enlargement which is always more or less observable at the same time in the superficial veins of the abdo. men. Something more, however, is probably necessary to consti. tute a dropsical tendency. It would be impossible, otherwise, to explain why ascites should be so common an attendant on ulcerated stomach and bowels, and such chronic disorganizations as denote a general *decay* of the whole frame. The constitutional origin of ascites is rendered still more evident, in the third place, by its aris. ing from causes exterior to the abdomen, such as produce dropsy generally, more especially structural diseases of the heart.

The treatment of ascites must of course to a certain degree vary with the cause which gives rise to it. When it depends upon or. ganic disease of the abdominal viscera, it is nearly beyond the reach of art. When it occurs along with extensive anasarca, it denotes so great an extent of constitutional disturbance as almost to preclude the hope of permanent recovery. That form of ascites which par. takes of the character of a *local* dropsy, and is connected with in. flammatory action in the peritonæal membrane, is the most under our control. The application of leeches, blisters, and fomentations, with the liberal use of mercury and of saline aperients, has in many of these cases succeeded perfectly in removing the complaint. The diuretic powder No. 104, containing nitre, is well adapted for these as for all other cases in which general inflammatory action takes place. Where our object is merely to afford temporary relief, the best system of treatment consists in the occasional use of hydra. gogue cathartics, especially jalap with cream of tartar (Nos. 9 and 103,) and elaterium (No. 11 ;) employing in the intervals such drugs as combine a *deobstruent* with a diuretic quality, more partie. ularly squills and mercury (No. 105,) and assisting their operation by the free use of any simple diluent.

When the accumulation of water becomes so great as to inter. fere with the breathing, or to create distress by distension of the ab.

dominal parietes, recourse must be had to the *paracentesis abdomi-
nis.* It is a commonly received opinion, that tapping, once performed, is a complete bar to the permanent recovery of the patient ;
but I doubt the correctness of this notion, and I am sure it has often proved hurtful by inducing practitioners to delay the operation
too long. I am far from wishing to advocate a hasty employment
of the trocar, but I have seen more danger from inordinate distension than I could ever trace to tapping.

2. HYDROTHORAX, or dropsy of the thoracic cavity. The diagnosis symptoms of this form of dropsy are very fallacious. Sometimes we are confident of finding water in the thorax, when that
cavity is perfectly free from disease. At other times we observe
the thorax full, when we had no suspicion of the complaint existing.* The symptoms usually set down as denoting the presence
of water in the chest are of two kinds—those that indicate dropsy
generally, above all œdema of the feet and ancles, and those that
mark mechanical impediment to the function of respiration. In
some instances, it may be possible to detect the presence of fluid
in the thorax by percussion and external examination ; but I am
well convinced this can never be held out as a certain means of
judging of the disease. Of the general symptoms of dropsy I have
already spoken. The local symptoms are difficulty of breathing
aggravated by exertion, and by the recumbent posture ; a sense of
weight or oppression, referred to the pit of the stomach, and referable probably to the pressure of the effused fluid upon the diaphragm ; starting from sleep in a fright ; cough ; a livid or mottled
colour of the lips, such as may be observed whenever respiration is
obstructed by a mechanical cause, and the blood imperfectly oxygenated. In the latter stages of the complaint, it is not uncommon
to find the expectoration tinged with blood.

Many attempts have been made to ascertain the symptoms peculiar to hydropericardium. This form of dropsy generally exists
along with hydrothorax, but sometimes it is present in a degree to
which other appearances do not correspond. On the 5th February
1823, I examined the body of a woman, in whom the pericardium
was so enormously distended as to contain eighteen ounces of serum, besides an enlarged heart. In this case there were no symptoms by which the locality of the effusion could have been foretold.

---

* Vide Morgagni, letter xvi, passim. This chapter contains some valuable
remarks on the symptoms of thoracic dropsy, and deserves an attentive
perusal.

It is commonly stated indeed, that in dropsy of the pericardium the pulse is intermittent and irregular, with an unusual *oppression* at the heart, palpitation, and that kind of paleness and anxiety of counte- nance observable when the heart labours exceedingly in its func- tions. The early appearance of the œdema of the face has been also adduced as indicating dropsy of the pericardium.

Of the causes of thoracic dropsy I have nothing to state beyond what was urged in the preceding chapter. In its treatment, the only peculiarity worthy of note is, that here the influence of diu- retic medicines is more decided than in any other form of dropsy, and that digitalis is of all others the most generally successful. The infusion, beginning with the dose of three drachms three times a day, and gradually augmenting it to six, is upon the whole the best form. It may be advantageously united with aromatics, espe- cially capsicum, and the spirit of nitrous ether (R No. 101). Pa- racentesis thoracis has been often proposed, but seldom practised, owing, I presume, in a great degree, to the uncertainty in the signs of hydrothorax. There is no reason to believe that it would afford less relief than the corresponding operation on the abdominal ca- vity, or that any particular danger attends it.

3. ANASARCA, or dropsy of the cellular membrane. This mem- brane, so extensively diffused throughout the body, is moistened by a fluid thrown out by its arterial exhalants. In various ways the quantity of this fluid may be increased, constituting the disease called anasarca. The *pathognomonic* symptom of it is the pitting of the skin on pressure. The affection usually commences in the feet and legs, perceptible perhaps at night only. As the disease advances the swelling becomes general over the body. The skin is dry and parched. There is a peculiar sallowness of counte- nance to be observed, with torpor, and disposition to sleep. In se- vere cases the cuticle gives way, and serum oozes through the pores of the skin. When the *habit* of body is bad, erysipelatous inflammation and gangrene are apt to follow. In worn-out, dehili- tated constitutions it is not uncommon to find anasarca associated with petechiæ ecchymoses.

Pathologists in all ages have occupied themselves in enumera- ting the several causes from which anasarca may originate. With- out following them into details, it may be useful to point out those which are most frequently observed to operate.

1. Local anasarca, or œdema sometimes arises from pressure ac- cidentally made on veins, as by the gravid uterus, swelled glands

in the groins or armpits, or a tight garter. The same result occasionally follows, even in healthy states of the system, from a too
long continuance in the erect posture.

2. General anasarca arises from a variety of causes which concur
in producing a debilitated state of the whole body, and more particularly perhaps of the venous system.   Hence it is that anasarca
succeeds severe hæmorrhagies (natural or artificial,) fevers, and
fluxes ; and that it occurs so frequently in the latter stages of diabetes, phthisis pulmonalis, and amenorrhœa.   Under such circumstances the dropsical symptoms commence slowly, and as it were
imperceptibly. There are instances, however, in which the disease
comes on suddenly ; and to the causes of this *acute* form of anasarca I shall next advert.

3. Exposure to cold and damp has frequently been followed by
dropsical swellings. I have known them to commence within forty-
eight hours from the application of the exciting cause. In this variety of the disease the pulse will commonly be found full and
strong, with perhaps some degree of hardness. There will be present at the same time symptoms denoting an affection of the thoracic organs—tightness across the chest, with cough and dyspnœa,
aggravated by exertion and the recumbent posture, and producing
head-ache.

4. General anasarca arises, in the fourth place, from excess in
the use of spirituous liquors. When the attack is sudden, this
dropsy is of the *arterial* kind, and attended with the symptoms just
described as accompanying hydropic effusion from cold.

5. Another cause of anasarca is disturbance in the uterine functions. I have already had occasion to notice, that amenorrhœa exhibits itself in two different habits of body, and is accompanied by
two opposite trains of symptoms.   The dropsy which attends this
state of disease is sometimes of the true *atonic* kind, but occasionally it is observed along with an *incompressible* pulse, hæmorrhages
from the nose and stomach, apoplectic symptoms, and others denoting plethora and increased arterial action.

6. The only other circumstance requiring attention in the pathology of anasarca, is its connection with some of the febrile eruptions.
It has long been known, that dropsy, particularly in the form of
anasarca, occasionally follows scarlet fever.   The same phenomenon is sometimes observed as a sequel of measles, small-pox, and
erysipelas.   It has been conjectured, that the dropsical tendency
is here dependent on a morbid condition of the *cutaneous exhalants,*

the consequence of the eruption ; and there are sufficient grounds for this notion. The accompanying symptoms occasionally point out some obscure affection of the heart and lungs existing at the same time. Under all circumstances the practitioner will do right to view this form of disease as of *constitutional* origin, and to be more solicitous about the state of the *system* than of the skin.

From the remark now offered it will appear, that the pathology of anasarca is closely connected with that of hydrothorax. In ma. ny cases these forms of dropsical effusion coexist, and the reme. dies are the same for both.ʼ ꝫ Blood-letting is better adapted for an- asarca than for any other variety of dropsy. Where it occurs sud. denly from exposure to cold, or excess in the use of spirits, blood. letting is often not only useful, but actually indispensable. The blood drawn is sometimes cupped and buffy, but more commonly it will have the appearance (hardly, however, less satisfactory) of great firmness of coagulum. The effects of blood-letting will be matèrially aided by the employment of purgatives (R Nos. 9, 14, 22, 103,) saline and antimonial medicines, and the relaxant diuret- ics, especially digitalis, nitre, and the acetate of potash (R Nos. 101 and 104.) The student will of course understand, that neither these nor any other diuretic medicines are likely to be of service without very copious dilution, and I have found nothing to answer this end so effectually as luke-warm barley water. There cannot be a greater error than to imagine that dropsical accumulations may be lessened by *withholding* liquids.

It is unnecessary to say that this plan of treatment is adapted only to one variety of anasarca. In all cases, the practitioner, by tracing the origin of the disease, and weighing accurately the accompanying symptoms, must form for himself some idea of its *proximate* cause. He will thus occasionally find the necessity of *supporting* the system, instead of lowering it ; and to effect this, he will have recourse to the use of tonics (bark, camphor, bitters, and aromatics,) in combination with the stimulant diuretics. The for- mula No. 102 will be found useful, to which ten drops of tincture of digitalis may with propriety be added.

Considerable diversity of opinion has prevailed regarding the propriety of scarifications in anasarca. By some they are utterly condemned, as leading to erysipelatous inflammation and gangrene, while in the hands of others they have proved eminently servicea- ble. This may partly be attributed to differences in the mode of operating. It has been stated, that a single deep scarification,

69

penetrating the cutis vera, is more efficacious, and less likely to produce unpleasant consequences, than the numerous but slighter punctures commonly made. It cannot indeed be denied, that in languid habits of body, scarifications of all kinds are occasionally dangerous. The relief which they afford, however, is often surprisingly great, and compensates the degree of risk which they bring with them.

Blisters and issues have been recommended in the cure of anasarca, but they are not advisable. Frictions, oil-skin stockings, and bandages, are useful where the effusion of serum arises from local obstructions; but they are unimportant in that more numerous class of cases, in which dropsy of the cellular membrane is associated with a disposition to effusion in the great serous membranes of the thorax or abdomen.

† See Appendix; Note Z.

CHAP. VIII.

Outline of their Pathology. Causes operating generally in the production of Chronic Cutaneous Diseases. Causes operating locally. General System of Treatment. Division of Affections of the skin into constitutional and local. General Character of the Remedies employed. Willan's Classification. Arrangement of Mr. Plumbe. Notice of the leading varieties of Chronic Cutaneous Diseases. ORDER 1. *Acne. Tinea Capitis. Psora.* ORDER II. *Lepra. Psoriasis.* ORDER III. *Strophulus. Eczema. Porrigo. Prurigo. Impetigo.* ORDER IV. *Pompholyx. Ecthyma and Rupia.*

A GREAT variety of affections are comprehended under the head of *chronic cutaneous diseases.* Expanded as they have been by some authors into a nosological system, and each made the subject of distinct investigation, it may appear impossible, consistently with the design of this work, to enter upon a discussion of them with any prospect of advantage to the student. I am indeed fully sensible, that in acquiring a knowledge of these affections, attention to detail is requisite. Still it behooves the student to be aware, that there are certain general principles which connect all the chronic diseases of the skin together, and link them in with the great chain of constitutional disorders. To point out these, although in a very summary manner, may possibly be useful. I shall attempt further to direct the attention of the reader to the leading *natural* divisions of chronic cutaneous disease, hoping thus to lay before him the elements of a study which the detailed descriptions of authors may hereafter assist him in pursuing, but a complete knowledge of which can alone be attained by constant attention, and extensive opportunities of observation.*

* We have two works in our own language expressly dedicated to cutaneous affections, *viz.*—Bateman's " Practical Synopsis of Cutaneous Diseases," and Plumbe's " Practical Treatise on Diseases of the Skin." To

Considering the diversity in the aspects of chronic cutaneous disease, there is less variety than might have been expected in their *exciting causes*. They may be distinguished into such as operate *generally*, and such as act through the medium of the skin itself.

1. In the first class may be ranked the presence of a poison in the system. This is very often the poison of lues, which, in common with other secondary effects, produces every possible variety of *cutaneous* disease. At other times, the poison is that of mercury. Hence it is that cutaneous eruptions constitute so important a part of that complaint to which modern pathologists have given the title of pseudo syphilis. Sometimes the poison is of a more familiar kind, such as shell-fish, bitter almonds, and other indigestible articles of diet, the influence of which, however, is only partial and transitory.

2. The next source of cutaneous disease is simple *debility*. To this we attribute the cutaneous eruptions bearing the character of *ecthyma* and *rupia*, which are observed in persons convalescent from tedious diseases, very remarkably in those of a naturally scrofulous habit, who are recovering from confluent small-pox. Closely allied to it is the state of *cachexia*, the consequence of bad food, want of air and exercise, and irregular modes of living. It has been conjectured, that in these cases the *blood* becomes altered in its qualities, and probably loaded with saline particles, which irritating the cutaneous capillaries produce different varieties of eruption. This doctrine is of the old pathologists, although but little talked of in modern times, still preserves its influence on practice, as will be apparent by considering the extensive use now made of the alterative vegetable decoctions, the principal effect of which is to improve or sweeten the condition of the blood.

3. A weakened or cachectic state of the system is not, however, the only one in which chronic cutaneous disease occurs. In some instances a degree of plethora is present. In the language of the humoral pathologists the blood is too rich, and stimulates too strongly the vessels through which it passes. This is particularly observable in the pustular eruptions to which young persons are subject about the period of puberty (*acne simplex* and *punctata* of Willan)

4. A disordered state of the stomach and bowels is one of the most common causes of chronic cutaneous disease. Sometimes

these useful volumes I am indebted for many of the remarks which have a place in the present chapter.

this consists merely in the lodgment of crudities in the alimentary canal. At other times, the presence of acid in the stomach appears to be the direct occasion of the cutaneous affection. Hence the use of purgatives and of absorbents in the chronic diseases of the skin.

5. Chronic cutaneous disease is sometimes observed in combination with symptoms denoting disorder of the thoracic viscera. I have already had occasion to illustrate this pathological principle when treating of purpura.

6. Lastly, I have seen a few cases which point to a connection between *lepra* and an affection of the brain and nervous system. I am well convinced that a disordered state of the cerebral functions has given rise to *erysipelas* ; and I have therefore no difficulty in imagining, that the same principle may possibly operate more extensively in the production of cutaneous disease.

Besides these *general* sources of cutaneous affections, there are others whose influence is very extensive, which may be referred more immediately to the skin itself. 1. The first I shall notice is a peculiar *irritability*, or delicacy of the skin. This is the probable cause of those numerous cases of *strophulus* which occur in infants, whose skin is as yet unaccustomed to the stimulus of air and soap. This irritable state of the skin often exists through life ; and hence it is that leeches and blisters produce in such habits very unpleasant effects. It is in some instances *hereditary*. The principle appears to be one of very general application in the pathology of cutaneous complaints.

2. The next cause of chronic cutaneous disease which requires attention, is want of cleanliness. It is doubtless on this account that obstinate cutaneous affections are so much more common among the lower than the higher classes of society. Hence too the great value of warm ablution in their treatment.

3. The third is local irritation. Its influence in the production of cutaneous disease is generally acknowledged, and is indeed very extensive. The principle is fully shown in the common effects of blisters, plaisters, and antimonial lotions ; but it is chiefly exemplified in those eruptions which follow the long-continued stimulus of the sun's rays, of flour, sugar, lime, or soap, constituting some of the species of eczema and psoriasis.

4. The last source of chronic cutaneous disease which I shall notice is contagion. There are not many cases, however, to which

it applies. Psora and tinea capitis are perhaps the only unequivocal proofs of it which can be adduced.

In laying down a few general principles applicable to the treatment of these affections, I must first advert to the necessity of distinguishing them according as they are constitutional or local.
Chronic cutaneous diseases may, in fact, be divided into two classes, such as implicate the constitution to a greater or less degree,
—and such as are decidedly local, arising from local causes, remediable by local means, and in the ordinary course of events not
influencing the system at any period of their progress. There
is a foundation in nature for this distinction ; but in other respects
these two classes of diseases are too intimately connected to make
it possible to discuss them separately. In practice, however, it
must be remembered, that where the disease is essentially local,
topical remedies are required. On the other hand, where the constitution is in fault, local measures are of little or no avail. It is
true, that in the treatment of the latter kinds of cutaneous disease
we are often glad to have recourse to local means (even though
their influence be but insignificant), for a large proportion of such
affections are unaccountably obstinate.

Of those kinds of cutaneous disease which are connected with
constitutional disturbance, many are set up by nature as a relief
to internal oisorder, and their *cure* would often be followed by
some serious mischief. Thus the crusta lactea of infants suddenly
suppressed has been succeeded by hydrocephalus ; the psoriasis of
elderly persons, by apoplexy ; the drying up of an old ulcer, by a
paroxysm of asthma. In connection with this subject we may
mention also the curious but well-ascertained fact, that very obstinate cutaneous diseases have sometimes been removed in the
course of a fever. Warts and scaly diseases of the skin, which
had resisted all remedies, have especially yielded in this manner.

In the treatment of cutaneous affections an attempt should always be made, in the first instance, to determine the cause of the
complaint ; for this, if successful, will at once point out the proper
remedy. When the origin of the disease cannot be ascertained,
the general system is to be looked to ; and according as a state of
fever, of cachexia, of debility, or plethora be present, remedies are
to be employed of a febrifuge, alterative, tonic, or evacuant quality. Attention is to be paid, in the third place, to the functions of
the brain, the heart, the stomach, and the bowels, and any irregularities in them corrected by appropriate means. Lastly, the condition

of the skin is to be carefully examined, with a view to determine whether the superficial vessels are *irritable*, requiring *soothing* medicines, or in that state of *torpor* which will be benefited by *sti. mulating* applications.

The constitutional remedies applicable in cases of chronic cuta. neous disease are, purgatives, absorbents, tonics, alteratives, febri. fuges, and lastly, such medicines as exert a peculiar effect upon the vessels of the skin. This class of drugs will naturally be re. sorted to whenever we fail in detecting some obvious cause for the complaint; and they ought frequently to be varied until we find one that fulfils our expectations. Those which experience has shown to be the most efficacious are dulcamara, sulphur, pitch, mercury, antimony, and arsenic.

The local applications employed in cutaneous diseases are di. visable into three kinds;—the mild, the cooling, and the irritating. To the first belong cold cream, pomatum, simple ointment, and the vapour of warm water. To the second, lotions of goulard, of vin. egar, of the muriate of ammonia ; and the ointments of zinc and of sugar of lead. Of the irritating applications, the variety is infinite. Those in most general use are citrine ointment, sulphur ointment, the decoction of white hellebore, spirituous lotions, and lotions containing either lunar caustic or corrosive muriate.*

There is still another class of remedies employed in the treat. ment of chronic cutaneous complaints, which may be considered to possess a double influence, that is to say, to act both generally and locally. Of this kind are sulphureous baths, mineral waters, and the warm and cold sea-water bath.

A brief sketch of the principal varieties of chronic cutaneous dis- ease will conclude the view which I proposed to take of this sub. ject, and complete at the same time the design of the present work.

Dr. Willan has divided cutaneous diseases into eight orders ac- cording to the appearance of the eruption in its most perfect state. This classification is now so generally adopted in this country, that it may be useful to the student to place it before him.† He will perceive that many of the diseases arranged by Willan as cutane. ous have been already discussed in this work, either as febrile or

* See Appendix ; Note Aa.

† See Bateman's Synopsis, page 1.

as constitutional disorders. These I have distinguished by *italic* characters. The remainder constitute the genuine affections of the skin.

ORDER I.

PAPULÆ.   (*Pimples.*)

Papular Eruptions.

Genus.
1. Strophulus.
2. *Lichen.*
3. Prurigo.

ORDER II.

SQUAMÆ.

Scaly Eruptions.
4. Lepra.
5. Psoriasis.
6. Pityriasis.
7. Icthyosis.

ORDER III.

EXANTHEMATA.

Efflorescences.
8. *Rubeola.*
9. *Scarlatina.*
10. *Urticaria.*
11. *Roseola.*
12. *Purpura.*
13. *Erythema.*

ORDER IV.

BULLÆ.   (*Blebs.*)
14. *Erysipelas.*
15. Pemphigus.
16. Pompholix.

ORDER V.

PUSTULÆ.

Pustular Eruptions.

Genus.
17. Impetigo.
18. Porrigo.
19. Ecthyma.
20. *Variola.*
21. Scabies.

ORDER VI.

VESICULÆ.

Vesicular Eruptions.
22. *Varicella.*
23. *Vaccinia.*
24. *Herpes.*
25. Rupia.
26. *Miliaria.*
27. Eczema.
28. *Aphtha.*

ORDER VII.

TUBERCULA.

Tubercular Eruptions.
29. Phyma.
30. Verruca.
31. Molluscum.
32. Vitiligo.
33. Acne.
35. Sycosis.
35. Lupus.
36. Elephantiasis.
37. *Frambœsia*

ORDER VIII.

MACULÆ.

Congenital Marks.

Genus.
38. Ephelis.

Genus.
39. Nævus.
40. Spilus.

I have already had occasion to express my distrust of some of the principles on which this classification is founded; and as it is clearly inapplicable to our purpose, I shall avail myself of a different arrangement, suggested in a great degree by Mr. Plumbe.* It has the merit of resting on principles strictly pathological, and is well calculated, therefore, for elementary instruction. The exclusion of the febrile exanthemata equally fits it for our purpose. It distributes chronic cutaneous diseases into four orders.

Order 1. Diseases strictly local, deriving their characters from local peculiarities of the skin:

1. Acne and Sycosis.
2. Tinea Capitis, or porrigo Scutulata.
3. Psora, or Scabies.

Order 2. Diseases marked by chronic inflammatory action of the vessels forming the cuticle, producing morbid growth of that structure. Constitutional causes or influence uncertain:

4. Lepra.
5. Psoriasis.

Order 3. Diseases having a decidedly constitutional origin, and characterized, in their progress, by local and constitutional excitement:

6. Strophulus.
7. Eczema.
8. Porrigo.
9. Prurigo.
10. Impetigo.

Order 4. Diseases dependent on debilitated states of the constitution, and characterised by diminished tone of the vessels of the cutis:

11. Pompholyx.
12. Ecthyma and Rupia.

* Plumbe's "Practical Treatise." London, 1824.

70

On these twelve genera of cutaneous disease I shall now offer a few remarks, referring the student to the works already quoted for such *detailed* information concerning them as may complete his knowledge of this very necessary branch of medical literature.

1. ACNE consists essentially, in its original form, of simple obstruction to the free passage of the sebaceous matter to the surface of the skin; in consequence of which, that substance accumulates, hardens, distends the follicles which contain it, and ultimately causes inflammation and small abscesses. It is a very frequent complaint from the age of puberty up to the twenty-fifth year of life. It is characterized by an eruption of papulæ in the face (especially on the forehead and chin,) as well as on the neck, shoulders, and breast. It never descends to the lower parts of the trunk, or to the extremities. It is common to both sexes, but the most severe cases of it are seen in young men. Persons labouring under it enjoy for the most part good general health, and are often unable to refer the complaint to any obvious exciting cause. The eruption occasionally recedes for a time, and recurs, more especially after violent exercise, great heat of the weather, a more liberal use of wine, or any unusual excitement of the cutaneous circulation. Except in females this complaint seldom calls for the attention of medical men. It is altogether a local disease, and neither requires nor is benefited by a low diet, purgatives, nor alteratives, or other internal medicines. At the same time it is to be remarked that external applications are equally without influence. The disease, therefore, usually proceeds to its natural but distant termination. Sycosis is nothing more than acne occurring in parts covered by hair, especially the chin.

2. TINEA CAPITIS (the porrigo scrutulata of Willan,) commonly called ringworm of the scalp, or *scald head*, is an affection of a very peculiar kind. Its leading feature is the falling-off of the hair, arising (according to Mr. Plumbe, who has paid great attention to the subject) from excessive excitement of the vessels of the scalp, which deprives the structure secreting the hair of its due nourishment. It undoubtedly originates in the application of an infectious matter, and spreads by the secretion of the pustules which are formed. It is a singularly obstinate complaint, and resists, in many cases, for a great length of time the best directed exertions of medical art. The treatment consists in shaving the head, carefully washing away the matter that has formed, and subsequently stimulating the affected parts. Lotions of the sulphate of copper,

and of lunar caustic ; the ung. hydr. nitr. and the ung. hydr. præ-cip, albi are the applications generally resorted to, and for the most part with good effect. Internal remedies are not required except to allay constitutional irritation which may *accidentally* have arisen.

3. Psora or scabies, so well known under the familiar denomination of *the itch*, is a very troublesome complaint, which usually assumes the form of small vesicles intermixed with pustules ; but its aspects are very various and deceitful. It may at all times, however, be distinguished by the incessant and importunate itching which attends it, the constitution being perfectly unaffected. It appears occasionally on every part of the body, the face alone excepted. Its most usual seat is about the wrists and fingers, the fossa of the nates, and flexures of the joints. The itch is highly contagious. There is every reason to believe that it consists essentially in the presence of a minute insect burrowing and breeding in the skin. This insect was first accurately described by Bonomo, in 1683, and is now called the acarus scabiei. To this, as to all other insects, sulphur is a complete poison, and, therefore, beyond all other remedies, entitled to the character of a *specific*. There are few cases of *genuine* scabies which will not yield to the steady employment of the sulphur ointment. Five or six applications, assiduously made, are usually sufficient to effect the cure. In very obstinate cases, the ung. sulphuris compos. containing the white hellebore, may be substituted with advantage.

4. Lepra is the most common, the most obstinate, and upon the whole the most formidable of all the varieties of chronic cutaneous disease. In its simple form it is recognized by its circular patches, about the size of half a crown piece, covered with small shining scales, encircled by a dry, red, and slightly elevated but well-defined border. It occurs at all periods of life, and under every variety of external circumstance. Except when very severe, it is not attended with uneasiness in the part, and hardly ever with constitutional disturbance. The pathology and treatment of lepra have long been the opprobria of physic. In some cases an hereditary origin may be traced ; but beyond this little is known regarding its causes. Females are certainly more subject to this disorder than males, and the periods of commencement and cessation of the menstrual discharge are those during which it chiefly shows itself. The system of treatment in lepra is quite empirical. Dulcamara is perhaps the only remedy which practitioners have agreed in recommending and yet its influence is often slight, and seldom permanent. The

bath waters externally applied are in great esteem throughout England, and to a certain degree have established their claim as a remedy of power.

5. PSORIASIS is closely allied to lepra, both in its appearance and general pathology. It chiefly differs from lepra in the *irregular* shape of the patches, and their being frequently accompanied by *rhagades*, or fissures of the skin. Psoriasis is not less difficult of cure than lepra. It is sometimes benefited by the application of dilute citrine ointment, and some advantage may be derived from the internal use of sulphur combined with the carbonate of soda ; but, like lepra, it often continues, even through life, in spite of every effort of medical art.

6. STROPHULUS is the earliest form of chronic cutaneous disease ever observed. It comprises several papular affections peculiar to infants, and known by the name of *red gum* and *tooth rash*. The affection is attributable to the very vascular and irritable condition of the skin in infant life, and is in some cases, perhaps, connected with indigestion. In its ordinary form, however, it is consistent with a state of perfect health, and requires little, if any, medical treatment.

7. ECZEMA is characterized by a diffused eruption of vesicles without inflammatory bases. It has for its local causes the direct rays of the sun (eczema solare), and for its constitutional causes the irritation of mercury in habits peculiarly predisposed (eczema mercuriale.) The constitutional disturbance attending this disease usually takes the form of slight feverishness. Its duration is very uncertain, seldom continuing longer than a month. Mild saline aperients, a spare diet, soft spunging of the affected parts, and occasionally a warm bath, appear to comprise all that is important in reference to treatment.

8. PORRIGO (*favosa* of Willan) is a very familiar form of chronic cutaneous disease. It chiefly affects children from the period of dentition up to the fourth or fifth year of life, but sometimes occurs much later. It is characterized by an eruption of straw-coloured pustules, scattered at times over the whole body, principally however observable on the scalp, the face, behind the ears, and about the ancles. A porriginous state of the *scalp* frequently accompanies the process of dentition, and is then perhaps rather salutary than otherwise. By neglect this disease assumes a most frightful aspect. The pustules discharge a viscid fluid, which concretes into scabs, and the face (when that part is attacked) be-

comes enveloped in a mask, the *crusta lactea* of old authors, the *porrigo larvalis* of Willan. Porriginous eruptions occur in different states of the system. They are, I believe, chiefly attributable to a *gross* diet, and connected with plethora; but at times they arise in feeble and flabby habits, and appear in combination with cachexia and marasmus. The treatment of this form of disease must be regulated by the varying circumstances under which it occurs. In general, purgatives are indispensable; and the combination of scammony and calomel (R No. 10) is well adapted to the class of children among whom it chiefly prevails.

9. PRURIGO is a papular disease of a more chronic nature, distinguished by the excessive, the uncontrollable itching which attends it. The papulæ do not differ in colour from that of the adjoining cuticle, and hence are often overlooked by superficial observers. This disease differs from psora in the circumstance of its never advancing to vesicle or pustule. Prurigo in some cases affeets the whole surface of the body: at other times it is *partial*, the generative organs and the back being its most usual seats. It often proves to elderly persons a most formidable ailment, interfering with every enjoyment of life. The pathology of pruriginous affections is very obscure. They are sometimes connected with general debility and visceral obstructions, at other times with richness of blood, and a preternaturally excited state of the cutaneous capillaries. Cleanliness and the warm bath are the most important remedial measures; but the occasional use of purgatives should never be omitted. Lotions containing vinegar afford some relief. The Harrowgate waters have obtained celebrity for the cure of this complaint. Mercury is sometimes useful.

10. IMPETIGO exhibits considerable diversity of external character. Vesicles, pustules, and regularly formed scales may be observed at different periods of its progress; but it is at all times distinguishable by the violent cutaneous irritation which accompanies it. High inflammatory action, extensive pustulation and scabbing, with deep fissures or *rhagades*, are its leading features. These are of course succeeded by a proportionate degree of relaxation in the vessels of the affected part. The causes of impetigo are very little known, and its treatment therefore is uncertain. Frequent ablution, gentle alteratives, and the sulphur vapour bath have occasionally proved serviceable.

11. POMPHOLYX is characterized by the eruption of *bullæ*, or vesicles of the size of walnuts, which appear in successive crops,

occupying different parts of the body, but more especially the extremities. This disease is unattended by fever.* It frequently
proves very tedious, lasting from six weeks to three or four months,
and is peculiarly obstinate and severe in old people. It produces
in them great itching and inconvenience ; and from the extent of
surface occupied by the eruption, and the occasional intermixture
of livid vesicles, presents on some occasions a very formidable as-
peet. Pompholyx however is certainly to be considered a rare
form of cutaneous disease. It appears to depend upon some *cachectic* (by which is understood a depraved and debilitated) state of
the whole system. Medicine, as far as I can judge from my own
limited observation, exerts very little power over it. Tonic and
alterative medicines appear to be called for, with a generous diet,
and an allowance of wine. The irritation of the skin admits of
some relief from the use of the lotion R No. 113.

12. ECTHYMA and RUPIA are different grades of that form of
pustular eruption which occurs in debilitated habits. The system
being weak, the vessels of the skin easily give way, either spontaneously or from very slight causes, and there is no sufficient energy
in the constitution to repair the injury. Obstinate ulcers, and scabs
resembling limpet shells (the true rupia) follow. Such a diseased
state of the surface is very common in scrofulous persons of all
ages after severe small-pox, and is occasionlly observed in children
succeeding measles. The disease is met with also in young persons
who, with constitutions not originally strong, imprudently indulge
in great excesses and irregularities. It frequently appears in the
first instance upon the legs, but extends in course of time to every
part of the body, proving, in very many cases, exceedingly tedious
and obstinate. The appropriate treatment consists in change of
air, cold bathing, and the internal use of sarsaparilla, bark, and other alteratives and tonics.

* The febrile vesicular eruption, to which nosologists have given the name
of *pemphigus*, is probably nothing more than pompholyx with fever *accidentally* combined with it.

APPENDIX.

FORMULÆ MEDICAMENTORUM.

I. EMETICA.

No. 1.

℞. Pulveris ipecacuanhæ scrupulum,
Aquæ menthæ sativæ drachmas
decem;
Misce. Fiat haustus,

No. 2.

℞. Pulv. ipecacuanhæ grana sede-
cim,

Vini antim. tartariz. drachmas
duas,
Aquæ pulegii unciam;
Misce. Fiat haustus.

No. 3.

℞. Pulveris ipecacuanhæ grana
quindecim,
Aceti scillæ drachmam,
Aquæ menthæ sativæ unciam
Misce. Fiat haustus emeticus.

H. PURGANTIA FORTIORA.

No. 4.

℞. Hydrarg. submuriatis grana
tria,
Extracti colocynth. compos.
grana quinque;
Misce, et divide in pilulas duas.

No. 5.

℞. Extract. coloc. comp. grana
quinque,
Hydrarg. submur. grana quin-
que,
Opii granum;
Misce. Fiant pilulæ duæ.

No. 6.

℞. Hydr. submur.
Pulveris antimonialis sing. gra-
na quinque,
Extr. papaveris grana tria;
Misce, et forma in pilulas duas.

No. 7.

℞. Hydrarg. submuriatis grana
tria,
Pulveris antimonialis grana
quatuor,
Extr. colocynth comp. grana
tria,

71

———hyoscyami grana duo;
Tere diligenter, et forma in pilulas
duas.

No. 8.

℞. Pulveris jalapœ grana viginti,
Hydrarg. submuriatis grana
quatuor;
Misce. Fiat pulvis.

No. 9.

℞. Pulveris jalapæ. scrupulum,
Supertartratis potassæ drach-
mam,
Pulveris aromatici grana tria;
Misce. Fiat pulvis catharticus.

No. 10.

℞. Hydrarg. submur. grana duo,
Pulv. scammoneæ grana qua-
tuor,
Sacchari purificati grana duo;
Misce. Fiat pulvis (basilicus) alter-
na nocte sumendus.

No. 11.

℞. Elaterii grana duo,
Mastiches,

Extractiœ glycirrhiz sing. grana
sex;
Misce intime, et divide in pilulas
quatuor æquales. Sumat unam
omni nocte.

No. 12.

℞. Hydrargyri submuriatis grana
tria,
Rhei pulveris grana septem :
Misce. Fiat pulvis.

No. 13.

℞. Hydrargyri submuriatis grana
quatuor,
Pulveris ipecacuanhæ compositi
grana decem;
Misce. Fiat pulvis.

No. 14.

℞. Infusi sennæ comp. uncias
quinque,
Potassæ tartratis unciam,
Tincturæ jalapœ,
——— sennæ sing. semunciam,
Syrupi rhamni drachmas tres;
Misce. Sumat partem quartam pro-
dosi, et repetatur quarta qq.
hora donec alvus plene soluta
sit.

III. PURGANTIA MITIORA.

No. 15.

℞. Extracti colocynth. comp. gra-
na duo,
Pilul. hydrarg. grana tria;
Fiat pilula omni nocte sumenda.

No. 16.

℞. Pilulæ hydrargyri grana duo,
Pulveris antimonialis grana

quatuor;
Misce. Fiat pilula quartis horis cum
haustu salino adbibenda.

No. 17.

℞. Pil. hydrarg. grana quindecim,
Pulv. ipecacuanhæ grana tria;
Misce et divide in pilulas sex. Sumat
unam omni hora donec alvus
responderit.

No. 18.

℞. Pulveris rhei scrupulum,
Potassæ sulphatis grana quinde-
cim,
Aquæ menthæ piperitæ sescun-
ciam;
Misce. Fiat haustus aperiens.

No. 19.

℞. Pulv. rhei grana viginti,
Confect. arom. grana quinde-
cim,
Aquæ menthæ piperitæ unciam
cum semisse;
Misce. Fiat haustus.

No. 20.

℞. Aquæ menthæ piperitæ sescun-
ciam,
Magnesiæ sulphatis drachmas
sex.
Conservæ rosæ drachmam ;
Misce et cola. Fiat haustus aperiens.

No. 21.

℞. Infusi sennæ compositi unciam,
Magnesiæ sulphatis drachmas
duas,
Tincturæ sennæ,
Tincturæ jalapæ,

Syrupi sing. drachmam ;
Misce. Fiat haustus.

No. 21.*

℞. Infusi sennæ compos. drachmas
decem,
Pulveris jalapæ grana quinde-
cim,
Potassæ supertartratis scrupu-
lum,
Syrupi aurantiorum,
Tinct. sennæ sing. drachmam ;
Misce. Fiat haustus.

No. 22.

℞. Infusi sennæ compositi drach-
mas novem,
Pulveris colchici grana octo,
Tincturæ jalapæ drachmas du-
as,
Syrupi mori drachmam ;
Misce. Fiat haustus catharticus.

No. 23.

℞. Infusi sennæ comp. uncias duas
cum semisse,
———— gent. comp. uncias tres,
Liq. potassæ sesquidrachmam,
Tincturæ cardam. compos.
drachmas tres ;
Misce. Sumat unciam bis die.

IV. PURGANTIA MITISSIMA.

No. 24.

℞. Fructus tamarindi unciam,
Foliorum sennæ drachmas du-
as.
Seminum coriandri semidrach-
mam,
Sacchari semunciam,
Aquæ bullientis uncias octo ;

Macera in vase clauso, et post horas
duas cola. Sumat cochlearia
tria majora omni hora ad al-
vi solutionem.

No. 25.

℞. Confectionis sennæ unciam,
Sulphuris loti semunciam,

Syrupi tolutani quantum sufficit;
Fiat electuarium, cujus sumat cochlearia duo (vel tria) mino-
ra omni mane.

No. 26.

℞. Olei ricini semuncium,
Mucilaginis acaciæ drachmas
tres,
Aquæ pimentæ drachmassex,
Syrupi drachmam,
Tincturæ opii guttas decem;
Misce. Fiat haustus sextis horis su-
mendus.

No. 27.

℞. Olei ricini drachmam,
Mann drachmas duas,
Pulveris acaciæ grana decem,
Aquæ drachmas decem;
Misce. Fiat haustus quartis horis
sumendus.

No. 28.

℞. Pil. hydrargyri,
Extracti rhei sing. grana
quindecim,
Olei anthemidis guttas duas;

Divide in pilulas sex. Sumat unam
nocte pro re nata.

No. 29.

℞. Magnesiæ sulphatis drachmam,
Infusi rosæ compositi unciam,
Syrupi aurantiorum drachmam;
Misce. Sumat haustum tertiis horis.

No. 30.

℞. Infusi rosæ comp. unciam,
æagnesiæ sulphatis drachmas
duas,
Tincturæ cardamomi compositæ drachmam,
Acidi sulphurici diluti guttas
decem,
Syrupi drachmam;
Misce. Fiat haustus semel vel bis
die sumendus.

No. 31.

℞. Infusi rosæ comp. drachmas
decem,
Magnesiæ sulphatis drachmam,
dimidiam,
Tincturæ opii guttas quatuor,
Syrupi rosæ drachmam;
Misce. Fiat haustus sextis horis su-
mendus.

V. STOMACHICA.

No. 32.

℞. Decocti aloes compositi drachmas sex,
Aquæ cinnamomi drachmas quatuor;
Misce. Fiat haustus omni meridie
sumendus.

No. 33.

℞. Infusi gentianæ comp. drach-
mas quinque,
Aquæ cinnamomi drachmas tres,
Carbonatis sodæ grana decem,
Rhei pulveris grana duo,
Spt. lavandulæ comp. semi-
drachmam;

Misce. Fiat haustus bis die sumendus.

No. 34.

℞. Infusi cascarillæ,
———— rhei sing. drachmas tres,
Aquæ cinnamomi semunciam,
Confectionis aromaticæ grana
decem ;
Misce. Fiat haustus semel (vel bis)
indies sumendus.

No. 35.

℞. Pulveris rhei grana duo,
———— capsici granum,

Extracti anthemidis q. s. ut fiat
Pilula omni meridie (vel ante pran-
dium) sumenda.

No. 36.

℞. Pulveris myrrhæ,
———— rhei, singulorum scrupulos duos,
Aloes socotr.
Extr. chamæmeli, singulorum
semidrachmam.
Olei anthemidis guttas decem ;
Misce. Divide in pilulas triginta ;
sumat duas omni nocte (vel
pro re nata) hora somni.

VI. SALINA DIAPHORETICA.

No. 37.

℞. Potassæ nitratis grana quinde-
cim,
Aquæ unciam,
Pulveris acaciæ grana decem,
Syrupi limonum drachmam;
Misce. Fiat haustus quartis horis re-
petendus.

No. 38.

℞ Potassæ nitratis grana quinque,
Aquæ menthæ pulegii drach-
mas quatuor,
Vini antim. tartariz. guttas
quinque,
Tincturæ digitalis guttas quin-
que,
Mucilaginis acaciæ,
Syrupi sing. drachmam ;
Misce. Fiat haustus, tertia quaque
hora sumendus.

No. 39.

℞. Subcarb. potassæ grana octode-
cim,
Succi limonum semunciam.
Spt. myristicæ guttas decem,
Aquæ destillatæ drachmas sex,
Sacchari albi scrupulum ;
Misce, et effervescentia finita, fiat
haustus, tertia quaque hora
repetendus.

No. 40.

℞. Liquoris ammoniæ acetatis drachmas tres,
Aquæ menthæ sativæ drachmas
sex,
Syrupi aurantiorum drachmam ;
Misce. Fiat haustus quartis horis
repetendus.

No. 41.

R. Liquoris ammoniæ acetatis un-
ciam cum semisse,
Vini antimonii tartariz. drach-
mas duas,
Spt. myristicæ drachmam,
Syrupi croci drachmas tres,
Aquæ destillatæ uncias qua-
tuor;
Fiat mistura cujus sumat partem sex-
tam quarta quaque hora.

No. 42.

R. Misturæ camphoræ unciam,
Liquoris ammoniæ acetatis dra-
chmas duas.
Spiritus ætheris sulphurici se-
midrachmam,
Mucilaginis acaciæ,
Syrupi mororum, sing. drach-
mam;
Misce. Fiat haustus quartis horis
repetendus.

No. 43.

R. Misturæ camphoræ drachmas
decem,
Liquoris ammoniæ acetatis
drachmas duas,
Ammoniæ subcarbonatis grana
sex,
Tincturæ opii minima quinque,

Syrupi croci drachmam:
Misce. Fiat haustus sexa quaque
hora repetendus.

No. 44.

R. Magnesiæ sulphatis drachmam,
———— ustæ grana quindecim,
Vini colchici minima triginta,
Aquæ menthæ sativæ drachmas
decem;
Misce. Fiat haustus sexta qq. hora
adhibendus.

No. 45.

R. Misturæ camphoræ drachmas,
sex,
Liquoris ammoniæ acetatis
drachmas tres,
Pulveris ipecac. compos. grana
sex,
Pulveris acaciæ grana decem;
Misce. Fiat haustus sextis horis sumendus.

No. 46.

R. Misturæ camphroæ unciam,
Vini colchici semidrachmam.
Liquoris ammoniæ acetatis
drachmas duas;
Misce. Fiat haustus sextis horis su-
mendus.

VII. ANODYNA (Irritationem Sedantia.)

No. 47.

R. Misturæ cretæ unciam,
Confect. aromaticæ scrupulum,
Tinct. cinnamomi semidrach-
mam,
Tincturæ opii guttas quinque;
Sumat haustum post singulas dejec-
tiones liquidas.

No. 48.

R. Misturæ amygdalæ unciam,
Tincturæ opii guttas viginti,
Syrupi drachmam:
Misce. Fiat haustus.

No. 49.

℞. Pulv. cretæ compositi scrupu-
lum,
Aquæ unciam,
Syrupi papaveris drachmam ;
Misce. Fiat haustus, sextis horis re-
petendus.

No. 50.

℞. Extr. conii grana viginti,
Pulv. ipec. comp. semidrachmam ;
Misce. Divide in pilulas decem. Sumat unam tertia quaque hora.

No. 51.

℞. Extracti conii grana tria,
Magnesiæ sulphatis scrupulum,
Aquæ carui drachmas quinque,
Syrupi rhæados drachmam ;
Misce. Fiat haustus ter indies su-
mendus.

No. 52.

℞. Misturæ camphoræ unciam,
Tincturæ opii minima triginta,
Liquor. antimon. tartariz. mi-
nima quindecim,
Syrupi croci drachmam ;
Misce. Fiat haustus hora somni su-
mendus.

No. 53.

℞. Confectionis opiatæ scrupulum,
Aquæ cinnamomi unciam,
Syrupi tolutani drachmam ;
Misce. Fiat haustus tertiis horis ad-
hibendus.

No. 54.

℞. Extracti conii drachmam,
Pulveris digitalis
Hydrarg. submuriatis, sing, grana quinque ;
Tere, et divide in pilulas quindecim
æquales, quarum sumat unam
ter die.

No. 55.

[tuor,
℞. Extracti hyoscyami grana qua-
Hydrarg, submuriatis granum :
Fiat pilula omni nocte sumenda.

No. 56.

℞. Succi spissati lactucæ virosæ
drachmam dimidiam,
Pulv. tragac. comp. scrupulum,
Potassæ nitratis scrupulos duo,
Misturæ amygdalea uncias qua-
tuor ;
Misce. Capiat cochl. unum amplum
ter die.

VIII. DEMULCENTIA.

No. 57.

℞. Mucilaginis acaci unciamæ,
Aquæ destillatæ uncias tres,
Syrupi tolutani,
Aquæ cinnamomi, singulorum
unciam ;
Misce. Sumat cochleare unum am-
plum quartis horis.

No. 58.

℞. Olei amygdalæ unciam,
Acaciæ gummi drachmas duas,
Aquæ destillatæ uncias sex,
Syrupi papaveris semunciam :
Tere oleum diligenter cum gummi,
dein adde gradatim aquam, et
syrupum.

Sumat cochl. duo ampla quater indies.

No. 59.

℞. Cetacei drachmas duas,
Vitellum ovi,

Syrupi althææ semunciam,
Aquæ cinnamomi semunciam,
—— destillatæ uncias quatuor
cum semisse;
Misce. Sumat cochleare unum amplum frequenter.

IX. STIMULANTIA SIVE CALEFACIENTIA.

No. 60.

℞. Infusi armoraciæ compositi unciam,
Spt. ammoniæ aromatici semidrachmam,
Syrupi zingiberis drachmam;
Misce. Fiat haustus sextis horis adhibendus.

No. 61.

℞ Misturæ camphoræ drachmas
decem,
Spiritusæ theris sulfurisi drachmam,
Confectionis aromaticæ serupu-
lum,
Spt. lavandulæ comp. semidrachmam,
Misce. Fiat haustus quartis horis
repetendus.

No. 62.

℞. Misturæ camphoræ drachmas
sex,

Tinct. guaiaci ammoniatæ
drachmas duas,
Mucilaginis,
Syrupi, singulorum drachmam
Misce. Sumat haustum bis die.

No. 63.

℞. Bals. copaibæ guttas quindecim,
Vitelli ovi q. s.
Aquæ cinnamomi,
—— destillatæ, sing. drachmas
quinque,
Spt. lavand. comp. semidrachmam;
Syrupi drachmam;
Misce. Fiat haustus ter die sumendus.

No. 64.

℞. Olei terebinthinæ drachmam,
Mellis drachmas duas¹
Aquæ carui drachmas sex;
Misce. Fiat haustus bis vel ter die
sumendus.

X. TONICA CUM FERRO.

No. 65.

℞. Ferri subcarbonatis,
Calumbæ pulveris, sing, grana
quinque;

Misce. Fiat pulvis bis die sumendus

No. 66.

℞. Ferri subcarbonatis drachmas
tres,

Syrupi aurantiorum unciam,
Pulv. cinnamomi comp. drachmam ;
Misce. Fiat electuarium. Sumat
drachmam bis die.

No. 67.

℞. Carbonatis ferri drachmam cum
semisse,
Rhei pulveris grana quindecim.

Olei anthemidis guttas quinque.
Conservæ rosæ q. s. ut fiat
massula, in pilulas viginti
æquales dividenda.
Capiat tres mane et meridie quotidie
superbibendo guttas quindecim elixir vitrioli acid. sulphur. aromat. Pharm. Edin.)
incyatho aquæ vel infusi zingiberis.

XI. TONICA AMARA.

No. 68.

℞. Decocti cinchonæ,
Infusi rosæ comp. singulorum
drachmas sex ;
Misce. Fiat haustus ter indies repetendus.

No. 69.

℞. Decocti cinchonæ drachmas decem,
Acidi sulphurici diluti guttas,
duodecim,
Tinct. cardam. compos.
Syrupi aurantiorum, ana drachmam ;
Misce. Fiat haustus ter indies sumendus.

No. 70.

℞. Decocti cinchonæ sescunciam,
Extracti cinchonæ grana quin-
decim,
Tincturæ ejusdem drachmam ;
Misce. Fiat haustus.

No. 71.

℞. Decocti cinchonæ drachmas decem,
72

Confectionis aromaticæ scrupulum,
Tincturæ cinchonæ compositæ
drachmam ;
Misce. Sumat haustum quarta quaque hora.

No. 72.

℞. Quininæ sulphatis grana tria,
Acidi sulphurici aromatice (Ph.
Edin.) guttas decem,
Infusi aurantii compositi drach-
mas decem,
Tincturæ cinchonæ compositæ,
Syrupi zingiberis sing. drach-
mam:
Misce. Fiat haustus tertiis horis ad-
hibendus.

No. 73.

℞. Quininæ sulphatis grana duo,
Infusi rosæ compositæ drachmas
decem,
Syrupi aurantii drachmas duas;
Misce. Fiat haustus quartis horis
bibendus.

No. 74.

℞. Infus. gentianæ comp.

Aquæ cinnamomi, sing. semunciam,
Sodæ carbonatis grana quindecim,
——— tartarizatæ drachmas duas;
Misce. Fiat haustus.

No. 75.

℞. Infusi gentianæ comp, uncias
duas,
Liquoris calcis uncias tres cum
semisse,
——— potassæ drachmam cum
semisse,
Tincturæ aurantii drachmas
tres ;
Misce. Fiat julepium, de quo sumat
cochl, tria majora bis die.

No. 76.

℞. Extracti taraxaci drachmam
dimidiam,
Aquæ menthæ sativæ sescunciam ;
Misce. Fiat haustus meridie, et vespere sumendus.

No. 77.

℞. Infusi cuspariæ unciam,

Carbonatis ammoniæ grana sex,
Tincturæ cinnamomi compositæ
drachmam ;
Misce. Sumat haustum bis die.

No. 78.

℞. Cascarillæ cort. contusi,
Calumbæ radicis incisæ, sing.
drachmam,
Aquæ ferventis uncias sex,
Liquori frigefacto et colato
adde
Tincturæ calumbæ drachmas
tres,
Spt. amm. aromat. guttas tri-
ginta,
Syrupi aurantiorum drachmas
tres,
Sumat drachmas sex pro dosi bis vel
ter die.

No. 79.

℞. Infusi cascarillæ drachmas octo,
Ammon. subcarbonat. grana
quinque,
Conf. aromat. grana decem,
Spt. armoraciæ compos. drach-
mas duas ;
Misce. Fiat haustus ter de die su-
mendus.

XII. CARMINATIVA.

No. 80.

℞. Spiritus ammoniæ aromatici,
——— lavandulæ compositi,
singulorum unciam ;
Misce. Sumat drachmam ex aqua,
urgente languore.

No. 81.

℞. Aquæ carni unciam,
Tinct. cardam. comp. drachmam,
Spt. ammon. aromat. guttas decem,

Syrupi croci drachmam ;
Misce. Fiat haustus.

No. 82.

℞. Misturæ camphoræ unciam,

Spt. ammon. aromat. guttas vi-
ginti quinque,
Spt. lavandulæ comp.
Syrupi sing. drachmam ;
Misce. Fiat haustus, urgente lan-
guore sumendus.

XIII. ANTISPASMODICA.

No. 83.

℞. Misturæ camphoræ drachmas
decem,
Tincturæ opii guttas quadra-
ginta ;
Spiritus ætheris sulphurici drach-
mam,
Syrupi rhæados drachmam ;
Misce. Fiat haustus.

No. 84.

℞. Valerianæ radicis semunciam,
Macera per horas duas vase
clauso in
Aquæ ferventis unciis octo.
Dein
℞. Colati liquoris uncias sex.
Tincturæ castorei,
Syrupi croci, ana semunciam ;

Misce. Sumat cochl. duo majora urgente spasmo.

No. 85.

℞. Misturæ camphoræ uncias quinque,
Spt. ammoniæ fœtid. drachmas
tres,
Syrupi croci drachmas quatuor ;
Misce. Fiat julepium antispasmodi-
cum, cujus sumat cochlearia
duo pro dosi.

No. 86.

℞. Misturæ assafœtidæ uncias
quinque cum semisse
Tincturæ valerianæ ammoniatæ semunciam ;
Misce. Sumat partem quartam ter
die.

XIV. EXPECTORANTIA.

No. 87.

℞. Extracti conii semidrachmam,
Pulveris scillæ grana decem,
————— ipecacuanhæ grana
quinque ;
Misce. Divide in pilulas decem
æquales. Sumat unam bis vel
ter die.

No. 88.

℞. Misturæ camphoræ drachmas
quatuor,
Tincturæ digitalis minima decem,
Oxymellis scillæ drachmam dimidiam,

Tincturæ camphoræ compos.
guttas decem

Misce. Fiat haustus tertiis horis sumendus.

Tincturæ opii minima quinque,
Syrupi drachmam;

Misce, et fiat haustus ter die sumendus.

No. 89.

℞. Pulveris ipecacuanhæ grana
tria,
Aceti destillati drachmas tres,
Aqæ menthæ pulegii drachmas
quinque;

Misce. Fiat haustis quartis ad quartam vicem repetendus.

No. 93.

℞. Tincturæ scillæ guttas decem,
Acidi nitrici guttas sex,
Extracti hyoscyami grana tria,
Aquæ puræ unciam cum se-
misse;

Misce, ut fiat haustus, tertiis horis
repetendus.

No. 90.

℞. Creœtæ preparatæ grana decem,
Pulveris ipecacuanhæ grana
tria,
Aquœ menthæ sativæ drachmas
decem;

Misce; et fiat haustus tertia quaque
hora repetendus.

No. 94.

℞. Misturæ ammoniaci drachmas
sex,
Aceti scillæ drachmam,
Tincturæ opii guttas sex,
Aquæ carni drachmas tres;

Misce. Tertia vel quarta quaque
hora sumendus.

No. 91.

℞. Sodæ subcarbonatis grana vi-
ginti quinque,
Vini ipecacuanhæ drachmam,
Tincturæ opii minima sex,
Syrupi drachmas tres,
Aquæ puræ unciam;

Misce. Sumat partem sextam quarta
vel sexta quaque hora.

No. 95.

℞. Oxymellis scillæ,
Tincturæ camphoræ compos.
Spt. ætheris nitrosi, sing. se-
munciam,
Infusi lini compositi uncias
sex;

Misce. Sumat cochlearia duo ampla
pro dosi.

No. 92.

℞. Infusi gentianæ compos. semunciam,
Aquæ cinnamomi drachmas
quinque,
Carbonatis sodæ grana decem,
Vini ipecacuanhæ minima decem,

No. 96.

℞. Oxymellis scillæ semunciam,
Aquæ menthæ sativæ uncias
duas,
———— destillatæ uncias tres,
Syrupi tolutani semunciam;

Fiat mistura, cujus sumat cochlearia
duo ampla ter die.

XV. ASTRINGENTIA.

No. 97.

℞. Aluminis scrupulum,
Cons. rosæ caninæ drachmam;
Mis. Fiat bol. sextis horis sumendus.

No. 98.

℞. Plumbi superacetatis grana duo,
Extracti hyoscyami grana tria;
Misce. Fiat pilula mane et nocte sumenda,

No. 99.

℞. Infusi rosæ comp. sescunciam,

Acidi sulphurici diluti minima quindecim,
Syrupi drachmam;
Misce. Fiat haustus quartis horis repetendus.

No. 100.

℞. Infusi cascarillæ uncias sex,
Pulveris kino compositi drachmam,
Syrupi papaveris semunciam;
Misce. Fiat mistura restringens, cujus sumat partem sextam sextis horis.

XVI. DIURETICA.

No. 101.

℞. Inf. digit. drachmas quatuor,
Aquæ cinnamomi drachmas quinque,
Potassæ acetatis scrupulum,
Spt. ætheris nitrosi drachmam;
Misce. Fiat haustus sextis horis repetendus.

No. 102.

℞. Infusi cascarillæ drachmas sex.
Spt. juniperi compos,
—- ætheris nitrosi, ana drachmam,
Confectionis aromaticæ grana quindecim;
Misce. Fiat haustus quinta quaque hora sumendus.

No. 103.

℞. Pulv. jalapæ grana viginti,

Potassæ supertartratis drachmas duas,
Oxymellis scillæ quantum sufficit:
Fiat bolus omni mane devorandus,

No. 104.

℞. Nitratis potassæ,
Supertartratis potassæ,
Pulveris acaciæ, sing. grana decem,
Sacchari albi scrupulum;
Misce. Sumat ex cyatho aquæ vel decocti hordei (tepidi) tertia quaque hora.

No. 105.

℞. Pil. hydrarg. grana tria,
Pulveris scillæ granum,
——— digitalis granum;
Misce. Fiat pilula meridie et vespere sumenda.

XVII. MEDICAMENTA EXTERNE ADHIBITA.

No. 106.

℞. Inf. rosæ comp. uncias novem,
　Mellis rosæ semunciam,
　Tinctuæ capsici semunciam;
Misce. Fiat gargarisma.

No. 107.

℞. Mucilaginis amyli uncias octo,
　Tincturæ opii drachmam;
Misce. Fiat enema astringens.

No. 108.

℞. Unguenti sambuci,
　Pulveris gallarum, sing. se-
　　munciam,
　Liquoris plumbi subacetati,
　　drachmam;
Misce Fiat unguentum.

No. 109.

℞. Liquoris ammoniæ acetatis un-
　　cias tres,
　Spiritus vini unciam,
　Aquæ fontanæ uncias 'duode-
　　cim;
Misce. Fiat lotio.

No. 110.

℞. Antimonii tartarizati scrupulos
　　duos.
　Tincturæ cantharidis unciam,
　Aquæ rosæ (calidæ) uncias duas;
Solve antimonium tartariz. in aqua
　　rosæ, dein adjice tincturam,
　　Fiat embrocatio.

No. 111.

℞. Linimenti saponis unciam cum
　　semisse.
　Olei succini semunciam;
Misce. Fiat embrocatio.

No. 112.

'　Linimenti saponis uncias duas.
　Camphoræ drachmam,
　Liquoris ammoniæ,
　Tincturæ cantharidis.
　———— opii ·sing. drachmas
　　duas,
Misce. Fiat linimentum.

No. 113.

℞. Plumbi acetatis.
　Camphoræ, singulorum semi-
　　drachmam,
　Aquæ ferventis octarios duos;
Misce, et liquorem frigefactum cola.
　Fiat lotio.

No. 114.

℞. Antimouii tartarizati drach-
　　mam,
　Unguenti cetacei drachmas octo,
　Hydrargyri sulfureti rubri scru-
　　pulum. Misce.

No. 115.

℞. Aquæ rosæ uncias decem,
　Sulfatis zinci scrupulum;
Solve, Fiat collyrium.

APPENDIX.

PROPOSITIONS IN MEDICINE.

BY M. BROUSSAIS.

SECT. I.

PHYSIOLOGY.

I. Animal life is only maintained by external stimuli (*Brown.*) And whatever augments the phenomena of life is a stimulant.

II. Caloric is the principal and most important of all stimulants ; and when it ceases to animate the economy, all other stimuli cease to exert their powers upon it.

III. Caloric is necessarily and constantly furnished to the fœtus by its mother : to the animal after birth by its lungs ; but it is also supplied incidentally by all other avenues.

IV. If caloric is deficient for a certain length of time, all the pre-servatory, restorative and sanitary powers lose their energy.

V. Caloric calls into play that power which composes the organs. This power forms them out of nutritive materials, and conducts free fluids through their interstices : The organs, or solids, as well as the fluids, are denominated animal matter.

VI. The composition of solids and fluids is a Chemistry peculiar to living beings. The power which developes this chemistry gives to the organs, in the act of forming them, the faculties of sensation and of contractile movement. Sensibility and contractility are, then, the evidences of life.

VII. Certain bodies in nature, besides Caloric, increase the sensibility and contractility of those parts of the system with which they are placed in contact. This is stimulation or irritation, and these bodies are stimulants.

73

VIII. Sensibility and contractility being increased in any given part, are soon increased in several other parts. This is Sympathy.

IX. Sympathy takes place through the medium of a particular form of the living tissue, or animal matter, which is termed nerve.

X. All the phænomena of association take place through the agency of nerves, which transmit stimulation from one part to another, or to more parts. These then are sympathies.

XI. The objects of primitive, as well as sympathetic stimulation are always nutrition, the removal of destructive or noxious materials, and reproduction; and the movements which effect these objects are termed functions. Now for the exercise of the functions, the fluids must concur with the solids : wherever, then, there is stimulation, there must be an attraction and accumulation of fluids.

XII. Sensibility and contractility are distributed, in different degrees, to the various tissues which compose the living system. Those which possess them in the highest degree receive the impression of stimulants directly, and transmit it to other organs. They are, then, the natural *mobiles* of the sympathies.

XIII. The tissues which may be considered as the natural prime-movers of the sympathies, are those in which the nervous matter is found under a pulpy form, mixed with the sanguineous capillary vessels, and also with other vessels which contain albuminous or gelatinous fluids. They are the skin, and the cerebral senses, which are distinguished as the external; also the mucous membranes, which constitute the internal senses.

XIV. All the organs of sense are exposed, by their very nature, to the action of external agents, and also of those which are internal; and the stimulation they receive from either is transmitted to the brain, their common centre. Besides, from these different points, stimulation is transmitted to the other tissues. And it is thus that the functions are mutually supported.

XV. Every stimulation, capable of transmitting a perception to the brain, pervades the entire nervous system of relation. It is then reflected to the mucous membranes, whence it is once more transmitted to the centre of perception, which judges of it according to the impression received from the viscus to which the mucous membrane belongs, and is determined to action according to the pleasure or the pain it receives, and this action always tends to prolong and repeat the impressions, or to remove the cause.

XVI. The action instituted by the cerebral centre of relation is

performed by means of the muscular locomotive apparatus under the command of the brain ; and the same nerves which served
to transmit the impression, serve also to execute the will of the
centre of perception, by that portion of their tissue which commu.
nicates with the locomotive muscles.

XVII. Whilst an impression, or rather the stimulation which
results from an impression, traverses the nervous system of the
viscera, it gives rise to movements in the muscles forming part
thereof, modifies the circulation of all the fluids which pass through
them, and produces even involuntary contractions in the locomotive
muscles.

XVIII. Whilst the stimulating influence of the brain is exerted
voluntarily or the reverse, upon the locomotive muscles, stimula.
tion is also communicated, but involuntarily, to the muscular and
vascular tissues of the viscera; because the nerves of relation are
common to the muscles of locomotion and the viscera.

XIX. The voluntary movements having brought the nutritive materials in contact with the organs of assimilation, these last assimilate them to the wants of the individual.

XX. Assimilation is a phenomenon of the first order which
cannot be accounted for by the action of sensibility and contrac.
tility ; it can be attributed only to the creating power, and is one
of the acts of the living chemistry.

XXI. Absorption depends, in the first place, on the affinities of
the living chemistry ; in the second, on the exercise of sensibility
and contractility.

XXII. The circulation is under the dominion of sensibility and
contractility in the heart and blood-vessels, so far as a certain point
of decrease which it is difficult to ascertain : beyond this point,
and at that where the extravasated fluids run between the fibres,
these fluids are moved partly by the heart, partly by the contrac.
tility developed by the local sensibility, and partly by the affinities
of the living chemistry which are constantly directed by the crea.
ting power. The same observation is to be applied to the causes
of the motion of the fluids in the organs called secretory.

XXIII. Whilst the fluids move in the tissues, the composition and
decomposition of those tissues, as well as the formation of the
fluids which are to remain for a greater or lesser time in their interstices, take place. These three phenomena, of which nutrition
is composed, essentially belong to the living chemistry, because
sensibility and contractility do no more than present to the organs

the assimilated materials, and eliminate the fluids unnecessary to the process of composition, as well as those disengaged by that of decomposition.

XXIV. Whilst the fluids move through the tissue of the glands, there occur, besides nutrition, changes in the form of those fluids which are not made use of in that process ; these changes, which belong to the living chemistry, are such that every gland has its own characterised by phenomena peculiar to each. Sensibility as well as contractility are of no other use than to eliminate the newly formed fluids, in order to conduct them externally if useless, or to deposit them on the mucous surfaces if intended to concur in a particular function.

XXV. Embryogeny is a product of the living chemistry. Sensibility and contractility carry the embryo into the uterus ; the vital chemistry causes its development and gives it its particular sensibility and contractibility ; its expulsion is effected by the sensibility and contractility of the mother. (*vide* Prop. 6.)

XXVI. There exists an order of nerves situated along the vertebral column, having for their centre ganglia peculiar to themselves ; the whole order bears the name of the great sympathetic : It is better to call them ganglionic nerves.

XXVII. The ganglionic nerves penetrate through the viscera and muscles along with the nerves of relation and the blood-vessels of those organs; they exist in great number in the viscera and muscles of the trunk, but there are very few in the muscles of the limbs.

XXVIII. A wound of the ganglionic nerves developes neither pain nor convulsion in the first instance ; they do not transmit sensations to the brain, nor the commands of the brain to the organs.

XXIX. The ganglionic nerves can only preside over the internal actions that are not directed by the cerebral centre. Blended with the capillary system of the viscera, their use is to regulate and transmit stimulation from one part to another, according to the wants of the creating power ; that is to say, they are particularly subservient to the vital chemistry.

XXX. The ganglionic nerves concentrate the stimulating influences of the cerebral nerves, and make them subservient to the actions that are independent of the centre of perception. Hence the will can neither withdraw nor even controul the stimulation it has once transmitted to them through the agency of the functions of relation.

XXXI. The ganglionic nerves render the vital force of the animal subservient to the living chemistry, notwithstanding the influence of the will ; and when the amount of this force is no longer sufficient to the performance of the two great orders of functions, these nerves divert it from the functions of relation and coneentrate it in those of nutrition : they operate this diversion by accumulating the vital force and the fluids along with it in the vessels of the viscera, and especially in those of the brain ; this is what produces sleep.

XXXII. When irritation is predominant in the viscera, the ganglionic nerves cause it to flow back to the organs of relation through the medium of the cerebral nerves with which they communicate in these same viscera ; and it is no more in the power of the will to prevent this irritation, than to take back from the viscera that which it has once transmitted to them.

XXXIII. The centre of relation, under the influence of the viscera, excites, with or without the concurrence of the will and the knowledge of the animal, certain actions in the locomotive organs which are in direct proportion to the visceral irritations, and which terminate only in the cessation of those irritations, or in the engorgement, compression, and disorganization of the brain.

XXXIV. .Whenever a stimulation is excited in the economy capable of giving a shock to the cerebral nerves, it is transmitted to the centre of relation, which may, in consequence, execute certain movements, without the consciousness or will of the animal. The phenomena, therefore, which give the idea of consciousness are discontinued, whilst the perception and reaction of the centre of relation are continued.

XXXV. The perceptions of the cerebral centre, attended by consciousness, are known by the name of *sensibility*, and the movements it directs are called voluntary. But the perceptions of the cerebral centre unaccompanied with consciousness, and the motions it unconsciously determines, are not referred to sensibility, nor to the will ; they are a particular species of organic phenomena. The nervous cerebral apparatus presents, then, two forms in its functions.

XXXVI. Whenever consciousness (*le moi*) experiences a perception, it feels at the same time in the brain and externally to the brain. Now the extra-cerebral points in which consciousness experiences sensations are not the external and internal senses only, they are also the accidental *foci* of inflammation ; because inflammation reduces the extremities of the nerves of relation of most of the tissues to a state pretty analogous to that of the nervous extremities which form part of the natural sensitive surfaces. These foci of phlegmasia become, then, accidental or occasional senses.

XXXVII. The will (*le moi**) can refuse to execute certain acts solicited by sensations excited by the natural and accidental senses. There are others which it can only retard for a longer or shorter period.

XXXVIII. The will does not enjoy the power of retarding or preventing the execution of actions demanded by the sensations except when the encephalic apparatus is already developed, enjoys a state of health, and is wakeful. This faculty has no existence, then, in early life ; it subsequently improves by the exercise of the intellect. In sleep, in mania, and other morbid conditions, it presents a host of modifications.

XXXIX. The actions which the will can only retard are solicited by sensations which proceed from viscera essential to life, and which have relation to the indispensable performance of their functions.

XL. Among the actions which the will can refuse to perform, some are solicited by the wants of viscera essential to life, but these wants are not urgent ; when they become so, either the will consents, or the reason is destroyed, or death supervenes. Others, again, have connection with the performance of functions which are not necessary to the preservation of life, and here too, the refusal of the will may engender madness.

XLI. When the animal suffers and undergoes death for having refused to satisfy the wants of the viscera, it betokens the triumph of the understanding over instinct. But if reason is alienated by this resistance, that is by the super-irritation which the wants have excited in the brain, then instinct triumphs over intellect.

XLII. Instinct consists in sensations developed by the viscera, and which solicit the cerebral centre to cause to be performed the actions necessary to the exercise of the functions.

XLIII. The actions solicited by instinct are often performed

---

* It will be seen that a varied translation of the uncouth and vague expression " *le moi*" is given in different paragraphs, modified by its application to the context. Consciousness and will obviously comprehend all the ideas involved in the term.—[*Translator.*]

without the participation of the will, and even in its absence; in-stances occur in the fœtus, in the sleeping state, &c.

XLIV. The actions solicited by instinct predominate in the in-fant, and diminish in proportion to the development and advance-ment of the understanding.

XLV. The intellect displays its actual influence over the sys-tem by the modifications which it produces in the sensations deter-mined by instinct, and also in the actions by it solicited.

XLVI. The Passions are sensations awakened, in the first in-stance, by instinct, but afterwards quickened and exalted by the attention bestowed on them by the intellect, so that they gain the ascendancy, and produce acts more or less remarkable, and always calculated to satisfy the instinctive wants, to which they owed their origin.

XLVII. The passions, like mania, evince the triumph of the vis-cera, and consequently that of instinct over intellect. So do they produce mania itself.

XLVIII. The passions always combine instinct and intellect.

XLIX. Instinct may operate either with, or without the aid of the intellect.

L. Intellect never operates without the blended aid of instinct.

LI. The intellectual faculties may operate without passion, but never without a sensation of pleasure or of pain.

LII. The pleasure and the pain which accompany the exer-cise of the intellectual faculties have the same seat as the pleasure and the pain attending the passions ; because the centre of relation cannot experience a sensation in the brain without also experien-cing it in the viscera : and it is always in these last that it feels the most.

LIII. Whilst the intellect is occupied with ideas relating to the wants of a viscus, or to the functions of a sense, the nerves of this viscus or sense are always in action, and they transmit sensations to the centre of relation ; it follows that the destruction of the nerves of a sense involves the gradual loss of the ideas to which they were wont to give origin.

LIV. An acephalous fœtus may live : It dies as soon as it is born, because it then requires the influence of respiration, which depends on the brain.

LV. Those organs which lose their communication with the brain, soon lose their vitality and their nutrition ; they wither and die. This state seldom occurs, because in palsies the sequelæ of affections of the brain, there is still a communication kept up with this viscus. But as the principal connection is through the medium of a diseased point, and the others by anastamoses with nervous cords rather inconsiderable, their influence is not able to maintain action in the organ to the requisite degree.

LVI. It is not by the defect of a peculiar principle of which the brain may be supposed to be the source, that the moving apparatus when paralysed withers; but from the want of excitement and exercise.

· LVII. The want of action in paralysed muscles does not proceed from the inaptitude of their nerves to excite motion, but from the absence of sufficient communication with the brain. After nutrition has been languid for some time in the paralysed part, its nerves deteriorate and are no longer capable of exciting action.

LVIII. The presence of oxygenated blood may preserve nutrition in paralysed parts, because there is yet some communication with the brain, but deficiency of exercise renders this nutrition more and more languishing, without always producing death in the part.

LIX. An uninterrupted and constant communication of excitement kept up in all directions between the different parts of the body, is indispensable to a preservation of an equilibrium of all the functions.

LX. In warm seasons and hot climates, excitement is imparted to animals by the external, more than by the internal, surfaces: In cold seasons and climates, excitement is chiefly derived from the latter. The gastric surface becomes then the principal medium of excitement; hence nutrition is more abundant.

LXI. Excitement is never uniform in the animal economy; it is always above par in certain parts, and below in one or more other parts; and successively predominates in various regions. This irregularity often terminates by destroying the balance of the functions.

LXII. Health is never disturbed spontaneously, but always because external stimulants, destined to preserve the functions in their integrity, have accumulated excitement in some part, or because they have been deficient in supplying the wants of the economy, or because it has been stimulated in a manner repugnant to the exercise of the vital laws; because there exist relations between the external modifiers, and the whole, or several parts of the system, of which some are friendly, others repugnant to the vital laws ; and these last are poisons.

LXIII. Certain external modifiers diminish the phenomena of life in the organs with which they have relation ; but the pain, which is developed in a debilitated part, performs the office of an excitant, which invites back the vital phenomena, sometimes favourably, sometimes injuriously to the preservation of the animal.

LXIV. The excess of hæmatosis or sanguification, augments the sum of vitality ; but this increase has a limit beyond which excitement is accumulated in an organ, and disease takes place by the over-irritation of this organ.

LXV. Excitement is also accumulated in organs by the influence of stimulant modifiers, although the sum of the general vitality is very much diminished ; and this condition may continue even unto marasmus and unto death.

L XVI. The economy never undergoes over-excitement with impunity ; and all those who appear the most habituated to stimuli of too much power, sooner or later experience local super-irritation.

SECT. II.

PATHOLOGY.

LXVII. Health implies the regular exercise of the functions ; disease results from their irregularities ; death from their ceasing altogether.

LXVIII. The functions are irregular, when one or more of them are performed with too much or too little energy.

LXIX. The energy of a function is in excess, when it hurries, or suspends, or deranges other functions, so that one or more of the organs which are engaged in the performance of the excited function, and of those which it has disturbed, are menaced with destruction.

LXX. The energy of a function is weak, when one or more of the organs charged with it do not enjoy a degree of vitality necessary to perform the function properly.

LXXI. The vitality of organs may have been exalted previously to its diminution, and vice versa.

LXXII. There is neither exaltation nor diminution of the vitality of organs which is general and uniform.

LXXIII. Excitement always commences in one organic system, and is communicated to others either in the same apparatus* or elsewhere.

LXXIV. The nature of the communicated exaltation is the same as that of the primitive. It is always an augmentation of the phenomena which evince vitality.

LXXV. The exaltation of one or more organic systems, or of one or more apparatuses always produces languor in some other system or apparatus.

LXXVI. The diminution of vitality in any system or apparatus involves *often* its increase in one or more others, and *sometimes* its diminution.

LXXVII. The exalted vitality of a system, (and *a fortiori* of an apparatus) always implies an action of stimulating modifiers, superior to that proper for the maintenance of health, that is to say, a super-stimulation, or super-excitation.

LXXVIII. A partial super-excitement always implies a too great flow of fluids ; there is then congestion, prejudicial to the exercise of the functions, in every over-excitement. It is a morbid congestion.

LXXIX. The combination of partial over-excitement and morbid congestion induces always an increased or irregular partial nutrition ; which constitutes active congestion that tends necessarily to disorganization.

LXXX. Active and partial over-excitement and morbid congestion are compatible with a general diminution of the amount of vitality.

LXXXI. Partial diminution of vitality involves always that of nutrition, although it often induces a morbid congestion ; but then this last is passive.

LXXXII. Passive morbid congestion may produce disorganization, but much less so than active.

---

* To understand this proposition fully, it may not be amiss to recur to the following definitions of the same author : " By the word *organ* we are to understand a portion of animal matter, arranged in such a manner as to render it capable of performing at least one of the acts which contribute in a manifest degree, to the maintenance of life."

" Whenever several organs are united together, and associated for the accomplishment of the same object, they constitute an apparatus.—*Broussais' Physiology*, p. 13, 14."

LXXXIII. Active morbid congestion being always accompanied with over-excitement or super-irritation, it is enough to name this last to be understood in tracing the progress of diseases. We may even rest content with the term irritation, provided we attach the same ideas to it as to the above two expressions : but the adjunct morbid is always implied.

LXXXIV. Irritation may exist in a system, without any other system's participating in it ; this takes place only when it is inconsiderable. It bears, then, on the local organic movement only, and on the nutrition of the part. As soon as the local irritation is increased to a certain degree, it is extended to other systems and other apparatuses more or less distant and always without changing its nature.

LXXXV. The nerves are the only agents in transmitting irritation, which constitutes morbid sympathies. These last act, then, in the same manner as the sympathies of health. They do not differ except that in the former case the nerves transmit more irritation, or a mode of excitement repugnant to the vital laws.

LXXXVI. Morbid sympathies are of two sorts : the first manifest themselves by organic phenomena ; to wit, increase of fibrillar movement, congestions, alterations in the secretions, exhalations, absorptions which are either augmented, diminished, or deranged, changes in the temperature, and vices of nutrition ; these are organic sympathies. The second by pains, convulsions of the voluntary muscles, and mental aberrations ; these are the sympathies of relation.

LXXXVII. Organic sympathies may exist without the sympathies of relation : These last always involve the former ; but the two orders of sympathies most frequently exist simultaneously.

LXXXVIII. The more considerable the sensibility of an irritated organ, and that of the individual, the more the sympathies are multiplied, and *vice versa*.

LXXXIX. The more numerous and active the sympathies, the more serious the disease.

XC. The excess of the sympathies of relation suffices to produce death, which then seems to depend on the disorganization of the centre of relation. The excess of the organic sympathies may also cause sudden death, which is then owing to the congestion and disorganization of several viscera.

XCI. The organ primitively irritated is sometimes the only one to undergo congestion and disorganization, the sympathising organ not receiving sufficient irritation to participate.

XCII. The organs sympathetically irritated may experience a higher degree of irritation than the organ from which they derived it. In this case, the disease changes its place and name. These are *metastases*.

XCIII. The organ, which has become the seat of a metastasis excites forthwith sympathies peculiar to itself; and these may, in their turn, become predominant. Such are the wandering phlegmasiæ, &c.

XCIV. If the sympathetic irritations, which the principal viscera produce in the secretory and exhalant organs, and in the periphery, become more powerful than that of these viscera, these last are freed from theirs, and the disease terminates by a speedy cure. These are crises. In these cases, irritation travels from the internal to the external parts.

XCV. The congestions of crises are always relieved by an evacuation either secretory, or purulent, or hæmorrhagic; without this, the crisis is incomplete.

XCVI. If irritation proceeds from the external to the internal parts, or from one viscus to another of greater importance, the disease is aggravated. These are the false crises of authors.

XCVII. Irritations have no fixed duration or progress; both the one and the other are regulated by the idiosyncracy, and by the influence of the modifiers which act upon the sick.·

XCVIII. Irritation has a tendency to propagate itself through similar tissues, and organic systems; this is what constitutes diathesis. Nevertheless, it passes sometimes to tissues altogether different from that in which it took its origin and this oftener in acute, than in chronic diseases.

X CIX. When irritation accumulates the blood in a tissue, with swelling, redness, and heat beyond what is ordinary, and capable of disorganizing the irritated part, it receives the name of inflammation.

C. Local pain is not inseperable from inflammation, even when intense.

CI. Local pain in inflammation offers many varieties, which are subordinate to the mode of sensibility of the part, and to the extent of that possessed by the individual.

CII. Inflammation often excites more pain in the parts where sympathetic irritations are manifested, than in its own focus.

Daily examples of this are to be found in the inflammations of the mucous membranes of the stomach, small intestines and bladder.

CIII. When inflammation causes no pain, it only excites organic sympathies.

CIV. Inflammation always brings on an alteration in the fluids of the part inflamed.

CV. Inflammation may exist without suppuration.

CVI. Inflammation is often followed by a form of irritation bearing a different name, and produces a cacochymy which has been reputed essential.

CVII. Inflammation not unfrequently brings on sympathies of relation which authors have considered as the predominant phenomena, and consequently designated by the appellation of *neuroses*.

CVIII. Inflammation does not change its nature in consequence of the diminution of strength which it occasions.

CIX. The irritations of all organs are transmitted to the brain if they acquire a certain degree of intensity, and especially if they be inflammatory ; the result of this complication is a derangement of the mental and affective faculties, and a state of pain and uneasiness which is referred to the locomotive organs ; the excess of this sympathy terminates in encephalitis.

CX. The violent irritations of all organs are always transmitted to the stomach at the moment of their invasion ; the result is inappetency, alteration in the colour of the tongue and of its mucus ; if the irritation imparted to the stomach attains the degree of inflammation, symptoms of gastritis come on ; and as the brain is always more irritated, it developes, in a still greater proportion, the sympathies proper to itself, and may even become inflamed.

CXI. All intense irritations of the organs are transmitted to the heart ; its contractions then become more frequent, the circulation is accelerated, and the increased heat of the skin creates an unpleasant sensation. This is what must be called *fever*, which is here considered in a general and abstract manner.

CXII. Fever is always the result of an irritation of the heart either primary, or sympathetic.

CXIII. Every irritation, sufficiently intense to produce fever, is one of the forms of inflammation.

CXIV. Every inflammation which is capable of producing fever by reaching the heart, is thereby sufficiently intense to be transmitted at the same time to the brain and the stomach, at least in its commencement, and as in order to its transmission, it does not undergo a change in its nature, it is always a form of inflammation which is developed in these three organs.

CXV. Irritations transmitted to the brain and the stomach by an inflamed organ sometimes diminish, notwithstanding the continuance of the inflammation from which they have proceeded, and both these viscera resume their functions, whilst the heart continues to be violently irritated, and to keep up the fever.

CXVI. Although both the stomach and the brain continue their functions during the inflammation of another organ, they are, nevertheless, organically irritated; their irritation always borders on inflammation; and not unfrequently attains that degree, if the focus from which it proceeds persists until death.

CXVII. If the irritation excited, by sympathy, in the stomach and brain, instead of diminishing, becomes more intense than that of the focus from which it proceeds, there occurs what we have seen in the propositions on metastasis. (Vide CII. et seq.)

CXVIII. Inflammation of the brain *always* involves that of the digestive organs, and *sometimes* that of their appendages; this is organic sympathy.

CXIX. Inflammation of the brain is more frequently the sympathetic effect, than the cause, of gastric inflammations.

CXX. The congestion of blood in the stomach, in cases of drunkenness, typhus fevers of a bad character, &c. is necessarily reflected to the brain and its envelopes.

CXXI. Inflammation of the brain gives rise to nervous phenomena which have often been deemed essential.

CXXII. All irritations of the brain which are prolonged unto death terminate in inflammation or hemorrhage; such are epilepsy, catelepsy, excessive struggles of the mind, &c.

CXXIII. Mania always implies an irritation of the brain; this irritation may be kept up there for a long time by another inflammation, and disappear with it; but if it protracts its duration, it always terminates in true encephalitis, either parenchymatous or membranous.

CXXIV. No extra-cerebral inflammation can produce mania without the concurrence of that of the stomach and small intestines. Here the liver is only secondarily affected.

CXXV. Arachnitis is more frequently consecutive to gastroenteritis, than a primitive inflammation; but the delirium, loss of sleep and convulsions, by which it is often characterised, may be

kept up by the gastro-enteritis, and disappear with it, or leave after death, in the arachnoides and pia-mater, some marks of phlegmasia which are either insignificant, or less prominent than those
found in the stomach, &c. &c.

CXXVI. Every acute suffering, either in consequence of the inflammation of an organ, or proceeding from the stimulation of the
branch of a nerve, or from a moral cause, engorges the brain, and
tends to develope inflammation in its substance, in the pia-mater,
and in the arachnoides. Now, the suffering of the stomach is the
most intense, and it is produced by all the others ; ergo, there can
never be gastro-enteritis without some degree of cerebral irritation.
All this applies also to encephalic hæmorrhages.

CXXVII. Tubercles, cancers of the brain, &c. are produced by
chronic inflammation of that viscus.

CVXXIII. All encephalic irritations may end in apoplexy.

CXXIX. The term apoplexy implies a cessation of the phenomena of relation. Two principal degrees of this disease may be
recognized according to the absence or presence of partial paraly-
ses ; but it cannot be classified upon a foreknowledge of the forms
of organic alteration in the brain.

CXXX. Inflammation of the internal or mucous membrane of
the stomach, is termed *gastritis* ; but it is never discovered in the
body after death uncombined with that of the mucous membrane of
the small intestines. It is best then to term it *gastro-enteritis*.

CXXXI. The inflammation of the mucous membrane of the small
intestines is termed *enteritis*. Autopsia sometimes exhibits it uncombined ; but it cannot be so recognized before death, and
moreover gastritis is always its origin. It is also best then to term
it *gastro-enteritis*.

CXXXII. Gastro-enteritis presents itself under two forms ; with
the gastric inflammation predominating, or the enteritic. Pain in
the stomach, nausea, vómiting, or difficult retention of the ingesta characterize the first ; the power of satisfying thirst, the rapid
absorption of any liquids introduced are the signs of the second.

CXXXIII. Acute inflammation of the mucous membrane of the
small intestines, without any affection of the peritoneum, does not
occasion colic in the majority of cases. It is almost always unaccompanied with circumscribed pain, but often with a general diffused burning and uneasiness, and with constipation. The invagin-
ation of these intestines, far from causing ileus, does not, in ordinary cases, produce even colic.

CXXXIV. Colic, frequent dejections and tenesmus are the pe-cnliar signs of mucous inflammation in the colon.

CXXXV. The word enteritis being appropriated to inflamma-tion of the small intestines, cannot serve to designate that of the colon, which must be termed Colitis. But the two blend with and succeed each other.

CXXXVI. Gastro-enteritis is unattended by pain in any parti-cular point, so long as the inflammation does not predominate with violence in the stomach or duodenum ; and even pressure of the abdomen does not occasion pain.

CXXXVII. Gastro-enteritis is recognized by the sympathies which it developes ; to wit : 1st. the organic, redness and heat of the apertures of the mucous membranes, and of the skin, change in the secretory ogans of the bile, of the urine, and above all of the mucus : 2dly. those of relation, which are pain in the head and limbs, disordered faculties of perception and judgment. The influence exerted upon the heart is common to several other phlegmasiæ.

CXXXVIII. Acute gastro-enteritis when aggravated, terminates in stupor, fuligo, lividity, fetor, prostration, and constitutes what is called putrid, adynamic, typhus fever : that in which the irritation of the brain becomes considerable whether or not it progresses to phlegmasia, produces delirium, convulsions, &c. and receives the name of malignant, nervous, ataxic fever.

CXXXIX. All the essential fevers of authors, are resolvable in-to gastro enteritis, simple or complicated. Writers have failed to recognise it when it is present without local pain, and even when this last has been present, they have always regarded it as an ac-cident.

CXL. Authors have sometimes expressed the idea that certain fevers depended on an inflammation of the digestive organs, but they never maintained that the pretended essential fevers can have no other cause, or that they were produced by the same agency as the fever of pneumonia, &c. never, in short that these are not essential fevers. All this was never thought of until the physiolo-gical doctrine.

CXLI. Authors, ignorant that the internal membrane of the small intestines may be inflamed wtthout local pain, have all attri-buted to enteritis the symptoms of peritonitis.

CXLII. It is by an acute gastro-enteritis, first effect of the con-tagious agent, that the small-pox breaks forth. The cutaneous phlegmasia replaces it, and terminates it when the pustules are few in number ; but reproduces it if the pustules are numerous, by the erysipelas which results from the confluence of the pock. Such is the *secondary fever* of variola, called also the *fever* of suppuration.

CXLIII. It is by gastro-enteritis, and by acute catarrh of the eyes, nose, throat or bronchiæ, that scarlatina and measles commence ; and these phlegmasiæ constitute all the danger of those diseases, aggravating them, and involving the brain and the whole of the viscera. The angina of scarlatina often becomes fatal, and attention must be paid to the bronchial catarrh of measles, which produces from the beginning a puriform expectoration, and which, even when it is not converted into a pneumonia, may produce strangulation by intercepting the passage of the air.

CXLIV. Hypochondriasis is the effect of chronic gastro-enteritis, which acts violently upon a brain predisposed to irritation.

CXLV. The greater number of cases of dyspesia, gastrodynia, gastralgia, pyrosis, cardialgia, and all those of bulimia are the effect of chronic gastro-enteritis.

CXLVI. Umbilical colics, intermittent or remittent, with constipation and without tenesmus, characterize certain varieties of the inflammation of the mucous membrane of the small intestines especially in a chronic state, if the symptoms of peritonitis are not present ; but this enteritis is more often indolent, than painful.

CXLVII. The lymphatic ganglia of the mesentery do not inflame except through the medium of enteritis, and this double phlegmasia, when prolonged, constitutes tabes mesenterica.

CLXVIII. The ganglia of the mesentery are not inflamed in simple peritonitis.

CXLIX. Hepatitis is always consecutive to gastro-enteritis, when it does not depend on external violence.

CL. Chronic gastro-enteritis is the cause of hepatic engorgements, of yellow and fatty livers, even among the phthisical.

CLI. The dropsy of persons who have abused alcoholic drinks and purgatives, is the effect of a chronic gastro-enteritis which has invaded the whole thickness of the digestive canal, of the liver, &c. and also slowly penetrated the peritoneum.

CLII. Bulimia is the effect of a chronic gastro-enteritis, with predominance of gastro-duodenal irritation ; This phlegmasia may in fact exist in a form which permits the assimilation of a quantity of aliment far superior to the wants of the economy, whence re-

75

sult plethora, polysarcia, and, subsequently, the extension of the irritation to the brain, the joints, the kidneys, in a word to all
the points where an accidental stimulation may invite it.

CLIII. The bulimic gastritis often depends upon the abuse of
stimulant ingesta, and above all of *stomachic* medicines, administered while the gastritis is still slight.

CLIV. The exuberant assimilation of bulimic gastritis is always
attended with more or less local and sympathetic pains; these
pains, progressively increase until they render digestion frightful to
the patient even when his appetite is still excessive; they finally
destroy hunger, produce emaciation, vomiting, &c : sometimes the
gastritis assumes an acute form.

CLV. When a long employment of stimulants has too much
exalted the sensibility of the stomach, the case is long, difficult,
and the relapses very easily induced; it is seldom that in these
cases there is not a degree of cerebral irritation capable of producing hypochondriasis; and scirrhus or perforation of the stomach
often closes the scene.

CLVI. Inflammation often passes from the digestive mucous
membrane to the peritoneum in the acute form.

CLVII. Acute hepatitis is never mortal except it is complicated
with gastro-enteritis, peritonitis, or in the inflammation of the organs of the thorax or cranial cavity.

CLVIII. Acute nephritis is not mortal except it is complicated
with inflammation of the principal viscera.

CLIX. The acute peritonitis of women in child-birth commences ordinarily with inflammation of the internal membrane and
whole thickness of the uterus.

CLX. The prolonged irritations of the mucous membrane of the
vagina produce, almost always, inflammation of the neck of the uterus and of the ovaries; thence scirrhus, cancers, &c.

CLXI. Scirrhus of the neck of the uterus is often the effect of
violence suffered by the neck in parturition.

CLXII. Painful menstruation announces a permanent focus of
irritation in the neck of the uterus, and the cancer of this part is
often the consequence at the period termed critical, if the irritation of the neck has not been allayed for a long time before this
pe riod.

CLXIII. Peripneumony often commences by catarrh or inflammation of the mucous membrane of the bronchiæ. The superior
lobes of the lungs are then the principal seat of the inflammation;

and if this inflammation is chronic, it developes tubercles in the parenchyma and produces phthisis.

CLXIV. Peripneumony of the middle and inferior lobes fo the lungs commences often without being preceded by bronchial catarrh : If it becomes chronic, tubercles are developed, and phthisis supervenes.

CLXV. Pleurisy, by the purulent collection which it occasions, gradually wastes the lung of the side affected, and most commonly without inflaming it ; but, at the same time, pneumonia is sometimes developed in the opposite side ; and if this condition is prolonged, phthisis appears in this last.

CLXVI. Pleurisy, seated in the pulmonary pleura, unattended by effusion or atrophy of the lung which it envelopes, inflames this lung and may, if it become chronic, develope tubercles in it.

CLXVII. Tubercles which succeed to inflammation of the internal membrane of the bronchiæ and bronchial vesicles originate in the same manner as in those in the mesentery in chronic enteritis.

CLXVIII. I have never seen pulmonary tubercles unpreceded by inflammation.* Those which are coeval with birth in new-born infants do not appear to me to be independent of this phenomenon.

CLXIX. Tubercles may occur in all constitutions attacked by chronic inflammation of a lung or of the intestines ; but they are more frequent in subjects predisposed to irritation of the lymphatic system.

CLXX. Cartilaginous, bony, calcareous granulations, melanoses, scirrhus, encephaloid growths, cancer of the lungs, &c. are productions developed in the same manner as ordinary tubercles.

CLXXI. The term *pulmonary phthisis* expressing disorganization only, which is a product of the inflammation of the parenchyma of the lungs, should not be applied to this last affection. A better appellation is chronic pneumonia, as it specifies in which tissue of the viscus the disease had its origin.

CLXXII. The heart is often inflamed in its serous membrane ; this is what is termed pericarditis. It is recognised by the seat of the pain, and by the depression and irregularity of the circulation, which produce suffocation, fainting, and fear of imminent death.

CLXXIII. The heart is also inflamed in its internal membrane,

---

* It is somewhat singular that in the very imperfect English version of these Propositions which appeared in the American edition of Johnson's Review, the translator either says, or is made to say the very reverse !

this is ordinary carditis. This inflammation attacks, in preference, the arterial orifices where it often becomes chronic, and causes obstruction to the passage of the blood, thickening, vegetations, ossifications, ulcers, and, subsequently, hypertrophy of the heart and aneurism. Irritation or inflammation which first invades the locomotive apparatus often produces carditis by seating itself in the interior of the heart.

CLXXIV. The irritation of any of the tissues which is sufficiently intense to reach the heart may inflame its two tissues. Inflammation of the internal coat of the arteries is effected by the same causes, and cannot alone keep up a violent fever.

CLXXV. Acute inflammation and suppuration of the muscular tissue of the heart is a very rare disease ; but this tissue always suffers after a long continued inflammation of its two membranes.

CLXXVI. The most serious consequences of aneurism of the heart arise from the impediment offered to the circulation ; hence result asthmas, various hæmorrhagies and dropsies ; but gastritis never fails to accompany the other symptoms, and the more so in proportion to the extent of the stimulating treatment.

CLXXVII. Ossification of the proper arteries of the heart is the consequence of inflammation of its internal membrane, or of that of the large arteries.

CLXXVIII. Dilatations of the arch of the aorta are often the effect of chronic inflammation of its tissue. This affection may produce an obliteration of the mouths of the arteries which bring the blood from the head and superior extremities. The same inflammation occasions friability in other arteries, and aneurisms which Scarpa has well described.

CLXXIX. Scrofula is an irritation of those external parts in which the albuminous part of the blood predominates ; but as it possesses little heat, and is without redness it may receive a particular designation. Will *subinflammation* be proper ?

CLXXX. Inflammation, either as cause or effect, accompanies this subinflammation, and sometimes as long as it continues.

CLXXXI. Subinflammation of the lymphatic tissues is not developed before inflammation, except in those parts which compose the skeleton, and the soft parts which envelope it ; it is excited by cold applied to the skin, in the manner that rheumatisms are by accidental irritations. As to the viscera they are not affected by it except after they have been inflamed. The same must be said of syphilitic subinflammations.

CLXXXII. The skin is susceptible of a chronic irritation, which exerts a special influence on its excretory tissues and ab-sorbent vessels, and which disorganizes this envelope by engorg-ing it with deteriorated albumen. Is this not still a species of sub-inflammation, to which inflammation may be joined in different de-grees of violence ? When irritation is communicated from the sub-inflamed skin to the viscera, it does not extend to the lymphatic ganglia, unless preceded by inflammation of their membranes.

CLXXXIII. The lymphatic ganglia do not tumefy, or harden, or soften in any case except by an increased exaltation of their irri-tability and contractility, that is to say, by their irritation, which is a subinflammation.

CLXXXIV. Tumours, analogous in appearance to those of sub-inflamed ganglia, but which occur in tissues, that in health present no appearance of lymphatic glands, must be regarded in the same light as lymphatic ganglia developed by irritation. All these bear the name of *tubercles.*

CLXXV. Whenever the absorbent glands chronically irrita-ted, degenerate into tubercles, some of their lymphatics may be dila-ted by a passive engorgement produced by the obstruction to the course of the lymph. This dilatation is to the absorbents, what va-rices are to the veins.

CLXXXVI. The cellular tissue is, after the mucous membranes, the most susceptible of acute inflammation ; it then suppurates, but it may do so without its inflammatory condition having been recog-nised by any external signs.

CXXXVII. The occult foci of phlegmonous suppuration with reabsorption of pus do not keep up the fever termed hectic, unless it is by an irritation imparted to the principal viscera, either through sympathy with the permanent focus of inflammation, or the stimu-lating impression of the re-absorbed pus. This fever is then no more essential than the others.

CLXXXVIII. When the cellular tissue, slowly engorged with lymph or fat, becomes hardened, without presenting symptoms of inflammation, or after inflammation has been subdued, it is always indebted for this condition, to an increase of irritability and con-tractility, and never to a contrary cause ; this is also a species of subinflammation.

CLXXXIX. The fat and lymph, which compose cellular engorge-ments attended by hardness, are always deteriorated ; and if soft-

ening supervenes, inflammation is developed.   This is what occurs in encephaloid growths, in melanosis, scirrhus, &c : hence
cancers which also supervene upon tubercles, &c.

CXC. When irritation has existed under the form of inflammation
or subinflammation in the tissues of the articular or arterial membranes, and other tissues naturally dry and little extensible, there
is extravasation of albumen ; and this fluid is dried by means of absorption, and converted into calcareous concretions: as, for instance, the gouty.   These concretions are, then, the effect of irritation.   The same thing occurs with those which are formed in
the lymphatic ganglia that have become tuberculous, and sometimes
in the follicles which secrete mucosity.

CXCI. A black colour often predominates in lymphatic swellings : This is what is termed melanosis.

CXCII. External cancer, produced by an irritative deterioration
of the tissues in which albumen and fat predominate, is always
accompanied with inflammation ; it is not incurable, so long as it
is local.

CXCIII. The inflammation which accompanies external cancer
is extended, by sympathy, to the principal viscera ; but cancer is
not developed in them excepting as a consequence of the inflammation.   It may even be not produced at all ; the cancerous diathesis is not so frequent, then, as is generally supposed.

CXCIV. The progress of cancer is always proportionate to the
degree of inflammation present.

CXCV. All inflammations and subinflammations may produce
cancer.

CXCVI. Inflammation of the serous membranes presents but
two forms, the one acute, very painful and febrile ; the other chronic, very indolent and without fever.   The last is confounded with
subinflammation.

CXCVII. Inflammation of the mucous membranes presents forms
and degrees much more multiplied than that of the serous ; because
the former as internal senses and continual incitants of the sympathies, possess a sensibility and irritability more varied and intense
than the latter, which, in health, have neither sensibility nor sympathies.

CXCVIII. All hemorrhagies, which are not caused by external
violence, and are spontaneous, are active, whatever be the degree
of strength of the patient.

CXCIX. Spontaneous hemorrhagies depend upon an irritation

of the sanguineous capillaries ; but they are rendered more frequent by hypertrophy of the heart.

CC. Spontaneous hemorrhagies depend upon the same remote causes as inflammation ; so also may they be complicated with it, produce it, and be developed with it in the same organ ; they may supplant it, and be supplanted by it in different parts.

CCI. The neuroses are active or passive, whilst inflammation and subinflammation are necessarily active.

CCII. The passive neuroses consist in diminution or abolition of muscular sensibility and contractility ; they cannot be complete except in the locomotive and sensitive apparatus.

CCIII. Active neuroses consist in an exalted sensibility of the nerves of relation, and a like condition of the muscular and vascular contractility under the influence of these nerves. They may occur in the locomotive muscles, in the viscera, and in all the capillaries in which the nerves of relation predominate. Such are the neuralgiæ.

CCIV. Both the active and passive neuroses are most frequently caused by a phlegmasia seated in the cerebral apparatus or in the other viscera ; the passive, sometimes, depend on a sedative influence acting upon the nerves affected.

CCV. In the active neuroses of the apparatus of relation, the capillary circulation is excited ; there is congestion ; inflammation or subinflammation threaten to appear in the tissues in which the neuroses manifests itself, and also in that point of the cerebral apparatus whence proceed the nerves of these same tissues; whilst the intermediate nervous cords are limited to the transmission of sympathetic influences from one point to another.

CCVI. When, in the neuroses of the viscera of the chest or the abdomen, there occur wandering pains or convulsions in the locomotive muscles, there are two points of irritation which are either inflamed or show a tendency to it ; the one is in the viscera, the other in the encephalic apparatus.

CCVII. Obstacles to the circulation do not disturb the functions of the principal viscera, unless they occur in the heart and large vessels.

CCVIII. In cases of obstruction to the circulation, dropsy is produced by the stagnation of the blood in the veins.

CCIX. The sudden increase of dyspnœa in aneurism of the heart, after locomotion, proves the influence of the muscular system over the venous circulation.

CCX. Inflammatory congestions and the secretions prove the influence of the capillary system over the circulation of the blood.

CCXI. Absorption proves the influence of the capillary system over the course of non-sanguineous fluids.

CCXII. The uneasiness and anguish which occur in cases of impeded circulation, sooner or later, develope gastritis: Stimulating medicines hasten its approach.

CCXIII. Scurvy is a peculiar condition of the solids and fluids produced by an imperfect assimilation ; its causes are numerous ; but cold, want of light, grief and bad food are the principal. Extravasation of the fluids is one of the principal effects of scurvy, because it renders all the tissues fragile ; but the viscera, and, above all, the encephalic apparatus resist it longer than the tissues in which the bones of the trunk and limbs are enveloped.

CCXIV. The phlegmasiæ are easily complicated with scurvy, but they are not essential to it ; they are produced by general causes. Such is the inflammation of the gums.

CCXV. External violence, powerful emotions, stimulating medicines, and the phelgmasiæ readily produce rupture and disorganization of parts affected by scurvy, because the vital chemistry is languid and the powers of life generally diminished in the scorbutic.

CCXVI. Dropsy enumerates, as its physiological causes, obstacles to the course of the blood and the lymph, the sympathetic influence of chronic inflammation, a want of action in the depuratory capillaries, imperfect assimilation, and debility.

CCXVII. Irritation presents natural intermissions in a state of health.

CCXVIII. Morbid irritation may be intermittent in all the apparatuses and organic systems.

CCXIX. Morbid irritation may be continued in an apparatus to a moderate extent, and be periodically exasperated to return again to its ordinary degree. In these cases, when it is moderate, it excites few sympathies ; when aggravated, it developes many : these are the remittent and intermittent *fevers* of authors.

CCXX. Intermittent and remittent irritations are always accompanied with exaltation of the sensibility and contractility, and by consequence, with congestion, either in the principal seat of the disorder, or in those parts which are sympathetically irritated.

CCXXI. Intermittent and remittent irritations are, always, phlegmasiæ, hæmorrhagies, neuroses, or subinflammations, which change their seat* and terminate spontaneously by critical metas. tases ; if they do not change their seat, they are converted into con. tinued phlegmasiæ, hæmorrhagies, neuroses, or subinflammation, either of an acute, or chronic character.

CCXXII. Intermittent and remittent fevers are periodical gastro-enterites ; but the brain and other viscera are sympathetically irritated as in those of a continued form, and may even become the principal seat of the irritation, and be inflamed in a periodic or continued form.

CCXXIII. Every regular accession of an intermittent fever is the sign of a gastro-enteritis, of which the irritation is transferred to the cutaneous exhalants, which produces a crisis ; if the irritation is not completely transferred, the fever is remittent ; if not at all, the fever is continued.

CCXXIV. The masked fevers of authors are periodical irritations of the different systems or apparatuses, internal or external, in which the heart is little affected, and the general heat little or not at all increased.

CCXXV. Fevers termed pernicious do not differ from the others except in their violence and in their dangerous congestions.

CCXXVI. The Dropsies, which follow intermittent fevers, depend always upon one of the five causes or physiological conditions indicated in proposition CCXVIII.

CCXXVII. The most ordinary external causes of intermittent fevers are alternations of atmospheric heat and cold; but all that impresses the economy in the same manner as these vicissitudes may engender, and, above all, reproduce them.

CCXXVIII. The cause of periodicity in certain painful and convulsive affections which are for a long time repeated at intervals is not known.

CCXXIX. Rheumatism is a fibrous or synovial phlegmasia, produced by vicissitudes of external heat and cold ; it is not surprising, then, that it is often intermittent and periodical.

CCXXX. Periodical inflammations of the joints become wandering by means of the sympathies, and terminate in crises, or by fixing themselves on some part, under an acute or chronic form, in the manner of visceral phlegmasiæ when left to themselves.

CCXXXI. Gout does not differ from inflammation of the joints

---

* The term used by Broussais is " *se deplacer.*" This is translated in Johnson's review " exhaust themselves."

except in circumstances connected with the age or idiosyncracy of the patients.

CCXXXII. Articular phlegmasiæ, when chronic, are converted into subinflammation ; hence nodes, concretions, &c.

CCXXXIII. The form of articular phlegmasia, termed gout, is often, but not always, complicated with chronic gastro-enteritis, which modifies its course, and invites the irritation to the viscera.

CCXXXIV. The liver is not affected in gout excepting in consequence of an accompanying chronic gastro-enteritis.

CCXXXV. The irritation of gastro-enteritis is communicated to the joints, by means of sympathy, under the form of arthritis, or gout ; this does not however happen until the influence of atmospheric vicissitudes or some other external irritants has previously predisposed the joints to be so affected.

CCXXXVI. The irritation of articular phlegmasiæ developes, sympathetically, that of the stomach ; and this last becomes sometimes predominant.

CCXXXVII. The multiplied infirmities, which torment old gouty subjects (gouty diathesis and cacochymy,) are sympathetic irritations of the stomach, encephalon, &c. which have grown up and been transformed into phlegmasiæ, neuroses, or subinflammations ; or these phlegmasiæ may even be primitive.

CCXXXVIII. In chronic and renewed articular phlegmasiæ, irritation always proceeds from the circumference to the centre. It is the same with all inflammations occurring in the periphery.

CCXXXIX. The transformation of gout into another disease is nothing else than a change of the principal seat of irritation, which produces effects modified by the structure and vitality of the different organs it invades.

CCXL. It is absurd to term an affection gout which has not been preceded by articular inflammation ; it is equally so to give this name to one which has been so preceded ; for to say that gout has been transferred to the brain, when mania supervenes on an articular inflammation, is the same as to assert that mania has been transferred to the great toe, when gout follows a paroxysm of delirium.

CCXLI. In retrocession of gout, it is useless to have in view the seat of primitive irritation, except so far as to decide upon the point of the circumference to which it is most proper to invite revulsion.

CCXLII. Revulsion is not possible in what is called misplaced gout, unless the viscus last attacked has not yet undergone disorganization.

CCXLIII. Acrid vegetables, which, in small doses, are emetic, purgative, drastic, diuretic, &c, will when administered in large doses, excite inflammation and ulceration in the mucous membrane of the digestive organs, and, secondarily, pains and convulsions, which differ according to idiosyncracy.

CCLXIV. Vegetables, which are astringents in small doses, become causes of gastro-enteritis in large doses.

CCXLV. Narcotic vegetables and alcoholic substances excite gastro-enteritis, if administered in large doses, at first without ulceration ; and they engorge the brain with blood producing convulsions and various forms of delirium ; they also gorge the lungs.

CCXLVI. Those acrid vegetables, which are termed antiscorbutics if given in large doses, excite gastro-enteritis.

CCXLVII. Corrosive or escharotic mineral substances in small doses, produce gastro-enteritis, and subsequently ulceration: in large doses, they develope the same inflammation around the eschar they have formed. In every instance they cause delirium and convulsions considerably varied in character.

CCXLVIII. If arsenic does not prove speedily fatal, it excites inflammation of the primæ viæ in different degrees according to the dose and the idiosyncracy ; from these result engorgement and inflammation of the brain and lungs, and, sometimes phenomena analogous to those of the pretended putrid and typhus fevers.

CCXLIX. Saturnine substances produce, in small doses, a constriction of the gastro-intestinal mucous membrane and painful convulsions in the muscular layers of the digestive canal, whence result colic, vomitings, and, sympathetically, spasms of the limbs ; but, in large doses, or favoured by individual predisposition, they incite gastro-enteritis, more or less allied to the convulsive state. Hence the great discrepancies which occur in the action of emetics, drastics, opium, and sudorifics given to counteract lead-colic.

CCL. Mineral astringents, the sulphate of alumine, of zinc, of iron, act nearly the same as the preparations of lead.

CCLI. Corrosive sublimate inflames the primæ viæ in a moderately large dose ; given in excess, it ulcerates by producing phlogosis and causes a variety of pains and convulsions in the gastric canal, and in the muscles of relation.

CCLII. All the preparations of mercury and copper are exciting, and a large dose of them always produces gastro-enteritis.

CCLIII. Cantharides produce gastro-enteritis, at the same time with phlegmasia of the urinary organs.

CCLIV. Putrefied meat, which the stomach cannot digest, produces gastro-enteritis, with irritation and engorgement of the brain, and developes symptoms of typhus by the intensity of the nervous symptoms; but ulceration does not supervene except secondarily, and after a certain duration of the inflammation.

CCLV. Tainted fish, and poisonous mushrooms cause gastro-enteritis with sense of suffocation, meteorism, colic, &c. imitating the symptoms of typhus, and often cutaneous inflammation; the delirium and convulsions (under which must be concluded the tremor or subsultus tendinum) are, in this case, at least as prominent as in that of poisons from putrid meat.

CCLVI. All inflammatory and escharotic poisons whether vegetable, animal, or mineral, when applied to the skin, in large quantities, develope in the digestive mucous membrane, in the brain, and some of them in the lungs, an inflammation analogous to that excited externally, by the transmission of the irritation to the interior.

CCLVII. Poisons of all kinds being injected into the blood-vessels, soon develope gastro-enteritis, &c, if they are not sufficiently powerful to cause immediate death.

CCLVIII. Putrid meat inserted into living flesh, or the sanies from it introduced into the blood-vessels, act on the primæ viæ as if they had been swallowed, unless a sudden death anticipates the gastro-enteritis.

CCLIX. The stings and bites of venomous animals, which leave poison in the wound they inflict, cause a local phlegmasia which passes into gangrene with a readiness proportionate to the intensity of the irritation. The most dangerous of these poisons cause distress and death by the deleterious influence which they exercise over the nervous system. Should life, however, be preserved, the inflammation they cause is extended to the principal viscera, to the primæ viæ more especially, and always with a tendency to mortification. Gangrene is, then, in this as in other cases, the result of a too rapid exaltation of the vital phenomena. Finally, the mildest of these poisons produce simply a local phlegmasia.

CCLX. The bites of rabid animals always cause a gastro-enteritis, and the inflammation is often extended to the pharynx, the brain, the lungs, and the genital organs. The delirium and convulsions which attend are always the sympathetic effects of these phlegmasiæ, and they vary according to the susceptibility and the idiosyncracy.

CCLXI. Worms are most frequently, but not always, generated in the primæ viæ, by depraved mucus and heat, the consequences of gastro-enteritis, more or less intense : Hence the discrepant ope‧ration of irritating anthelmintics.

SECT. III.

THERAPEUTICS.

CCLXII. It is ever dangerous not to arrest inflammation at its onset ; because crises are always violent, sometimes dangerous ef‧forts which nature *deploys* to relieve the system from imminent danger ; it is wise then to anticipate them and imprudent to wait for them.

CCLXIII. There are four kinds of means by which we may arrest the progress of inflammation : debilitants, revulsives, fixed tonics, and stimulants more or less diffusible.

CCLXIV. The debilitants proper to arrest inflammation are blood letting, abstinence, emollient‚ and acidulated drinks ; but bleeding is the most efficacious of them all.

CCLXV. General blood-letting is indicated in those sanguineous engorgements, which are rapidly formed in the parenchymata un‧der the influence of irritation ; local or capillary bleeding, practi‧sed as near as possible to the principal point of irritation, that is, on the portion of skin corresponding with the seat of the inflamed organ, should enjoy the preference in all other cases, whilst the disease is still recent.

CCLXVI. There is no danger or impropriety in bleeding to syn‧cope in recent inflammation, occurring in persons who enjoyed health previous to the present attack of disease ; in cases of a con‧trary character, the patient would be made to undergo a sacrifice for which it would be doubtful if he would recover indemnity. The same may be asserted of a complete abstinence from food, espe‧cially if prolonged. Hæmorrhagy from leech-bites often becomes excessive in infants and young people, whose skin is surcharged with blood, and the action of whose hearts is very powerful. The flow of blood should be stopped, therefore, as soon as weakness is felt.

CCLXVII. Local bleeding is often injurious in long standing inflammation of the principal viscera, when there is not a supera-bundance of blood in the system. It is seldom that it does not, in this case, increase the congestion; it is far better to abstain from it altogether, or, at least, to practise it at a remote point from the seat of irritation.

CCLXVIII. General or local bloodletting, performed upon an individual who has not much blood, causes always great uneasiness, increases visceral congestions, and produces, thereby, convulsions and fever.

CCLXIX. When a very recent inflammation, occurring in a previously healthy subject and having yielded to local bloodlet-ting, is suddenly rekindled, it may be attacked repeatedly by the same measures; convalescence will be more prompt and easy. But if a chronic phlegmasia have preceded the acute, such practice would be dangerous. It would be equally so if the inflammation were general* in one, or more viscera; in these cases the bleeding must be arrested whenever the pulse loses strength, even if it has not lost its frequency.

CCLXX. Moderate inflammations of the encephalon readily yield to leeches applied over the epigastrium, especially if gastri-tis has preceded: but more serious congestions in the brain re-quire bleeding from the arm and from the jugular veins, also arteri-otomy, and leeches applied to the upper part of the neck; it is necessary, afterwards, to apply cold to the head, whilst heat is made to act upon the lower extremities.

CCLXXI. Cerebral congestions attended by feebleness of pulse require the application of cold to the head and of rubefacients to the lower extremities, before recourse is had to blood-letting.

CCLXXII. Leeches applied to the lower part of the neck, be-tween the insertions of the sterno-mastoid muscles, remove bron-chial catarrh, and prevent phthisis pulmonalis. This remedy is ef-ficacious in the catarrh which attends upon measles, and which would without its employment, produce a fatal strangulation. The purulent appearance of the expectoration offers no contra-indica-tion.

* A very unpardonable error occurs in the translation of this section fur-nished by the Medico-Chirurgical Review. Broussais is made to say that " if the inflammation had been general, or," &c. Now the whole scope of these propositions aims to establish the fact that there is no general disease whatever.

CCLXXII. Leeches applied around the clavi. les and under the axilla, arrest the progress of catarrh which has attacked the supe- rior lobe, and which would infallibly induce phthisis. A dull or less clear sound, altogether recent, announces that the catarrh has penetrated into the parenchyma, and indicates the indispensable necessity of local blood-letting.

CCLXXIV. Leeches applied to the epigastrium sooner arrest gastritis, than those applied to the anus. These last are, however, most efficacious in subduing colitis.

CCLXXV. When colitis resists leeches applied to the anus, and there can be perceived pain and swelling in some point in the course of the colon, a new application of leeches to this point, or of cups will put an end to the disease.

CCLXXVI. To arrest incipient colitis by the application of leeches to the appropriate spot is to annihilate epidemic dysentary.

CCXXVII. Tonsillitis, pharyngitis, laryngo-tracheitis or croup, hooping-cough, &c. yield sooner to local bleeding than to emetics, which frequently aggravate them, especially if there exist pletho- ra, gastric inflammation, &c.

CCLXXVIII. Bilious, mucous, and other symptoms termed gas- tric derangements, are more speedily and surely removed by leech- es applied to the epigastrium, or simply by abstinence and by wa- ter, than by emetics.

CCLXXIX. Jaundice depending in almost every case upon gas- tro-duodenitis, or hepatitis, is removed by the application of leech- es between the epigastrium and hypochondrium, provided it is fol- lowed by the use of emollients and an appropriate regimen.

CCLXXX. Inflammation of the joints will yield to leeches pro- vided they are not complicated with gastro-enteritis ; in this latter case, local bleeding at the epigastrium becomes necessary.

CCLXXXI. The fever which ushers in the acute cutaneous phlegmasiæ being the sign of a visceral inflammation preceding that of the skin, local bleeding, performed as nearly as possible to the principal internal point of irritation, promotes the eruption and diminishes the danger.

CCLXXXII. The *secondary* fever of confluent small-pox, being the effect of an erysipelas induced by the pustules, may be moder- ated and sometimes obviated, 1st by bleeding in the eruptive fe- ver ; 2dly by leeches applied to the neck immediately before the development of the erysipelas of the face.

CCLXXXIII. The fever termed *adynamie* which supervenes

upon confluent small-pox being no more than a gastro-enteritis produced by the erysipelas of the skin, may be prevented by those
means which arrest the march of this erysipelas. (See the last
proposition.)

CCLXXXIV. The worms, which accompany acute gastro-enteritis being the effect thereof, do not require specific remedies,
and are expelled by nature after the removal of this inflammation.

CCLXXXV. Worms do not require a specific treatment, unless
they occur without gastro-enteritis acute or chronic, or unless they
continue after such inflammation has been subdued.

CCLXXXVI. The *sequelæ* of measles are inflammations of the
bronchiæ, of the lungs, or of the primæ viæ ; they require no treatment distinct from that proper to these affections.

CCLXXXVII. Emetics do not cure gastro-enteritis excepting
by the revulsion and the critical evacuations they induce ; their effect is therefore uncertain in slight cases ; and in severe ones, they
are always dangerous, because they never fail to aggravate the inflammation when they do not succeed in subduing it. It is the same
with purgatives, but those which are bitter increase the heat, whilst
the saline disguise the phlegmasia, rendering it chronic. Such is
often the effect of calomel and of the neutral salts which do not allay the distress in gastro-enteritis, except by instituting a diarrhœa which terminates in marasmus and dropsy.

CCLXXXVIII. Blisters often aggravate gastro-enteritis, because
the inflammation they produce adds fuel to the digestive mucous
membrane instead of creating a revulsion ; they do not therefore
render the service expected of them in that degree of the disease
which has been designated as *adynamic fever*.

CCLXXXIX. Blisters aggravate, most generally, the inflammations of the different pneumonic tissues, whether acute or chronic,
when they are applied before the antiphlogistic treatment has been
employed ; but after repeated bleeding, they produce a very efficient
revulsion.

CCXC. The stomach is an organ which requires stimulation, in
order to maintain the sympathies by which it awakens the degree
of irritation necessary to the exercise of the functions ; but it should
be in a degree and mode adapted to its degree of vitality, because
this organ is the seat of the internal regulating sense of the economy.

CCXCI. When the sensibility and irritability of the stomach
are too much excited, all stimulants injure it and precipitate the

action of the functions, even to their destruction. Such is the case in aggravated gastritis, in cholera, in yellow fever, &c.

CCXCII. Excessive irritability of the stomach not manifesting itself always by pain, nor vomiting, but oftener by fever more or less violent, by delirium, stupor, and convulsive movements, these sympathetic affections should be sufficient to induce the practitioner to reject the employment of stimulants.

CCXCIII. The stomach, when tormented by stimulants, relieves itself sometimes of the irritation by transferring it upon the exhalent and secretory vessels, through the medium of its natural sympathics with them; this explains why gastro-enteritis, even when treated by excessive stimulation, does not always prove fatal.

CCXCIV. When the stomach is affected with chronic inflammation of a certain intensity, and occupying the whole extent of its mucous membrane, all stimulants prove injurious to it, and it can only throw off the irritation they induce by assuming acute inflammation, and thus eliciting those organic sympathies by which it may effect a crisis; because the sympathies of relation are inadequate to its relief.

CCXCV. The stomach affected with gastritis and still more irritated by stimulants is exposed to great danger if the inflammation is too intense to be relieved by revulsion, because it is likely to undergo disorganization. Hence results either the cure, or the aggravation of chronic gastritis, from the use of mineral waters, &c. The irritation transferred to the lungs, the brain, or the extremities, is often converted into phthisis, mania, apoplexy, or gout.

CCXCVI. If chronic gastritis is circumscribed to a small part of the stomach, which is always pointed out by the seat of the pain in the viscus and in the muscles surrounding it, and by the period of the digestion in which it is more prominent, stimulants injure it, increase the pain, and produce uneasiness and fever; but when the irritation of the diseased part has been allayed by emollients, the rest of the organ which has been too much relaxed craves stimulants; these will procure ease, renew strength, and augment nutrition, until they renew the local inflammation which was only smothered. As soon as this last effect is produced, the symptoms are renewed and stimulants again rejected.

CCXCVII. In partial phlogosis of the stomach, several years will often elapse in alternate states of excitement and calm, induced by the variations of treatment, until the inflammation has reached the point of disorganization producing either scirrhus, softening or

77

perforation : There arrives, in short, a period when nothing can be taken into it, and death is inevitable.

CCXCVIII. Partial irritations of the stomach, distinguished by the history laid down in the two last propositions, are removed by perseverance in rejecting all stomachic medicines and by furnishing sufficient nourishment to maintain the strength, but of such a nature as while it yields nutritive material, is not too stimulating ; and, lastly, by allaying, by means of emollient drinks, the irritation which always supervenes after digestion. This treatment may require years for its success, but it is the only durable one ; it may succeed even when a certain degree of disorganization has already taken place ; it is particularly important not to debilitate the system by sanguineous depletion, or by abstinence which might involve the loss of the assimilating powers of the viscera.

CCXCIX. In chronic gastritis and gastro-enteritis, not complicated with colitis, a cure is sometimes obtained by overcoming the constipation by means of calomel and the neutral salts ; This occurs in those cases only in which the inflammation is slight ; because if it is aggravated and deep seated, especially if the integrity of the viscus is threatened, this treatment can only be palliative, like that procured by all other stimulants.

CCC. Hemorrhoidal irritation is frequently the effect of a chronic gastritis or gastro-enteritis, and must be treated like these affections. An aggravation of the gastric disease may suppress this flux, as it does menstruation ; it is very imprudent to have recourse to stimulants to restore it. It is most safe to attend to the gastritis, because when this is removed, either the piles are cured with impunity, or they return should their flow be necessary to the system.

CCCI. When the stomach is not supplied with food sufficiently stimulating, all the functions are rendered languid ; but hunger soon excites an irritation that revives several of them, in a manner unfavourable to the preservation of the individual ; Such are the mania and mental fury of starved persons.

CCCII. Hunger, unallayed, excites gastritis, and this its accustomed train of sympathetic affections.

CCCIII. Heat at the pit of the stomach, pains of the head and limbs, and redness of the tongue produced by hunger, disappear on the administration of food, provided they are not too intense. When they have become so, they are aggravated by food, and will only yield to emollients, followed by graduated nourishment; yet bleeding would be improper.

CCCIV. When the stomach allows food to pass into the intestines, which was not sufficiently stimulating to excite its assimilating powers, there will supervene colic and diarrhoea which will yield to time and alcoholic drinks: If these substances are administered as soon as the colic is felt, digestion is re-established and the diarrhœa obviated. This fact proves that assimilation is continued in the intestinal canal.

CCCV. Imperfect digestion often takes place during the emollient treatment of partial chronic gastritis; but the sympathies resulting from this cause must not be attributed to the inflammation. In this case the treatment pointed out in proposition CCXCVIII must be pursued.

CCCVI. The digestion of unstimulating food becomes imperfect, during the treatment of general chronic gastritis, about the period when a cure has commenced.

CCCVII. He who does not know to manage irritability of the stomach will never know how to treat any disease. A knowledge of gastritis and gastro-enteritis is then the key of all pathology.

CCCVIII. When pulmonary inflammation resists the antiphlogistic treatment and blisters, it may still be efficiently overcome by cautery, setons, and moxas applied as nearly as possible to the seat of the disease. This will not always apply to inflammation of the digestive mucous membranes.

CCCIX. Acute hepatitis, at its commencement, must be subdued by means of local bleeding which acts at the same time upon the gastro-enteritis which almost always accompanies it. This complication renders emetics more dangerous than useful.

CCCX. Chronic hepatitis is sometimes palliated by emetics, purgatives, calomel, and saponaceous medicines; but it is rarely cured otherwise than by perseverance in a mild regimen, and by revulsives and issues placed near the affected organ.

CCCXI. Jaundice, unattended by fever, even that of newborn infants, being most generally the effect of gastro-duodenitis is more efficiently combated by the remedies adapted to this phlegmasia than by purgatives and pretended solvents; and much more so when it is accompanied with fever, and depends upon hepatitis.

CCCXII. Peritonitis is easily subdued at its commencement, by leeches applied to the abdominal parietes; but when it has contin-

ued for several days, it is frequently beyond the reach of any treatment. General bleeding seldom effects a cure.

CCCXIII. Puerperal peritonitis being ordinarily the effect of inflammation of the uterus must be arrested, at its very onset, by
leeches applied in large numbers over the hypogastrium ; it does
not yield to emetics except by revulsion, that is to say, it is often
aggravated by their use.

CCCXIV. The warm bath does not effect a cure of peritonitis
except by a revulsion on the skin, and if this revulsion fails, the
disease is rendered worse. The bath also frequently causes a return of peritonitis which has been subdued by leeches. This is not
the case with emollient fomentations.

CCCXV. The warm bath often aggravates acute gastro-enteritis, because the stimulation of the skin is ordinarily extended to
the internal parts and the primæ viæ. Cold applications to the abdomen, and even the cold bath is more useful when the lungs are
not inflamed. These means sometimes obviate the necessity of
recurring to repeated bleedings.

CCCXVI. When inflammation attacks the mucous membranes
of the lungs and of the gastric canal at the same time, cold may be
applied to the abdomen after venesection, provided a warm cata-
plasm is also laid upon the thorax ; but if the cough increases, the
cold must be withdrawn.

CCCXVII. Typhus being a gastro-enteritis produced by a miasmatic poison, that is by putrid gases, and frequently complicated
with some other phlegmasia especially of the encephalic cavity,
may be arrested by the treatment appropriate to these affections,
provided it be employed at the onset of the disease.

CCCXVIII. When the inflammation of typhus is not attacked at
its commencement, bloodletting is frequently attended with danger ; because the putrid gaseous poison enfeebles the vital power
and the living chemistry, to such a degree that the loss cannot be
repaired.

CCCXIX. The excessive exaltation of the phenomena of life
is the most powerful cause of their diminution, and heat is the most
proper agent to induce this exaltation : It is for this reason that the
typhus of warm climates, where the putrid gases are also more
poisonous, is more dangerous than all others, and proves fatal to
the robust more readily than to the weak. It is right to conclude
that cold is more efficacious than repeated bleeding in this disease ;

but it must be employed at its very commencement, as soon as possible after bloodletting, and internally as well as externally.

CCCXX. The slightest stimulation increases very much the intense violence of the typhus of the tropics, when it is employed in the first stage. Emetics are then very dangerous; for instance in yellow fever.

CCCXXI. As acute inflammation is more rapid in its course when lighted up in a tissue already affected with chronic inflammation, the most efficacious means of diminishing the ravages of yellow fever, is to obviate the development of chronic gastro-enteritis, which is the frequent prelude to the acute, and to induce acclimation.

CCCXXII. Acclimation in hot climates is procured by general bleeding, by considerable abstinence from food, and by repose; but excess in vegetable diet and refrigerant drinks must be avoided, as they cause indigestion, which induces an irritation that becomes the source of the very gastro-enteritis that is so redoubtable.

CCCXXIII. Heavy meals are dangerous to new comers in hot climates; because they require too prolonged an action of the stomach, and induce too abundant sanguification. Abuse in spirituous liquors also offers much danger; these two excesses retard acelimation, and facilitate the action of miasmatic poisons.

CCCXXIV. The use of aromatic drinks, rendered stimulating by the addition of alcohol, and likewise acidulated, will supply the loss of fluids, induced by excessive perspiration in hot climates, in northern subjects; but if the quantity of solid food be sufficiently reduced, thirst and perspiration will become considerably less.

CCCXXV. Concentrated stimulants are always injurious to the inhabitants of northern climates who emigrate to the tropics, at least until they are acclimated.

CCCXXVI. When debility succeeds to over-irritation in yellow fever, the principal remedies are to be found in acidulated drinks and enemata, and in cold applied to the external parts of the body, provided the heat of the skin is considerable.

CCCXXVII. When acute gastro-enteritis, whether typhoid, or not, resists local bleeding practised over the epigastrium, and afterwards over the chest and skull, if the inflammation has extended itself to these cavities, and when livor, stupor, and enfeebled pulse are present, we must nourish the patient with gummy, sweetened and acidulated drinks; but if the mouth becomes clean and appetite is manifested, nourishment must be supplied by milk and

water, and afterwards by very light broths ; otherwise the patient may die of inanition before the termination of the phlegmasia.

CCCXXVIII. The nausea and vomiting which accompany the
invasion of acute gastro-enteritis, do not indicate the employment
of emetics, but of leeches tô the epigastrium, and of emollient
and pretty warm fomentations to the lower extremities.

CCCXXIX. Constipation is favourable in acute gastro-enteritis,
because it denotes that the colon does not participate in the inflammation. It indicates the employment of no other remedy than an
emollient enema daily ; if it continues for some time, and if the
heat is considerable, this enema must be administered cold.

CCCXXX. The diarrhœa of acute gastro-enterito-colitis is removed, at first, by leeches applied to the anus in numbers proportioned to the strength of the patient. But if the prostration is great,
and the sanguineous apparatus little supplied, we must rest contented with giving gummy rice water, and enemata composed of a solution of starch with some drops of the watery solution of opium.

CCCXXXI. Should an excessive discharge from leech-bites induce great debility in the commencement of an acute gastro-enteritis, care must be taken not to restore the strength by stimulants ;
the patient must be let alone, provided the circulation is not interrupted, because it is ordinarily followed by a prompt cure, and an
extremely rapid convalescence. Should the syncope and asphyxia
persist, we must administer some spoonsful of wine and water, and
as soon as the circulation is re-established.

CCCXXXII. When the flow of blood from leech-bites continues
notwithstanding the occurrence of syncope and asphyxia it must
be arrested, especially in young infants who are the most exposed
to death from hemorrhage, and therefore require particular watching.

CCCXXXIII. Local bloodletting, abstinence, and watery drinks,
always break up incipient phlegmasiæ, so long as the inflammation
has not extended itself far among the viscera ; but if several organs are inflamed at the same time and to a great extent, which is
evinced by excessive anxiety, prostration, and very frequent pulse,
all the blood might be withdrawn before the disease would be arrested. In this case, the frequency of the pulse continues notwithstanding copious bleedings. We must, then, spare this fluid
and rest satisfied with nourishing the patient with watery drinks,
to which may be added gum and milk as soon as the sordes and
dark colour are removed.

CCCXXXIV. Meteorism commencing in gastro-enteritis is dissi-pated by one application of leeches to the abdomen; it is also re-lieved by that of ice; if not removed, or stimulants be given, it may be converted into peritonitis.

CCCXXXV. Subsultus tendinum and delirium supervening upon acute gastro-enteritis are signs of an extension of the irritation to the brain, and are removed, at their onset, by the application of leeches to the abdomen; but if these symptoms have continued for some time they must then be attacked by leeches to the tem-ples, or better still to the course of the jugulars, because the sym-pathetic irritation of the brain has already assumed the form of in-flammation.

CCCXXXVI. When appetite manifests itself with energy in gastro-enteritis, the patient having recovered from his stupor, broths should be allowed, notwithstanding the continued frequency of pulse, the acrid heat and the red tongue; otherwise the hunger would render the gastro-enteritis more intense, and bring back the stupor, the dark livor and the prostration; but more substantial ali-ments would be hurtful.

CCCXXXVII. When, during convalescence from acute gastro-enteris, there arise pain of the head, foul breath, nausea, uneasi-ness, and frequency of pulse, it is from the patients having eaten too much. In this case it is necessary to restrict, for one day, the use of nourishment, instead of administering emetics and purga-tives. The convalescent will, on the next day, be better.

CCCXXXVIII. When, during the course of a gastro-enteritis, there arises a difficulty of passing water, it is owing to the irrita-tion having extended itself to the bladder. A prompt application of leeches to the hypogastrium will remove this additional affection and obviate a great number of symptoms.

CCCXXXIX When inflammation of the parotid gland super-venes upon gastro-enteritis, it must be removed, or at least check-ed in its course by leeches, if the patient be not too anemic; oth-erwise this external phlegmasia, would rekindle the internal, or produce a fatal congestion in the brain.

CCCXL. Epistaxis, occurring in gastro-enteritis, is favourable, provided the pulse lessens in its frequency. If the flow of blood should be excessive, it is overcome by a blister applied to the back of the neck or between the shoulders.

CCCXLI. If hemoptysis occurs during acute gastro-enteritis, notwithstanding the use of bleeding, it indicates the necessity of a blister applied to the top of the sternum.   Intestinal hemorrhagies require a blister to the abdomen, and mucilaginous drinks, or rice water with the addition of sulphuric acid, because these hemorrhagies produce a loss of blood in the viscera which obviates the injurious effects of blisters.

CCCXLII. Phthisis pulmonalis may be prevented by removing as early as possible, by antiphlogistic means and by revulsion, all irritation in the respiratory organs.

CCCXLIII. Hypochondriasis is cured, and scirrhus of the digestive canal prevented, and even phthisis obviated, by the same means which overcome chronic gastritis.   Muscular exercise and moral diversion exert, in this case, a most powerful influence.

CCCXLIV. Congestions of the liver are cured and prevented by the means adapted to the treatment of chronic gastro-enteritis.

CCCXLV. Chronic gastritis is cured by means of a light diet, and especially by refrigerating drinks administered in small doses, from the first hour after the introduction of food until the next repast, or the hour of sleep.

CCCXLVI. Unless it occurs in robust subjects, chronic gastro-enteritis is not to be treated by repeated local bloodletting, and entire abstinence; because this treatment would in feeble subjects, induce a debility that would require years for its removal, during which time the predisposition to disease is extremely great, and relapses very frequent.   Perseverance in a mild regimen and in the use of watery drinks during digestion, always answers for these patients and effects their cure, provided the viscera are not disorganized.   They should always be apprised of the length of time necessary for their radical restoration to health.

CCCXLVII. Riding is dangerous in chronic gastritis attended by a considerable increase of gastric sensibility.

CCCXLVIII. The atmosphere of large cities is injurious to persons labouring under chronic gastro-enteritis; that of the country is beneficial, especially if they employ exercise; because these agents shorten the period of digestion, the slowness of which always keeps up the irritability of the stomach.

CCCXLIX. Emetics, purgatives, and tonics employed in gastritis and chronic gastro-enteritis effect palliative cures only, and render the radical cure more difficult.

CCCL. Mineral waters, whatever be their composition and temperature, do not cure chronic gastritis except by the revulsive evacuations they produce, but then it is always after having aggravated it; these cures, accordingly, are seldom radical, and after having undergone them for several consecutive years, the patients generally remain incurable.

CCCLI. Chronic congestions of the liver, spleen, or mesentery being, almost always, the effects of chronic gastro-enteritis, cannot be completely removed except by the treatment proper for this affection.

CCCLII. Those medicines and mineral waters which procure an evacuation of bile, of mucus, of urine, or which produce perspiration, hemorrhage, and cutaneous inflammation, diminish, for the moment, by this revulsion, the congestion of the liver and spleen so long as the gastric irritation is not very great; but they seldom effect a decided cure. This is only obtained by a long perseverance in the regimen proper for chronic gastro-enteritis.

CCCLIII. Mucous congestions of the lungs, or chronic catarrh attended by difficult expectoration of bronchial mucosity, are palliated by the expectorants and incisives of authors; they are only cured by antiphlogistic means, by the influence of heat, and by revulsion.

CCCLIV. If we are desirous of preventing scirrhus of the neck of the uterus to which females who have laboured under dysmenorrhœa are subject at the turn of life, we must allay the irritability of the organ long before this period takes place.

CCCLV. The abuse of venereal indulgences, and the violence which the uterus suffers in consequence, being frequent cause of uterine cancer, we must limit ourselves to allay the chronic inflammations which are their effects, in order to prevent the development of this cancer.

CCCLVI. Calculus in the kidneys and gravel do not require a long time for their formation. They are best prevented by applying leeches over the region of the kidneys and administering emollient drinks as soon as the first symptoms of nephritis manifest themselves, and the very habitual permanence of this disease may be entirely removed.

CCCLVII. Powerful diuretics, such as the saponaceous, the alkaline, uva ursi, turpentine, &c. procure the expulsion of calculi already formed, but they often keep up the latent phlegmasia which led to their formation.

CCCLVIII. Recent catarrh of the bladder yields easily to local bleeding, to cooling drinks, to abstinence, and to the restoration of any external irritations which may have disappeared; but if it has

78

become chronic, it is frequently incurable, and diuretics only palliate it. The means which procure most relief in this last case
are almost always to be found among antiphlogistic measures.

CCCLIX. Madness never exists without some degree of cerebral irritation, accompanied with and always dependant on chronic
gastritis, and these affections must be treated by local bleeding,
by antiphlogistic measures, and by revulsion. If abandoned to nature the patients,become liable to epilepsy, paralysis, and apoplexy,
which are the sequelæ of inflammatory disorganization of the brain.
They are also exposed to organic alterations in the abdomen which
are always the terminations of neglected gastritis.

CCCLX. Phthisis pulmonalis, peritonitis, rheumatism and gout
are only incidental to mania; not so the inflammations of the mucous membranes of the abdomen and the congestions of the viscera
of this cavity. It may hence be inferred what is necessary to obviate and remove these incidental affections.

CCCLXI. The principal differences to be established between
'cases of mental alienation must not be drawn from the character
of the delirium, but only from the degree of organic irritation of
the brain and gastric organs. The most inflammatory are the most
severe; the others take their rank under these according to the intensity of the inflammation and also according to their duration
and the probable chances of their inducing disorganization; hence
are derived the indications of the physical treatment; but the nature of the delirium must guide our choice in the employment of
moral remedies.

CCCLXII. Laryngeal and tracheal phthisis are ever the effects
of a local phlegmasia, which has not been arrested at its onset,
and they do not become fatal unless they induce pneumonia or gastro-enteritis; this misfortune may be obviated, then, by early subduing the inflammation of the trachea, or it may be retarded when
far advanced, by counteracting that of the lungs or digestive organs.

CCCLXIII. Hypertrophy of the heart, if not congenital, being
often the effect of a latent inflammation of this organ, may be prevented by general and local bloodletting, by digitalis, and by revulsion practised upon the seat of any external irritation that may
have been displaced; these means must, however, be employed as
soon as the pulsations of the heart acquire extraordinary violence.
Antispasmodics are, then, but impotent palliatives.

CCCLXIV. Digitalis does not produce an abatement of the action

of the heart, unless administered to a stomach unaffected by inflammation, and in a system of which the principal viscera are also
thus exempt ; otherwise it accelerates the contractions of the heart,
by adding fuel to the phlogosis.

CCCLXV. Digitalis weakens the contractile power of the locomotive muscles. It may, then, be rendered useful in convulsions, provided there is no inflammation present in the. viscera ;
but in no case is it prudent to administer large doses, or to continue its use long.

CCCLXVI. Spontaneous hemorrhage must be attacked, like inflammation, by general and local bloodletting, by refrigerants, and,
above all, by revulsion, whatever be the strength of the patient :
this last means is our best resource when there is considerable
weakness.

CCCLXVII. Spontaneous hemorrhagy being often kept up by inflammation, either local, or distant, the attention of the physician
must always be directed to this cause.

CCCLXVIII. Spontaneous hemorrhagies often coexist with hypertrophy of the heart. Digitalis may, then, be useful, provided the
condition of the stomach permits its employment.

CCCLXIX. Spontaneous hemorrhagy very often succeeds inflammation, or takes on its character in the same locality. That
of the lungs should therefore be combated by the antiphlogistic
and revulsive treatment, unrestricted by the fear of pre-existing tubercles.

CCCLXX. Mineral waters actively irritate the heart and sanguineous system generally, increase the hemorrhagic diathesis, induce it even where there is no predisposition to it, and often give
rise to aneurism, paralysis, and apoplexy.

CCCLXXI. Spasms and convulsions of all kinds being always
the effect of a local irritation, fixed or wandering, yield to the
treatment of this irritation, in other words to antiphlogistic means,
and to revulsions sometimes provided the irritated organ is not dis-
organised.

CCCLXXII. Antispasmodics* never cure convulsive diseases,
unless the stomach bears them without being over excited, and
the focus of irritation, from which these affections arise, has not at-

---

* The reader must bear in mind that by antispasmodics I designate
stimulating medicines, according to the acceptation of the vulgar; and
not mild, soothing remedies, which are most generally the best antispasmodics.

tained the height of inflammation. Hence they often prove inju-
rions in hypochondriasis and hysteria.

CCCLXXIII. Antispasmodics may suspend nervous symptoms,
notwithstanding the inflammation of the tissue from which these
symptoms proceed ; but the disease is thereby exasperated, and a
cure is to be obtained only by means of antiphlogistics and revulsion.

Exercise of the muscles of locomotion is the most effectual
means of destroying a convulsive diathesis for it displaces the visceral irritations, exhausts the superabundant activity, and diverts
the vital powers to the functions of nutrition, and to the exhaling
and secretory tissues.

CCCLXXIV. Abstinence from all spirituous liquors is essential
to the cure of spasmodic and convulsive phenomena.

CCCLXXV. Scurvy unattended with inflammation readily yields
to wholesome food, either vegetable or animal, provided its effect
be promoted by a pure and dry atmosphere, by light, and by exciting the agreeable passions, and here active stimulants may accelerate the cure ; but if it be complicated with the phlegmasiæ, then
gelatine, albumen, milk, and all substances containing mucus and
saccharine principles must be given without any stimulants. Acrid
antiscorbutics, bitters, and alcoholic drinks are eminently injurious.

CCCLXXVI. Since the affection of the gums which sometimes
accompanies scurvy is an inflammation, it must be treated first by
antiphlogistics, and, at a later period of the disease, by gently irritating topical remedies, but it is indispensable to remove the tartar
of the teeth. This is also the case with inflammation of the gums
unattended with a scorbutic diathesis ; these latter are more common than scorbutic affections.

CCCLXXVII. There are five ordinary modes of treating intermittent and remittent inflammations, 1st by antiphlogistics during
the hot stage ; 2nd by stimulants and tonics given during the apyrexia ; 3rd by stimulants given during the hot stage ; 4th by stimulants on the invasion of the cold stage ; 5th by antiphlogistics during the apyrexia.

CCCLXXVIII. Intermittent inflammations give way to bleedings and cold applied during the hot stage in the spring of the year,
when the subject is robust and plethoric, and the disease recent ;
in these cases, leeches must be placed as near as possible to the
main point of irritation.

CCCLXXIX. Intermittent inflammations are safely removed by

bark and other tonics administered during the apyrexia, if there be no plethora, and if the principal viscera, and especially the organs of digestion exhibit not the least trace of inflammation after the excitement ; that is if the fever is not remittent.

CCCLXXX. Intermittent irritations are seldom cured by stimulants given during the period of excitement ; this method rather tends to make the inflammation continued or remittent.

CCCLXXXI. Intermittent irritations are seldom cured by stimulants administered on the invasion of the chills, because the irritation they produce increases the intensity of the hot stage. This method seldom succeeds excepting after the use of antiphlogistics, and in robust subjects in whom the apyrexia is complete.

CCCLXXXII. Inflammations accompanied with periodical exasperations are cured by antiphlogistics, administered during the remission, if some degree of inflammation still remains in the viscera after the sweating stage, and especially if that inflammation is sufficiently intense to keep up some degree of pyrexia, I mean, if the fever is truly remittent.

CCCLXXXIII. The best and surest mode of curing inflammations attended with periodical exacerbations consists in administering antiphlogistics during the excitement so as to render the apyrexia complete ; if this effect be not produced, the same treatment must be continued after the paroxysms. If apyrexia is induced, bark and tonics are to be given, as well as diffusible stimulants at the commencement of the chill. But we must recur to cooling drinks, when excitement is again developed.

CCCLXXXIV. Bark and stimulants administered while any inflammation remains in the alimentary canal induce the phlegmasia with the acute and continued form or maintain it in a chronic form owing to its having cut short the paroxysms ; then irritation and congestion are developed in the parenchymatous viscera. It is in this manner that bark produces *obstructions*.

CCCLXXXV. Intermittent inflammations will spontaneously disappear when they are slight, and their exciting causes cease to operate ; under other circumstances, they assume an acute or chronic continuity which is finally attended by obstructions and dropsy.

CCCLXXXVI. Obstructions of the parenchymatous viscera (the liver, spleen, lungs) sometimes accompany intermittent fevers although the inflammation of the gastric mucous membrane is not continued ; they are then cured by bark administered during the apyrexia.

CCCLXXXVII. When bark arrests the paroxysms of intermittent fever, and there supervene uneasiness, visceral engorgements, loss of appetite and slow fever, they are owing to the development of a chronic gastro-enteritis induced by the too early administration of the medicines. In this case a cure is obtained by antiphlogistic measures.

CCCLXXXVIII. When the suppression of the paroxysms of intermittent fever is followed by a diseased condition unattended by fever, the recurrence of the paroxysms excited by the cold bath and by purgatives is favourable, provided the critical termination of the paroxysms is accompanied by the removal of the gastric irritation, so that the apyrexia is complete ; otherwise such recurrence is bad. In the former case bark must be given during the apyrexia ; in the latter antiphlogistics must be employed, which will cure the disease, and render the apyrexia complete, so that the bark may be given.

CCCLXXXIX. If the stomach cannot retain bark in intermittent fever it must be administered by means of enemata ; but if the large intestines are inflamed, it can only be externally employed, either as a local application or by means of friction in the form of the alcoholic tincture. In this case, emollients must be simultaneously given internally. Rubefacients are also proper during the apyrexia.

CCCXC. Intermittent fevers, termed pernicious, must be treated in the same manner as those to which this epithet is not applied, excepting only that more promptitude is to be observed.

CCCXCI. Dropsy sometimes occurs during the early paroxysms of intermittent fevers ; but it is more generally the result of their long continuance.

CCCXCII. Dropsy produced by obstructions to the circulation yields to bleeding and mild diuretics, unless the cause of the obstruction is incurable ; digitalis is useful, if this cause depend on hypertrophy of the heart.

CCCXCIII. Dropsy induced by the sympathetic influence of a chronic phlegmasia is rarely curable, because it is rarely so induced excepting the organ which is the seat of the phlegmasia is already disorganized. The treatment is composed of that proper for the phlegmasia, and of diuretics administered so as to spare the gastric organs.

CCCXCIV. Dropsy, which depends on an accidental aberration

of the serous fluids, that is, on a cessation of action in the depuratory capillary vessels, yields on the restoration of healthy transpiration and of the flow of urine. Hot and dry vapours applied to the
skin, dry and stimulating baths, (as hot sand, &c.) diuretics and
even purgatives will effect a cure; care must be taken, however,
to reduce the plethora, and not aggravate any co-existent phlegmasia.

CCCXCV. Dropsies which depend upon an imperfect digestion
yield to tonics, a warm, dry, and well lighted atmosphere, wholesome nourishment, and to the remedies for scurvy, if this last affection co-exist. But those which originate from an abuse of mercury
or other mineral substances, are frequently obstinate on account of
the gastro-enteritis which accompanies them, and which often assists in their development.

CCCXCVI. Dropsies arising from starvation, from excessive
losses of blood, or other causes of exhaustion, are cured by tonics,
wholesome nourishment, wine, alcohol, and active diuretics, provided there exist no point of disorganization in the viscera; great
care must, however, be taken to restore the strength by degrees.

CCCXCVII. Scrofula, which makes its first attack, under what
ever form, on the external surface may be removed by leeches boldly applied. In this manner the formation of a strumous diathesis,
which is merely the extension of the irritation from one to another
similar tissue, may be prevented.

CCCXCVIII. The scrofulous habit (which always developes itself externally) if not inveterate, is overcome by a dry, warm, well
lighted atmosphere, in other words, by those conditions of this fluid
opposite to those that produce the disease. It also yields to exercise in the open air.

CCCXCIX. Stimulants administered internally do not overcome
the scrofulous diathesis except by exciting the depuratory organs,
that is by revulsion; if they do not effect this, they exasperate the
scrofulous irritation as they do all others.

CD. If stimulants, internally administered, do not produce revulsion, they give rise to gastro-enteritis so as to complicate it with
the external scrofulous irritations; [this is the tabes mesenterica
of authors; and if the lungs become irritated, then a scrofulous
phthisis is the consequence.

CDI. The inveterate scrofulous diathesis confined to the external parts of the body is gradually removed by exercise in the open
air, by temperance and healthy nourishment, provided these stimu-

lating means are so employed as not to occasion visceral inflammation.

CDII. In the same disease diaphoretics are proper, provided a sufficient quantity of exercise is employed, and the irritation is not determined to the interior by excessive stimulation.

CDIII. Malacosteon is an irritation of the osseous system, depending on the same causes as scrofula, and cured by the same means.

CDIV. Chronic pneumonia (phthisis) occurs less frequently than chronic gastro-enteritis (tabes mes :) in scrofulous habits and rickety infants ; because the lungs are in these subjects, less disposed to inflammation than the digestive organs ; this predisposition is not, then, to be encouraged.

CDV. Syphilis is an irritation, which, like scrofula, affects the external parts, and its extension throughout the system is prevented by attacking it at its very commencement, with local antiphlogistic means, and, above all with numerous leeches.

CDVI. Syphilitic irritation, even when inveterate, will yield to antiphlogistic measures and to abstinence ; but as this method is troublesome and slow, mercury and sudorifics are preferred.

CDVII. Mercury, sudorifics, and other stimulants do not cure syphilis except they effect a revulsion in the depuratory capillaries, and then they must be assisted by abstinence ; because too great plethora keeps up the syphilitic irritation.

CDVIII. Those stimulants which are termed antisyphilitic must be administered internally with great caution, or they will give rise to gastro-enteritis, which, reacting on the external syphilitic irritation, prevents revulsion, or maintains the irritation in the viscera and produces their disorganization.

CDIX. If antisyphilitic stimulants give rise to gastro-enteritis, before the syphilis has been cured, it can only yield together with this to a long continued antiphlogistic treatment ; but if the gastric viscera are disorganized, or the patient too much enfeebled, then a cure is impossible.

CDX. Gastric phlegmasiæ, cured by the abuse of antisyphilitic remedies are easily extended to the lungs, and phthisis is the consequence, if the antiphlogistic treatment be not promptly and energetically pursued.

CDXI. Mercurial stimulants, applied locally to external syphilitic irritations always render them worse if they are severe ; but if they are moderate, they may succeed, by opposing one irritation to another. This applies to all external phlegmasiæ, and also to hemorrhagies.

CDXII. Predisposition to syphilis is the same as that to scrofula; thus patients affected by it are more difficult of management.

CDXIII. Patients predisposed to gastritis must be treated, when attacked by syphilis, with antiphlogistic remedies, both externally and internally ; if the stomach is stimulated, and over-excited, the venereal is not cured.

CDXIV. Cutaneous irritations, such as herpes, must be treated by local bleedings, emollients externally applied, and refrigerants internally administered, so long as the skin is inflamed ; when a sub-inflammatory condition alone remains, stimulants may be applied to the skin, especially preparations of sulphur, and revulsion may be attempted by means of sudorifics, diuretics and purgatives ; but the internal stimulation must not be carried so far as to induce gastro-enteritis, because this affection will cause a recurrence of the herpes, or at least produce a disorganization of the digestive organs. This is what is termed herpes introversa. All this will apply to the Grecian or tuberculous leprosy.

CDXV. In the cure of phlegmasiæ, subinflammations, ulcerations, in a word, of all irritations occurring in the external parts of the body, effected by means of astringents, narcotics, rubefacients, caustics ; in erythemata, ophthalmies, blenorrhagies, itch, herpes, scrofula, syphilis, &c. ; in all these cases we can only recognise morbid irritations, which yield to new irritations induced by the treatment. But these cures obtain only when the diseases are not intense. If they are so, they are aggravated by these means, and disorganization may be the consequence. In this manner are developed phagedænic and cancerous ulcerations. The treatment of one irritation by another must therefore be always preceded by antiphlogistic measures ; otherwise a perfect game of hazard (double or quitts) is played.

CDXVI. When an external irritation treated by stimulants is intense, long continued and attended with a copious discharge of fluid, or when it is aggravated without changing its seat, or is supplanted by an increased action of the secreting depurating vessels, *we should recollect that* these two last conditions are cases of revulsion of which one is favourable, the other injurious.

CDXVII. The cure of intense inflammations, such as puerperal or simple peritonitis, acute rheumatism, pneumonia, &c. by tartarized antimony, by calomel, by mercurial frictions, by opium, by

79

oil of turpentine, or by drastics, is not a direct sedative effect ; it results from the development of a great number of organic sympathies, which cause a revulsion; this is not effected unless critical
evacuations take place, and if the stimulant remedy has not been
sufficiently powerful to produce these, or if the morbid irritation is
too intense to be removed, the disease is aggravated, and acute or
chronic disorganization is the consequence.   These plans of treatment should, therefore, be preceded by the antiphlogistic, and,
with even this precaution, great hazard is incurred.

CDXVIII. It seldom happens that the cure of acute morbid irritation, obtained by stimulant and active revulsives, is not followed
by chronic morbid irritation, or more especially by gastro-enteritis.
It is thus that hypochondriasis is often produced, because active
stimulation of the stomach accumulates sensibility in this organ and
gives force to the sympathies which connect it with other organs.
In these cases one disease is merely substituted for another.

CCXIX. The effects of poisoning by acrid vegetables, corrosive
minerals, concentrated acids, alkalis and cantharides, are gastro-
enteritis tending to ulceration unless this last be immediately produced by the eschar, formed by the first application of these
poisons.   Their treatment should be the same as that of ordinary
inflammations, but acids must be prohibited.

CDXX. The effect of narcotic poisons is gastro-enteritis unattended by corrosion at first, but followed by encephalic irritation
which produces congestion, inebriation, delirium, convulsions, &c.
It must be treated by acidulated drinks, and without bleeding so long
as the stupor is considerable ; but when it is removed, the inflammation which remains must be overcome by the same means, which
are proper for that produced by corrosive poisons, because it may
be productive of the same results.   Madness is a frequent sequela.

CDXXI. The poisonous effects of lead (colica pictonum) is gastro-enteritis differing in intensity.   In the least degree, unattended
by fever, it may be cured by the revulsion induced by emetics and
purgatives, in the same manner as ordinary inflammation of the
same kind : but this treatment often leaves behind it a chronic
phlegmasia of the digestive mucous membrane ; In the higher degree, accompanied with fever, these lead-colics must still be treated as similar degrees of the ordinary gastric inflammation.   It follows from all this that the antiphlogistic method is the only safe
one of treating these affections.

CDXXII. The poisonous effects of putrid meat, or fish, or of mushrooms when introduced into the stomach, are gastro-enteritis attended by cerebral congestion, and stupor, which are soon followed by general debility ; it must be treated by emesis induced by mild liquids, and by mild laxatives such as the mucous and sacharine and the neutral salts, provided the poison is still present in the primæ viæ ; afterwards by acidulated drinks, cnemata, and lotions, and by leeches applied to the epigastrium and neck, proceeding always with great circumspection and watching narrowly the effects. The antiphlogistic regimen must perfect the cure.

CDXXIII. Debility is, *most frequently*, the result of irritation, but *sometimes* constitutes the whole disease.

CDXXIV. A deficiency of respiration is the most powerful cause of debility ; it necessarily induces defective stimulation ; but it is sometimes preceded by irritation.

CDXXV. In spontaneous and excessive hemorrhagy, even if unaccompanied with inflammation, debility is always preceded by irritation ; it becomes, subsequently, the principal disease. In traumatic hemorrhagy, it does not depend on irritation, but furnishes in itself the principal indication.

CDXXVI. Palsy succeeding to cerebro-spinal affections is always the result of irritation ; it furnishes but partial or local indications.

CDXXVII. Palsy succeeding to great losses of non-sanguineous fluids always depends on irritation ; but it only furnishes partial indications.

CDXXVIII. Whatever degree of debility attends irritations, these last are alone to be attended to so long as they are sufficiently intense to be aggravated by food and stimulating medicines. As soon as this condition is reversed, then the debility offers indications which must be fulfilled in combination with those presented by the irritation ; and, finally, when this last has ceased altogether, then the debility becomes the prominent disease ; but the irritability of organs requires great management and prudence in the employment of stimulants.

CDXXIX. Convulsion and pain, whatever name they receive, leave after them a debility which furnishes the only indications; they are more often combined, because some irritation will remain in the organ, which has excited the convulsion and pain.

CDXXX. The debility which follows venereal excesses is almost

always accompanied with the irritation of one or more of the viscera.

CDXXXI. External cold, when excessive, produces a debility,
which is extended from the skin to the locomotive apparatus, as well
as to the vessels and nerves of the periphery, and from them to the
viscera, whence death may ensue ; debility constitutes, in these
cases, the principal disease. But if the cold is moderate, the powers of life excite, in the periphery or in the viscera, an irritation
which becomes the principal disease, and furnishes the only indications when the action of the cold hath ceased.

CDXXXII. Paralysis of the limbs depending on concussion is
the product of irritation ; if this last continues, it furnishes the
proper indications ; but if not manifest, then debility is the princi
pal disease.

CDXXXIII. There are some external agents, which extinguish
life without producing any appreciable reaction ; but such effects
are more rare than has been, for a long time, supposed.

CDXXXIV. Miasms arising from the decomposition of dead animal and vegetable matter, and from the emanations of diseased or
healthy animals confined in a too crowded spot, are sometimes sufficiently deleterious to produce debility, or even death without the
intervention of reaction ; but whenever they produce pain and fever, then an irritation is already established in the digestive mucous membrane, and frequently by sympathy, in other viscera, and
this last offers the principal indications. It is this which constitutes
typhus, and it is, then, produced by infection. (See the propositions
respecting the treatment of acute gastro-enteritis.)

CDXXXV. Every patient affected with typhus may become, in
himself, a focus of infection and communicate his disease to all
healthy persons, if he is confined in a small apartment, and if his
emanations stagnate around him ; this is febrile contagion ; but if
he be removed to a healthy, well aired and clean room, this communication will be difficult. Are the pestilential typhus and variola
the only diseases which are contagious, in spite of these precau.
tions ?

CDXXXVI. Delivery is sometimes followed by a debility which
progressively increases until death, and which furnishes the only
indication, although it is the product of irritation.

CDXXXVII. Syncope is the effect of an interruption to the cir.
culation of the blood towards the head ; it always indicates stimu.

lants; but after it has ceased, it presents opposite indications, if the cause of the interrupted circulation is an irritation.

CDXXXVIII. Asphyxia produced by the inhalation of deleterious gases is an abirritation; but when it is removed, an irritation always remains in the principal viscera.

CDXXXIX. The debility, induced by the depressing passions, such as terror, &c. always evinces the existence of an irritation in the principal viscera, which becomes the principal disease.

CDXL. The debility attending scurvy does not furnish the principal indications of treatment, unless unattended by any co-existent inflammation.

CDXLI. When the most violent gastro-enteritis is continued beyond a certain point, the debility occasioned by it presents indications requiring the administration of nourishment, lest the patient die from exhaustion, because there is a period in which digestion is practicable without causing any aggravation of the inflammation present.

CDXLII. Those who have, for a long time, been under the degree of fulness and strength which is consistent with their constitution, require a long time to be restored to this point. They cannot bear a certain quantity of blood without experiencing the injurious effects of plethora and the consequent predisposition to inflammation.

CDXLIII. The strength is lessened in diseases of irritation, because the overhurried organic movements cause decomposition and elimination to prevail over composition and absorption; certain bulimie gastrites should be excepted, in which the fulness and strength increase, notwithstanding the existence of irritation.

CDXLIV. The indication to restore the strength by an abundant nourishment, is derived neither from emaciation nor weakness, but solely from the rapidity with which assimilation takes place, and from the predominance of composition over decomposition.

CDXLV. The indication to excite the stomach by tonics is derived neither from feebleness, nor emaciation, but rather from the paleness and breadth of the tongue, as also from the feeling of languor and the slow digestion, when too stimulating food has been taken. It may be also drawn from pains of the stomach, the eructations, borborygmi, and colic which accompany this kind of digestion, if these symptoms disappear on administering food of a more irritating quality.

CDXLVI. General debility unattended with inflammation requires only good nourishment and a moderate dose of wine, provided the digestion is good. If this function is painfully performed bitters are necessary.

CDXLVII. Debility, attended with inflammation situated elsewhere than in the digestive canal requires light nourishment, and which produces little feculence, provided the inflammation is acute; but it proscribes the use of stimulants which might increase irritation in the inflamed organ; if the phlegmasia is chronic, the debility indicates substantial, but easily digested food. As to tonics, they are only proper occasionally and in small doses.

CDXLVIII. Debility attending upon catarrh, which exhausts by a too copious expectoration, and is unaccompanied with fever, requires nourishment which is substantial and easy of digestion, as also astringent tonics cautiously administered, such as bark, lichen, and acetate of lead. It also requires revulsives, but without prolonged suppuration.

CDXLIX. Debility accompanying acute gastric inflammation requires the same treatment as this last affection; but if complicated with chronic gastritis it requires farinaceous nourishment, and even milk and white meats, also careful attention to lessen the heat of the stomach by small quantities of bland drinks, whenever it undergoes the process of digestion.

CDL. Debility attending upon acute colitis requires no other treatment than that necessary for this last affection; but if upon chronic it indicates the employment of farinaceous nourishment divested of whatever materials will leave feculence in the colon, and likewise the moderate use of red wine to enable the stomach to retain its contents; because the irritated colon attracts them before they have undergone the process of digestion, and thus converts them into purgatives.

CDLI. Debility induced by excessive hemorrhage requires the employment of gelatinous, albuminous, and farinaceous nourishment together with a little red wine, astringents, and permanent stimulants; but it rejects high seasoned food and diffusible stimulants.

CCLII. Debility, induced by violent convulsions, and unattended with gastritis requires the same treatment as that caused by hemorrhage; but diffusible antispasmodics must also be employed.

CDLIII. The debility and exhaustion, which are produced by excessive muscular exercise, require food which is highly nutritions in a small volume, a moderate use of wine and even of alcohol, because the sensibility is considerably diminished in the nervous system of relation; but if the fatigue has likewise induced gastric irritation, the debility must then be treated by nutritious drinks which are not stimulating.

CDLIV. If debility predominates in gastro-enteritis induced by excessive muscular exercise, or by the abuse of stimulants too often had recourse to in this case, blood-letting must be very sparingly employed, and should always be practised locally.

CDLV. The extreme debility consequent upon long continued fasting, must be treated by very small quantities of farinaceous decoctions, milk porridge or light broths, which must be very slowly increased, because indigestion and gastritis are very easily induced.

CDLVI. Debility induced by cold is successively treated by the external application of snow, ice, cold and then lukewarm water, &c. and by the internal administration of diffusible stimuli, alcohol, and distilled liquors in graduated doses; but as soon as febrile heat is developed, recourse must be had to emollients, and even to bleedings; otherwise visceral phlegmasia may be developed.

CDLVII. Debility occasioned by deficient respiration is removed on the restoration of this function; hence there are several methods to be pursued according to the causes of the obstruction to the passage of the air. Thus bleeding is proper in pulmonary phlegmasiæ, in mechanical strangulation, in angina, aneurism, &c.; whilst stimulants, as well internal as external, are useful after drowning and in all cases of asphyxia, which require however, at the same time, the introduction into the lungs, of respirable air.

CDLVIII. When, at the very onset of an acute affection, there are present extreme debility and depression of spirits, we are to infer that the inflammation occupies a large space either in the respiratory, or in the digestive organs, or in both. Then, if one general or local bleeding, proportioned to the strength and to the intensity of the symptoms lessens the strength instead of raising it, it must not be repeated, because it is a proof that these viscera, the natural introductors of the preservative materials of life, have failed to perform their functions, and that the economy has, in consequence, no more means of repairing any abundant losses. Emollients internally, cold and revulsion externally, are the feeble resources of medicine in these unfortunate cases. (See the propositions on typhus and on gastro-enteritis.)

CDLIX. Cyanosis is sometimes produced by gastro-enteritis and is cured along with it.

SECT. V.

COROLLARIES.

CDLX. Empirical medicine, consisting in the recollection of symptoms already observed, and of remedies which have been beneficial or hurtful, without any attempt at physiological explanation, is impracticable ; because the injury of a single organ presents a crowd of symptoms, which, combined with those depending on other organs, and innumerably diversified, render it quite impossible to meet,'in nature, with groups of symptoms altogether similar to those which are assumed as models.   This confusion can only be remedied by referring symptoms to peculiar organs.

CDLXI. To practise medicine with success, it is not sufficient to refer symptoms to particular organs, but it is necessary to determine in what respect these organs differ from a state of health, in other words, to ascertain the nature of the disease.

CDLXII. The nature of the disease must alone furnish the physician with his curative indications.   It is ascertained by a knowledge, 1st of the agents which have excited, depressed, or deranged, somehow or other, the action of the organ primarily affected ; 2dly of the influence of this organ upon the other organs ; 3dly of the means by which an equilibrium may be re-established in the system, or the intensity of the disease be, at least, diminished.

CDLXIII. The groups of symptoms, which are pointed out as diseases, without being traced to the organs on which they depend, or even, if so traced, without ascertaining the character of the physiological deviations in these organs, are metaphysical abstractions which do not represent a constant and invariable morbid condition, of which the prototype is to be found in nature ; they are then factitious entities, and all those who study medicine by this method are *ontologists*.

CDLXIV. To consider imaginary morbid entities as evil doing powers which act upon the organs and modify them so as to develope this or that disorder, is to mistake effects for causes : it is to erect an ontology.

CDLXV. To consider a succession of symptoms once observed as the necessary and invariable march of a disease, and to deduce from it essential characters for diagnosis, and by consequence for its treatment, is to create an imaginary entity ; because organic affections differ in their appearances according to the agents which produce them ; it is, in short, rendering the treatment of the disease impossible until after its termination, except in contradiction to principle. This is still ontology.

CDLVI. To apply remedies to an imaginary morbid entity, without estimating their effects on the organs which receive their primary impression, as also upon those which sympathise with these, is to cure or aggravate a disease without knowing the rationale.

CDLXVII. He who cures a disease without first appreciating the physiological agency by means of which the cure has been effected, has no surety that he will recognise or cure the same disease when it shall present itself anew ; whence it necessarily results that neither the success nor reverses of ontologists avail to render them good practitioners, or to enable them to teach others to be such.

CDLXVIII. The seven last propositions will explain why medicine has remained uncertain and fluctuating until the present time.

80

NOTES.

NOTE A—PAGE 14.

Is there any fever truly *idiopathic*?

Such a question, proposed some fifty years since, would have convicted the rash inquirer of madness or folly. What! Fever—a disease so common that two thirds of mankind are supposed to perish by its instrumentality, and eight out of nine by its superaddition to other severe affections,—difficult indeed to be defined, but about which " mankind, whether professional or laical" are the least likely to be mistaken,—is its very existence, as a distinct disease, to be doubted and denied? Can scepticism reach so far as to impugn the records of centuries faithfully transcribed from the pages of nature by Hippocrates, by Sydenham, and by Boerhaave? Even so : Medical genius and learning, ambitious to inscribe its name on the tablets of an imperishable fame, had rested, hitherto, satisfied with framing successive hypotheses to explain the hidden nature of fever, or, in other words, to generalize, after the most ingenious methods, the accumulated facts, which had been faithfully, and cautiously, and patiently gleaned from observations made at the bedside of the sick. These hypotheses were, for a long time, ' few and far between ;'—Hippocrates governed the medical world for centuries, and Galen, in assuming the empire, only confirmed and extended the sway of his illustrious predecessor, and triumphantly maintained its supremacy for thirteen hundred years. Wrested partly from his grasp by the audacious, eccentric, and original Paracelsus, it was still divided between these two rulers, until both were finally hurled from the throne by the successful efforts of Stahl, Hoffman, and principally, of Boerhaave. Great as was the learning, profound the genius and sagacity, and apparently eclectic and consistent the theory of this last incomparable physician, his unbounded dominion was successfully usurped by his disciple Cullen. A similar fate awaited this elegant scholar and eloquent teacher whose pupil, Brown, gave the first shock to his power and finally, struck at its very root by his novel, simple and captivating views. And now the aspect of medical history underwent a change. No single individual appeared any longer, destined to hold absolute power over the medical world.—The sensorial theories of the poetical Darwin, the *convulsive vascular reaction* of RUSH (and indeed of Armstrong, and all the essentialists or *ontologists* of the present day) participated, with the vis medicatrix naturæ and spasm of Cullen and the excitability of Brown, in the divided rule. This multiplication of authorities naturally weakened the force, and lessened the influence of all, and an eclectic spirit was fast engendering in the profession, which threatened to demolish all exclusive systems, and to rest contented with a simple induction from facts, recommended by the example of Hippocrates, and enforced by the philosophy of Bacon. Genius was threatened in its pride of place, and extraordinary efforts were now called for, suited to the venturous spirit of the age. The Gordian knot had not been untied,—universal empire was the aim,—and it was cut. M. Broussais, possessed of an acute genius, versed in the lore of his profession, and trained to combat in the camp, is the bold adventurer, who aspires to mastery in medicine, and who, by this Alexander-like achievement hopes to effect the great design. Professing to have divested himself of the spirit of system, and to have communed with nature alone in the very depths of her mystery, he steps forth to inform the world, that her former interpreters were false prophets, and that they had either misunderstood or betrayed her. Their facts had been ill observed ; their conclusions were false and delusive ; and even their success in the practice of the healing art had been, in every age and in every clime, merely ideal,—it was all an imposition.* Fever, more especially, was a chimera, the offspring of ignorance, the fosterchild of antiquated prejudice. Here, then, is a glorious discovery, which will blot out all former impressions from the records of medicine, and leave a *tabula rasa* on which the great reformer's name shall pre-eminently appear as the *new* father of medicine.

* See the introduction to " L'examen des Doctrines Medicales." page 4
The disputed priority of M. Broussais' claim to his own views of fever is not here taken into the account, Baglivi, Rega, Rahn, Bordeu, and even Senac point out the stomach as the source of fever. But Broussais has the true claim to be considered the founder; he alone having condensed, analysed, and perfected the system.

What are the results of this discovery, of this successful communication with the *Egeria* of Medicine?

The first and most important conclusion to which the physiological school, or that of M. Broussais, has arrived, is that all disease consists in irritation, or abirritation, but specially in the former.

The *second* is, that irritation is invariably an exaltation of the vital forces.

The *third*, that irritation, when intense, constitutes inflammation.

The *fourth*, that fever considered in an abstract manner is always the result of irritation of the heart, in consequence of which this organ quickens its contractions.

The *fifth*, that irritation of the heart constituting fever is never primitive, but always the result of sympathy with the irritated gastro-enteric membrane.

These five points constitute, if I mistake not, the bases on which the Broussaian doctrine rests, and on their strength depends its durability.

The evidences in favour of these points, so far as they relate to fever, are the following :

1st. All the causes of fever act locally ;

2dly. In all fevers there are unequivocal symptoms of local irritation of the stomach and small intestines.

3dly. Post mortem examinations invariably prove the existence of gastro-enteritis in fever.

A formal discussion of these several views will not be expected in this place. As they have however been embodied in the present volume for the benefit of the medical student, it would seem appropriate to accompany them by a few desultory remarks, such as would most readily suggest themselves to the mind of a practical physician.

I. It will be perceived that M. Broussais maintains that disease consists in irritation principally, that irritation is always an exaltation of the vital forces, and that this action carried to a sufficient extent constitutes inflammation. Increase or diminution of action is alone regarded in this system, and identifies it thus far with that of Brown. *Altered* action, independently of excitement or depression of the vital powers, is not admitted. Irritation or exalted action constitutes inflammation, fever, syphilis, scrofula, gout, and even the gravel. A difference in its intensity and seat alone gives rise to these various expressions of disease. The question here arises how happens it that the same organ or part shall be affected

at different times with different expressions of disease, each equally severe, yet altogether dissimilar. Thus a joint shall at one
time be a prey to gout or rheumatism, at another to white swelling ; the kidney to simple inflammation now, and again to calculus &c. Is the action, in these different instances, the same, differing only in intensity of violence, that is, either simple iritation or
subinflammation, or inflammation ?

If this question be answered in the affirmative, then the conclusion is irresistible, that all diseases are only grades of the same
morbid condition, and should therefore present a certain uniformity
in their symptoms, in their post mortem appearances, and, not
least, in their indications of treatment. This they are far from doing, however, to the satisfaction of the clinical observer at least, not
overanxious to simplify doctrines, but desirous of rendering his
knowledge and experience subservient to the great object of ascertaining the characteristic features of disease, and discovering
the most appropriate and prompt means for its removal. He finds
that irritation, so far from being accompanied at all times with exalted action, is frequently productive of depression and even destruction. Many fevers might be adduced in proof, which leave
no traces of inflammation after death, and even the most corrosive
poisons, as arsenic, corrosive sublimate &c. frequently destroy life
without leaving any impressions of inflammation or even fluxion
upon the stomach. There is, in these instances, a depraved action, a disturbance of function independently of mere increase or
diminution. And the effects of different remedies go far to establish this point. Were disease to consist simply in excitement or
the reverse, two simple remedies would suffice for its cure ; the
one calculated to diminish, the other to restore action. In accordance with this required simplicity, the new doctrine almost expun-
ges the materia medica from the face of medical science, and places its chief reliance on those means only, which impart strength,
or debilitate. Whatever success may attend such a limited me-
dication at the Val de Grace, it is found inapplicable in this country. Many physicians, who have embraced the physiological doctrine in its broad outlines have nevertheless frankly told me, that
they are still compelled to use the old fashioned remedies, calomel, antimony, &c. notwithstanding their misgiving of the practice being empirical. Now the employment of these medicines,
and of all the immensely varied articles comprising the different
classes, can, in no manner, be explained except on the supposition,

that, in different diseases or in different stages of the same disease, the morbid action, whether sthenic or asthenic, changes its form and mode, and accordingly indicates a corresponding modification in the treatment. Neither does the simple intensity of irritation constitute inflammation, as is evinced in the neuralgiæ and many purely nervous disorders, as tetanus, &c.

It will likewise be perceived, that the fluids are entirely over-looked in the Broussaian theories. This omission can scarcely be defended in the present state of medical science. Undue importance was undoubtedly attached to their derangement in the humoral pathology, but the opposite extreme has been the equally great and no less injurious error of the solidists and the phlogotics. Abundant proofs exist of the depravement of the fluids in almost all diseases. M. Broussais himself tells us, in his 104th proposition, that inflammation always alters the fluids of the affected part. But he evidently considers this alteration a mere effect of this one disease, not adverting to it in any other view—as a cause of disease, or as constituting disease itself. Yet that it is often such does not admit of a doubt in the mind of any well informed physician not blindly wedded to exclusive hypotheses.

II. Fever is a local disease, because, 1st, its causes act locally, and, 2dly, its symptoms and post mortem appearances give evideuces of local inflammation, i. e. of gastro-enteritis.

That some of the causes of fever act locally or upon a single organ in the first instance, there cannot be a doubt ; such are the ictus solis, cold applied to the surface, indigestible food and intoxicating liquors, with many others which might be enumerated. But these do not excite fever unless in an individual, whose system has been predisposed for its reception by a remote cause, the operation of which is *general*. The other and the principal causes of fever, as marsh and animal miasmata, make their primary impression upon the whole nervous system. To reach the nerves they must indeed penetrate by some avenue ; the skin, the internal mucous membrane, or the lungs. But their action rests not in these organs, as maintained by the Localists. It pervades the whole nervous system of relation, and is, by sympathy, communicated to the heart and large bloodvessels. The object of the Localists is farther to demonstrate that the local action of these causes is exerted upon the stomach ; and marsh miasma is supposed to be swallowed with the food and thus to exert its direct action upon the gastro-enteric mucous membrane. This supposition, doubtful at best, is rendered very improbable by the following considerations.

First, morbid poisons, as they have been not very aptly termed, such as variolous matter, &c. are generally received into the stomach without exerting any deleterious effects, and it is scarcely to be supposed that so subtle an effluvium, as that which generates fever, and which has hitherto escaped the most delicate Eudiometrical tests would exert any influence upon that organ.

Secondly, why should this miasm, pervading the atmosphere, delay its specific operation, until it was formally introduced by the intervention of a meal into the digestive organs, when it is constantly in contact with the sensitive schneiderian membrane, with that lining the mouth and fauces, with the vastly extended surface of the pulmonary tissues, and, not least, with the skin. It is urged by one of the eloquent defenders of this system,* that these membranes are destined to specific purposes, the schneiderian has exclusive cognizance of odours, &c. If we admit this reasoning, we must infer that the mucous membrane of the stomach has no other function to fulfil than that of digesting febrific effluvia. But, contends the writer, the administration of food previously to entering the district infected by morbid effluvium, is a preventive against its effects. That it is invariably so, he does not, and cannot contend ; and, surely, its prophylactic agency, in any case, may be far more satisfactorily and philosophically explained by the general tone and vigour imparted by nourishment to the frame, enabling it to resist successfully the impressions of external agents. The debilitated and the irritable are always most susceptible of malarious diseases, and it is at night when the system is exhausted by the labours of the day and when the damp and chilly air exerts an unfriendly influence on the surface of the body, that these affections are most readily contracted.

Thirdly, the suddenness, with which the febrile, miasm frequently operates, would seem to favour the belief, that its impression is made simultaneously with that of the air inspired into the lungs, acting, perhaps, like the poisonous fumes which induce asphyxia.

These remarks are not intended to convey the idea that the digestive mucous membrane *may not* be, at times, the avenue through which the febrile miasm makes its inroad into the general system, but simply to point out the fact, and the probability, that it is not so exclusively.

* Chapman's Therapeutics, vol. 1, p. 116.

Let us next inquire whether the symptoms of fever are invariably indicative of local inflammation. No fact has been more
clearly established in the whole range of medical learning; no
position more incontestibly advanced, than that there is *no one*
symptom pathognomonic of fever, no one which is not occasionally
present, occasionally absent. All writers, whatever has been the
complexion of their theories, and how much soever they may have
differed in their peculiar views of the treatment, or causes of this
disease, admit that fever is proteiform, assuming the most discrepant and variegated characters. To assert then that symptoms of
gastric inflammation are always present, is at least a solecism in medical history. Were the epithet *local* substituted for gastric it would
at least not have been a novelty, as Erasistratus some two thousand years ago advanced the same idea; in other words, identifi-
ed fever with inflammation. The error of this view has long since
been pointed out. It is exceedingly simple and captivating in
speculation, but carried out into practice has been productive of
great and irreparable mischief.

To be consistent, it should inculcate the employment of the same
measures in fever as are proper in inflammation, and their more
or less bold employment in proportion to the violence of the disease. What says experience to such treatment?—In typhus gravior, in yellow fever, in dysentery, has active depletion, general
and local, been found advantageous to the almost unlimited and
universally acknowledged extent that it has in phrenitis, gastritis,
and enteritis?—No—far from it.—Yet if these latter affections are
identical with the former, why should their treatment be found so
different? Are the symptoms however similar? Let the history
and descriptions of the several diseases be carefully studied in the
writings of the most experienced and unbiassed physicians who
have contributed to the stock of professional knowledge by recording the result of their observations, and the answer will be clearly
in favour of the idiopathic character of fever.—But if it is contrary to recorded observation and tried experience to confound fever
with inflammation generally, how much more so with that of *one*
particular organ? The symptoms of fever are confessedly various
and multiform; those of local phlegmasia are well defined.

There obtain in fever almost invariably two states of the system,
which do not occur in local phlegmasia, unless it has become intense, or in other words become an exciting cause of fever. These
states are, a loss of balance in the circulation and in the nervous

81

excitement, as has been well shown by our illustrious Rush, and subsequently, by Armstrong, Johnson, and others.

Every practical observer will admit that these two states frequently occur without any demonstration of local inflammation. The mind will be confused or irritable, or indisposed to thought ; there will be wandering pains flying from part to part, general sense of soreness in the muscular system, oppressed breathing, quickened pulse, loss of appetite, interruption of *all* the secretions. Is this condition of the system induced by local disease ? If so, where shall we fix it ? All the important tissues and systems seem equally overpowered. The result is reaction, not local, but general ; and general treatment only, directed to every part of the frame, will overcome this reaction. Thus, rest and the removal of all stimulating impressions relieve the brain, abstinence the stomach, and the warm bath or affusions the surface, whilst emetics, purgatives, and diaphoretics restore the obstructed secretions, or invite the fluids from the large bloodvessels, and perhaps the spleen in which they have been stagnant, to the internal and external capillaries. This is frequently effected by nature herself, as in intermittent fever, and it is only where she is not competent to the task that the judicious physician interposes his artificial aids to accomplish the same object.

It may be asked then, whether inflammation is never present in fever ?—The prompt answer will be, that it often is, nay, that it frequently forms a very prominent feature of the disease. It must be regarded, however, as an incidental or contingent, not an essential, phenomenon. It will be developed in a phlogistic diathesis, or where any one organ is predisposed, by previous debility however induced, to assume the inflammatory action. This development does not, in indiopathic fever, take place until the stage of excitement has commenced. Then the blood, rushing with violence from the heart towards the outposts of the system, and meeting with the excitable organ, becomes arrested there, and inflammation is the consequence. Far different is the history of a pure, an undisguised phlegmasia. Here the local affection first makes its appearance, and the fever is only lighted up as a secondary and sympathetic affection. To present this subject in a clearer point of view it may be well to designate a few characteristic differences between idiopathic and symptomatic fevers,—differences, which can only be explained by the admission that the one are purely general, the other sympathetic of local diseases.

1. Idiopathic fevers owe their origin to causes which act gene-rally on the nervous and circulating systems, such are malaria, contagion &c.—

Symptomatic fevers to causes which act upon particular organs, such are cold, intemperance, study, the passions, &c.—

2. Idiopathic fevers commence without the previous develop-ment of any local affection ; such affections may indeed arise du-ring their course, but it is as a contingent casualty, and may occur in any part of the system indiscriminately, but does not invariably attack the same organ.

Symptomatic fevers are always preceded by a local irritation or phlegmasià, and never arise until this last has become intense.

3. Idiopathic fevers run a certain course. In some countries, as in Greece, &c. this course is very clearly defined, and hence the critical days of the ancients, of Cleghorn, of Jackson, &c. Local affections, arising during this course, exercise no influence upon it, although they may aggravate the general disease in some instan-ces, and mitigate its violence in others.

Symptomatic fevers are dependent for their duration and intensity on the local affection which gives them birth. With it they appear, by it they are modified, and its removal puts an end to their ex-istence.

4. Idiopathic fevers observe periodic movements, are intermit-tent, remittent, or continued.

Symptomatic fevers run an uninterrupted course, modified by the increase or diminution of the pabulum which sustains them.

This distinction has been attempted to be overruled by M. Broussais by the broad and gratuitous assertion that irritation and inflammation are intermittent, remittent, &c. This is a mere de-duction from his own premises, and cannot prove their validity.— Simple gastritis, pleurisy, and pneumonia, were never suspected to present quotidian, tertian, quartan, or septan exacerbations, until the rise of the physiological doctrines.

5. Idiopathic fevers require modified methods of treatment, ac-cording to the reigning character of the epidemic, the season of the year in which they occur, and the peculiar complications attending them, such as inflammation, congestion, nervous irritation, &c. Even the local affections which may be superadded to them require a similar modification of treatment.

Symptomatic Fevers invariably require the treatment adapted to the removal of the local affection to which they owe their development. Induced generally by visceral inflammation, they are uniformly relieved by bold antiphlogistic measures.

7. Idiopathic fevers present innumerably diversified appearances after death. To this circumstance are we indebted for the varying local hypotheses of the present day. Thus Marcus, having observed in his autopsic examinations different organs exhibiting the traces of inflammation, and identifying, in theory, this affection with fever, locates it indiscriminately in any of the viscera. Clutterbuck, living in a country where the intellectual habits of the people predispose the brain to assume inflammatory action in fever, restricts it to this organ ; while Broussais in France, a country of which the peculiar diet renders the digestive organs peculiarly susceptible of irritation, confines his view exclusively to this quarter. It has been well observed of these theorists that they are all right and all wrong, because fever does sometimes leave traces of inflammation in one, sometimes in another organ, according as it is complicated with the one or other of these incidental affections. It is essentially linked with none, as innumerable cases of dissection have abundantly proved. These may be found recorded by Pinel, Fodere, Jackson, Good, Armstrong, and a host of other writers. Therefore, says Dr. Good, "a single example of fever terminating fatally without a trace of inflammation in any organ whatever, and such examples are perpetually occurring, is sufficient to establish the existence of fever as an idiopathic malady, and to separate the febrile from the phlogistic divisions of diseases."

Symptomatic fevers, it is scarcely necessary to add, will generally exhibit post-mortem traces of the local disease with which they have been complicated.

If the observations which have now been made have any force, the last argument in favour of the local and gastric seat of fevers, derived from port mortem appearances, must fall to the ground. In addition to the remarks already made, it may not be improper to observe that an undue reliance has been placed, by many of the physicians of the present day, on pathological anatomy. Its importance and value in throwing light upon the hidden nature of many diseases can never be questioned. Yet it is somewhat singular, that the therapeutical management of those affections the nature of which has been chiefly illustrated by the labours of modern pathologists, was well known centuries ago. Thus the treatment of inflammation was well established long before the dissector's knife had designated its numerous and diversified shades ;

and so also that of small pox and measles was as successful in the days of Sydenham, as it has been since the recent discoveries. Of chronic and nervous diseases, pathology has not as yet demonstrated the nature, nor led to any useful improvement in the treatment. With respect to the influence this science has exerted upon the doctrine of fevers, it is impossible to speak in the most favourable terms. Dissections are only useful in so far as they illustrate symptoms or signs existing previously to death. This they cannot, however, do in all cases.

Death frequently takes place so suddenly, as in the invasion of fevers, that it is impossible to trace its cause in the corpse.

The constitution may be so debilitated, that no reaction takes place, and a simple venous congestion remains perceptible after death.

Death frequently takes place from simple exhaustion, after the irritation, if any have previously existed, has altogether subsided.

The redness perceptible on the surface of the mucous membrane after death, is frequently owing to a stasis of the blood in the capillaries occurring in *articulo mortis*.

This last appearance, even if the result of irritation, subinflammation, or inflammation, may be an *effect* of some incidental cause operating during the course of the disease—perhaps near its final termination.

The fluids may have been morbidly changed.

The considerations now adduced, I think, throw strong doubts upon the correctness of the Broussaian doctrine in so far as it applies to fevers. Of its general merits, its great ingenuity, its successful explanation of many hitherto obscure points in medicine, too much cannot be said in praise.—Its great defect consists in its undervaluing symptomatology, and elevating pathological anatomy to an importance warranted neither by its application to the diagnosis nor to the treatment of diseases.—After all, it is to an accurate knowledge of the symptoms and the signs of diseases that a physician must mainly depend for their successful removal or mitigation. Post mortem appearances should never be neglected, as they throw considerable light on the state of the system previous to death. But they should ever be regarded as a subsidiary, not a principal, or infallible means of detecting such a state.

To conclude: This note has been extended not with an idle view to combat speculative doctrines, but from a sincere desire to preserve the ancient landmarks by which alone a rational and successful method of treatment in fevers can be attained. No exclusive doctrine can accomplish this arduous and delicate task, whether it be local, humoral, nervous, chemical, or Stahlian. The proud distinction of physiological may be assumed with about equal pretensions by any one of these. It belongs rather to that system of theory and practice of physic, which regards the human body, whether in health or in disease, as a *whole* compounded of parts, not insulated in themselves, but linked together by innumerable though inexplicable affinities, the derangement of any one of which may lead to general disorder and confusion. Such a view alone can lead the cautious physician to success in treating the endlessly varied forms of fever. So many foreign modifiers exercise the most unbounded influence upon this disease—climate, seasons, locality, epidemic constitution, and moral agents so protean ; are, in consequence, the shapes which it assumes, and so diversified the indications it presents, that the most eclectic spirit will experience occasional difficulty and doubt in attempting to struggle with, and overcome, its violence and insidious malignity. That view of it which, under whatever form it may be endued considers it either as simple general excitement, or as compounded of this state in complication with local inflammation, or congestion, or debility, will alone lead to a guarded and eventually successful practice.

NOTE B—PAGE 16.

Proximate cause.—It is somewhat curious to observe the revolutions and changes which medical theories undergo at different times : while Broussais, Mills, Clutterbuck, &c., regard fever as the effect of local affections, and thus reduce it to a mere symptom, RUSH, on the other hand, considered these very local affections to be, in all cases excepting when produced by local injuries, not primary diseases, but "symptoms of an original and primary disease in the sanguiferous system," in other words, of fever !—The doctrine of Rush has received no slight confirmation from the fact of its having been incorporated, tacitly, indeed and without acknowledgment, but not the less essentially, into the amplified systems that are most popular and current with the profession at the present day. To prove this claim of the illustrious father of American medicine, it is only necessary to recur to his " Outlines of the Phenomena of Fever," and in them the views of Armstrong and

Johnson and Parry will be found not darkly shadowed out, but palpably figured and delineated. A few extracts will suffice to es-tabilsh this point.

Fever, says Rush, is, " in common cases, seated in the blood-ves-sels, and particularly in the arteries."

" My theory places fever in excitement and excitability *unequally* diffused, manifesting themselves, at the same time, in morbid ac-tions, &c." " The business of medicine is to equalize excitement in the cure of fever, that is, to abstract its excess from the blood-vessels, and to restore it to the other parts of the body."

"Morbid action in the blood-vessels, whether it consist in pre-ternatural force and frequency, or preternatural force without fre-quency, or frequency without force, constitutes fever. Excess in the force and frequency in the pulsations of the arteries have been considered as the characteristic marks of what is called inflam-matory fever. There are, however, symptoms which indicate a much greater excess of irritating impressions upon the blood-ves-sels. These are preternatural slowness, intermissions, and depres-sions in the pulse, such as occur in malignant fevers."

The congestive fever of Armstrong, and its pathology, are well described in the section devoted to *malignant* fevers.

" They are the effect of such a degree of impression as to pros-trate the arterial system and to produce a defect of action from an excess of force. Such is this excess of force, in some instances, in this state of fever, that it induces general convulsions, tetanus, and palsy, and sometimes extinguishes life in a few hours by means of apoplexy or syncope.* * * * * The less violent degrees of stim-ulus in this state of fever produce palsy in the blood-vessels. *It probably begins in the veins*, and extends gradually to the arteries. * * * There are cases in which this palsy affects both the veins and arteries at the same time. It is probable from this simultaneous affection of the blood-vessels that the arteries are found to be nearly full of blood after death from malignant fevers."

Compare these extracts with the observations of Armstrong on the congestive typhus, and not a doubt will exist of the source of the latter.

The excessive momentum of the blood determined to particular organs, as taught by Parry ; the loss of balance in the blood-vessels and in the nervous excitement, insisted on by Johnson ; and the congestion and venous turgescence, as well as the remora of the blood in the spleen, beautifully illustrated by Armstrong ; were all

virtually comprised in the ingenious and too much neglected writings of Benjamin Rush. His acute mind and penetrating genius
conceived and sketched the outlines of the figure which has been
since so admirably developed by his able, but not always candid,
successors. The vindication of his fame should ever be dear to
the American physician.

---

note C—Page 18.

The doctrine of critical days, so strongly insisted on by the ancient writers, with the exception of Celsus, and also by Cleghorn
and Jackson, has received little or no support from the experience
of American physicians. The active treatment usually employed
at the commencement of fevers in this country has been supposed
by many writers to have changed their aspect and disturbed the
regular periodical harmonies of nature. But the observations of
those physicians who have pursued an expectant method, and interfered litle or not at all with the progressive developement of febrile symptoms, have been, alike with those of the most active
and bold practitioners, unfavourable to the supposition that fevers
in the United States observe regular critical periods. Thus the
late professor Nathan Smith, whose means of practical knowledge
were only excelled by his sagacity and general skill, disclaims their
presence in the typhus of the Eastern states, although his treatment of the disease was quite inert.—Fevers of simple excitement
will, however, run a certain course, if not arrested at their onset.
Those complicated with phlegmasiæ or congestions are very indefinite in their duration.

---

note D—page 24.

Epidemic influence.—There cannot be a doubt in the mind of any
attentive reader of history, ancient or modern, that particular diseases prevail in certain years more than in others, and are, at
times diffused over whole quarters of the globe, after having been
rarely observed for a long period preceding their general occurrence. To this extended prevalence of any disease, the name of
epidemic has been given from the remotest times. And to ascer-

tain the cause of such epidemy has been the ambitious and indus-trions object of research of every enlightened and philosophical physician from the age of the Coan down to the present century. That observant student of nature, despairing of ascertaining its cause, gave it the vague name of the divine agent.—And in one form or other, this title has pervaded the successive nomencla-tures of medicine ; its nature remaining still unsuspected and un-defined. Latterly Dr. JOSEPH M. SMITH, Professor of the Theory and Practice of Physic in the University of New-York has attempt-ed to illustrate its nature and has given it the name of "*epidemic meteoration.*" That he has succeeded in attaining the great ob-ject of elucidating the nature of the causes of epidemics, is not pretended, but by suggesting a simple and easily remembered name for an agent, of which, however occult the nature, the ex-istence is undisputed, he has rendered a valuable service to etio-logical nomenclature.

Under the term meteoration, are arranged " all atmospheric sour-ces of disease, such as the vicissitudes of temperature and mois-ture, and those occult influences of the air which are occasionally experienced in every climate and season of the year, and which affect in a peculiar manner the animal and vegetable creation."* Meteoration has no reference, therefore, to that insalubrity of the air, which depends upon infectious and contagious effluvia. It is divided into Sensible and Epidemic Meteoration.

The first embraces the diurnal vicissitudes of the weather and also those manifest qualities of the atmosphere which prevail in different climates and different seasons of the year.

The second comprehends all those insensible qualities of the general atmosphere, which produce, or favour the prevalence of popular diseases, The same forms of disease produced by this last cause will occur in very different and even opposite conditions of the former. Hence the natural differences of the two agents may be safely predicated.

It would be injustice not to mention in this place the names of RICHARD BAYLEY and EDWARD MILLER whose successful research-es have shed a flood of light upon the history, causes and mode of development of the epidemics of the United States. To them all sub-sequent writers on the same subject have been deeply indebted,

* Elements of the Etiology and Philosophy of epidemics, &c. by J. M. Smith, M. D. &c.

82

and New-York may be proud of ranking them among her enlightened and scientific ornaments.

NOTE E—PAGE 37.

Contagion.—" A contagious disease is a disease which is capable
of being communicated from person to person. An Epidemic disease is a disease which at certain periods prevails generally over
the whole, or over a large portion of the community. A sporadic
disease is one which arises in a single instance only, or of which
the cases at one time are few and scattered. The cause of a contagious disease is a specific animal poison. The cause of an epidemic
disease is, or rather is supposed to be a certain condition of the air.
A contagious disease prevails by the communication from person
to person of that specific animal poison from which the malady derives its existence. An epidemic disease prevails through the influence of the atmosphere. The specific animal poison which gives
origin to a contagious disease must have existed in some person
and have been communicated by that person to another, by actual
contact, before such a disease can be propagated. The application by contact of its own specific virus is indispensable, as a first
step to the progress of a contagious disease ; it is essential to every subsequent step. For the extension of an epidemic disease, on
the contrary, it is only necessary that a person (provided he be
predisposed to receive the malady) be surrounded by the noxious
air from which the epidemic arises. A distinction has, indeed, been
made between a contagious disease which is communicable by pal-
pahle matter, and one which is communicable by invisible effluvia :
the distinction is truly unphilosophical whether the contagious matter be visible or not, it must still be matter : whether its application
to any part of the body of the individual who receives, can be distinctly traced or not, it must come in contact with some part of his
body. The small-pox is communicable by the application to a
healthy person of the matter contained in its pustules ; it is also
communicable by placing a healthy person within a certain distance
of the diseased ; in the former case, the application of the morbid
matter is palpable ; in the latter case, it is not palpable ; it is too
subtle to be appreciated by the senses, it is conveyed through the

medium of the air, but its application is as real, and as really by contact, as when it is applied by the lancet of the inoculator."

The statements contained in the above extracts are adduced in this place that they may be applied, in all cases, as tests of the fact whether any given disease be contagious or not. That they are correct so far as they go, no one will dispute. And they tend to overthrow an ingenious, but indefensible attempt at the classification of contagious diseases, which aimed at undermining one of the most powerful arguments against the contagious character of certain epidemic diseases.* Let every case of fever be subjected to a rigid scrutiny based on the above definitions and views, and the conclusion will be irresistible that epidemic idiopathic fevers are not contagious. The former vary in so many essential respects from diseases universally acknowledged to be contagious, that it does seem incredible they ever should have been confounded. Thus the symptoms of contagious fevers are determinate and uniform, never varying except in degree, preserving their specific character under the influence of every possible modification in the external agents which surround them. The symptoms of epidemic fevers are the reverse, varying according to climate, season, constitution of the air, &c.—Contagious diseases, likewise, observe certain periods of accession, duration, and termination. Not so with epidemic, which are indefinite in their progress. It may be doubted whether the former are ever generated *de novo*; the latter are sometimes regularly, and sometimes irregularly, but constantly renewed. The former seldom attack the same individual more than once; the latter may attack it at every period of their recurrence.

Dr. Gregory attributes much of the confusion which has been introduced into this subject to the employment of the term infection, &c. If reference were had to the very lucid distinction proposed by Dr. Richard Bayley between infection and contagion, this confusion and even the erroneous views of the author himself on the subject might have been obviated. His assertion that the contagion of typhus is denied by " a few, and happily a very few" is certainly incorrect. In this country such denial is almost general, and even in England, the recantation of the contagious doctrine by so high and popular an authority as that of Dr. Armstrong, the most experienced observer and historiographer of typhus, is no slight evidence of the doubts generally entertained of its accuracy.

* See Letter to Dr. Chisholm by DAVID HOSACK, M. D. F. R. S., &c. &c.

The same arguments which have been enforced time after time against the contagiousness of typhus, have been advanced with respect to Yellow Fever, and with no less dexterity and temporary success.

By a very large majority, however, of the physicians of the United States, and of the British naval service, who have had the most ample opportunities of studying fever in its every phase, it has been positively denied that contagion is an attribute of any idiopathic fever. The facts upon which this absolute contradiction of a belief sanctioned by time, and almost consecrated by the fears, the prejudices, and the superstitions of mankind, are simple, and not easily set aside.

Every fever yet known arises at times from causes independent of contagion. These causes are generally pervading, and require only a peculiar combination of circumstances to awaken them to action. If this general fact be not controverted, and it can scarcely be done with any shadow of plausibility, the inference ensues that those cases supposed to depend on contagion as their source are the product of the same general cause, as those in which this last is admitted to act, but with this difference that its immediate presence is either not palpable, or remains unsuspected or unnoticed. For instance: in seasons when typhus prevails epidemically to a great extent, it will be conceded even by the believers in contagion, that a great number of the cases arise from cold, fatigue, or from the constitution of the atmosphere. And if so, why may not all the cases arise from the same cause? If it be replied that this question in the abstract will apply to both sides of the question, the argument still recurs that the other causes, independent of contagion, must be admitted to originate the fever in the first instances which occur, and its continned agency appears at once more probable and conformable to the principles of a simple etiology, than the intervention of an adventitious and at best doubted cause.—That general causes do give rise to fevers appears satisfactorily established by the evidence of the very best writers who have described epidemics. The sources of pestilential disorders, of dysenteries, and of some of the worst cutaneous diseases have been sieges, camps, jails, and hospitals. The plague itself appears to originate with the crowded inhabitants of the villages of the East.* To prove, therefore, the superaddition

* Ferriar's Medical Histories, vol. i, p. 124.

of contagion to the influence of the original causes of an epidemic disorder, it should be incontestibly proved, that the disease can be engendered *without* the sphere of the latter. This has been often attempted, but without the success always claimed.

It has been well observed by Dr. Mills, in his comparative view of Fever, that as Typhus originates spontaneously, it must be proved that it is transmitted, under other circumstances, than those, to the operation of which it owes its birth, before we can possibly admit its contagiousness.

A peculiar circumstance attending the production of typhus deserves notice, as tending to throw some light on its supposed contagious character. This disease may be produced by vitiated effluvia from human beings sick of any disease, as yellow fever, plague, and even typhus, or even from those in health, if they are crowded in ill ventilated apartments, wherein no cleanliness is observed and the excretions become putrescent and offensive. "In this manner typhus produces typhus, and hence the erroneous conclusion that the disease is propagated by means of a specific contagion."* The mistake which is committed in these cases consists in not distinguishing between specific secreted poisons or contagion, and excreted matter which acts like other general causes of disease.

General facts, it may however be urged, are after all inconclusive. Details alone will suffice, and such details as are well authenticated and do not admit of ambidexter construction. To these then let us recur, and a stronger case could scarcely be made out, than one selected from Yellow Fever, a disease of the contagion of which the dread is still so great in the popular mind of this country, notwithstanding the labours of Miller, Mitchill, Bayley, Rush. Irvine, Moseley, Bancroft, and a host of others to prove its nonentity.

The last epidemic Yellow Fever which visited New-York occurred in 1822. Several interesting accounts of the disease were drawn up. The most able, so far as the question of its contagiousness is involved, was presented to the public in an elaborate review which appeared in the eighth number of the New-York Medical and Physical Journal. It was drawn up by my friend Dr. JOHN B. BECK, now Professor of Materia Medica in the University of New-York, and is a masterpiece of clear and philosophical argument. My limits will not allow me to extract the whole of this very valuable arti-

* Philosophy of Epidemics, p. 30—1.

cle. I can only quote those sections which are more immediately
calculated to throw light on the subject under consideration.

"The believers in the doctrine of the contagious character of
Yellow Fever, may be divided into two classes. 1. Those who
contend that the disease is contagious under all circumstances, and
that it may as readily display this character in the pure and healthy air of the country, as it does in the confined air of our cities.
2. Those who admit that in the pure air of the country it is seldom if ever contagious, while in the impure and vitiated atmosphere of our cities it proves extensively so. Both classes, however, agree in this ; that every case of the fever which occurs, must
result from contagion, as they do not admit the existence of any
other cause capable of producing the disease. * * * *

"As we wish to meet both these views of contagion, the following
facts shall be arranged under two heads ;—Those which prove that
the Yellow Fever of 1822 was not contagious in the pure air of the
country :—Those which prove that it was not contagious in the vitiated and impure air of our city."

"I. From the official returns of Dr. Joseph Bayley, Health Offi-
cer of the port, it appears that during the prevalence of the Yellow
Fever in this city during 1822, seventy persons sick with that disease were sent down to the Marine Hospital,* on Staten Island.
Of this number thirty-seven died, eighteen of whom had black vomit. The first of these patients was received into the hospital on
the 13th of August, and died on the 15th. From that period until
the final cessation of the fever, patients were almost daily carried
down to this place. These cases were regularly attended by the
physicians and nurses of the establishment, not one of whom became affected with the disease, nor has a single case came to our
knowledge of any person taking it, who was engaged in transport-
ing the sick from the city to the hospital."

Into details I shall not enter, but, refering to the article itself,
go on to the other general facts.

"II. We now proceed to state the second fact in proof of the
non-contagious character of the yellow fever. At the distance of
about three miles from the city, at Kip's Bay, a spacious two-story
dwelling house was provided at the public expense, for the reception of such of the inhabitants from the infected district as were
unable to provide a refuge for themselves. From the official ac-

* Situated at the quarantine establishment, about six miles below the
city of New-York, on the west side of the bay.

count* given to the Board of Health by the attending physician, Dr. Drake, it appears that during the season ten persons lay sick of yellow fever in this establishment, two of whom died. Of the physicians and nurses in attendance, not one contracted the disease. But to render the facts connected with this building still more conclusive, it is stated that " besides the above sick, the house was occupied, during the unhealthy season, by the family of Mrs. Roberts, consisting of four persons ; the family of Mrs. Thompson, of eight persons, and three children of the Coit family ; all of whom continued in good health, with the exception of two children of Mrs. Roberts, and two of the young Coits, who suffered from intermitting fever, which was doubtless to be attributed to the low wet grounds in the neighbourhood of the house."†

" III.' During the prevalence of the fever, six persons lay sick of it at Greenwich, a village about a mile from the city. All of these had contracted the disease in the infected district. Five of the six died. In no instance did they communicate the disease to physicians, nurses, attendants, or friends. To give additional weight to this fact, it should be recollected, that to this place had been transferred the seat of business—that in consequence of this, almost all the merchants of the city had retired to it, and that to accommodate them, hundreds of temporary buildings had been erected. From this influx of inhabitants, it may naturally be inferred that the village was crowded to excess ; and from this circumstance, as well as the want of comfortable accommodations, every thing seemed favourable to the propagation of the disease. Still, although a number of very decided cases of the fever were carried to this place, lay sick, and died there, it was not in a single instance, communicated. It only remains to add, that the body of one of the patients who died here, was dissected by two physicians, Drs. Donaldson and Torrey, neither of whom suffered from it the slightest indisposition."

" IV. In addition to the cases already recorded, there were a large number of persons, who after having contracted the seeds of the disease in the city, had the disease developed in them after their removal into different and distant parts of the country. There occurred about thirty-six cases of this sort, and at the following places, viz. three at Newark, N. J. ; one at Harlaem ; three in the

---

* History of the Proceedings of the Board of Health, &c. p. 63.
† History of the Proceedings of the Board of Health, &c. p. 130

city of Jersey ; one at Tappan, N. Y. ; six at Bloomingdale ; one at Albany ; three at Middletown-point, N. J. ; four in different parts of New Jersey ; one at Newtown, L. I. ; one at New-Canaan, Conn. ; two at Amboy, N. J. ; one at Hempstead, L. I. ; one in Westchester ; one at Bloomfield, N. J. ; one at Woodbridge, N. J. ; one at Saugatuck, Conn. ; two at Bushwick, L. I. ; two at Elizabethtown, N. J. ; and one at Boston. Of this number there were twenty-seven deaths. From the very extraordinary propor-tion of deaths among these cases, it is evident that they must have been very decided and malignant in their character, and yet not in a single instance was the disease communicated. In relation to the case at Boston, we have the recorded testimony of the editors of the New-England Journal of Medicine and Surgery, who state that the patient " lodged at one of the largest hotels in that place, filled at the time with persons from all parts of the country, and there sickened and died of the Yellow Fever ;" and although " he was constantly watched and attended in a small and badly ventila-ted apartment, no one was in the slightest degree affected by his sickness."*

" Let us now pause and reflect upon the amount of testimony al-ready advanced. It appears then, from the foregoing facts and state-ments, that upwards of one hundred persons, sick of Yellow Fe-ver, (about one fourth of all the cases,) lay in different parts of the country, without a in single instance, communicating the disease. If it had been previously proposed to settle this question by actual experiments, we cannot conceive that any could have been sug-gested which would have been more satisfactory to all parties, than the very ones which actually transpired during the summer and autumn of 1822. That one hundred persons, sick of a disease highly malignant and contagious, located in different parts of the country, should not, even in a solitary instance have communica-ted it to a second person, seems to us literally impossible ; and we believe, that were it not for the influence of preconceived opinions, and long-cherished theories, facts of this sort would come home to the mind of every man with a force perfectly irresistible. Aware of these facts, the contagionists, so far from abandoning their fa-vourite theory, have invented new schemes for upholding it. One of the most popular of these, at present, is this, that Yellow Fever, although it may not prove contagious in the pure air of the coun-

* New-England Journal of Med. and Surg. vol. vii. p. 384.

try, yet is eminently so in the impure atmosphere of cities, &c. Whether any countenance was given to this doctrine, by the facts which were developed during the Fever of 1822, we now propose to investigate.

· " We cannot, however, refrain from first making a few remarks upon the theory itself, which asserts that a disease may be contagious in one sort of air and not so in another. Notwithstanding this doctrine has received the sanction of some very distinguished names, we have never been able to convince ourselves that it is correct in fact, or philosophical in principle. That it is not correct in fact, so far as it relates to Yellow Fever, we shall show directly. The grounds upon which it is conceived to be unphilosophical, are these.

" If contagious effluvia emanate from the body of a person sick of a peculiar disease, they can be influenced by the surrounding air in only one of two ways. First, the surrounding air may serve simply as a medium of transmission. In this way the effluvia are diffused more widely than they would be in vacuo. It is evident, however, that here the contagion remains unchanged in its character, and produces its specific effects without any aid from the atmosphere, except that of enabling it to act at a greater distance from the sick body. Second the contagious effluvia may enter into chemical combination with the surrounding atmosphere. An entirely new compound then is formed, the effects of which upon the human system, must necessarily be different from those of the original contagion.

" These are the only possible methods in which contagious effluvia can be influenced by the surrounding atmosphere. Now, if we apply these propositions, and push them to their conclusions, they will be found to destroy completely the theory of which we are speaking. If the contagious effluvia enter into chemical union with the air, and form a new poison, then the same specific disease cannot be reproduced ; this supposition, therefore, is inadmissible. If, on the other hand, the air serves merely as a medium for transmitting the poison to a greater distance, then no reason can be assigned why if you approach near enough to the sick body, contagion should not display itself in a pure as well as an impure atmosphere.

Let us take another view of the subject. If a disease be contagious in one kind of air, and not in another, then it must acquire its contagious character from some peculiarity in the air in which it

83.

is so. And if this be the case, then the principle of contagion must exist in the air, and no reason can be assigned why the air tself should not, under these circumstances produce the disease, independently of all sick and diseased bodies. This seems to us to be an inevitable conclusion f om the premises ; and to our minds, it appears most satisfactorily to do away the necessity of resorting to contagion, to account for the origin and propagation of yellow fever. On these grounds we think the popular doctrine which supposes that this disease may be contagious in one species of atmosphere and not in another, is unphilosophical."

Abundant testimony is adduced to prove this admirable train of reasoning, the perusal of which is calculated to satisfy every mind not warped by prejudice or interested motives.

Dr. Beck finally comes down to the infected district, where the principal stand in favour of contagion must, after all, be made.

"Our reasons for believing that the contamination of the air was not owing to any exhalations from the sick, are the following :

1. It has already been shown, that not merely in the pure air of the country, but even in the most impure and unhealthy parts of our city, patients sick of the yellow fever, in 1822, were uniformly approached with perfect impunity. The *air*, therefore in the infected district, must have been much more venomous than the contagious poison itself, coming off directly from diseased bodies. That is, the poison diluted in atmospheric air, must have been more powerful than the pure unmixed poison itself; a proposition absurd in itself, and contrary to all analogy. We infer, therefore, that as the *air* of the infected district was more deleterious than actual contact with the sick, the poison existing in the air must have been some other than effluvia from the bodies of the sick.

2. If the infection of the air depended upon emanations from the sick, then it should have extended *pari passu* with the sick and the dead. That this was not the case is notorious. That it was not so out of the infected district, is proved by the fact, already established, that no case of communication was known ; and that it was not so in the infected district, is equally evident from the circumstance, that the limits of the district were only known and defined from persons being taken unexpectedly sick, without, in many instances, any sort of intercourse with those already affected.

3. The gradual and measured extension of the limits of infection, proves conclusively that it must have originated from some

other cause than contagion. So regular was this extension, that attempts were made and with apparent success, to calculate its daily progress. From the point at which i first commenced, it extended very nearly to equal distances in all directions, Can any man of common reflection contend, that such an effect could follow from patients scattered in different directions?

4. But what settles this beyond peradventure, is the fact that by far the largest number of the sick did not lie in the infected district at all. From the official list published by the Board of Health it appears, that in all not more than about one hundred and thirty lay sick in both infected districts during the whole of the prevalence of the fever, while about one hundred and seventy-two lay sick in different parts of the rest of the city. As therefore one hundred and seventy-two patients did not infect the air in which they lay sick, it is reasonable to conclude, that a *less* number would not produce such an effect, and therefore that the infection of the district was not owing to the sick.

From all these reasons we conclude, that the infection of the air was not owing to contagious exhalations from the sick, but to some other cause. What this cause was, it is not our business at present to inquire. That it was a gaseous poison, is evident—that it was permanent in its action is also clear from its gradual extension until the uppearance of frost. Whence or how it originated, is a question very far from being settled."

There are two arguments which have been much relied on by Contagionists as establishing the truth of their doctrine; the one is that a *number* of cases of the disease suspected of possessing a contagious character occur in individual houses; the other that these causes occur in *succession* and not simultaneously.. These arguments are thus irrecoverably laid at rest.

The *number* of persons attacked in *individual* houses does not prove the existence of Contagion:

1. Because all the cases alluded to occurred in the infected district, where every person was exposed to the same *common cause* which produced it in the first patient. Under such circumstances, the fact of half a dozen persons sickening in one house does not prove contagion any more than it does their exposure to the same general cause, producing the same effects upon each. When, however, it is recollected that in houses where the sick lay in the city *beyond* the infected district, no such fact was known to occur,

the conclusion is not only legitimate but inevitable, that when it did occur in the infected district, it was *not* owing to contagion.

2. Another very satisfactory reason why so large a number of cases occurred in a comparatively small number of houses is, that almost all the houses of the district were deserted by their former inhabitants. In some streets not a single one remained inhabited —in others only one or two. It is evident, then, that if any cases occurred at all, they must have taken place in those solitary buildings which were occupied. If this general and almost total desertion of the district had not taken place, victims to the disease would have been found without difficulty in almost every other house.

3. Because persons inhabiting the same house, from equal predisposition—equal exposure—and similar modes of living, were most likely to be similarly affected by the common poison pervading the atmosphere ; hence it was to have been expected, if one was seized with the disease, others in the same house would also be liable to it."

The second argument regarding the *succession* in which cases occur, does not, any more than the first, prove contagion.

1. Because, even admitting it to the fullest extent contended for, the simple fact of succession is no test of a disease being contagious. This we think may be proved satisfactorily by a very simple and obvious illustration frequently occurring. Suppose a person living in the neighbourhood of a marsh, is seized with bilious remittent, a disease universally admitted not to be contagious ; he is visited by a friend, who continues with him, and attends upon him during his sickness. In a few days, this friend finds himself beginning to sicken, and is also taken with bilious remittent fever. Now here, we have actual communication with the sick—precisely the same disease reproduced—and the one taken *in succession* to the other. What more can be wanting to make out a case of contagion? And yet all this apparent proof, conclusive as it appears, amounts to nothing. It merely proves, that *both* patients were exposed to the influence of the miasms from the marsh, *the common cause* producing precisely similar effects in all who are so exposed.

2. Because the fact of persons taken sick in succession may be explained satisfactorily without resorting to contagion. It is admitted on all hands, that certain states of the system predispose persons to be acted upon by the poison of yellow fever. The depressing passions have uniformly been considered as producing this effect. Hence cautions on this subject are laid down by al-

most every practical writer. Now, we cannot imagine any situation more truly depressing or one more calculated to excite fear and anxiety than that of a family remaining in a pestilential district, and accordingly none more likely to prepare the system for being assailed by the disease. More especially would all this be the case, if one of the members of a family thus situated were taken sick, and it would rather be a matter of surprise than otherwise, if with all these predisposing and exciting causes operating upon them, persons did not take the disease."

I have made free use of this admirable argument against the contagiousness of Yellow Fever, because it will serve as a model by which to analyze the histories of all diseases that either are, or are supposed to be contagious. It recommends itself the more strongly to the attention of the medical critic ; because it is divested of all speculation. The question respecting the *origin* of yellow fever is, with logical propriety, left out altogether, the writer's aim having been simply to sift the question whether the epidemic of 1822 was, or was not, contagious. To this object, so important every way to the interests of the community at large, and of mercantile cities in particular, the author restricted himself, and he has accomplished it in a manner which has forbidden all reply or contradiction.

NOTE F—PAGE 72.

Intermittent Fever. The causes of the frequent failures experienced by practitioners in the management of intermittent fevers may, in general, be traced to the affections with which they are very liable to be complicated. These must always be removed, before a cure of the original disease can be accomplished ; in other words, the complicated must be reduced to the simple intermittent, before it can be successfully encountered by its own specific remedies. As these complications offer themselves to the frequent notice of physicians, it may not be amiss to enumerate a few of the most important. It may be observed of all these forms, that the *superadded* symptoms, as they would be termed by Dr. Gregory, will generally be more or less present and may easily be recognised, by the attentive observer, during the apyrexia.

1. Intermittent fever may be attended by plethora, and general excitement, or by visceral inflammations, their frequent effects. Such complication forms the angeiotenic intermittent of the school

of Pinel, who consider it a combination of inflammatory with intermittent fever. This form is not of very frequent occurrence, because the circumstances which favour the development of periodical or miasmatic diseases, do not often exist in combination with the sthenic diathesis. When it takes place, it is observed in the quotidian type, and in robust subjects who live well. The signs which designate this complication are, a full, strong, and chorded pulse, pain of the head, occasional discharges of blood especially from the nose, deficient secretions, a hot and dry skin, and an aggravation of all the febrile symptoms, if tonics or stimulants are administered. If local inflammation be present, the symptoms peculiar to the affected part will of course be developed. The indications to be fulfilled in the treatment of this form are sufficiently obvious. Blood-letting, general and local, evacuants suited to the individual requisitions of the case, and external counter-irritation furnish the appropriate means. When the fever is reduced to its simple form, it is to be treated by the ordinary means. The hot stage is sometimes fatal in this variety.

2. Extreme prostration of strength sometimes accompanies intermittent fever, giving it the form of an adynamic fever. This combination rarely occurs in our climate and country. It is met with chiefly in high north latitudes. Pinel cites instances of it in his very admirable Nosography. When it does make its appearance in temperate latitudes, it is most apt to attend upon the quartan type, and attacks persons enfeebled by age, excesses, previous diseases, &c. It is in this variety that the cold stage occasionally proves fatal. General and partial tremors, livid spots like petechiæ upon the extremities, utter prostration of all the vital functions characterise this form. The treatment must be adapted to the exigencies of the case, consisting of diffusible, as well as fixed stimulants; carbonate of ammonia, wine, alcohol, and a rich nutritious diet. Care must however be taken not to confound apparent, with real debility, and attention should always be paid to the presence of any visceral congestion. Costiveness is of course to be obviated, and a pure and healthy air chosen for residence.

3. Gastric and biliary derangements are very often complicated with intermittent fever. This complication is very prevalent in autumn after a very warm summer, and offers the most frequent obstacle met with by practitioners in the United States to the safe and speedy cure of intermittents. Depression of spirits, great physical languor, head-ache, a yellowish tinge in the complexion, a

foul yellow, or brown tongue, bitter taste in the mouth, thirst, inappetency for food, nausea, uneasiness about the præcordia, occasional vomiting, and diarrhœa alternating with costiveness, high
coloured urine depositing a pink sediment, are the distinguishing
features of this variety. To restore the functions of the stomach
and hepatic system to their healthy condition, by means of emetics,
purgatives, the warm bath, and particularly by alteratives, is the
great object to be accomplished.

4. Alibert has bestowed the epithet *penicious* on a variety, or
rather a number of varieties of intermittent fever, marked by complication with diversified affections, chiefly of a nervous character.
The term ataxic has been prefered by other authors, whilst the physiological school condemns all these distinctive appellations, and
substitutes one single word for them all—gastro-enteritis !—The very existence of intermittents is denied by Dr. Mills. So far will human prejudice go !—The prominent affections of which the complications under this head consist, are, excessive stupor (observed by
Morton in his pyretologia cap. 9. hist. and Torti in his Therapeu-
tic special ; &c.*) constant delirium, epilepsy, convulsions, syncope, (Riverius and Sennetrus relate cases) asthma, aphonia (M.
Double,) catarrh, excessive cold (Riverius and Pinel,) and many
others all denoting derangement in the nervous system.—The
treatment of these different complications must be modified by their
respective natures, but Cinchona is, according to Alibert and the
best writers, the great specific for all.

Masked Intermittent. Febres Larvatæ.

Intermittent fever sometimes makes its appearance without developing any general action of the heart and arteries, but confines
its attack to a periodic irritation of some one part of the body.
Thus apoplexy, cephalalgy, chorea, mania, asthma, rheumatism,
gout, toothach, &c. will return at periods exactly corresponding
with those observed by intermittent fevers. When they occur simultaneously with these last, and owe their origin evidently to miasmatic causes, there is little doubt of their being intermittents in disguise. To these the appellations at the head of this article have
been appropriately given. In vain shall we attempt to remove
them by other remedies than those indicated in intermittents. It
requires therefore all the sagacity and attention of the practitioner
to recognise them. The greatest physicians have acknowledged
their occasional mistakes on this point. FODERE, in his valuable

history of Epidemics, informs us, that in an ophthalmia which prevailed at the college of Strasburgh in the spring of 1818, and with
which his own son became affected, he at first used the ordinary
means for its removal, such as antiphlogistic measures, local depletion, &c. These succeeded, indeed, in subduing the disease,
even causing it to disappear altogether. Every second day the
same symptoms would, however, return, and this for a successive
number of times, until the learned Professor, ascertaining the true
nature of the disease, had recourse to cinchona, which entirely
overcame it and put an end to its reappearance.

Treatment of Intermittents. In addition to the means described
by Dr. Gregory, there are two somewhat novel methods of subduing this fever which have lately been recommended upon high
authority.

1. The first is proposed by Dr. Mackintosh of Edinburgh, and
consists in the detraction of blood during the cold stage. He considers this plan conjoined with the subsequent use of laxatives and
the sulphate of quinine, to be as " certain a remedy for intermittent
fever, as any remedy for any known disease." Bleeding in the
cold stage will generally cut it short, and frequently prevent the
return of the disease altogether. The quantity of the blood to be
drawn varies according to circumstances, from one ounce and a
half to twenty four ounces. Some difficulty may attend the operation at first on account of the tremulous motions of the patient:
this vanishes as he is relieved. Dr. Mackintosh was once successful by bleeding in a cold stage which had endured twenty six
hours. The relief is evinced by the ease with which the patient
breathes, the subsidence of the tremors, and an abatement of the
sensation of cold. It acts probably by relieving the heart and large
bloodvessels, the brain, and the lungs, from the accumulations of
blood which oppress them. For the safety of the practice Dr. M.
refers to Dr. Haviland, Professor of the theory and practice of
physic in the University of Cambridge ; to Dr. Malden of Worcester; Dr. Buller of Cork ; Dr. Allison of Edinburgh ; and also
to the work of M. Bailly.*

II. The second plan which I shall relate is that pursued by my
very excellent friend JAMES FOUNTAIN, M. D. of Yorktown, N. Y.
whose clinical experience has only been equalled by his unremtting
study and application. It consists in administering *large* doses of

---

* NewYork Medical and Physical Journal Vol. i, New Series, p. 325—6.

arsenic, so large indeed as to strike with astonishment all those who have not courage to make use of a similar bold expedient. Were his own testimony however not sufficient, that of numerous practitioners might be adduced in its confirmation. My pupil, Dr. Carver of Carmel, Putnam county, has repeatedly witnessed its successful and perfectly safe employment not only in intermittent fever, but in other diseases of aggravated irritation. Dr. James Hubbel now practising in the western part of this state has likewise informed me that he constantly employs arsenic in the doses recommended by Dr. Fountain and with perfect impunity. I shall quote the passage in which Dr. F first published his views on this medicine, together with his mode of administering it.

"*Arsenic.* This is almost the only article I ever employ for the cure of intermittent fever. I have administered the bark, quinine, and the prussiate of iron. But arsenic is certainly the most prompt, efficacious, convenient, and cheap medicine with which I am acquainted. Properly managed, it is perfectly safe for old and young invalids, and pregnant women, as well as for the phthisical. The swellings so much feared are the effects of mismanagement or of the disease. Dr. Parr says of arsenic, "It is undoubtedly a very active and powerful medicine; nor have we found any disadvantage from its use. It has succeeded where bark in every form and with every addition, failed." And I can safely add that I have administered it to more than a thousand people, and I never saw any injury arise from its use in my practice. Besides the dropsy, it has been accused of producing rheumatism; but this opinion partakes too much of vulgar prejudice to merit a serious reply.

"Arsenic is usually directed to be administered in very small doses at first, beginning with three, five, or six drops of Fowler's solution, morning and evening, increasing the dose one drop every day until a cure is effected. In this manner two or three times the quantity which was originally sufficient to accomplish a cure, is introduced into the system, and yet the disease continues. In the meantime the patient's face swells, and the medicine is discontinued as the physician should be, who prescribed it. Dr. Paris observes that great and dangerous accumulations of medicines sometimes take place in the system, especially mercury, lead, arsenic, &c.; and this would be the most easy and efficacious method of introducing it to effect that object. As was observed of bark, arsenic should be administered during one apyrexia *only*, and it may be given in substance or in solution. The following are the combina-

tio is I have always used. Neither undergo decomposition by time ;
I therefore prepare enough to last several years.

Arsenical Solution.

℞ White oxide of arsenic three drachms,
    Carbonate of Potass one drachm,
    Powdered Rhuba-b do. do.
    Rain Water one pint,

Boil half an hour. Remove it from the fire ; then add immediately brandy half a pint and water enough to make the whole
amount one pint and a half; lastly, filtrate.

Arsenical Pills.

℞ White oxide of Arsenic, one scruple,
    Powdered Rhubarb, two and a half drachms,
    Oil of Caraway, ten drops,
    Molasses q. s. M.

Make a mass to be divided into eighty equal pills.

From eight to fourteen of these pills may be administered according to the obstinacy of the complaint and the urgency of the
case. In tertians they are all to be given during one apyrexia. In
quotidians one half of what is intended to be administered may be
exhibited during one apyrexia, and the other during the next ;
and, in quartans, they are to be given within the eighteen or twenty
four hours previous to the expected attack. They should be always administered at as equal distances of time as convenient, not
disturbing the hours of sleep, as that would derange the harmony
of order amongst the functions.

" When the drops are preferred, from sixty to a hundred may
be taken, as the case may seem to require ; dividing them in the
same manner as the pills ; eight or ten may be administered every
two hours during the apyrexia, beginning in the morning at six and
continuing until ten o'clock in the evening ; the remainder may be
taken the next morning. * * *

Six or eight hours after the last dose of arsenic a cathartic
should invariably be prescribed. This is an injunction not to be
neglected on any pretext whatever. Cathartics act as specifics in
removing any unpleasant consequences which might arise from the
use of arsenic. I have not, in a single instance, where they have
been administered, known any swelling of the face to succeed, even
where four grains of arsenic had been exhibited. The most troublesome effect of the medicine is the nausea which it will sometimes

create. This is however of short duration, and does not interrupt the cure.

By this plan of treatment the expected paroxysm may be pre-vented in ninety-nine cases out of a hundred; the diseased habit is thereby thoroughly broken up, and a cure is the result."

For further interesting remarks on the same subject I refer the reader to the nineteenth and twentieth numbers of the New-York Medical and Physical Journal.

My own experience with arsenic is limited. Quinine usually succeeds in the intermittents of this city, unless some complication or untoward circumstance in the system of the patient counteract its useful influence. The formula I have used is the following,

> R Sulphate of Quinine eighteen grains
> Elixir Vitriol fifteen drops
> Simple syrup, and
> Water, each one ounce. Mix.

A teaspoonful or more may be taken every hour during the apy-rexia.

I have sometimes administered eight grains of the sulphate of quinine in substance one hour before the expected paroxysm, and with the happiest effects.

Latterly, I have advantageously used, in obstinate cases, the quinine combined with small doses of tartrate of antimony and potass as recommended by Dr. Dominique Gola.* The following is the form of the combination.

> R Tart. Antim. and pot. three grains,
> Sulph. quinine, three grains;

Mix accurately and divide into six equal parts. One of these parts is to be taken every two hours during the apyrexia. The first dose sometimes produces vomiting of bitter fluid, sometimes alvine evacuations, sometimes no evacuation at all. The fever is gene-rally arrested. I have seen it answer in those cases more especially which are attended by a dry husky condition of the skin.

NOTE F—PAGE 72.

Bilious Remittent Féver. The proper autumn endemic of the Uni-ted States is the bilious remittent fever. This prevails more or less generally every year and is particularly rife in the country in marshy districts. When it occurs as an epidemic, it often proves

* Annali Universali di Medicina 1825, (Magendie.)

speedily fatal, and is then confounded with yellow fever. That it is however distinct from this latter affection will shortly be made to appear. I shall first enumerate some of the prominent symptoms of the disease, and allude to the more successful methods pursued in its treatment.

The disease is generally preceded for a few days by a disagreeable sense of lassitude and languor, inappetency, and occasional slight rigors. It generally makes its attack, between eight and eleven o'clock in the morning, with a distinct chill followed by great heat, acute pain in the head, back and limbs, occasional delirium, frequent and full pulse, uneasy respiration, nausea succeeded by bilious vomiting and diarrhœa, thirst, yellow furred tongue, hot and dry skin, high coloured spare urine, jactitation, &c.

In cases complicated with high inflammatory action, the pulse will be chorded, and obstinate constipation attends. The stomach and præcordia are generally affected with a sensation of tightness, and the disposition to vomit, so urgent in the first stage, frequently ceases in that of excitement. This stage lasts through the night till near morning when an evident remission ensues. The exacerbation is renewed the second day on the same hour as on the first, but the cold stage is not developed. The fever often puts on the form of the *hemi-tritæus*, and is worse every second day, the remissions being very obscure. This fever, like the typhus of Armstrong, has three varieties : the simple, the inflammatory, and the congestive. A regard to this fact will explain the success of the discrepant methods of treatment which have been pursued in different years and by different practitioners, and likewise the cause of its having been confounded with so many other diseases. When the fever has continued for some time, a yellow suffusion will generally overspread the eyes and skin, and tinge the secretions, more especially the urine. Typhomania is then frequent, and the pulse becomes small and sometimes slow. The symptoms of the latter periods of the disease are a frequent small pulse, great uneasiness and sighing, a dejected and anxious countenance, pungent heat and stricture of the skin, faintness, subsultus tendinum, low delirium, a dark brown and sodden tongue, offensive dark and involuntary evacuations from the bowels, dark coloured urine, insensibility to external objects, colliquative sweats, hiccough, accumulations of mucus about the trachea, death.

This fever may be protracted from one, to five or six weeks. Currie observes that when it terminates favourably, it is generally on the fifth, seventh, ninth, eleventh, or thirteenth day. The signs of a favourable issue are a full development of the remissions, warmth and moisture on the skin, lateritious sediment in the urine, and a gradual restoration of appetite and strength.

The causes of this fever may be summed up in the word *malaria*, operating in warm and moist seasons, on constitutions predisposed by debility however induced.

It is somewhat singular, that Dr. Gregory, in describing the treat. ment of remittent fever, should omit any mention of emetics, the most useful class of medicines in this affection. They are gene. rally indicated early in the disease, and should always follow the employment of bloodletting, wherever high arterial action indicates the previous use of this latter measure. They are useful, not only in unloading the stomach of the foul contents which the incipient in. disposition has allowed to accumulate in that organ, both mechani. cally and sympathetically, but also in exciting the action of the bil. iary organs, which is usually languid at the commencement of all bilious diseases. They are likewise useful in equalizing the circula. tion, as they unload the portal and intestinal circulations, and excite action in the capillaries of the mucous membranes, as well as in the exhalants of the skin. They are never contra-indicated in bilious c. vers excepting in cases of great prostration, or where there is an in. ordinate determination to the head, complicated gastric inflamma. tion, pregnancy, &c. The emetic which will best fulfil these seve. ral indications, is a combination of tartar emetic with ipecacuanha.

Purgatives, diaphoretics, and alteratives, constitute the next most important resources of the physician in this fever. Mercury should enter largely into his prescriptions. In severe cases, it must be used with a bold and decisive hand, after vascular excitement has been overcome. In milder cases, the ordinary cathartics, neu. tral salts alone, or combined with senna and manna, are sufficient. Where there is great irritability of the stomach present, Rhubarb combined with the alkalies, or taken in combination with the draught of Riverius is an excellent article :

    ℞ Rhubarb powdered, thirty grains,
        Carbonate of soda, one scruple ;

Mix in a table spoonful of mint water, add a like quantity of fresh lemon juice, and then let the draught be swallowed in the act of effervescence.

The soda or seidlitz powder furnish a refreshing beverage in this fever.—Great attention should be paid to ventilation and cleanliness both as regards the atmosphere of the apartment in which the patient lies, and his clothing and bedding. Tepid ablutions with rum and water prove admirable detractors of heat and remove the sordes so apt to collect about the skin.

Convalescence in bilious fever deserves the most watchful attention of the practitioner. Stimulants, tonics, and a rich diet of oysters and beefsteak diluted with porter and brandy and water, are, excepting in very rare and extraordinary cases of debility and old age, to be *sacredly forbidden.* It has repeatedly and even lately fallen to my lot to see persons who had been safely carried through three and four weeks attack of bilious fever, suffer irrecoverable relapses from an overabundant or too stimulating meal taken stealthily or perhaps allowed by the improvident facility of the medical attendant. I am aware that Dr. Daniell of Savannah treats this fever with capsicum and brandy, and dreads the administration of a cathartic. *Such treatment answers not in the State of New-York.*

Before quitting the subject of this fever, I cannot omit noticing what I conceive a capital error, into which many physicians have fallen, by confounding the Bilious Remittent with the Yellow Fever. Believing them to differ specifically in their origin and symptoms, and that the belief of their identity has an unfavourable influence on medical police and the laws of quarantine, I shall be excused if I state the reasons of my opinions somewhat at large. This is the more necessary, because some of the highest names which have adorned our native medical literature are to be found on the other side of the question.

The fact, that the contagionists have espoused the contrary doctrine, and that they have, for very obvious and interested purposes, made no small efforts to associate it with the great question of contagion itself, has lent no little force to the spirit with which the identity of the two diseases has been maintained by many of the non-contagionists. It is not the contagionists alone, however, who contend for a specific difference between bilious remittent and yellow fever. Some of the earliest, most zealous, and most powerful opposers of contagion have supported the same opinion, and, to my apprehension, with indisputable power of fact and argument. That this may not seem to rest on my mere assertion, I shall, in the first place, quote two or three writers who have treated on the subject, and whose authority will not be disputed, and, in the second place, mention those points of distinction, which the recorded experience of others and my own in both diseases have enabled me to trace with marked accuracy.

. One of the most enlightened and forcible writers on the yellow fever, and one to whom subsequent authors have been much indebted for their knowledge of the character and method of treating this afflicting disease, is Moseley. Intimately acquainted with the yellow fever of the West Indies, and possessing a powerful and discriminating mind, he was early led to reject the belief in contagion which had been before his time so prevalent, and also to draw the decided line of demarcation between the ordinary remittent of all hot countries and climates, and the yellow fever. Thus in one place he states, that "the *bilious remittent fever* is a common disease with which the *endemial inflammatory fever*, (called the *yellow fever*,) has been so confounded by writers." In another, speaking of two unfortunate physicians, Williams and Bennet, who terminated their disputes on yellow fever by killing each other in a duel, he says "both adopted the opinion that the yellow fever was a bilious fever, and gave it that appellation, and though William's indications of cure were rational, he was not able to distinguish it from diseases *really* bilious. This want of discrimination," Moseley adds, "had always existed in the West Indies, and the consequence was, that cardiacs, and refrigerants, evacuants and bark, emetics and bleeding, *frequently* and *fatally* usurped the place of each other." Again: in defending his opinion that yellow fever is a species of the *causus* of Hippocrates, Aretæus, and Galen, and he does it with no small degree of plausibility, he says, " it is *totally* different from the remittent bilious fever to which all habits of body are subject in hot climates, particularly after rains, and in the fall of the year." On the symptoms and treatment, this same author observes, that " they who have mistaken the bilious remittent for the causus, consequently speak of remissions, which do not happen in this disease," and "that emetic tartar, however useful it may often be in bilious diseases, will be fatal in this."

I shall next adduce the opinion of Dr. Robert Jackson, so well known by his masterly treatises on the fevers of warm climates and latterly by his full and accurate description of the yellow fever of Spain. This justly celebrated physician offers to the world the interesting spectacle of a man of science, who was engaged, for half a century, in the investigation of disease, and who, at the advanced age of seventy-five, promptly quitted the sweets of retirement, and fearlessly undertook a distant voyage to the sources of a raging pestilence, in the hope of ascertaining its character, and shedding additional light on the long agitated question of conta-

gion. It is no small confirmation of the truth of the non-contagious
doctrines, that the enlarged and prolonged experience of such an
observer is strongly enlisted in their favour, and it will not be denied that his opinion with respect to the specific difference between
yellow and bilious fevers is equally entitled to our respect. He
expressly discriminates the yellow fever from the *endemic remitting
fever*, inasmuch " as it has no remissions, nor exacerbations, does
not attack the same person twice, unless accidentally on his return
from a colder region ; attacks lately arrived Europeans, and not
those who are climatized or natives ; while the remittent does not
cease to attack those who have resided long in warm climates."*

In our own country, two of the latest writers on epidemics, Dr.
Chapman of Philadelphia, and Dr. Joseph M. Smith of this city,
have both defended the opinion, that there is a specific difference
between the two diseases.

It is an error therefore to suppose, that it is to contagionists
alone that the belief in a specific difference between bilious and
yellow fever is confined. Having satisfactorily shown this, I
shall next proceed to offer a few reasons, which induce me independently of the opinion of others, to maintain the same doctrine.
This I shall do under four distinct heads, and for obvious reasons,
be brief and summary in my remarks under each.

1. The yellow fever differs from the bilious remittent in its *history.* The former prevails in places near the sea-coast only, and
has never yet appeared farther north than 44° N. The bilious fever, on the contrary, appears equally in the interior of countries,
and on the coast, and is constantly occurring in places situated as
high as 55° N. Nor is the appearance of yellow fever confined to
the sea-coast in temperate latitudes only ; this rule holds equally
good in the tropics themselves—in the West Indies, and on the
continent of South America.

The yellow fever occurs at indefinite periods, marked frequently
by no traceable resemblance in their general character as to moisture and heat ; the bilious fever always appears where heat, moisture, and miasmatic exhalations concur. Thus the yellow fever
did not prevail in New-York or Philadelphia from 1760 to 1793, although in the meantime the bilious fever was repeatedly observed as often as its appropriate causes had an opportunity of action.

The yellow fever in the tropics does not attack natives or sea-

* Jackson on Fevers, p. 163.

soned foreigners, but is confined to strangers within a year or eighteen months after their arrival. Hence it may be laid down as a general position, that yellow fever does not, under the same circumstances, attack the same individual twice. The exceptions to the rule are furnished by those, who, after having lived in a warm climate, visit a cold region, and then return again to the tropics. Under this exception are included the permanent residents of temperate climates, whose systems assume a new predisposition for the disease under the agency of a winter's cold.

The bilious fever, on the contrary, attacks the natives, and seasoned inhabitants, and one attack, so far from imparting an exemption from future attacks, rather predisposes to them. This observation applies to temperate, no less than tropical countries.

2. These fevers differ in their *cause.* It is scarcely necessary to say more under this head than what will not be denied, that while no one disputes the agency of moisture heat and malaria in the production of bilious fever, the causes of yellow fever are still matter of dispute, not between contagionists and non-contagionists only, but among these respective parties themselves. The truth is, that the causes of yellow fever are hidden in obscurity. Some of the causes of bilious fever appear indeed accessary to the production of yellow fever, but that there must be others entirely distinct is abundantly proved by the fact that they are not alone sufficient to its production, else why are these fevers not simultaneous in their occurrence?

If the causes differed merely in grade, is it not a singular circumstance that the lesser grade shall continue to produce its effects on acclimated individuals, in the tropics for instance, while a more powerful and concentrated grade shall be inert; that is, the same cause in less quantity shall continue to produce bilious fever, perhaps annually, while in greater quantity, it cannot act so as to produce yellow fever?

3. These fevers differ in their *symptoms.*

The yellow fever consists of one paroxysm of fever only. This is followed by a total cessation of febrile symptoms, not a remission, and this again by a state of collapse; no distinct exacerbation ever re-appearing. Lest we should be supposed to be unsupported in this statement, we refer to the descriptions of yellow fever by Lining, Mosely, M' Arthur, &c., as describing the disease truly called yellow fever.

Valuable as the New-York Medical Repository undoubtedly is in

85

other respects, it is calculated to diffuse much error with respect to the true character of yellow fever, there being multiplied instances of ordinary remittent fever described in it, under the appellation of yellow fever. A careful analysis will expose the error in almost every instance.

The yellow fever most usually runs its course in a short time, say from three to five, or to seven days.

The bilious fever generally continues from nine to twenty-one days.

The stomach is always and essentially affected in yellow fever, as is evinced by the burning heat about the præcordia, the pain at the pit of the stomach, the vomiting of matter not bilious, but evidently a secretion from the stomach itself, or whether a secretion or not, proceeding from this organ alone.

In bilious fever the stomach may indeed be affected, but it is in a milder degree, and this organ cannot be considered the seat and throne of the disease.

The pulse and temperature, in yellow fever, are frequently natural; in bilious fever, they are never so. The appearance of the eyes is very different in the two diseases, as is that of the suffused skin.

The muscular system always suffers under great debility as bilious fever advances, while the arterial system is more and more excited. In yellow fever on the contrary, the muscular strength is frequently retained to the very hour and moment of death.

The appearances on dissection differ also very materially in the two diseases. To sum up all the points of difference will scarcely be expected of us in this place. It is enough to mention the different conditions in which the stomach is found, after death, in the two diseases.

4. The *treatment* required in the two diseases differs essentially. Bleeding, emetics, cathartics, &c., are obviously indicated in bilious fever, and, if properly directed, seldom fail to produce their intended effects, and relieve the patient. In yellow fever, it is still matter of dispute what treatment is most proper, and of the measures proper for bilious fever, some are improper in yellow fever, and others seldom produce any effect at all. Thus bleeding is still considered a doubtful remedy in yellow fever, and emetics, which are indispensable in bilious fevers, are positively contra indicated."

It is unnecessary to extend this article further. I have advanced enough to show that the lines of distinction between the two diseases are pretty well defined, and that the error of blending them does not merely affect a question of speculative theory, but is actually fraught with danger in practice.

NOTE H—PAGE 80.

Yellow Fever. The symptomatology of this interesting and so often terrible malady as furnished in the text, is so jejune that I deem it my duty to extend it. To do so I shall avail myself of a description of the disease* which I drew up after my return from the West Indies, where I had enjoyed repeated opportunities in 1818. 21.22, of witnessing of it in its most severe forms. In the latter year I studied its character as developed in the epidemic of Rector street, and was struck with the striking features of identity displayed with the tropical fever in all its more aggravated cases.

" The disease generally invades the patient with the ordinary symptoms of fever: slight rigors, seldom amounting to a chill; pain in the head and loins; uneasy sensation about the stomach, and a general sense of weariness. Sometimes these symptoms are altogether wanting, and pyrexia seizes the patient suddenly: at other times they continue for several hours, and then are succeeded by increased arterial action, quick, full, and chorded pulse; great, and even pungent heat of skin; increase of the pain of the head, more particularly across the eye-balls; soreness and pain in the loins, stretching forward to the umbilicus, or shooting down to the thighs and settling in the calves of the leg, in which the patient likewise complains frequently of a sense of weakness. The countenance has a sad and characteristic appearance: the eyes are inflamed and watery; the tongue is slightly covered with a whitish mucus, and is most frequently moist. The skin is sometimes of a dingy hue, mostly not altered in its appearance, and frequently it is covered with a slight moisture. The stomach is very uneasy, experiencing a sense of vacuity, sometimes of hunger, and is generally painful on pressure from without; in some cases it retches even at this early period, and if vomiting be superadded, the prognostic is fearfully certain. The bowels are

---

* Observations on the climate and diseases of the is'ard of Curaçao; published in the first volume of the N. Y. Med. and Phys. Journal.

costive, and respond with difficulty to the action of purgatives.
The urine is scanty, and what is voided is reddish and clear. The
mind in general is serene, but fearful of the event.

The symptoms continue increasing for forty-eight or sixty hours,
when relief seems approaching in a temporary alleviation of the
more violent symptoms. The febrile heat and pain yield and frequently go off altogether, But when the stomach has once been
disordered, there is no cessation of its sufferings. This second
stage has not inaply been termed, by Mosely, *Metaptosis*; it is the
token that re-action is exhausted, and the system is undergoing a
rapid change, form a state of excitement to one of collapse and
passive suffering. The third or last stage accordingly developes
itself sooner or later in the sunk and irritable pulse, though in
some cases it is little changed, the low temperature of the body,
constant sighing, burning sensation in the œsophagus, occasional
delirium, the approaching coldness of the extremities, and yellowish suffusion appearing first about the angles of the mouth, and on
blistered surfaces, particularly in moments when the patient either
from vomiting or any other exertion is exhausted, and then diffusing itself over the neck, breast, and whole body. The patient
complains now of increasing uneasiness about his stomach, and is
urgent for cold drink, which is no sooner taken than it is rejected
and accompanied with increasing quantities of black membrana-
ceous flocculi swimming in the fluid, and of a slate coloured sediment at the bottom. He is frequently free from all disturbance, and
inclines to doze, but he no sooner falls into a slumber, than the
perturbation of his stomach becomes perceptible, and vomiting is
brought on. He now lies on his back, with his knees drawn up in
the bed, and is intolerant of any covering about his head : he occasionally sighs, and tosses his hands to and fro ; is anxious for
something hard upon which to press, and frequently leaves his bed
with insane violence, and grasps the floor or the bed and seems
to experience relief from the indulgence. Hiccough, increase of
black vomiting, dark and fetid stools, hemorrhage, and perhaps a
convulsive fit end his acute sufferings.

Such is a general outline of the train of phenomena characterizing this disease, whose mortal progress it is the severe duty of a
humane physician to watch with scarce a hope of any other reward to his labours and anxiety, except an addition to his melancholy experience.

All cases are not, however, thus distinctly marked. Patients sometimes labour for a day or two under no other symptoms than those attending on ordinary cold, for which a dose of salts from the medicine chest is prescribed ; their eyes are watery, they feel disinclined to move about, and lie down listless and unconcerned of what is passing about them, when, of a sudden, retching and vomiting come on, and, perhaps, before the physician has time to appear they are in the agonies of death.

On the treatment I have nothing new to offer. Emetics were, however, proscribed, and blisters were by some thought hurtful. In two cases, which threatened to put on the most violent forms of the disease, the most active depletion by the lancet, and brisk cathartics led me to flatter myself that I succeeded in arresting the disease."

The authorities against emetics are so numerous that it appears idle at the present day to denounce their use. From Lining, who practised in South Carolina in the last century and who wrote an exceedingly interesting history of the Yellow Fever in the Edinburgh Physical and Literary Essays, down to Mc Arthur, Jackson, Dickson, Wilson, Musgrave, all writers who have been most experienced in this disease dissuade their readers from the use of vomits. A few American physicians have indeed recommended them, but as the fevers they have treated occurred in the interior, they were probably the bilious remittent with which they had to deal.

Dr. Gregory lays much stress in favour of the contagiousness of Yellow Fever, on "the obvious arguments suggested by its appearance in Cadiz, Gibraltar, and, still more lately, at the Island of Ascension." It would appear that the author has not consulted the obvious arguments and facts developed on the *other* side of the question by the labours of Jackson, O' Halloran, Deveze, Bancroft, &c. The fever occurring at Ascension Island among the crew of the Ship Baun was evidently the product of local malaria engendered on board that ship. For a more ample discussion of this last fact I will take the liberty to refer to an anonymous article which appeared in the New-York Monthly Chronicle of Medicine and Surgery for July 1825.

The answer, to the question whether the yellow fever may be taken a second time is not, in my opinion, so 'short' as Dr. Gregory seems to suppose. The permanent inhabitants of nothern latitudes udoubtedly contract it more than once, provided they have been predisposed by a preceeding winter's cold to its renewed attack. So likewise those who have become acclimated in the tropics may lose their immunity by visiting high latitudes in winter, and then returning again to a warm climate. Of these facts instances have occurred within my knowledge.

NOTE I—PAGE 107.

Small-pox, Varioloid, Vaccination. From a very full and interesting dissertation on the value of vaccination as a preventive of small-pox, written by my friend and former colleague, JOHN BELL, M. D. now of Natchez, Miss. I extract the following conclusions respecting this important subject. They are the result of ample research and extensive personal acquaintance with the subject.

"1. Small-pox proves fatal one in about five cases, when contracted naturally.

2. The eruptive diseases known under the names of sheep-pox, swine-pox, water-pox, wind-pox, horn-pox, &c., are all varieties of small-pox, produced by atmospheric influence, constitutional peculiarities, or some other unknown causes.

3. Varicella, or chicken-pox, formerly regarded as a variety of small-pox, but since the year 1767 considered a distinct disease, must be again restored to its former situation, and classed with the varieties just mentioned.

4. Small-pox is modified in three several ways: 1st, by a previous occurrence of the same disease; 2d, by inoculation; and, 3d, by vaccination.

5. Though it is difficult to form even a tolerably accurate estimate of the degree of protection which the first of these cases offers, from the want of sufficiently extensive data, yet it is evident from those which we have, that though cases of this kind are more rare, they have proved more fatal than those succeeding inoculation.

6. Small-pox, communicated by inoculation under favourable circumstances and in a proper manner, does not prove fatal in more than one in three hundred cases, though its former mortality was much greater.

7. Inoculation should be discouraged in every manner possible, since its performance serves to keep up and diffuse the small-pox emongst those who, from ignorance or negligence, possess no protection against it.

8. Vaccination furnishes, in a great proportion of cases, a complete and perfect immunity against the attacks of small-pox.

9. It modifies the access of small-pox in a slight degree, usually rendering the febrile stage somewhat milder, although the stomach and respiratory organs are often more strongly affected than in its ordinary course.

10. It possesses a controlling power over the progress of inflammation in the eruption, shortens its course in the majority of cases, prevents its reaching the pustular stage, and, in almost every instance, obviates the occurrence of secondary fever.

II. The varioloid disease, or small-pox after vaccination, does not endanger life; there being no case on record in which it has proved fatal, after the system has been thoroughly subjected to the influence of the cow-pox.

12. That reason and probability are highly in favour of the truth of Dr. Jenner's opinion, that the security which vaccination offers is in a direct proportion to the degree of perfection of the vaccine process; and that in consequence, it is advisable to re-vacinate as long as any effect is produced.

13. The vaccine virus, which has now been employed upwards of twenty years, in every civilized part of the globe, has suffered no deterioration; and it now confers all the security against the small-pox which it ever has done.

14. There are no grounds for believing that time weakens, in any degree, the protection which an individual receives from having been once properly vaccinated.

15. It cannot be considered otherwise than the duty, not only of all medical men, but of the public authorities and all interested in the public health, to encourage as far as is practicable, the practice of vaccination."

NOTE J—PAGE 130.

Is the appearance of the blood abstracted as a remedial means, just criterion in considering the propriety of repeating the operation of blood-letting ? This question was discussed by Dr. John Davy of Malta in some very interesting observations published by him in the Edinburgh Medical and Surgical Journal for April 1829, and as it is a subject of paramount practical importance, I shall offer in this place a short abstract of his views.

The appearances and qualities of the blood commonly supposed to be indicative of inflammation, and to warrant further venesection are, an unusual degree of fluidity of the blood the moment it is drawn ; unusual slowness in coagulating ; and when coagulated, being covered with a buffy coat, and cupped.

Although these appearances are generally met with in cases of local inflammation there are exceptions occurring which deserve special notice.

1. When the inflammation is violent, running rapidly on to suppuration, and very extensive, so that it attacks more than one texture, or the same texture but in different organs, the blood drawn is, often, according to Dr. Davy's observations, neither cupped nor buffy. In peritoneal inflammation, this is more especially the case.

2. In diffuse cellular inflammation, the blood often coagulates rapidly, even as in health, and yet being very liquid, exhibits a slight buffy coat.

3. In pleurisy and pneumonia the blood drawn at the commencement of the disease is occasionally not cupped nor buffy, although it puts on these appearances subsequently.

4. In inflammations of the mucous membrane, whether of the respiratory or digestive passages, the blood does not always exhibit these appearances.

5. There is no relation yet established between these appearances and the intensity of the inflammation. Sometimes they are very prominent when the diseased action is not violent, and vice versa.

6. Fibrinous concretions are found in the heart and large bloodvessels in the great majority of fatal cases, whether the lancet has been freely used, or only very moderately, or not at all.

These considerations and facts are calculated to weaken our confidence in the importance formerly attached to the appearance of the cupped and buffy blood as indicating sanguineous depletion. Nor will the supposed opposite appearances of the blood, a very soft crassamentum, little if at all contracted,—or the blood remaining liquid—or the proportion of crassamentum to the serum being unusually small, lead to any more unexceptionable or certain indications.

1. In the remittent fever of hot climates, in epidemic cholera, &c. the crassamentum is often softer than natural and little contracted ; yet bloodletting is often beneficial even when repeated.

2. Blood without fibrine is very uncommon. Dr. Davy has only witnessed it in pulmonary apoplexy, and that, after death in the

heart and large vessels, it could not however have been a post mortem change.

3. The absence of a due proportion of crassamentum is often witnessed in the advanced stages of acute diseases, or in acute diseases supervening on chronic of long duration, or occurring in very delicate persons. Yet the lancet must often be used in these cases.

Lastly; In many very important affections, as the continued summer fever, in tetanus, apoplexy, and other neuroses, the blood is not apparently altered, and bleeding may yet be indispensable.

The result of Dr. Davy's researches is that the practitioner should pay more attention to the state of the patient, than to that of the blood. In this he was long since anticipated by the experienced Dr. Heberden, whose observations merit careful attention.

NOTE K—PAGE 143.

Treatment of Inflammation. 1. The most direct and powerful means of subduing inflammatory action is the abstraction of blood. No measure is accordingly more frequently resorted to, and, as might be expected, no one is employed with so little discretion. Capable, when skilfully managed, of subduing disease more promptly than any other remedy we possess, it is frequently, nay daily converted into one of the most noxious agents by which disease is protracted, health permanently impaired, and even life itself put into jeopardy. Its indiscriminate employment, on all occasions when inflammation is only suspected of being present, and when the practitioner is at a loss perhaps what else to do ; the excessive quantity often abstracted without regard to effect but merely to adhere to an abstract standard measure adopted as an undeviating rule ; and finally, its injudicious use in cases attended by great exhaustion and irritability are the besetting sins of modern practice. They are the extreme perhaps, to which the profession have fled from the formerly prevalent doctrines of debility and putrescency, and they are equally injurious and fatal. It is to be regretted that Rush, amidst the immense benefits which he conferred on the profession of his country, should have been led, by his overweening attachment to a favourite hypothesis, to establish an ultra system of vascular depletion, to which too many admirers of his eloquence, his ingenuity, and his undisputed merits have become blindly enslaved.

At the onset of visceral inflammation bleeding should be promptly and efficiently employed. The extent to which it **is to be** carried must be regulated not by any abstract measure, eight, **or** sixteen, or thirty ounces, but by the effect it produces, in subduing arterial excitement and relieving the sufferings of the patient. In all inflammatory attacks of vital organs, it is desirable to produce syncope. This can be most readily accomplished by observing a rule laid down by Pemberton in his invaluable and practical treatise on the inflammatory diseases of the abdominal viscera. It consists in so regulating the size of the orifice of the punctured vein that eight ounces of blood shall flow in three minutes. Twenty or twenty four ounces thus drawn will in general suffice to produce relaxation and a mitigation of the symptoms. A decided and efficient conduct at the onset of phlegmasiæ will frequently cut short their existence, while irresolution and timidity will allow them to advance so far that neither venesection nor any other antiphlogistic measures can arrest their march to disorganization. The employment of active measures at this period will frequently obviate the necessity of a recurrence to the repeated bleedings so much in vogue with certain practitioners.

2. It has been well suggested in the text " as a matter deserving of inquiry how far the nerves are concerned in inflammatory action." That they become deeply implicated in the disease, especially after the development of sympathetic fever, even if they are not primarily affected, there cannot be a doubt. To them we may refer the irritability which so generally accompanies visceral inflammation, which so far from being subdued by vascular depletion is often augmented by it. and which by reaction in the heart and the arteries becomes the principal cause of the frequent renewal of the inflammatory symptoms. It is by allaying or wholly overcoming this nervous irritability that opium proves such an admirable auxiliary to venesection in the treatment of inflammation. To prove effective, it should be given in *full* doses immediately after depletion. Dr. Armstrong has pursued this method for years and with the greatest success. The late Dr. Wright Post of this city also employed opium in phlegmasial affections, and in subacute cases, as a substitute for depletion.*

In acute peritonitis Dr. Armstrong orders the patients to be bled, in the first stage, so as to produce the most complete relaxation, whatever quantity may be necessary to produce this effect. As

* New-York Medical and Physical No. XXXIX. New Series No. I. p. 31.

soon as the patient recovers from his faintness, *three grains* of opium in the form of a soft pill are given and absolute rest is enjoined. In some irritable habits, less of the solid and some fluid opium is prescribed in order that the anodyne effect may be more quickly produced. "The effects of the opium, thus administered, are to prevent a subsequent increase in the frequency and force of the heart's action, and a return of the abdominal pain, while it induces a tendency to quiet sleep and a copious perspiration over the whole surface. In many instances, this simple procedure will remove the inflammation at once, nothing being afterwards necessary, when the patient awakes, but spare diet absolute rest, and and quietness with an occasional mild laxative. But on all occasions I visit the patient, if possible, about three or four hours after the administration of the opium, and if there be pain on pressure in any part of the abdomen, with a hot skin, a quick, jerky pulse, I order the patient, in my presence, to be promptly bled in the same decisive manner as before."* Opium is then again administered as before, combined perhaps with Calomel. A third bleeding is sometimes necessary, after which opium may be given in smaller doses. Leeches to the abdomen are occasionally very useful, as are likewise glysters of warm water.

3. Mercury was first used as an antiphlogistic remedy in this country. Dr. Armstrong claims the merit of its first employment in inflammatory affections for Dr. Hamilton of Lynn Regis, who wrote a valuable essay on the subject in 1783.† A reference to the letter of the late venerable Dr. Holyoke, published in the first volume of the New-York Medical Repository will establish the priority of claim in favor of the physicians of New-England. It was extensively used in 1735 in a very malignant distemper of the throat, and was afterwards much employed in pleurisies, quinsies, inflammatory rheumatisms, and other phlegmasiæ. Its combination with opium, camphor, &c. was not unknown. Dr. Holyoke tells us : "The preparation of mercury most commonly made use of was mercurius dulcis, or calomel ; in large doses joined with some purgative when designed to act as a cathartic ; and in smaller doses, of one or two grains as an alterant, or when the intention was to affect the system ; and then it was frequently combined with

* Transactions of the Associated Apothecaries and Surgeon Apothecaries of England and Wales. Vol. i. 1823.
† Medical Commentaries vol. ix.

camphor and sometimes with some preparation of *antimony*, and sometimes with small doses of opium; or with all of them together as the prescriber judged most proper; though in some cases the native mercury, rubbed down with terebinth, &c. was preferred."*

Of the modus operandi of mercury little is known. Its effects are however well ascertained. "Confessedly" says Dr. Chapman, "there is no article of the materia medica so diffusive in its effects, which pervading the whole system, enters into every recess, and acting on every part leaves no morbid impression untouched. It is by virtue of this general and revolutionary action, that it is calculated to meet such a vast variety of indications."* In fever and local inflammation it undoubtedly acts by restoring the obstructed action of the secreting vessels, by equalizing the circulation, and perhaps creating new points of irritation which relieve the diseased organs.—Its action on the salivary glands is by no means indispensable to its curative action, and it were well if it could be altogether obviated. It is at best but an index of its more general operation. The best method of administering mercury in inflammatory diseases is to give it after the entonic action and plethora of the bloodvessels have been removed by suitable depletion, in large and purgative doses at first, and then in smaller doses combined with diaphoretics, &c.

4. Antimony offers another valuable means of reducing vascular action, and subduing inflammatory diseases. It has been long used with this view, and either alone or combined with other agents proves an efficient sedative and diaphoretic. In ordinary cases the tartrite of antimony and potass dissolved in the spiritus mindereri or aqua acetitis ammoniæ is an invaluable remedy. Two grains, of the former added to eight ounces of the latter form a good combination of which half an ounce may be given every two hours.

The Italian school place their exclusive reliance on antimony, and administer it in doses which seem almost incredible. Rasori treats pneumonia, for instance, with this remedy alone, discarding bloodletting and other evacuants, and he gives it to the amount of

---

* Medical Repository vol. i. page 492.

† It is somewhat singular that although the author of the Elements of Therapeutics admits of this all pervading influence of mercury, he should ridicule the idea of its entrance into the circulation. His exclusive doctrines of solidism are ably and unanswerably refuted in a review written by Dr. J. B. Beck. in the first volume of the N. Y. Med. and Phys. Journal.

a scruple and even some drachms in the course of twenty-four hours. Neither vomiting nor purgation follow—but the phlogistic action is subdued by the direct *contra-stimulant* operation of the antimony. The facility with which patients bear such huge quantities of tartar emetic is attempted to be explained by the fact that the susceptibility to its impression is overcome by the morbid process going on in the system, and it is further stated that a return to health renews the sensibility to its action.

NOTE L—PAGE 149.

It is recommended in many of our most popular elementary treatises on the practice of physic and therapeutics, that, in diseases attended by a great determination to the brain, blisters should be applied to the head. It has always appeared to me that this practice is directly at variance with the object aimed at, and inconsistent with the other measures simultaneously recommended, as ice, cold water, leeches, &c. applied to the same part. One of the strongest advocates for blisters in phrenitis and typhus admits that in mania they are hurtful while they are drawing, and they are therefore best applied to distant parts. (Elements of Therapeutics.) Now the same fact obtains in inflammation of the brain, and every argument drawn from analogy contra-indicates their application so near to the seat of the disease. Dr. John Clark in his admirable treatise on diseases of children deprecates their application to the scalp in phrenitis. He denies that they produce the same effect here in affections of the head, as they do in thoracic and abdominal phlegmasiæ, when applied to the parietes of those regions, because the connection between the external and internal parts in the latter is a *distant* one, in so far as bloodvessels, nerves, absorbents, &c. are concerned. In the former the connection is close and intimate: the supply of blood to the scalp and internal skull being derived from one and the same source. In the one case then a revulsion may be hoped for from blisters; in the other if they act, they must act by increasing the determination to the head which is the very object to be overcome. If they are ever successfully applied to the head is it not in the second stage or after effusion has taken place?

NOTE M—PAGE 152.

Delirium Tremens. Excepting in cases attended by very marked symptoms of inflammatory action, and which very rarely occur,
bloodletting is a decidedly injurious remedy in this diseases. I have
every reason to believe that in persons predisposed to this affection
bloodletting is one of its most frequent exciting cause. I have known
intemperate persons, who having been bled, and very unwisely too,
for pain in the head, fall victims shortly after of this affection.
Bleeding should always be used with great caution in persons habituated to the operation of powerful stimuli, as wine, strong mental emotion, &c. &c. When it is once formed, it is difficult of
removal, and, if subdued for the time, is very liable to return and
finally puts an end to the patient's life. Dissection has failed hitherto in elucidating the nature and seat of the disease. It arises
probably from an irritable and collapsed state of the nervous system, more especially that of perception induced by previous over-
excitement. Hence the utility of narcotics and diffusible stimulants.
The great object to be accomplished in the treatment is to procure
sleep, and great difficulty attends the attempt. Dr. Stephen Brown
of this city has given upward of thirty grains of opium in four hours
with this view before he could succeed.* Emetics, it is well known,
are highly recommended by Dr. Klapp of Philadelphia,† and they
do prove eminently serviceable on certain occasions. The tepid
and cold affusion have both been employed with advantage by
Dr. Armstrong ; the latter in those cases only in which there was
considerable vigour of the constitution present.

NOTE N—PAGE 160.

Hydrocephalus. If Quin originated the idea that dropsy of the
brain was the effect of previous inflammation in that organ, Rush
enjoys the rarer merit of having illustrated and established its
truth. His observations on this disease are among the most valuable of his writings, and it is gratifying to find their merit acknowledged by some of the latest writers on Pathological Anatomy. The
same candor has not been manifested towards him by practical wri-

---

* For a very valuable history of the disease, consult Dr. Brown's paper in
the fifth volume of the Medical Recorder.
† Medical Recorder, vol. i.

ters either in Europe or in this country. His method of treatment is, however, the most successful which has as yet been pursued. His condemnation of mercury is, however, not borne out by subse. quent experience. A highly interesting case of recovery from this disease is recorded in the Dublin Medical Transactions in which calomel was administered to a young child, after active depletion, to the extent of several hundred grains.

In connection with this subject I cannot refrain from reccom. mending to the reader the attentive perusal of an essay on certain affections occurring in children which stimulate hydrocephalus, but are in reality very different, and rendered fatal by depletion and evacuants. It is written by Dr. Gooch of London, and may be seen in the New-York Medical and Physical Journal for October 1829.

I have lately seen a highly interesting autopsic examination of a young man who had been a patient of Dr. John S. Bowron, of this city, and who had been from youth affeected with pain in the right ear. Until two weeks before death he had not been ill. He was then attacked by hydrocephalic symptoms. The following notes on the post mortem appearances were taken down by Dr. John R. Rhinelander, who conducted the dissection in the most scien. tific manner.

"*Autopsic Examination.* Patient aged about 20, body emacia. ted countenance expressive of great placidity. *Examination of the Brain and its Membranes.* The brain was exposed in the usual manner, the dura mater was found strongly adherent to the anterior table of the cranium; this membrane was not found much inject. ed; water was found between the parietal folds of the arachnoid membrane and that covering the pia mater, and also between the arachnoid and pia mater; so that it might be pushed by means of the knife from different parts of the cerebrum. The veins were greatly distended and the arteries somewhat injected, as in cutting the substance of the brain numerous red points could be seen. The substance of the cerebrum was in general firm except at its anterior portion, where it was soft and had the feel of fluctuation. The ventricles were pale and contained about four oz. of fluid, and the tunica arachnoidea could be raised from a portion of the ventricles, and from the plexus choroides with. out difficulty. The foramen Monronianum was large enough to ad-

mit the little finger. The thalami nervorum opticorum and the corpora striata and third ventricle were sound, upon raising the posteri-
or lobes of the cerebrum the tentorium cerebelli super-extensum
an abscess was found in the right posterior lobe, communicating
through the tentorium with the right lobe of the cerebellum, and in
it was found a large abscess occupying one third of its extent.
The dura mater was found separated from the posterior and superior part of the petrous portion of the temporal bone. The bone
was carious and opened into the semicircular canals, the portio
mollis being entirely destroyed before it entered the foramen
auditorium inturnum. The portio dura was perfectly sound.
The abscess in the cerebelli showed its secreting surface. The
pus was of a greenish appearance, and exceedingly offensive.
The tentorium cerebelli on the right side was covered with a
thick layer of lymph and hardened pus. (What was the proximate cause of this man's death? was it loss of the substance of the
brain by abscess, or superabundant quantity of water effused between
the different membranes of the brain? The effusion of this fluid was
evidently in part an action set up by nature to supply the loss of
substance created by the abscess, and to prevent hemorrhage of the
vessels of the brain. If it had been a diseased action, the symptoms
would have been manifested through the mind, as in all cases of Hydrocephalus.—(Vide Carson upon the circulation of the blood in
the head. Edinburgh Med. and Surgical Journal, vol. 123.")

NOTE O—PAGE 177.

Laryngitis. My attention was called to this disease some years
since by its occurrence in a case which presented most aggravated symptoms. The details were published in the eighth number
of the New-York Medical and Physical Journal, accompanied by
some reflections. Repeated venesection carried to syncope, emetics, and the specific action of calomel, effected a cure. The
subject of this case has since suffered three violent attacks of the
same disease, which were quickly subdued by active depletion and
full vomiting. It is strange, that Dr. Gregory, in describing the
treatment of the acute form of Laryngitis should make no mention
whatever of emetics. They deserve to rank side by side with venesection ; in the forming stage of the disease, they will frequently
arrest it altogether, and in old debilitated subjects they must
be mainly relied on, when bloodletting cannot be safely had re-

course to. Neither can I subscribe to the view taken of the disadvantages supposed to attend tracheotomy in this disease. So long as the affection has not extended to the trachea, I think it far more likely to prove serviceable in this disease than in tracheitis. Of its perfect safety and of the great success which has attended its employment, the reader may satisfy himself by consulting a valuable paper by Mr. Lawrence in the sixth volume of the Medico-Chirurgical Transactions of London. For some pertinent suggestions on this point, as well as for a very comprehensive and graphic history of the symptoms, causes, and treatment of this interesting affection. I cannot do better than refer to an admirable essay drawn up by Professor John B. Beck, which appeared in the third volume of the New-York Medical and Physical Journal. Dr. Beck has concentrated, in a few pages, the numerous and previously scattered facts which had been accumulating in foreign and domestic publications respecting the nature and methods of treatment of the disease, and, by careful comparison and analysis, systematised and rendered them available in practice. In this excellent monograph the opinion is advanced that Washington died of this disease, and not, as was generally supposed, of croup. *Vide in loco-citato.*

NOTE P—PAGE 178.

Croup. Dr. Hosack has furnished the profession in this country with the best *practical* essay that has yet appeared on this frequent and dangerous affection. This experienced physician recognises three stages in croup. The first he denominates the forming stage. In this the disease is purely local ; " the child sits laughing and playing upon its mothers lap, manifesting a very unusual but morbid degree of exhilaration ;" the circulation is as yet unaffected, the skin preserves its ordinary temperature. But the hoarse, hollow sounding and frequent cough, the wheezing inspiration, and the cries which it utters after each fit of coughing denote to the sagacious physician the existence of danger. The indication in this stage is to restore the suppressed secretions of the trachea and surface of the lungs, and to prevent the development of the febrile or second stage. The means to effect these objects are an emetic of tartarized antimony and ipecacuanha, an enema, and calomel in effective doses. Sometimes the emetic gives complete relief. The second stage is characterised by quickened circulation, heat and dryness of the skin, hurried respiration, white furred tongue indicative

of inflammation, flushed countenance, frequent cough attended by
a very acute sound. The wheezing is now almost uninterrupted,
the trachea and air passages are choked up by accumulations and
great oppression is the consequence. If the patient is plethoric
and not relieved, the countenance becomes livid, and stupor often
ensues.

The third stage is denominated the membranous or purulent. It
commences with the establishment of effusion from the exhalant
vessels opening into the windpipe, bronchiæ, and lungs. "In the
two former the effused matter assumes a membranous appearance,
probably owing to the forcible passing and repassing of the air
through those preternaturally constricted tubes, but in the lungs
themselves it appears in the form of a viscid fluid partly resembling
both phlegm and pus." After the effusion has taken place the febrile symptoms and pain often abate, but the paroxysms of coughing
and dyspnea are frequent and violent, and convulsions frequently
put an end to the suffering.

The treatment of the second stage of croup cunsists in the most
active depletion. Dr. Hosack prefers bleeding from the arm, or
the back of the hand to opening the jugular vein, because patients
are so restless that hazard may attend the latter operation. From
a child of two or four years of age as many ounces of blood should
be taken and so on. Immediately after the bleeding, an emetic is administered, and if the symptoms are not subdued, the bleeding is
repeated, the patient is immersed in a warm bath, a large blister is
applied to the throat, and a cathartic of calomel, of from five to ten
grains, is given to be repeated every two hours until it produces a
decisive effect. Should these means fail, small doses of calomel
and James' powder, from two to five grains each, are next administered every two hours. The antimonial wine or a solution of tartar emetic may be substituted, and laudanum is sometimes indicated
when the arterial excitement has been subdued, and diarrhœa or the
cough prove distressing.

In the last stage Calomel in small doses, squills, the syrup of on-
ions, seneka snakeroot, ammonia, assafœtida and the vapour of vinegar and water are the medicines most relied on. They are given
to excite tracheal and bronchial secretion, without weakening the
already exhausted system. If emetics are indicated in this stage,
and the polygala senega fails to produce vomiting, the vitriolic articles of this class should be preferred to antimony or ipecacuanha.
The sulphate of copper has been found singularly serviceable in

some very unpromising cases treated by Dr. J. W. Francis.   (See third volume of N. Y. Med. and Phys. Journal.)

<hr>

NOTE Q—PAGE 190.

Among the means which have been recommended as useful in subduing the action of the heart and arteries in thoracic inflamma. tion, the Sanguinaria Canadensis, or blood-root, merits a conspicu. ous place.   Dr. Wm. Tully thus sums up its remedial qualities.*
" Taken internally, in moderate doses, it increases the excitement of the sanguiferous system, augments the action of the lymphatics of the viscera, excites appetite, and promotes digestion.   In large doses, it nauseates, diminishes sanguiferous action, and still further increased, it vomits.   In proper quantities it vomits with much vio. lence, produces heartburn, faintness, dizziness, diminished vision, and great prostration of strength.   Snuffed into the nose it excites sneezing, and applied externally, in diseases of the skin, or to the surface of ulcers, it irritates, promotes absorption, and changes ac. tion.   It may therefore be considered as tonic, deobstruent, emet. ics, narcotic, sternutatory, antipsoraic, and escharotic.   It may, therefore be made to produce the most useful effects of squill and senega, without their tendency to vomit and purge ; of fox-glove without danger of prostrating the powers of life ; of ammoniacum and guiacum without their occasional irritation, and of the mineral tonics without their slowness."

Dr. Ansel W. Ives of this City considers its peculiar and chief remedial excellence to consist " in subduing phlegmasial diseases of the respiratory organs, after they have arrived at that period in their progress, when depletion with the lancet can be carried no far. ther ; when inflammatory excitement is suspended by excessive irri. tability."   In such a condition of the system he has witnessed the happiest effects from its use in every species of cynanche pneumo. nia, pertussis, and particularly in incipient pulmonary phthisis.†

My own experience with this article, although not very extensive, is decidedly in its favour, if it is employed promptly and early after bloodletting.   In cases of subacute bronchitis in children, which will not always bear very active depletion, I have found much benefit from its employment in moderating the excitement and restoring the

* New-England Journal of Medicine and Surgery vol 8th p. 160.
† Paris Pharmacologia Ives' Edition vol. ii.

secretions. I have generally used calomel simultaneously and, I believe, that as is the case with colchicum, this combination of two deobstruents promotes the respective action of each.

NOTE S—PAGE 207.

On the use of Purgatives in Thoracic Inflammation.* The administration of purgatives has been pronounced by some of the most eminent writers on the theory and practice of medicine, not only to be not beneficial, but even positively injurious in all inflammations of the viscera of the chest. Of these writers, some do indeed forbid their use in the second stage only of these diseases, or when expectoration is already freely established ; but there are not wanting others who condemn their employment altogether, throughout every stage of pulmonary inflammation. As my own experience has led me to form different and far more favourable views of the powers of this class of medicines in subduing inflammation of the lungs and its membranes, I have been induced to enter into a critical examination of the arguments upon which their indiscriminate denunciation is founded ; and, also, to inquire whether there is not sufficient authority to be found in their favour, to counterbalance the influence of the writers to whom I have alluded. The result is not uninteresting, and I proceed to offer it without further preface.

Cullen, with his usual moderation, observes in the 370th section of his First Lines : "Some practitioners have doubted if purgatives can be safely employed in this disease, (*pneumonia* ;) and, indeed, a spontaneous diarrhœa, occurring in the beginning of the disease, has seldom proved useful ; but I have found the moderate use of cooling laxatives generally safe, and have always found it useful to keep the belly open by frequent emollient glysters."† And again, in section 381, in speaking of peripneumonia notha : "Purging may indeed be useful ; but as it is seldom so in pneumonic affections, nothing but gentle laxatives are here necessary." It will appear from these extracts, that Cullen, although not inclined to use purges in pneumonic affections, does not, in this place, adduce any important objection against their use ; excepting indeed, we admit,

---

* It may not be irrelevant to state that the observations which follow were published several years ago in an anonymous form.

† Cullen's First Lines of the Practice of Physic, Vol. I. pp. 136 and 137.

that the supposed injury, from the occurrence of a spontaneous diarrhœa in the beginning of these diseases, constitutes one. I say, *supposed*, because it is by no means an established fact, that injury does arise from such an occurrence. Not to mention other instances, Cleghorn relates, in his account of the pleurisies which prevailed at Minorca, that diarrhœas, though not generally *critical*, did prove beneficial.*—Storck, in his Præcepta Medico-Practica, expressly tells us, that pleurisy is very often cured by the occur-rence of a spontaneous diarrhœa, or enuresis, without the aid of expectoration. " Nonnunquam pauca tantum in quantitate sputa prodeunt, sed diarrhœa simul mitis, mucosa, biliosa et male olens supervenit, aut multa excernitur urina, quæ copiosum sedimentum puriforme deponit, unde morbus *non raro* sine multis sputis *perfecte* sanatur."†

In his Materica Medica, however, Dr. Cullen assigns, as a reason for purging not being useful in the inflammatory diseases of the lungs, the fact that " by emptying the system of the descending aor-ta no considerable derivation can be made from the bronchial arte-ries, in the extremities of which the inflammations of the lungs are seated."‡ There seems to me to be little force in this argument. The institution of a new focus of irritation in so extensive a sur-face as that of the mucous membrane of the intestines, must relieve the affected organ both directly and indirectly : directly, by the abstraction of a large quantity of fluid, previously invited to it by the presence of an irritating cause ; and indirectly, by the lowered tone of the general system induced by the very evacuation from the descending aorta, through the agency of purgatives. It will afterwards be made to appear, that this view is amply confirmed by the practice and authority of no inconsiderable names in medicine.

Thomas, who attempts to follow Cullen as his guide, asserts, that purgatives are improper remedies in these diseases, because " they are found to determine the flow of blood to the internal parts !"§ It would be difficult, I conceive, for the most profound and acute reasoner in medicine to solve the difficulties involved in this ex-planation. I shall, therefore, let it alone, and pass over to the con-sideration of the objections offered by more intelligible writers.

* Cleghorn on the Diseases of Minorca.

† Anton. L. Baron de Storck, Præcepta Med-Practica, etc. tom. 1. p. 111. (1777.)

‡ A Treatise on the Materia Medica, by William Cullen, M. D. Vol. II. page 282.

§ Thomas' Practice of Physic, page 152. [1817.]

I should not, in fact, have noticed this author, had it not been that his book has received such extensive encouragement in this country.

Armstrong, whose practical illustration of diseases will remain as ever-during monuments of his medical skill and theoretical knowledge, condemns the use of purgatives in pneumonic inflammations in the following words: "As copious and frequent purging has a tendency to diminish expectoration, it should hardly ever be enforced in thoracic inflammations, but more especially when the mucous membrane of the bronchia is the seat of the inflammation; because very copious purging then not only checks expectoration, but it most frequently prevents a perspirable state of the skin, which is always most desirable in affections of the bronchia."* He adds, however, that the bowels should be moderately moved, &c.

Before noticing the objections of Armstrong, which comprise all that can be said against the employment of purgatives in thoracic inflammations, it may be proper to observe, that several writers in this country have concurred with the physicians already mentioned in denouncing purgatives. Most of them, as Thacher,† have been satisfied with barely recording their vote in the negative, without assigning any reason whatever for their decision: and even the ingenious Chapman has no more to offer than what is couched in the following extract: "It is a very curious fact, but one fully confirmed by experience, that urged to any extent, evacuations from the bowels are found, in the complaints of the lungs, always mischievous, and in some cases so injurious as to be wholly inadmissible. Even in pleurisy, we cannot purge with the same freedom as in other cases of acute inflammation." It is unnecessary to make any comment on this *curious* passage, except to observe that experience, so far from confirming this fact, actually contradicts it as will be presently shown.

To return, then, to Armstrong: His objections may be reduced to the two following heads: Purgatives are hurtful, first, because they diminish expectoration; and secondly, because they prevent

---

* Practical Illustrations of Typhus Fever, &c. by John Armstrong— from the last London edition, with Notes by an American Physician, p. 132. New-York, 1824.

† Thacher's Modern Practice of Physic, p. 420.

‡ Elements of Therapeutics and Materia Medica, by N. Chapman, 3d edition, Vol. I. p. 183.

perspiration, which is so desirable in pulmonary affections.   With respect to the first objection, if it were intended to apply to the impropriety of administering purgatives in the second stage only of these diseases, it would be allowed on all hands to be not without considerable weight.   But if it is meant to extend to the early stages likewise, it is assuredly unfounded and based on an erroneous view of the nature of these diseases.   It goes entirely upon the supposition, or rather the assumption, that expectoration is indispensable to the cure of thoracic inflammation.   Now that this is by no means the case, can be as clearly demonstrated as any the most undisputed fact in medicine.   Cases have repeatedly come under my observation, in which plentiful bleeding, at the very onset of an attack of pulmonary inflammation, followed forthwith by the most active purging, have in three days, brought about an entire solution of the disease.   It is only within a few days that a case of this kind fell under my notice, in which, after depletion the most active, cathartics were repeated, and with the happiest effect, no expectoration having been present throughout the disease.   I have also seen cases in which, owing to the debility of the patient, bleeding was thought inexpedient, and purging altogether relied on for the evacuant effect necessary to subdue the inflammation, nor was there any inconvenience felt as a consequence of this course of proceeding.   It is not thought proper to relate particular cases, as the history of the disease is too familiar not to render detail superfluous.

The correctness of this view, relating to expectoration, is by no means without support. Sydenham, after laying down his method of cure in pleurisy, adds with his usual simplicity and vigour, "If it be said here, that our method is defective because we are so far from treating amply of the means of promoting expectoration in the different stages of the disease, that we scarce mentioned them ; we reply, that this has not been omitted through negligence, but purposely after mature consideration, as having always thought those to be in great danger who trusted the cure of this disease to expectoration.   For not to mention the tediousness of this method, by which nature endeavours to expel the morbific matter, it is likewise unsafe ; for it often happens, that part of the matter being concocted, and perhaps expectorated, the remainder continues yet crude, and this successively : the most powerfully expectorating medicines having been been ineffectually used."* He afterwards adds, very pertinently, that whereas expectoration is not under his control, bleeding on the other hand brings " the morbific matter" under his own management, " and the orifice of the opened vein may be made to supply the function of the windpipe."

Johnson, when treating of pneumonia, in his very interesting work on the atmosphere, &c. recommends a diminution of the circulating mass of fluids; first, by bleeding from a large orifice, &c.; and " secondly, by purgations, which by acting on the intestinal canal, abstract from the general circulation a very considerable portion of fluid, besides clearing the bowels, and thereby allowing a freer course to the blood through the great vessels, distributed to the various abdominal viscera, as well as the lower extremities."+ Who will hesitate to adopt this view of the action of purgatives, in preference to the unsatisfactory and almost unintelligible one, which we have seen advanced by Cullen? As Johnson justly observes, in the same paragraph from which the above sentence is extracted, " it seems to be the aim of some practitioners rather to moderate than to subdue the inflammatory actions when they rely on the natural process of expectoration for the completion of the cure."

From what has now been offered, I think it must appear evident that the objection to the use of purgatives in pulmonary inflammation, because they prevent expectoration, or diminish its extent, is altogether untenable. It has been observed, that a cure may be effected without the aid of this natural process, and it becomes then equally clear that wherever this can be prevented or obviated, it should be done. Purgatives are then no more objectionable in this genus of the phlegmasiæ, than in any other; and if they are at any time improper, it is in the secondary stages, when expectoration has been permitted to take place. Then it would indeed be highly improper to administer them freely, and on the same principles which forbid their employment in similar stages of other inflammatory affections.

We have still to consider another objection advanced by Armstrong, viz.—that purgatives prevent a perspirable state of the skin, which is so desirable an object in pneumonic inflammations. This

---

* Rush's Sydenham, page 222.

+ On the Atmosphere, &c. embracing Practical Observations on Derangements of the Liver, Internal Organs, &c.—by James Johnson, M. D. page 19.

objection we do not consider more fortunate than the first. That perspiration is desirable in these affections, we do not deny; but we must contend that if relief can be obtained by any other more powerful derivation of fluids from the system at large, and from the particular organs affected, this last should unhesitatingly be preferred. Now that purgatives have this claim to preference, there is none to dispute. So far we seem to admit that perspiration is necessarily prevented by purgation; but is this indeed the case? Let us examine Dr Armstrong's writings for an answer. " The full operation of aperients sometimes reduces the morbid force of the pulse, almost as effectually as the affusion of cold water or venesection; consequences which surely indicate that their action extends further than the mere removal of mere fecal matter from the intestinal canal."[*] Dr. Armstrong will scarcely deny that calomel and the neutral salts, besides their purgative effects, produce a salutary action on the skin, inducing diaphoresis most generally during their operation on the bowels, by means of what Johnson denominates the cutaneo-intestinal sympathy. This sympathy may be daily observed in health, and in disease it is too frequently obtruded on our notice to escape the most ordinary attention. At the same time it will not be denied, that under particular conditions of the system, as where the balance between the ordinary functions of various important organs is destroyed or interrupted, these sympathies may not exert their usual play. And also where purgation is carried to an extreme, diaphoresis may in some instances be checked, but this is not an invariable effect. The debility induced by profuse evacuations more frequently produces a relaxation of the skin, simultaneously with that of the liver, &c. This relaxation may not be made evident at once, nay, a contrary effect may at times seem to result, but it will in general be found to be transient, and to give way sooner or later to the effect first mentioned. It is, therefore, not established by any means that al purgatives prevent perspiration from taking place; nay, some of them actually have a tendency to promote this excretion; and may, therefore, be additionally serviceable in relieving the inflammatory or congested condition of the lungs.

If the criticism which has now been attempted be just, it necessarily follows that the denunciation of purgatives in pneumonic inflammation is founded in error, and calculated to deprive the prac-

* Armstrong on Typhus, p. 93.

titioner of one of the most powerful means within his reach, of
wholly subduing this affection. Expectoration, it will have been
seen, may with advantage be wholly prevented, and can only be
desirable when early depletion and evacuation have been omitted
or neglected. When this process has been already established,
then indeed the use of active cathartics would not only be superfluous as to the cure of the disease, but likely to prove injurious, especially where there is much debility present or the complaint has
been protracted.

NOTE S—PAGE 207.

Diagnosis of pneumonic diseases. I regret to find that Dr. Gregory notices the invaluable labours of Læennec in a manner so
slight, as to induce the suspicion that he is either not acquainted
with their extent, or that he is wedded to the antiquated prejudices which reject any essential improvement because patience,
industry and perseverance, are required to attain a knowledge
of its practical application. In the present state of medical
science that practitioner who refuses to avail himself of the almost infallible means of distinguishing the different diseases of the
chest by means of auscultation and percussion commits a positive
breach of the duty which he owes to his fellow creatures and his
own moral and scientific reputation. How often are certain forms
of pulmonary inflammation mistaken for hydrothorax, and necessarily mismanaged. Drs. Graves and Stokes inform us in their valuable essays published in the fourth volume of the Dublin Hospital Reports, that numerous cases have been sent into the medical
wards of the Meath hospital by practitioners, who had named and
treated them as cases of simple hydrothorax ; but in no instance
did they find this diagnosis correct, and often did they succeed in
saving the life of such a patient by the bold use of the lancet. Difficulties of no ordinary nature obstruct the acquisition of a requisite
knowledge of the uses and application of the stethoscope in private
practice, but in our hospitals and our infirmaries the facilities are
great and should not be thrown away through indolence, incompe-
tency, or indifference. I conceive that the profession in the United
States is under special obligations to Dr. A. L. Peirson of Salem,
Mass. for the laudable and successful attempt he has made to promote and diffuse a knowledge of this all important subject by his
edition of Colin's valuable "manual for the use of the stethoscope

and by the very pertinent and lucid introductory remarks with which he has accompanied it.

To assist in this object I shall here introduce, from Martinets useful treatise of pathology, such extracts as will assist the student in understanding the terms and appearances so often made use of, and referred to, by writers of the present day.

METHOD OF EXAMINATION APPLICABLE TO DISEASES OF THE CHEST.

After having examined the external conformation of the thorax, and inquired whether pain is felt in any particular part, and learned its seat and character, we should proceed to investigate the phenomena which result—

1st, From the act of respiration ;

2d, Those which depend on the voice ;

3d, The product of expectoration ;

4th, The symptoms given by percussion ;

5th, Those which are referrible to the heart and its connexions.

OF THE PHENOMENA WHICH RESULT FROM THE ACT OF RESPIRATION.

In Health.—Inspiration and expiration are performed slowly and with ease, none of the muscles appearing to make any particular effort ; they succeed each other regularly, their rythm is constant and uniform; all the ribs are alternately elevated and depressed, and the dilatation and contraction are equal at both sides, except in cases of deformity of the thorax. Respiration in children is performed in a great degree, by the motion of the ribs alone ; in adults, by that of the ribs and diaphragm ; and by this last muscle alone, in old persons in whom the cartilages have become ossified.

The younger the subject is, the more frequent is the respiration. Thus, during the first year, an infant respires about thirty-five times in a minute, but an adult makes about eighteen or twenty respirations in the same time. Its frequency is greater in women and persons of a nervous or irritable habit.

In Disease.—The movements of the chest present many varieties, which may be referred to the following heads : They may be frequent or unfrequent, quick or slow, regular or irregular, great or small, equal or unequal, easy or difficult, complete or incomplete ; and, finally, the respiration may be abdominal or thoracic. All these phenomena are within the reach of the ordinary means of examination; but auscultation conducts us to the knowledge of others which we now proceed to detail.

Auscultation may be made either by applying the ear to the walls of the thorax, or by means of the stethoscope invented by Laennec.

Immediate auscultation is more particularly useful to persons who have not acquired much experience in this mode of examination; for when the phenomena havebeen rendered sensible by the application of the ear, and the observer has formed some idea of them, it becomes more easy for him to seize their minute shades, than if he had commenced in the first instance by employing the stethoscope. However, it should be remembered that there are cases in which the use of the instrument is altogether indispensible, where, in fact, the ear cannot be applied; for instance, immediately above and below the clavicle, in the hollow of the axilla, and beneath the mammæ in females. Besides, the head can scarcely follow the movements of the chest, as it is elevated and depressed; and even if it could, the friction it produces must render the sound somewhat confused.

When using the stethoscope, it should be held like a writing pen, the fingers being so placed on the instrument, as to feel at once its extremity, and the point of the thorax to which it is to be applied. · It should be also placed evenly upon the surface, and perpendicular to it.

Before we begin the examination, or at all events before we note its results, we should wait until any impression this process may have made on the patient shall have passed away; for if this precaution be necessary in examining the state of the circulation by means of the pulse, it is no less so when investigating the respiration by the stethoscope. The phenomena which exists in the healthy state of the organs should first be studied, in order that they be not confounded with those which are produced by disease; and that their various changes may be accurately estimated, or their absence determined, which is by no means an unusual occurrence.

Examination of the Respiration in the healthy State.—When examining the respiration, the funnel should be removed from the end of the cylinder. On applying its extremity to the chest, we perceive in a healthy adult, during inspiration and expiration, a slight, though distinct murmur, marking the entrance of the air into the cells, and its passage out of them. This murmur is loud in proportion to the depth and frequency of the respiraton—to the youth of the subject, to the thinness of the walls of the thorax, and completeness of their dilatation. In females it is more strongly marked than in males, and still more so in children, whence the term "*puerile*" is applied to respiration when it becomes very sonorous.

The respiratory murmur is most perceptible in the hollow of the axilla, in the space between the anterior border of the trapezius muscle and the clavicle, immediately beneath this bone, and at the inferior and posterior part of the chest ; for these are the parts in which the lungs are nearest to the surface. Opposite the trachea, larynx and root of the brochi, the sound of the respiration is much more loud and distinct ; it is not unlike that of a bellows, and gives the idea of a considerable column of air passing through a tube of large diameter; the air also appears as if sucked in from the cylinder, during inspiration, and expelled again during expiration. To this peculiar sound the term "*tracheal* respiration" is applied.

Examination of the Respiration in Disease.—The respiratory murmur may be stronger or weaker than natural, may be altogether suppressed or heightened, so as to resemble what we have described as the "*tracheal*" respiration ; and lastly, it may be pure, or mixed with some of those various sounds, to which the term "*rale*" has been applied.

When the respiration becomes more strong than natural, it assumes the character it manifests in children, and therefore is termed by Laennec "*puerile respiration.*" This intensity of sound is not owing to a lesion of the part of the lung in which it is heard ; on the contrary, it is heard only in the healthy parts, whose action becomes momentarily increased to supply that of the diseased parts. Thus in pneumonia, we usually find the "puerile" respiration, in those portions of the lung which are not yet attacked by the inflammation.

As the respiratory murmur presents a number of varieties even in the healthy state, it is only by comparing different parts of the lungs that we can judge of any diminution of its intensity that may occur. It is always easy to make this comparison; for the respiration is seldom weakened in the entire of the lung, or in both lungs at the same time. Bdt its degrees vary from a slight weakening of its natural intensity to total suppression. A diminution of the movements of the thorax seems to be the most usual cause of this weakening of the respiratory murmur ; it sometimes arises from a partial obstruction of the smaller bronchial tubes, either by a thickening of their mucous membrane, or by the presence of some viscid matter. It is also found to occur in cases in which false membranes are yet soft and just beginning to be organized.

Complete suppression of the respiratory murmur arises from various causes. It occurs when the lung becomes impermeable to the air, or when there is interposed between it and the walls of the thorax any liquid or gaseous exhalation, which prevents the sound from being transmitted. It seldom happens that the sound is suppressed through the whole extent of a side of the chest. Some trace of it can almost always be discovered near the clavicles, and opposite the root of the lung ; and probably it is never altogether inaudible at the latter of these points.

When treating of the natural phenomena, we described the "tracheal" respiration, and indicated the points in which it is heard. It sometimes happens that a similar sound is emitted from other parts, besides those in which it is audible during health. This occurs either when there are cavities of a certain extent communicating freely with the bronchi ; or when the tissue of the lung becomes indurated, and so transmits more readily the sounds which the air produces in passing through the large bronchial tubes. In the parts of the lung which remain unaffected, we find that the respiration has become "puerile."

The respiratory murmur, whatever be its degree of intensity, may be pure, which indicates that the air tubes are free from obstruction ; or it may be blended, and as it were disguised by other sounds, to which the term "rale" has been applied. By "rale" or rattle, is understood any sound produced by the circulation of the air in the bronchi and air-vesicles, different from that murmur which it determines in the healthy state.*

---

* Some seem disposed to use the English translations of these terms. It appears, however, preferable to adopt at once the terms devised by Læn-nec, which will save us from having new translations of them, according to the whim or the fancy of particular persons. The inconvenience of this practice should it become general, will soon be rendered apparent, as histo-ries of cases begin to be published, containing statements of the signs furnish-ed by the stethoscope. For all these consist of simple ideas, if each of them be not marked by a term precise and definite, it will lead to endless con-fusion and discrepancy. The terms devised by Laennec, are purely terms of art—and if we paraphrase or translate them, we can never be sure that they will excite in the minds of hearers or readers the precise ideas which he meant them to express, and which we seek to convey.—T.

The "rale" seldom occupies the entire extent of the lung ; they are usually audible only in a certain part of it, the respiration remaining natural, or becoming "*puerile*" in the rest. They indicate either a contraction of some part of the bronchial tubes, or the presence of a fluid which obstructs them or the air-vesicles. The " rales" are divided into four species ;—1st, the " rale muquex ;" 2d, " rale sonore ;" 3d, " rale sibilant ;" 4th, " rale crepitant."

The "rale muqueux," or mucous rattle, is produced by the passage of the air through sputa accumulated in the bronchi or trachea, or through softened tubercular matter. The character of the sound indicates that the fluid, which fills up the air-tubes, is unctious but not tenacious. Sometimes it is weak, and audible only from time to time, at others it is rather loud and continuous. In the former case the air meets only at intervals portions of mucus, which determine the sound ; in the latter the bronchi are almost entirely filled with it. When carried to a very high degree, it constitutes a gurgling, or, "*gargouillement.*" This is the term that has been applied to the loud murmur, which is produced by the agitation of the matter of tubercles, or puriform sputa, by the passage of air through them. This " rale" occurs in catarrh and in softened tubercle.

The "*rale sonore,*" consists of a sound more or less grave, and occasionally very loud, resembling sometimes the snoring of a person asleep, at others the sound of the base string of an instrument when rubbed by the finger, and not unfrequently the cooing of a dove. It seems to be caused by a contraction of the bronchial tubes, by a thickening of their mucous membrane, or by some change in the form of these canals, induced probably by the thickening of the spur-like processes or folds of membrane at the points of division of the bronchi ; at least this change is almost constantly observable in subjects that have died during the existence of chronic catarrh, of which this " rale" is characteristic.

The " *rale sibilant,*" consists of a slight, though prolonged, hissing sound, which occurs either at the termination or commencement of inspiration. It may be grave or acute, dull or sonorus. These two varieties may exist at the same time in different parts of the lung, or may succeed each other at variable intervals, in the same part. It is owing to the presence of mucus, thin, and viscid, but not abundant, which obsrtucts, more or less completely, the smaller bronchial ramifications, which the air has to pass through before it arrives at the air-cells. This "rale" seems to indicate a more serious affection of the lungs than the one last described, inasmuch as it is seated in the more minute bronchial ramifications; hence, when it extends to any considerable portion of the lung, it is attended by great difficulty of respiration. It is during the existence of this "rale" that the sputa present that aborescent appearance, which resembles so much the form, dimensions, and ramifications of the small bronchial tubes, from which they have been expelled by the efforts of coughing. It occurs in the first stage of bronchitis.

The "*rale crepitant*" resembles very accurately the crackling or crepitation of salt, when thrown into a heated vessel, or that emitted by a piece of dried lung, when pressed between the fingers. It depends on an exhalation of blood on the internal surface of the air-cells, such as occurs in the first stage of pneumonia, of which this "rale" is the distinctive sign. It occurs also in hæmoptysis and œdema of the lungs.

These are the different "rales" which the stethoscope enables us to recognize. It would appear from this description of them, that their characters are so strongly marked, that they cannot be confounded or mistaken one for the other; but still it frequently happens that their differences are not so striking, and that they glide into each other, by a sort of transition indicative of a mixed lesion, or one more nearly allied to one than the other. It is by habit and practice alone that we can learn to appreciate these shades; words cannot convey an adequate idea of them.

OF THE PHENOMENA WHICH DEPEND ON THE VOICE.

When examining the voice, the funnel should be retained in the extremity of the cylinder, and then the phenomena will be found to vary: 1st, according to the points at which they are examined; and, 2d, according to the natural character of the voice.

When a person speaks or sings, his voice thrills in the interior of the chest, and produces in its whole extent a trembling motion, which we can readily perceive on the application of the hand. This phenomenon is not of much importance, and seldom demands any particular attention. However, when a large cavity happens to exist, the trembling becomes so forcible, as of itself to make us suspect its existence. When the cylinder is applied to the thorax, we hear a confused resonance of the voice, the intensity of which varies in different points of its extent. It is most distinctly heard in the arm-pit, at the back, between the internal border of the scapula and the vertebral column, and anteriorly at the angle formed by the clavicle with the strenum. We do not hear any thing distinct or articulate, it is rather a sound more or less confused, which seems to waste itself against the walls of the thorax. In other parts of the chest, particularly posteriorly and inferiorly, the sound is much more weak, and produces only an indistinct murmur. It is in all cases rendered more manifest where old adhesions exist.

In persons whose voice is deep and grave, the degree of resonance is greater, but it is confused, and nearly equal at all points of the thorax; but in females and children, whose voice is acute, it is clear and distinct.

In Disease, the phenomena furnished by the voice are referrible to three heads; Resonance, Pectoriloquy, and Ægophony. By the term resonance, is understood a thrilling of the voice more loud than natural, or its existence in a part in which it is not heard during health. It sometimes becomes so strong as that the sound seems to be produced at the very extremity of the cylinder which is placed on the thorax, but it never conveys the impression as if it traversed the length of the tube to reach the ear of the observer. A thickened and hardened state of the lung, caused either by a mass of crud tubercles, or by inflammation, produces this phenomenon, by rendering the lung a better conductor of the murmur of the voice in the bronchi. Hence the origin of the term "*broncophony.*" This symptom, though not usually of much importance, becomes occasionally of considerable value : when it co-exists with phenomena furnished by other means of examination, and also as enabling us to make a comparison between the state of the two sides of the thorax.

Pectoriloquy.—This phenomenon is said to exist when the voice of the patient, distinctly articulated seems to issue from the point of the chest on which the cylinder is applied, and traverses its whole length to strike the ear of the observer, with its natural tone, or probably more strongly. These are the circumstances which constitute *perfect* pectoriloquy ; but it admits of two other degrees, namely, the *imperfect* and the *doubtful*. It is termed *imperfect* when the voice thrills strongly under the cylinder, seems to approach the ear, but never traverses the whole length of the tube. And, lastly, it is said to be *doubtful*, when the voice seems acute and suppressed like that of a ventriloquist, and is arrested at the thoracic ex-

89

tremity of the tube, thus approaching to the character of simple resonance.

Pectoriloquy presents some varieties, which depend on the tone of the voice, the size and form of the excavations, the firmness of their walls, the degree of facility with which the air can penetrate them; and finally, the existence or non-existence of adhesions with the pleura costalis.

The more acute the voice is, the more evident does the pectoriloquy become; hence in persons whose voice is grave and deep, the thrilling or vibration of the walls of the thorax may be sufficiently intense to mask it, and render it doubtful.

In cases of aphonia, the pectoriloquy is not entirely suppressed. It sometimes occurs that we can distinguish better what the patient endeavours to express, by placing the cylinder on the point corresponding to the excavation in the lung, than we can by the naked ear at the same distance.

The pectoriloquy is sensibly affected by the size of the cavities. Thus, when they are unusually large, it becomes changed into a very full and grave sound, similar to that of the voice transmitted to some distance through a tube, or cone of paper. In very small cavities, on the contrary, it bebomes doubtful, particularly when the parts of the lung which surround them, are still permable to the air.

The more dense and firm the walls of the excavation are, the more perfect is the pectoriloquy. It sometimes acquires even a metallic tone when the cavity has become lined by a membrane, whose structure approaches that of fbro-cartilage.

It is also rendered very distinct when the cavity is superficial, and its walls thin, and adherent to the pleura costalis; but when there is no adhesion, and the sides of the cavity become compressed together during expiration, the pectoriloquy becomes doubtful; the existence of the exeavation must then be ascertained by other symptoms.

Again, its force becomes increased, and the voice seems as if transmitted through a tube when new cavities begin to communicate with those already existing; but if the excavations become very numerous and tortuous, the sound is rendered somewhat confused and indistinct.

The less liquid the cavity contains, the more evident is the pectoriloquy, for then the communication with the bronchi is usually open, and allows a free passage to the air.

If this communication be obstructed for any time by the ac.
cumulation of matter in the bronchi, the pectoriloquy is rendered
doubtful, and acquires somewhat of an intermittent character.

It sometimes happens that we can find scarcely a single individual with pectoriloquy in the wards of a hospital, though at
the previous visit there had been several ; in such cases, we observe that in the greater number of the patients, the expectoration
had been very much diminished or altogether suppressed.

Ægophony.—This phenomenon consists of a strong resonance
of the voice, which is more acute and sharp than that of the patient, but never seems to traverse the cylinder as pectoriloquy
does ; its tone is thrilling and tremulous, like that of a goat ; whence
the term is derived.

Though its limits are usually circumscribed, they are not so
much so as those of pectoriloquy ; it is found between the base
of the scapula and the vertebral column, towards the inferior angle
and external border of that bone, and sometimes in the direction of
a line, which may be conceived to pass from its centre to the strenum, following the direction of the ribs. When ægophony exists at
both sides at the same time, it is difficult to determine whether it is
produced by disease ; for in some persons the natural resonance of
the voice presents this acute and tremulous character at the root of
the lungs. If old adhesions exist at one side of the chest, the
ægophony becomes much more evident.

Ægophony, though it may vary in its force and extent, always
indicates the existence, in the cavity of the pleura, of a moderate quantity of fluid, or of false membranes, somewhat thick and
soft ; it ceases when the effusion becomes too considerable ; hence
in the former case it indicates pleurisy in its first stage : and in the
latter, it marks its passage to the chronic state, if the general
symptoms still continue after the cessation of the ægophony ; but
it is not a sign of its resolution, if these symptoms cease as it disappears.

Ægophony does not prevent us altogether from hearing the
respiratory murmur, when it is not suppressed by hepatization of
the lung.

The *Metallic tingling— Respiration* and *Resonance* are very
remarkable phenomena, with which we shall conclude this account
of the signs furnished by the voice and respiration.

The metallic tingling, or " tintement metallique," resembles the
sound produced by any very small hard body striking against a

metallic or glass cup.   When the phenomenon is not so strongly
marked, it produces only the *metallic resonance* , lastly, the respiration also may assume this character, in which case it resembles the
murmur produced by air blown into a metallic vessel with a narrow
aperture ; these different sounds cease occasionally for a short time,
but recur soon after.

The metallic tingling occurs when there exists a large excavation filled with air and fluid, communicating with the bronchi,
and is heard when the patient coughs or speaks.

The metallic respiration occurs when there is a fistulous communication between the bronchi and the cavity of the pleura.

The metallic resonance and respiration indicate, in addition
to the fistulous communication between the bronchi and pleura, an
effusion of a gaseous fluid into the cavity of that membrane.

When the metallic tingling occurs together with the metallic resonance and respiration, it denotes the existence of a vast excavation, whose walls are thin, adherent and compact.

OF THE EXPECTORATION.

In the Healthy State, the expectoration consists of a viscid, ropy fluid, which is transparent, colourless, inodourous, insipid, and
exists only in sufficient quantity to moisten the inner surface of the
air passages.

In Disease, the sputa sometimes consist of a transparent, limpid, and slightly viscid fluid, the consistence of which gradually
increases, until it ultimately becomes changed into an opaque, yellow, or greenish mucous matter, such as usually occurs in pulmo
nary catarrh.

In other cases, the expectoration is composed of a transparent mucous fluid, so tenacious as to adhere closely to the bottom
of the vessel in which it is deposited, even when it is inverted.
This may be marked by bloody striæ, or the blood may be combined with it in greater or less quantity, so that its colour varies
from a yellow slightly tinged with red, to that of the deepest ma-
hogany.   These are the characters of the expectoration in acute
pneumonia.

We sometimes observe the product of expectoration to consist of a frothy, colourless fluid, containing, suspended, several
portions of a flocculent matter, or presenting on its surface some
yellow, rounded, purulent masses, in greater or less quantity : in
other cases it is composed of a mucous matter, marked by striæ of

a dull white colour. These varieties occur during the early stages of pulmonary tubercles. As the disease advances the quantity of the yellow diffluent fluid increases, and ultimately forms the whole of the matter expectorated. It sometimes contains bubbles of air, and presents more or less the characters of pus. Such is the expectoration in the last stage of phthisis.

In some cases the sputa are ejected forcibly, and in large quantity at a time, so that the patients seem to vomit them. This occurs when an effusion into the cavity of the thorax finds an exit through the bronchi.

Again, we sometimes observe portions of false membrane expectorated, either in the form of lamellæ, or moulded into that of the bronchial tubes, trachea, or larynx. This is characteristic of croup.

Lastly, the expectoration may consist of pure blood, sometimes of a bright, at others of a dark red colour, as occurs in hæmoptysis. When a large quantity is brought up at a time, we should take care to examine whether the blood is frothy, and accompanied by cough, as these are the symptoms which distinguish hæmoptysis from hæmatemesis.

In all cases the observer should ascertain whether the sputa exhale any particular odour, particularly when the general symptoms induce him to suspect the existence of gangrene of the lung, or of a tubercular cavity, or collection of pus, which may have opened a passage for itself from the pleura into the bronchi.

In cases of gangrene of the lungs, the sputa are as dark as the lees of wine, or greenish; and the odour is so strong as to prevent any mistake as to their real character.

OF PERCUSSION.

The value of percussion, as a mode of examination, has not been by any means diminished by the discovery of auscultation. It is still considered a very efficient means of distinguishing diseases of the chest. Though it appears to be a very simple operation, it requires some precautions in performing it, so as to obtain satisfactory results. The fingers should be semi-flexed, their extremities placed closely together, and so adjusted as to be on the same plane, none of them passing beyond the others. In this way they are made to strike the chest perpendicularly, the integuments being made tense by the fingers of the other hand. The percussion should be made alternately on the corresponding points of each

side of the chest, with the same degree of force and same angle of
incidence. The wrist should be free and unrestrained, so as not
to strike too forcibly and cause pain. Percussion may occasionally
be made, by striking the walls of the thorax with the hand flat and
extended ; but in this case allowance must be made for the sound
emitted by skin.

The position of the patient should also be properly adjusted.
He should be made to sit upright, his arms being carried backwards when the anterior part of the chest is to be examined ; elevated towards his head, when percussion is being made on the lateral parts, or crossed in front, whilst we strike the back. He should
at the same time be directed to bend forwards, so as to give the
back an arched position. These several measures are intended for
the purpose of rendering tense the muscles which cover the walls
of the thorax.

The condition of the external parts should be attended to ;
thus the sound will be more clear when the patient is thin and his
fibres dry, than when he happens to be very fat, or when the flesh
is soft and flaccid ; but if the integuments be infiltrated by a serous effusion, no sound will be emitted, on percussion.

The sound is more clear when we make percussion on those
parts that are covered merely by the skin, or by thin and tense
muscles; for instance, on the clavicles, or immediately below
them to the distance of two fingers' breadth on the sternum ;—
towards the cartilages of the ribs, within the margins of the axilla
as far as the third rib, and posteriorly on the angles of those bones ;
—on the spine of the scapula, and, in thin subjects, on its supra
and infra spinous fossæ.

The sound must obviously be dull at the region of the heart,
opposite the mammæ in females, and great pectoral muscle in
males ; and also inferiorly at the right side, in consequence of the
position of the liver ; at the left side, on the contrary, the sound is
rendered more clear by its vicinity to the stomach, particularly if
that viscus be distended by flatus.

In Disease, the sound emitted by the chest, frequently becomes altered, being rendered dull, obscure, or even totally suppressed ; or, on the contrary, may become more clear than in the
natural state ; so much so, as in some instances to give rise to a
gurgling, or even a metallic tingling. When this phenomenon occurs, it is observed most usually beneath the clavicles. This exaltation of sound occurs when the lungs contain a greater quantity

of air than is natural, or when this fluid is effused into the cavity of the pleura.

When the elasticity of the lung is diminished by its becom-ing infiltrated, without at the same time losing altogether its per-meability to the air, the sound is rendered dull or obscure, ac-cording to the degree in which the pulmonary tissue is affected. This change takes place in cases of intense catarrh, in the first de-gree of pneumonia, and in œdema of the lungs.

The sound is suppressed altogether in the second degree of pneumonia, when the substance of the lung becomes dense and heavy like that of the liver, and so is rendered impermeable to the air. The same effect is produced when the lung is compressed by a fluid effused into the cavity of the pleura, or by the development of any accidental production in its substance. This suppression is, however, but partial in most cases. Its extent depends on that of the effusion, hepatization, or tumour with which it is connected, the remainder of the side still emitting its natural sound on percussion.

When the lung contains an unusual quantity of air, or when an elastic fluid is effused into the pleura, the sound becomes more clear than natural. And lastly, its tone may be increased so as to resemble a metallic tingling, in cases of pulmonary excavations, or pleuritic abscess, which are circumscribed and filled partly with air, partly with fluid.

NOTE T—PAGE 233.

Dysentery. Although this affection is essentially complicated with inflammation, subinflammation, or irritation of the mucous mem-brane of the large intestines, it cannot with impunity be considered a purely local disease. The whole tenor of its history, as detailed by the best writers, Sydenham, Moseley, Pringle, and latterly Johnson, establishes its claim to be ranked among general febrile diseases. This view is still further confirmed by the fact of its occurring epi-demically, of its alternating with periodical fevers, of its varying, like them, in its aspect, in different years and requiring a correspond-ing modification in its methods of treatment. No other view, in fact, can explain the alternate success and failure of the same plans of treatment boldly employed to their fullest extent. The last of the authors above enumerated enjoys the merit of having written the most satisfactory essay which has yet appeared on a disease frequently so terrible in warm climates. The theory adopted by this writer in his valuable treatise on the diseases of tropical climates leads to indications, which, it appears to me, will apply to all the varied forms of dysentery in every season and climate. The disturbance in the functions of the skin and of the liver, the plethora in the cœliac and mesenteric circulation, fever, and finally a vicarious or transferred irritation to the intestines will furnish the rationale of almost every symptom of dysentery. This enlarged and comprehensive theory enables us to combine, or select the differing remedies which have all been recommended upon authority. Certain it is that the indiscriminate employment of any one remedy must be attended with hazard. There are two, however, which appear to have succeeded so often and under such apparently opposite circumstances as to be almost entitled to the character of specifics for dysentery. These are calomel and opium.

Purgatives so strongly insisted on in the text are positively injurious, and I cannot well see how their use is to be defended upon the supposition that dysentery is a simple enteritis. Laxatives are indeed proper and indispensable. Bleeding is frequently indicated but can never be employed to the extent required in ordinary inflammation. The great object of the physician must be to restore the lost balance of the circulation to divert the force of the disease from the internal organs, excite a healthful action in the liver and intestines, and allay the nervous irritability. Mercury and opium alternated with gentle cathartics will, in most cases, fulfil these indications more safely and speedily than all other medicines combined.

Mercury has indeed been denounced as a too irritating application to the inflamed surface of the intestines : But does this article exert no other than a local action on the mucous membranes and does it delay its alterative and deobstruent effects until it has reached the caput coli? Other remedies have, it is true, been occasionally employed with success in this complaint—emetics, sudorifics, ipecacuanha, and even bark. This victory is however seldom obtained except in mild and sporadic cases occurring in healthy seasons and climates, or produced by the agency of causes which are not general in their influence, such as bad food, damp lodging, &c. In severe and epidemic cases where the whole system is subjected to the influence of malaria, and the biliary organs become deeply implicated, these articles will disappoint the practitioner who trusts exclusively to their remedial powers. The most efficient plan of treatment is that which has regard to the epidemic character of the disease, to the state of the constitution and previous habits of the patients, and to the symptoms without regard to any *effects* which may, or may not, be developed after death. As a general rule, it will be advisable, in a subject previously healthy and robust, to abstract blood largely at the onset of the disease, and then to apply leeches to the abdomen and to the anus. The warm bath—calomel alone in scruple doses followed by castor oil,—or calomel and ipecacuanha in small doses with opium alternated by the same mild laxative, mucilaginous drinks, and occasional anodyne enemata will generally subdue this disease in three, five, or seven days. In cases attended by great fulness of stomach, an emetic should precede the use of the above measures. The following is an excellent formula:

> ℞. Submur Hydrargyri, gr. xxxii.
> Pulv. Ipecacuanha, vel,
> Pulv. Antim, gr. xii.
> Opii gr. vi. M.

Divide into eight pills and let one be taken every two, four, or six hours. A dose of the Ol. Ricini or of Epsom salts should be given after every second pill to procure a fecal evacuation. The bolder plan of giving scruple doses of calomel is perfectly safe in this country. I have repeatedly pursued it in this city with the happiest success. To Mr. Sawyer, in 1823, I gave nearly three hundred grains in five days, without any other effect than the complete removal of most aggravated sufferings. No salivation ensued.

NOTE U—PAGE 266.

Erysipelas. One of the best external applications in erysipelas that I have seen employed both in public and private practice is the unguentum hydrargyri. A strip of blistering plaster to the edges of the inflamed surface will often arrest its extension. The general treatment recommended by Dr. Gregory is admirable.

NOTE V—PAGE 335.

Mania. One of the most able authors who has yet written on this disease, so interesting to the intellectual interests of man, is Bayle of France. His work is entitled "Traité des Maladies du Cerveau et ses Membranes." In it are defended the following opinions :

1st. That mental alienation is. for the most part, a symptom of a primitive chronic inflammation of the membranes of the brain.

2. This inflammation is sometimes seated in the external surface

90

of the arachnoidean side of the dura mater ; and sometimes it commences in the pia mater, which is more or less injected, and in the internal or adhering surface of the arachnoid from which it may extend more slowly to its external surface and sometimes even to the arachnoidean side of the pia mater. It affects, almost always, in these cases, the arachnoid of the ventricles. This distinction, which may appear somewhat trivial, is nevertheless of the greatest importance. These two species of chronic inflammation of the encephalic membranes present different anatomical characters, symptoms altogether distinct from each other, and signs which it is impossible to confound. The first is termed, by Bayle, *chronic or latent arachnitis*, because its seat is principally in the arachnoid membrane ; and the second *chronic meningitis*, because it affects simultaneously the pia mater and the arachnoid.

A few very rare cases of mental alienation depend on a specific or sympathetic irritation of the brain.

4. Certain cases of monomania and of melancholy depend primitively on a durable and profound injury of the moral affections, and on a prevailing error, which governs more or less the will of the patient, and becomes the source of delirium. M. Bayle is far from admitting that these species of mental alienation are unconnected with physical disease. He refers simply to their origin which is purely mental, but there are hereditary and constitutional predispositions, and certain effects on the train resulting from these species of alienation which become, in their turn, causes of a particular train of symptoms. Thus there is a constant reaction between the moral and physical faculties.

6. Idiocy depends originally on an innate malformation in the brain, as has been established by the researches of many physicians, especially of M. Esquirol. The great feature, then, of M. Bayle's theory consists in attributing mental diseases to a chronic inflammation of the meninges of the brain.* I observe, with pleasure, that this eminent writer places the name of RUSH in the highest rank of those who have contributed to elucidate the symptomatology and history of maniacal disorders.

*Traite des Maladies du Cervau et de ses Membranes. Par A. L. J Bayle. D. M. &c. &c. A Paris.

Hooping Cough. Ingenious attempts have been made by several authors to identify this affection with inflammation. The attempt to ascertain its seat has however given rise to as much discrepancy as the local views of fever. Thus Watt and Gamage consider it bronchial inflammation, Robertson regards it as cephalitic, and the last of all the writers on the subject, Desruelles, an exclusive, pathologist and Broussaian, wishing to reconcile both parties, announces it to be cephalo bronchitis ! These differences go to prove that this epidemic affection may be complicated with inflammation of this or that organ, but may also exist independently of any one of them.—And this view will alone explain the discrepant views of its nature and the results of the differing and often opposite methods successfully pursued in its treatment. Dr. Gregory's chapter on this disease I consider to be invaluable. His opinion of its contagious character is however too dogmatical, as I hope to prove in my essay on the disease which is soon to be submitted to the public.

NOTE X—PAGE 394.

Diseases of the Heart. Laennec has referred the actions of the heart to four heads ;—1st the extent in which the movements of the heart are perceptible ; 2d, the impulse which they communicate ; 3d, the sound which accompanies them ; 4th, their rythm.

In a healthy man whose heart is properly proportioned, we can distinguish its pulsations only in the præcordial region ; that is, in the space between the cartilages of the fifth and seventh ribs ; and at the inferior part of the sternum. The movement of the left cavities is most perceptible in the former situation, that of the right, in the latter ; but if the sternum be very short, they are sensible even in the epigastrium.

In some corpulent persons we cannot by the hand distinguish the pulsations of the heart, and the space in which we can perceive them by the cylinder, is very limited, being not more than a square inch ; but in emaciated persons, particularly when their chests are narrow, they are heard in a much wider range, namely, in the inferior fourth, or probably three fourths of the sternum, or, occasionally, even along the whole length of that bone, under the left clavicle, and sometimes even as far as the right.

When the stroke of the heart is confined within these bounds, and when it is less strong under the clavicles than in the præcordial region, in persons of that conformation which has been just described, we may still consider the organ as retaining its proper proportions.

The stroke of the heart, will of course, be heard in situations different from those here stated, in cases in which a transposition of the viscera has existed from infancy.

The Impulse.—When one extremity of a stethoscope is placed on the cartilages of the ribs, or base of the sternum, and the ear is applied to the other, a sensation is communicated as if it were elevated by each stroke of the heart ; this is termed its impulse.

It is very slight in a healthy person, particularly if somewhat corpulent ; but even when altogether imperceptible by the hand, it is rendered distinct by the cylinder. In general, it is distinguishable only in the præcordial region, or, at farthest, along the inferior half of tne sternum.

It is most forcible opposite cartilages of the ribs, being the part which corresponds to the point of the heart. Its degree of strength is extremely variable ; we learn, however, by practice, to distinguish when it is more intense than it ought to be.

Of the Sound.—The alternate contractions of the auricles and ventricles emit sounds peculiar to each ; which, though imperceptible by the ordinary means of investigation are rendered quite manifest by the cylinder, no matter how small the volume and force of the organ may be.

In the healthy state, there are two distinct sounds ; one dull and lengthened, coincides with the arterial pulse, and sensation of impulse above described, and therefore indicates the contraction of the ventricles ; the other clear and sudden, somewhat like that of the valve of a bellows, corresponds with the systole of the auricles.

The sound of the right cavities is heard most distinctly opposite the base of the sternum, that of the left at the cartilages of the ribs.

When the walls of the heart happen to be more thin than usual, which may occur in persons who are enjoying uninterrupted health, the pulsations are heard in a greater extent of space than in persons differently constituted, but the sound is always louder in the region of the heart than in any other part. In such persons we also observe that the contraction of the auricles is more audible under the clavicles than that of the ventricles, which is not the case either at the base of the sternum, or cartilages of the ribs.

In some cases, the anterior border of the lung is prolonged in front of the pericardium, which renders the sound of the auricles more dull than that of the ventricles, but still not so much so as to make it indistinct. This evidently arises from its being masked by the murmur of respiration, or by that of the air forced out from this process of the lung, by the compression exerted upon it by the heart.

Rythm*.—The movements of the heart are performed in a determinate order, which constitutes their rythm. Each contraction of the ventricles coincides with the dilatation of the arteries, and is accompanied by a dull, prolonged sound ; this is instantly followed by a clear and rather quick sound, which is owing to the contraction of the auricles ; a moment of repose succeeds, when the ventricle again acts, and so the succession goes on.

OF THE PHENOMENA FURNISHED BY THE HEART.

In Disease.—When treating of the derangements of the heart, we shall follow the arrangement adopted when considering its actions in health.

Extent.—the pulsations of this organ are sometimes heard beyond the limits above assigned to them, or they may be restricted

---

* By means of the stethoscope, we can analyse the heart's action, and assign the time occupied by the contraction of each of its cavities. When the instrument is applied to the præcordial region, we hear first a dull, lengthened sound, synchronous with the arterial pulse, and therefore produced by the contraction of the ventricles, this is instantly succeeded (without any interval) by a sharp, quick sound, like that of a valve, or the lapping of a dog ; this corresponds to the interval between two pulsations, and therefore marks the contracsion of the auricles ; then comes the interval of repose. The relative duration of these three periods may be thus stated— one half or somewhat less may be assigned to the contraction of the ventricles—a quarter or a little more to that of the auricles—the remainder for the repose.—According to this statement, if we take any given period, say 24 hours, we at once are compelled to conclude that the ventricles are in action 12 hours, and therefore rest 12 hours, the auricles are in action 6 hours, and rest 18 hours.

This calculation is applicable to a healthy adult, whose pulse beats 70 strokes in a minute. It assumes, what some will be disposed to deny, that the heart is passive in its dilation—but opinions on the subject are so various that it would be impossible to give any summary of them in a note.— T :—See Laennec, Vol. 2.

and confined to a very limited portion of the walls of the thorax.

The increase of extent is perceptible, first along the left side from the axilla to the region of the stomach, then for the same space at the right side, next at the posterior part of the left; and, finally, but very rarely, in the same region of the right side; the intensity of the sound becoming progressively less in the order here indicated.

The possibility of thus perceiving the pulsations of the heart in these different points always indicates a diminution of the thickness of its walls, particularly those of the ventricles. It also marks a weakness or dilatation of the organ, which in the latter case strikes the sternum and ribs with a large surface. However, it should not be forgotten, that similar effects are occasionally produced by causes altogether independent of any affection of the heart; for instance, narrowness of the chest, emaciation, hepatization of the lung, or its compression by a liquid or gaseous effusion, the presence of an excavation with firm walls, nervous agitation, fever, or, in a word, by any thing that can increase the frequency of the pulse.

Sometimes the pulsations of the heart are distinguishable only in a very circumscribed extent of space. This is a more rare occurrence than the preceding, and is produced by an increased thickness of its walls.

It sometimes happens that we perceive the pulsations more distinctly at the right side than at the left, or more high or low than usual. These variations are determined by the existence of a fluid or tumour at one side of the thorax, in the mediastinum, or in the cavity of the abdomen; and finally, the seat of the pulsation may vary, being perceptible now in one place, now in another.

The Impulse.—As the intensity of the impulsion communicated by the heart varies very much during health, it becomes difficult to decide positively upon its absolute increase or diminution in disease, unless it be very strongly marked, or be more manifest at one side than the other, which is the deviation most usually found to exist. This increase is sometimes very slight, but in some cases becomes so great as to elevate the walls of the thorax so strongly, as to render this movement perceptible at a considerable distance. This is the pathognomic sign of hypertrophy of the heart.

The force of the impulse is directly proportioned to the thickness of the walls of the ventricles, and therefore, to the narrowness of the limit within which their contractions are audible.

When the ear is appiled to a stethoscope laid on the cartilages of the ribs, a jerking motion is communicated to it, which is strongly felt by the observer, and manifest to all around him.

Whatever increases the activity of the circulation, such as walking, running, fever, &c., may momentarily determine this state ; and causes of an opposite tendency, rest, bleeding, &c., produce the contrary effect: hence, when we want to examine a patient, we should wait until a perfect calm is established.

The diminution of the heart's impulse is never so strongly marked as its increase. It depends sometimes on the weakness of the organ and the thinness of its walls, and therefore occurs in ca-ses in which its contractions are perceptible in a wide extent of space ; at others, it is produced by extreme embarrassment of the respiration and difficulty of the pulmonary circulation, and then may co-exist with a well-marked hypetrophy ; we also observe this diminution to occur towards the close of this latter disease. Cer-tain emotions, such as fear and depressing passions, may also pro-duce it.

Of the Sound.—The sound of the heart's contractions may become more dull, or more clear and loud than natural ; or sounds altogether new may be produced, which bear no similitude to any that are emitted in the healthy state of the organ. A diminution of the intensity of the sound is caused by an increased thickness of the walls of the heart ; but if it occurs together with a weakness of the impulsion, it indicates a " ramollissement," or softening of its structure.

The alteration most usually observed, is an increased loud-ness and clearness of the sound, which always denotes a thinness of the walls of the heart. This may be emitted by the auricles or by the ventricles. The place in which it is audible marks its seat, and the time determines whether it arises from the contraction of the auricles, or that of the ventricles.

As to the sounds, which possess no similitude with any that occur during health, a knowledge of which is necessary as a means of distinguishing several of the derangements of the heart, they may be referred to the three following heads :—

" *Bruit de Souflet,*" or a sound like that of a bellows. Its name accurately expresses the character of this phenomenon. It may accompany the contraction of the ventricles, auricles, or large arteries : it may be continued or intermittent ; the slightest cause being sufficient to induce its return after it has ceased. It is observable sometimes in hysterical and nervous persons, and also in those disposed to hæmorrhagies, even though there is no alteration of the functions or struture of the heart; however, in other instances, it co-exists with affections of that organ.

"*Bruit de Rape,*" or sound of a file. This, like the former, may occur during the contraction of either of the cavities of the heart, but it is not intermittent; when once developed, it invariably continues with, however, some occasional changes in its degree of force. The contraction of the auricles or the ventricles, is more prolonged than natural, and emits a sound, hard, rough, and as it were, stifled.

This phenomenon indicates a contraction of the orifices by cartilaginous deposits or ossification of the valves. The place and time in which it is heard, indicate its situation. If it coincides with the systole of the ventricles, the contraction exists in the sigmoid valves: if, on the contrary, it occurs during the contraction of the auricles, it occupies the auriculo-ventricular opening.

"*Craquement de Cuir,*" or sound like the crackling of new leather, was observed by M. Collin in a case of pericarditis, of which he looks on it as symptomatic.

Rythm.—The contraction of the ventricles may be lengthened beyond their ordinary duration, so may that of the period of repose also; this indicates hypertrophy of these cavities which is the more considerable, as the time of the contraction is the more prolonged.

In other cases, on the contrary, the contractions are found to be more rapid, and the repose more short than natural, this variation may coincide with quickness, or even with slowness of the pulse, and is not considered as indicative of any morbid alteration.

The time of the systole of the auricles is rarely observed to be lengthened, or shortened. Their contraction seems sometimes, to anticipate that of the ventricles particularly during palpitation, the consequence of which is that the sound of the auricles is masked by that of the ventricles, and in cases of strongly marked hypertrophy becomes altogether imperceptible.

Sometimes, during one systole of the ventricles, the auricles may make two or three contractions, or, on the contrary, while the auricles are making one, the ventricles may make two, within the time of an ordinary contraction. These phenomena do not mark any particular lesion; the pulse even, does not participate in their anomalies.

We sometimes observe several equal contractions followed by one or more, which are shorter and quicker than the rest, or by a perceptible pause constituting an intermittence ;—this should be considered as indicative of disease.

Sometimes again, the contractions are so frequent and irregular, that it is impossible to analyse them; this is always connected with some organic affection.

After having examined the heart, attention should be directed towards the region of the sternum and the first ribs on the right side, to ascertain whether there are any pulsations determined by an aneurism of the arch of the aorta.

Having thus concluded our remarks on the method of examination, applicable to the heart as the central organ of the circulation, we shall, in the next place, proceed to consider the varieties which the pulse presents, though these are not confined to affections of the chest, more particularly than to those of the other cavities.

The Method of examining the Pulse.—The observer should wait until any emotion, which his presence may have caused, has subsided. He may then proceed to examine the pulse at the wrist, temple, lateral parts of the neck, or, in a word, in any other part where an artery of a certain size happens to be superficially seated. After having ascertained that the course of the blood is not interrupted in the arm, by tight clothes, or by a ligature, he takes the wrist of the patient, who ought to be either sitting, or lying in such a way as that the weight of his body may not incline more to one side than the other : the arm being placed in extension, and the fore-arm in pronation, supported by its ulnar border, while the radial is somewhat elevated, the artery is felt with the hand opposite to that of the patient.

The fingers should be laid in a right line on the course of the artery, the index finger on the anterior, and the thumb on the posterior or dorsal side of the wrist, furnishing a support to the others. The little finger, which receives the first impulse of the blood, should be applied to the vessel but slightly, but the others may compress it more or less. We should continue this process for a minute or two, and always observe the precaution of examining the pulse in both arms. The abdominal aorta and crural arteries may be examined by means of the stethoscope, which enables us readily to distinguish the circulation in those vessels. A watch, with

91

a second hand, is in general necessary, in order to ascertain exactly the number of pulsations that are made in a given time.

In Health the pulse is equal and regular, of a moderate degree of strength and frequency. The number of its beats vary according to the age, sex, temperament, stature, and idiosyncracy of each
individual. In the first months of life there are one hundred and
forty arterial pulsations in a minute; up to the completion of the
second year, there are about one hundred; at puberty the number
is reduced to eighty; in middle life we count from sixty to seventy-
five; and, finally, in old age, from fifty to sixty. The pulse is generally more frequent in females, and persons of a nervous temperament; it becomes quickened after meals and exercise, during pregnancy, or after any sudden emotion; but it is rendered slow by repose, fasting and bloodletting.

The observer should also recollect, that the pulse is subject
to variations, both as to the duration and order of its beats; it is
necessary to bear this in mind, lest he attribute to disease what may
be altogether independent of it.

In Disease the pulse may be quick or slow, strong or weak,
full or small, hard, contracted, resisting, or soft and compressible,
requiring a greater or less pressure on the artery to measure its
degree. It may also be frequent or the reverse, regular or irregular, in which latter case there are sometimes intermittences coinciding with the contraction of the auricles; and further, it may be
equal or unequal, distinct or confused, thready or insensible.

In general, the larger the artery is, the stronger is the pulse;
this should be taken into account when it happens to be stronger in
one arm than in the other. The strength of the pulse diminishes
gradually, when a tumour is developed near the trajet of the artery, as we observe in cases of aneurism of the arch of the aorta, when
the subclavian artery suffers compression against the walls of the
thorax.

The veins sometimes present pulsations synchronous with those
of the arteries. This may be observed in the jugular veins, when,
in consequence of an aneurism of the right cavities of the heart,
a reflux of blood is determined into them, which may occasionally
be perceived even as far as the superior part of the neck. When
a communication is established between an artery and vein which
are contiguous, it determinates a similar result.

There still remain to be described two other méans or proce.

dures, which are occasionally used in examining diseases of the chest.

OF THE MEASUREMENT OF THE THORAX.

This process may be performed as follows :—The patient being placed in a sitting posture, or standing upright, with his' arms hanging freely by his sides, or raised towards his head, a cord is drawn round his chest at any part of it ; if this be doubled upon it-self, we ascertain the natural extent of each side. The cord should then be applied successively to each side, beginning at one of the spinous processes of the vertebræ, and extending to the middle of the sternum, care being taken that it passes in a right line from one of these points to the other ; by comparing the result of this latter measurement with that given above, we ascertain the dilatation or contraction, that may exist at either side of the cavity.

In making this calculation, we should however recollect, that even in the healthy state, the two sides rarely present the same capacity, and that in persons who have been attacked by very se-vere pleurisies, the side that remained unaffected, acquires an in-crease of development, whilst that which had been the seat of the disease becomes narrowed and flattened ; the point of the shoulder is depressed, the side hollowed, and the muscles thin and wasted. Sometimes, also, in cases of phthisis we observe the upper ribs somewhat depressed, which is caused by adhesions between the pleura costalis and pulmonalis.

The thorax is dilated in cases of fluid or gaseous effusions, in-to the cavity of the pleura or pericardium, or of any considerable development of accidental tumours. It is contracted by original malformation, or after the termination of pleurisies, as has been al-ready stated.

OF SUCCUSSION.

This process consists in giving to the body one or more slight jerks, for the purpose of ascertaining the existence of a fluid supposed to be in the thorax. This motion determines a sound sim-ilar to that produced by shaking a bottle which is half full.

The sound is not emitted unless the effusion consists at the same time of air, or gas and liquid. For if the effusion be liquid only, then the lung will fill exactly all the rest of the cavity, and cannot be compressed by the fluid, sufficiently for the succus-sion to excite any sound ; and again, if the gaseous effusion be too abundant, or not sufficiently so, no result will be obtained. Hence these fluids must be combined in certain fixed proportions.

These are the principal indications which mark the different affections of the chest. The observer should also note the expression of the countenance, the colour of the cheeks and lips, their state of emaciation or injection, the manner in which the patient lies, the distribution of temperature in the limbs, the existence of partial sweats, and the state of the blood after bleeding, particularly in acute disease.

In phthisical cases, he should always inquire whether there be any hereditary predisposition. We shall recur to each of these points more in detail when treating of the diseases peculiar to each organ.

We may here briefly sum up the different points to which the observer should direct his attention. He should begin with examining the expectoration, as being of considerable value in distinguishing diseases of the chest. If limpid and viscid, it indicates acute catarrh ; if, after presenting this appearance, it becomes opaque, yellow, greenish or puriform, it marks chronic catarrh ; if it adheres firmly to the vessel in which it is received, and, is more or less tinged with blood, it announces pneumonia ; if round and opaque, masses float in a quantity of frothy fluid ; or if they are puriform, and streaked with white lines, and containing small white masses insoluble in water, we conclude that they are produced in a tubercular excavation. If the expectoration is fluid, purulent, and suddenly coughed up in great quantity, it should make us presume, that a fluid contained in the pleura, has made its way through the bronchi, and so is evacuated. When pieces of false membrane are expectorated, they are recognized at once as the product of croup ; and a dark green fluid, exhaling a fetid smell, marks gangrene of the lungs. I hæmoptysis, bright red and frothy blood is expectorated ; this should not be confounded with that which occurs in hæmatemesis, or with the bleeding which occasionally comes from the gums or the nares.

The effects of percussion should next be attended to, as they tend to direct the observer in the examination he is about to make with the assistance of the stethoscope. It should not be forgotten that, even in health, there are some parts of the chest which give a dull sound, as for instance the region of the heart, and the lower part of the right side ; there are others in which the sound is heightened as the lower part of the left side. Percussion indicates the parts in which the sound has become more dull, and those in which it is more clear than natural ; diminution and absence of the natural sound, characterize pneumonia,—accidental tissues developed in the lung or cavity of the pleura, hypertrophy of the heart, and effusions into the pleura or pericardium ; increased loudness of sound occurs in emphysema of the lung, or effusion of gaseous fluids into the pleura ; finally, the gurgling and metallic tingling indicate pulmonary excavations, or circumscribed cavities in the pleura, communicating with the bronchi.

Inquiry should next be directed to ascertain the state of the respiration, (whether it be painful and provokes cough, the character of the cough and also of the voice, which may be hoarse, croupal, &c. after which, by the stethoscope the observer may ascertain the parts of the lung which are or are not permeable to the air. The " rale crepitant" will indicate to him the first degree of pneumonia, œdema of the lung, and pulmonary apoplexy ; acute catarrh will be distinguished by the " rale sonore" or " sibilant,"— chronic catarrh, and the gurgling of softened tubercle by the " rale muqueux," and interlobular emphysema, by the peculiar sound described above, as the *murmur frictionis.*

The phenomena of the voice should be explored in the different parts of the chest. If pectoriloquy is heard under the clavicle, or in the hollow of the axilla, particularly at one side, it indicates phthisis ; œgophony is the proper sign of effusion into the cavity of the pleura ; finally, the metallic tingling announces a cavity communicating with the bronchi, and the metallic respiration, a simple bronchial fistula.

When any symptoms of effusion exist, it will be necessary to measure each side of the chest, and try by succussion to discover the presence of the fluid supposed to be present.

When the heart is supposed to be affected, the observer, after having ascertained that there is no unnatural enlargement in the præcordial region, and after making percussion, should proceed to examine the pulsations of the organ, between the fifth and seventh ribs, and at the base of the sternum. He should consider these in reference to their extent, impulsion, sound and rythm. If they are feeble, and heard in different parts of the thorax, he may suspect a dilation of the ventricles ; if, on the contrary, they are strong and circumscribed, they indicate hypertrophy ; if they emit a clear sound, it is a symptom of thinness of the walls of the heart. The disease is proved to exist at the right or left side of the organ, ac-

cording as these effects are more audible at the base of the sternum, or between the cartilages of the ribs, and the time at which
they are heard, marks whether it is the auricles or ventricles that
are affected. When the " bruit de rape," or sound like a file, is
heard at the left side, and is synchronous with the contraction of
the ventricle and the pulse, it indicates a narrowing of the sigmoid-
aortic, and mitral valves : when, on the contrary, it is synchronous
with the contraction of the auricles, the narrowing is at the auriculo-ventricular opening ; when it is heard at the base of the sternum, it is a sign of contraction of the tricusid or sigmoid valves of
the pulmonary artery.

The observer should examine the anterior part of the sternum,
to ascertain whether there be an aneurism of the arch of the aorta,
and the posterior part of the thorax, to determine that of the descending portion of this vessel. In all these cases, he should attend particularly to the state of the pulse, whether it be frequent,
small, irregular, contracted, or developed ; lastly, he should conclude this examination by noting the expression of the countenance, the appearance of the body, and the symptoms referrible to
affections of other organs.

NOTE Y—PAGE 460.

Infantile Fever and Marasmus. It is matter of deep regret that
so few dissections are on record of this formidable and intractable
complaint so prevalent in this country every summer and fall. For
full information on its history and its most sucsessful methods of
treatment, the student should study attentively the works of Miller,
Cheyne, Pemberton, Rush, and Currie.

NOTE Z—PAGE 546.

Dropsy. An attentive perusal of the luminous and original essays
of Rush " on Dropsies" will convince every impartial judge that to
him are we indebted for the improvements in theory and practice
which render dropsy so much less fatal now than formerly. Parry,
Armstrong, &c. have evidently borrowed their most valuable ideas
from our countryman.

ADDITIONAL NOTES.

MEDICAL TOPOGRAPHY.

The history of disease has probably received a greater share of the attention of physicians in this country, and been more success. fully cultivated by them than any other branch of medical learning. The writings of all our distinguished authors, and almost every num. ber of our successive and numerous periodical publications, might be safely appealed to in confirmation of this fact. Such an appeal would, at the same time, afford ample and gratifying opportunities of observing the rich and important contributions rendered by our countrymen to medical knowledge ; and if the observation of the illustrious Sydenham be not founded in error, that the improve. ment of physic depends upon collecting a genuine and natural de. scription or history of all diseases that can be procured, and laying down a fixed and complete method of cure, entitle them to a pre. eminent rank among the zealous promoters of science and the ef. fective benefactors of mankind. In claiming thus much for Amer. ican physicians, we trust we shall not be suspected of a disposition to indulge in idle national vanity. Our object in introducing these remarks is widely different, more elevated, and, we trust, more useful. It is, on the one hand to remind our professional brethren of the causes which have hitherto led to this direction of the med. ical mind of the country and which still continue to stimulate their inquiry, and elicit their talents and industry ; and, on the other, to offer a few observations on the best method to be pursued in the important investigations of the causes, nature, and treatment of disease. Difficulties beset the task, and but a very limited scope is afforded in these pages even to its partial accomplishment; but its importance will secure indulgence to our attempt.

1. Extending from the twenty-fifth to the forty-seventh degree of north latitude in length, and from the Atlantic to the Pacific oceans in width, the United States comprehend every possible di.

versity of climate and situation. To the tropical heats of the southern states may be opposed the artic cold of the northern, and to the
moist and variable atmosphere of the maritime coasts the equable
and dry of the interior and mountainous regions. Independently
of these more general features of difference, there exists every variety of locality which topographical situation can confer—hills,
valleys, and plains—sterile wastes and fertile tracts—sandy deserts
and marshy swamps—large rivers and ocean-like lakes—together
with all the minor shades of character arising from the peculiarities of vegetable and animal productions accommodated to individual regions.

Endowed to a certain extent with the power of resisting external agencies and enabled by reason and experience to prevent and
remedy their evil effects, man is nevertheless sensibly affected by
them, and sooner or later becomes moulded in his moral, no less
than his physical features, by the impressions of climate. An attentive view of the condition of the inhabitants of this country will
fully illustrate this fact, and, lead to an important step in the investigation of their diseases.—The northern and eastern inhabitants of
our empire will be found to differ essentially from their brethren of
the south and west ; and although this difference has not yet had
time to reach its maximum, on account of the too recent settlement
of the country, it is sufficiently striking to arrest attention. If it
be not, however palpable during health, it is most amply developed
in the hour of disease. The inflammatory and acute diseases,
which prevail in elevated, dry and cold situations, are forthwith ex-
changed on a removal to low, moist and warm places, for low and
chronic affections ; fevers, attended by the diseases of the chest,
for those in which the abdominal viscera are implicated ; and emigration from the sea-coast to the interior, removes, in a great degree, the liability to that fatal scourge of the Atlantic states—consumption. How great a variety of morbid phenomena must occur
under all these aspects of differing seasons, climates, and situations, is sufficiently apparent ; and to this circumstance we may
safely attribute, in part, the numerous and interesting histories of
disease with which the medical annals of our country are enriched,
and which have tended in no small degree to enlarge our knowledge of the relations subsisting between diseases and their more
general and pervading causes. This circumstance still continues
to operate, and as much remains to be done, it will open to the

medical inquirer an unbounded field for observation and reflection.

2. The political history and condition of the United States have exercised an important influence over the habits of the people, and consequently cannot have failed to modify the features of their diseases. The more immediate effects of the revolutionary war, and of the freedom which it so dearly bought and permanently secured, have been recorded in an interesting memoir, written by Dr. Rush, himself an active and zealous participator in the important events which led to the termination of the one and achievement of the other, and an acute observer of their influence over the minds and fortunes of his fellow-citizens.* If the stimulus of novelty, which operated so powerfully in the early periods of our history, has ceased to act, the invigorating influence of a sense of freedom continues still to put forth and display its healthful energies. The general diffusion of knowledge, the intelligence, the elevated tone of morality, the salutary restraints of religion, and the love of country—the mental and bodily activity, the ardent and indomitable spirit of enterprise, every where aroused and nurtured by the incitements of political, scientific, or literary ambition—by the desire of wealth, and the characteristic abhorrence of dependence— all combine to exert a powerful agency in moulding the temperaments, constitutions, and manners of our citizens. And it is scarcely necessary to point out the inseparable connexion which unites these moral agents with the causes and peculiar characters of the diseases of a people. While we enumerate the favourable constituents of our national character, let us not altogether overlook the unfavourable ingredients which unite with them and bring us to a level with all humanity, a mixture of good and evil. A spirit of licentiousness—the indulgence of malignant passions, and too great a fondness for excesses, especially in the use of spirituous liquors, are among the prominent vices, from the charge of which certain districts, more especially cannot be altogether exonerated. That they are peculiar to our form of government, or inseparable from our condition, in other respects so enviable and unparalleled, we do not believe, and are not in this place permitted to inquire. They are here exposed, with the simple view of citing their modifying influences upon the diseases incident to our countrymen.

3. Another important agent in modifying the diseases of the Uni-

* See Rush's Inquiries and Observations, vol i.

92

ted States, is the mixture of different varieties of the human species, which long-continued and extensive emigrations from remote
countries have here brought together in the anxious search for repose and happiness. The sanguine temperament of the northern
nations of Europe has amalgamated itself with the bilious constitutions of the southern, and both have not disdained to mingle their
currents with the lymphatic or phlegmatic disposition of the Hol-
lander, engendered in fogs and 'dull as his lake that slumbers in
the storm.' The diseases peculiar to each one of these distinct
varieties become, of consequence, subjected to great and frequently entire alterations in their nature and modes of treatment, presenting novel phenomena and indications, and requiring in the physician skill bold and original.

4. A fourth circumstance to be considered in the history of the
diseases of this country, is the more or less recent period in which
particular districts were first settled. All the gradations between
the most simple and the most refined conditions of life, from the
first faint dawn of civilization to the meridian splendour of luxu-
ry, may be discovered in glancing over the different portions of
the union—here resembling the oldest and most wealthy regions
of Europe—there approximating to the rude haunts of the helpless
and uninstructed savage.

The important influences of these different states of being on the
moral and physical character of man, have long been the subject of
philosophical investigation, and their power in modifying the phenomena of diseases will not be disputed. In connexion with this
subject that of emigration, as affecting health, will not be lost
sight of.

5. To the causes already enumerated, as offering particular
stimuli to the investigations of the medical philosopher, in this
country the prevalence of the fearful epidemic, known by the title
of yellow fever, deserves to be added. Few subjects have ever
presented such unbounded limits for inquiry, and awakened such
undiminished ardor for discussion and discovery as this. Arrayed
in a most awful form of malignity and destruction, setting ordinary skill at utter defiance, and laughing to scorn the antiquated prejudices of the schools and the prescriptive laws of an inadequate
and inapplicable police, this monster every where awakened the
spirit of curiosity, and provoked intellect and industry to a zealous
but patient investigation. Reformation in our medical theories, a
bold and original practice, and a host of illustrious names, at the

head of which let us gratefully remember that of RÜSH, have been the fruits of this contest and of the labours to which it gave rise.

Such are some of the leading circumstances which have influenced the direction medical literature has pursued in the United States, and their continued agency warrants the anticipation of still wider harvests of accession to science, and of renown to the fortunate labourers.

II. When Hippocrates was asked, who is the physician that is an honour to his profession? his reply was—" He who has merited the esteem and confidence of the public, by profound knowledge, long experience, consummate integrity ; who has been led through the whole circle of the sciences ; who has a due regard to the seasons of the year, and the diseases which they are observed to produce, to the states of the wind peculiar to each country, and the qualities of its waters ; who marks carefully the localities of towns and of the surrounding country, whether they are low or high, hot or cold, damp or dry ; who, moreover, neglects not to remark the diet and regimen of the inhabitants, and, in a word, all the causes that may produce disorder in the animal economy. Simple as these requisites to the formation of a skilful physician may appear, they are not to be attained but by an exquisite discernment, a sound judgment, and the most unwearied industry ; and where these are possessed, it is gratifying to know that they are, in general, accompanied by that liberal spirit, and that honourable love of distinction, which incite the possessor not to rest satisfied with hoarding up for his private use the accessions he makes to knowledge, but to communicate them to the world for the benefit of his contemporaries and of those who may succeed them. In the present age, and in the medical profession, this desire of communicating knowledge burns with an intensity of ardor that requires direction rather than incentive. There is, in fact, far greater inconvenience to be apprehended from the cacoethes scribendi, to which we owe the unnecessary multiplication of books, than from the grovelling passions which confine knowledge within the limited sphero of the owner's breast. In this country, where so many causes incite to authorship, we have, accordingly, no reason to complain of the want of *new books*. Within the last few years, more especially, our shelves have been literally crowded with text books, either original, compiled, or foreign, enriched with additions for domestic use, with histories of diseases that have appear-

ed in particular districts of our country, and with novel theories of
fever innumerable. To the second class of writings our attention has
always been carefully directed ; and however unequal we may have
found the productions, we always consider ourselves amply repaid
by the local information they convey. It has too often happened,
however, that authors, while writing expressly descriptions of endemic diseases, neglect to make their readers acquainted with
those important topographical details, without which their histories
are both unsatisfactory and void of interest. To obviate this deficiency is one object in these remarks and those which follow ; and we
shall, therefore, be pardoned if we dwell, perhaps tediously, on what
may be considered common places.

To render descriptions of endemic or epidemic disease a valuable accession to medical knowledge, the rules of Hippocrates, already quoted, must be carefully adverted to. A short amplifica-
tion of some of them and the enumeration of others, will point out
their importance.

1. *Celestial and terrestrial phaenomena.* The appearance of comets
and meteors, the periodical revolutions of the planets and their sa-
tellites, that of the moon more especially, the eruptions of volca-
noes, the convulsions of earthquakes, violent tempests, and extraordinary seasons, have all been supposed to have a direct influence
in the production and diffusion of epidemic diseases. Whether or
not this hypothesis be founded in truth, the numerous facts which
have been collected by the industry and research of our countryman, Webster, go far to show that there is an intimate association
between the occurrence of these phenomena and that of epidemics, and they deserve, therefore, a place in the records of every
medical inquirer.

. 2. *The sensible qualities of the atmosphere.* The essential constituents of the air we breathe, as oxygen, nitrogen, and carbonic
acid, are uniformly found, at all times and in all places, to exist in
the same definite proportions. Even the air of marshes has been
found by repeated experiments made by several distinguished physicians, and more recently repeated sixty times by professor Julia
of Lyons, not to differ from atmospheric air in any principle of
which chemical analysis can discover the existence. It is then to
the adventitious principles which combine with the atmosphere,
such as light, caloric, electricity, and aqueous vapour, that we
must look for the causes of disease. The innumerable variations
these elements are constantly undergoing, must inevitably exert a

more or less powerful agency on the health and lives of animated beings, and therefore form a prominent subject for examination.

The influence of light upon the animal economy has not yet received all the attention to which it is entitled. The general health of man, it has however been justly observed by Dr. Parr, one of the most learned physicians of our age, is apparently connected with light; and " the peculiar acid of the animal system the phosphoric, has a powerful attraction for this element, and appears to contain it, not only in a chemical combination, but, when in the form of an oxide, unites with and allows it to separate without decomposition."* Certain it is, that the complexion of a man, long confined in darkness, becomes sallow, his skin liable to foul exulcerations, and his whole system languid and not unfrequently dropsical. The consequences of long continued and intense light, emitted from the unclouded sun in Egypt and other similar situations, are well known.

Heat and cold exercise an influence not to be disputed in the production of disease, and their relative degrees deserve on this account, to be accurately noted. The tropics and the north of Europe are proverbially subject to the inroads of wide and devasting epidemics. The thermometer should be an indispensable part of the domestic furniture of a physician who resides in the country.

The opposite states of humidity and dryness in the atmosphere are not to be overlooked. Moisture, if not directly unpropitious to health, forms, nevertheless, a most ready vehicle for such poisonous substances as directly cause disease ; and dryness long continued, especially in hot climates and in hot seasons of temperate climates, has been known, from the days of Hippocrates, to produce the most deleterious effects. The operation of rains, in changing the character of particular districts for salubrity, will be sufficiently obvious.

The density and rarity of the atmosphere, and the prevalence of particular winds, will also deserve notice.

3. Next to the qualities of the air come to be considered *those of the soil, its geological history, and the chemical composition of its waters*—the general features of the country, whether it be hilly or low ground, fertile or barren, whether it contains marshes, and whether it is in proximity to the sea, &c.

4. The *botanical and zoological histories* of the region described are, on no account, to be omitted. No justifiable apology can be offered for a neglect of this important item at the present day, when

the opportunities for the cultivation of natural history are so numerous, and a knowledge of it become an indispensable requisite of medical education.

5th and lastly. We ascend to man himself, and ascertain, as far as we can, his physical and intellectual condition. His bodily constitution and strength ; his habits, as respects diet and regimen ; his moral propensities and sensibilities, the energy of his thinking faculties as developed by his moral political, and religious condition, will all tend to illustrate the etiology of the diseases to which he is subject, and explain the greater or less mortality of different portions of the earth. These subjects, it may be urged, are extensive and even difficult of investigation, but they are in proportion important and cannot escape the discrimination and perception of a skilful and observing physician. His previous liberal education, his acuteness and sagacity, cultivated by an intimacy with mankind in all the relations of life, his perseverance, lofty ambition of professional distinction, and an active and enlightened philanthropy, will smooth the path of labour and ensure value and success to his exertions. It may still be argued, that a knowledge of all these subjects has hitherto been found inadequate to the solution of the difficulties connected with the histories of disease. The fallacy of this argument will sufficiently appear, when it is considered within how short a period true principles of medical logic have been cultivated, and the sciences, which chiefly aid the researches of physicians, as natural history, chemistry, physiology, &c. attained their present improved state.

INDEX.

Moore